TOXICS A to Z

A GUIDE TO EVERYDAY POLLUTION HAZARDS

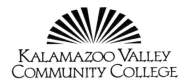

TOXICS A to Z

A GUIDE TO EVERYDAY POLLUTION HAZARDS

John Harte
Cheryl Holdren
Richard Schneider
Christine Shirley

UNIVERSITY OF CALIFORNIA PRESS · Berkeley · Los Angeles · Oxford

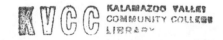

University of California Press
Berkeley and Los Angeles, California

University of California Press
Oxford, England

Library of Congress
Cataloging-in-Publication Data

Toxics A to Z: a guide to everyday pollution hazards /
   John Harte . . . [et al.].
      p.   cm.
   Includes bibliographical references.
   ISBN 0–520–07223–5 (alk. paper).—
ISBN 0–520–07224–3 (pbk.: alk. paper)
   1. Toxicology—Popular works.   2. Environmen-
tal health—Popular works.   3. Consumer education.
I. Harte, John, 1939–
RA1213.T76   1991
615.9—dc20   90–25860
                                                  CIP

Printed in the United States of America

      3   4   5   6   7   8   9

The paper used in this publication meets the minimum requirements of American National Standard for Information Sciences—Permanence of
Paper for Printed Library Materials, ANSI
Z39.48-1984 ∞

Contents

How to Use This Book ix
Ten Effective Ways to Reduce
    Toxics in Your Environment x
Preface xi
Acknowledgments xv
Cross-References to Entries
    by Exposure xvi

PART ONE

ALL ABOUT TOXICS   1

FUNDAMENTALS   3

1 Toxics in Perspective   5
A. Thinking about Risk 5
B. Causes of Death and
   Disease 8

2 The Language of Toxics   15
A. How Risk Is Described 15
B. Units Used to Describe
   Toxics 18

SOME BASIC MEDICAL ASPECTS OF
THE TOXICS PROBLEM   25

3 Testing and Classification
   of Toxics   27
A. Testing Toxics 27
B. Classification of Toxics 31

4 Toxics in the Body   34
A. Entry, Dose, and Exit: How
   Chemicals Harm the Body 34
B. Sensitive Groups 40
C. Nutrition and Susceptibility
   to Toxics 42

THE FOUR MAJOR SOURCES OF
TOXIC EXPOSURE   45

5 Toxics in Air   47
A. Air Pollution and Health 47
B. Smoking and Health 50
C. Indoor Air Pollution 51

6 Toxics in Water   55
A. Drinking Water and Health 55
B. The Threat from Below: Toxics
   in Groundwater 58

7 Toxics in Food   61
A. Food Additives and Health 61
B. Why Alcohol and Other
   Chemicals Don't Mix 63
C. Food and Cancer: How Much
   Is Nature to Blame? 64

8 Toxics in Consumer Products   67
A. Inert Ingredients 67
B. Hobbies and Crafts 68
C. Some Product Comparisons 69

TOXICS AND THE ENVIRONMENT   75

9 Movement of Toxics through
   the Environment   77
A. Air 77
B. Water 81
C. Soil 83

10 Toxics in the Biosphere   86
A. How Toxic Concentrations
   Build Up in Animals 86
B. Ecological Effects of
   Toxics 88

11 Three Global Environmental
   Hazards of Pollutants   91
A. The Greenhouse Effect 91
B. Stratospheric Ozone
   Depletion 94
C. Acid Rain 96

FOUR SPECIAL GROUPS OF TOXICS   101

12 Toxic Metals   103
A. Significance and Sources of
   Toxic Metals 103
B. Human Health Effects 104

13 Petrochemicals   106
A. Sources and Products 106
B. Solvents 108

14 Pesticides   112
A. Overview 112
B. Classification and Patterns
   of Use 115
C. Human Health Concerns 120
D. Environmental and Economic
   Constraints 126
E. Cotton: A Case Study 131

F. Alternatives to Conventional
Pest Control 132

15 Radiation 141
A. The Nature of Radioactivity 141
B. The Electromagnetic
Spectrum 143
C. How Radiation Affects Us 144
D. Nuclear Fission and Nuclear
Fusion 145
E. Units Used to Describe
Radiation 146
F. Background Exposure and
Radiation Standards 149
G. Estimating the Risk of
Radiation 150
H. Food Irradiation 151
I. Nuclear War 153

MANAGING TOXICS 155

16 The Waste Crisis: Sources
and Solutions 157
A. Overview of the Waste Crisis 157
B. Waste Disposal 159
C. Waste Processing 164
D. Recycling and Other Approaches
to Source Reduction 166

17 Regulating Toxics 171
A. The Regulations: An
Overview 171
B. Protection of Air Quality 175
C. Protection of Water Quality 177
D. Public Health and Safety 179
E. Waste Management 184
F. Additional Laws Recently
Passed or Under
Consideration 187
G. The Right to Know about
Toxics 188

PART TWO

A GUIDE TO COMMONLY
ENCOUNTERED TOXICS 195

acetic acid 197
acetone 198
acrolein 200
aflatoxins 201
alachlor 203
aldicarb 205
aldrin and dieldrin 207
aluminum 210
ammonia 214

arsenic 217
asbestos 222
aspartame 225
asphalt 226
azinophos-methyl 227
barium 229
benomyl 231
benzene 233
benzo[a]pyrene (B[a]P) 236
beryllium 238
BHT and BHA 241
bis(chloromethyl)ether 243
cadmium 244
caffeine 248
captan, captafol, and folpet 250
carbaryl 253
carbon black 255
carbon monoxide 257
carbon tetrachloride 260
carrageenan 262
cesium-137 263
CFCs 265
chlordane 268
chlorine, hydrogen chloride, hydrochloric
acid, and hypochlorite 270
chloroform 273
chromium 276
creosote 279
2,4-D 281
daminozide 283
DDT 286
diazinon 289
dicamba 290
dichlorvos 292
dioxane 294
dioxin 296
Di(2-ethylhexyl)phthalate 298
EBDCs: mancozeb, maneb, metiram,
and zineb 300
ethylene dibromide (EDB) and ethylene
dichloride (EDC) 303
ethylene glycol 306
ethylene oxide 308
extremely low frequency electromagnetic fields 310
fluoride 313
food colors 316
formaldehyde 318

fosetyl Al 322

glyphosate 323

heptachlor 325

hydroquinone 327

iodine-131 329

laser light 331

lead 333

lindane 336

malathion 339

mercury 341

methyl ethyl ketone 344

methylene chloride 346

microwave and radio frequency
    radiation 348

mineral fibers (nonasbestos) 350

monosodium glutamate (MSG) 351

naphthalene 353

nickel 354

nicotine 358

nitrates, nitrites, and nitrosamines 359

nitrogen oxides 365

noise 368

oxalic acid 370

ozone and other photochemical
    oxidants 372

paraquat 375

parathion and methyl-parathion 376

particulate matter 379

PCBs and PBBs 382

plutonium 386

pyrethroids (pyrethrum and
    permethrin) 388

radon 391

saccharin 394

selenium 395

sodium hydroxide 398

strontium-90 401

styrene 403

sulfites 405

sulfur dioxide and sulfates 407

2,4,5-T 411

tetrachloroethylene 413

toluene 415

trichloroethane 418

trichloroethylene 420

TRIS 422

tritium 424

ultrasound 426

ultraviolet radiation 428

vinyl chloride 430

vinylidene chloride 432

warfarin 433

xylene 435

zinc 436

Glossary 439

Commonly Used Abbreviations
    for Units 449

Abbreviations for Environmental
    Laws and Institutions 450

Annotated Suggested Readings 451

Sources for Home Testing
    Equipment 453

National Hotlines 455

Index 457

How to Use This Book

This book is divided into two major parts. In Part I, All About Toxics, you will find a vast amount of information on general issues concerning the hazards of toxics. Many commonly asked questions about toxics are answered here: "Is there a cancer epidemic?" "How reliable are tests to determine if a chemical causes cancer?" "What is happening to the ozone layer and the global climate?" "Do existing laws really protect us?"

Part II, A Guide to Commonly Encountered Toxics, contains specific information about individual toxics. Information found here includes how to identify the substance, symptoms of exposure, and how to reduce or prevent exposure. The individual toxics in Part II are arranged alphabetically for easy access.

Following the preface, you will find a cross-referenced list of all the individual entries. Its purpose is to identify all the toxics in this book that are likely to be encountered in particular places or as a result of particular activities. Suppose, for example, you want to know which of the substances discussed in this book are likely to be encountered in the course of garden and lawn work. Turn to the appropriate cross-reference heading (Garden and Lawn Activities) to find such a list and then turn to the alphabetical listing of entries in Part II.

Throughout the book, certain words appear in **boldface**. These refer to toxics that are listed as entries in Part II. Other words appear in *italics*, to indicate that they are defined in the Glossary. Abbreviations for scientific units used throughout the book are explained in Commonly Used Abbreviations for Units, which follows the glossary. Acronyms and abbreviations for laws and agencies are given under Abbreviations for Environmental Laws and Institutions, also at the back of the book.

Ten Effective Ways to Reduce Toxics in Your Environment

1. DO NOT SMOKE (See pages 50–51, 358–359.)

2. READ LABELS ON CHEMICAL CONTAINERS AND FOLLOW DIRECTIONS CAREFULLY Do not believe that if a little of a chemical is good, then a lot of it is better.

3. CONSERVE ENERGY Plug heat leaks in your house. Purchase energy-efficient appliances. Carpool. Avoid unnecessary lighting, driving, and other uses of appliances.

4. REDUCE, REUSE, AND RECYCLE Use products made from recycled materials; use nondisposable or reusable items rather than disposable; recycle newspapers, bottles and cans. Give away used toys, clothes, appliances, and furniture; don't throw them away. (Consult your yellow pages for information; see also pages 166–170.)

5. FIND SUBSTITUTES FOR HAZARDOUS CHEMICALS WHEN POSSIBLE Substitute "elbow grease" for hazardous solvents and cleaners. Try out alternative methods for controlling pests in the home and garden (see pages 166–170).

6. TEST YOUR HOME FOR RADON If you have reason to believe you live in an area with high radon levels, conduct a home test (see pages 391–393, 453).

7. TEST YOUR HOME'S WATER QUALITY If you have reason to believe your drinking water is hazardous, conduct a home test (see pages 55–60, 453).

8. DON'T IGNORE WORKPLACE SAFETY GUIDELINES Use appropriate gloves, clothing, eye protection, respirators, exhaust fans and hoods whenever required.

9. SUPPORT SOUND ENVIRONMENTAL LEGISLATION (See pages 171–193 for a discussion of existing and proposed legislation.)

10. SHARE YOUR KNOWLEDGE WITH OTHERS

Preface

Purpose and Scope

Public awareness of the hazards of toxic chemicals has mushroomed in recent years. Headline stories grimly describe such events as the tragedy at Bhopal, India, where the accidental release of gas from a pesticide factory killed several thousand people and imposed lingering illness on tens of thousands more. Closer to home, the U.S. government relocated the entire town of Times Beach, Missouri, because of contamination of the soil with dioxin. To the myriad fears facing the modern world, humanity has now added the fear that a truck or train carrying a toxic material may crash, exposing numerous people to its potentially lethal contents, or that a child playing in a vacant lot may return home dusted with some unrecognized powder that escaped from a disintegrating barrel buried there.

While such dramatic events deservedly capture newspaper headlines, an equally important aspect of the toxic chemicals problem has usually been relegated to the back pages or, more likely, has remained unpublicized: even small recurring exposures to chemicals are capable of causing cancer and other diseases. Such long-term exposure is called *chronic,* in contrast to briefer exposure resulting typically from massive spills and other accidents, which is called *acute.* Chronic exposure can occur with each mouthful of food or each glass of water we ingest and with each breath of air we inhale; it occurs daily as we work in the garden or office or as we repair a child's toy.

This book originated with the conviction that people need reliable and easily understandable information about the most frequently encountered toxic dangers; where such dangers are most likely to be found; how to recognize them and the symptoms

that exposure to them can cause; and above all, how chronic and acute exposure can be reduced or avoided altogether. We provide information on over 100 of the most common and potentially hazardous toxics in our environment. The format is designed for the lay person who feels confused about the potential dangers posed by eating, drinking, and breathing and by using everyday consumer products.

In our discussion of governmental regulations and the politics of toxics, we emphasize toxics found in the United States, but most of these can be found throughout the world. We have not included the toxic side effects of medicines nor of poisons found only in nature.

Our society is hooked on chemicals of its own making. Each year during the past few decades, approximately 1000 new chemicals have been manufactured and introduced into the marketplace. In the United States today there are approximately 50,000 such chemicals in commercial use. Virtually every aspect of our lives is touched by these substances, from food production to recreation. No matter how carefully we use these, some fraction inadvertently ends up in our food, water, or air. And not all exposure is inadvertent; a great number of commercial chemicals, such as food preservatives and pesticides, are deliberately introduced into our environment.

Although not all of these pose risks, the variety of new chemicals now showing up in the environment is huge. Because we could not include all such substances here, we think it useful to explain how we selected the entries. The most important characteristic qualifying a chemical for inclusion is widespread public exposure at levels known or strongly suspected to be harmful. We are primarily concerned with those substances believed to cause cancer, birth defects, genetic mutations, and other serious human health problems, such as liver damage or respiratory stress. Nevertheless, a few substances, such as DDT, were selected because they damage the environment. Toxics that are widely distributed geographically and found regularly in water, food, air, or common household products are given preference over those that are found only in a few small areas of the nation or that show up rarely. Toxics encountered primarily in the workplace are also included, provided that workplace exposure is not limited to a few people in specialized industries. Several toxics that are not currently a significant hazard are also included because they have the potential to become a serious problem if the present increase in their use continues. A few that pose little threat to the public were selected because of a widespread misconception that they are a serious threat.

We did not restrict ourselves to substances that are regulated by the U.S. government. The slow process of formulating and enacting regulations is not capable of keeping up with the stream of new chemicals produced each year. Thus, the absence of a regulation for any particular substance is no guarantee that the substance is safe at levels ordinarily encountered. We describe the major regulations that do exist for a given substance, but we caution the reader that the existence of a regulation does not imply that exposure at or below allowed levels is necessarily safe.

Structure of the Book

Part I of this book entitled "All About Toxics" is a collection of short essays organized to form a "book within a book," giving the reader the broad picture and highlighting the general issues. Included are 17 chapters covering such topics as the nature of risk, the methods used to learn more about whether particular chemicals cause cancer, the problem of indoor air pollution, the threats that chemical pollutants pose to our global environment (including the climate and the ozone layer), the threat of pesticides in our foods, existing governmental regulations and how

they work (or in some cases, why they don't work), and tips for disposal of toxic substances found in the home. These chapters are arranged into six groups that lead the reader in a natural progression from fundamentals, basic medical information, and sources of toxics to environmental issues, the main types of toxics, and how they are managed. Some readers may want to read Part I cover to cover before turning to Part II, entitled "A Guide to Commonly Encountered Toxics." Others may find Part I more useful as a reference and seek out only particular chapters for further insight into subjects briefly mentioned in Part II.

Over 100 toxics are described in Part II. They are arranged in alphabetical order in the likely event that the reader has heard the name of a toxic, or has read it on the label of a package, and wants to learn about its hazards. In some cases, however, a reader might want to know what toxics will be encountered in a particular situation, such as in the use of garden pesticides, but does not know the name of the substances. To help the reader quickly locate this information, all entries are cross-referenced according to types of activity or types of products that could lead to exposure in a special listing called "Cross-References to Entries by Exposure," which follows this preface.

In Part II, each entry title is the most commonly used name of the toxic. Thus, the substance technically known as 2,3,7,8-tetrachlorodibenzo-*p*-dioxin is found under dioxin. (We list chemical elements under their full name rather than their chemical symbol.) If the most commonly used name is an abbreviation, such as DDT, then this is used instead. If the substance is commonly referred to by several names, we list them in the entry following the entry title. Following that are trade names of common products containing the substance.

In the Index, we include all common and technical names and abbreviations that might reasonably be used to characterize each toxic. If you do not find something alphabetically in Part II under what you think is its common name, check the Index and you may find that it is covered in an entry under a different name.

Each entry of Part II is broken into a number of sections. The Introduction gives an overview of the threat posed by the toxic. The reader will also find here helpful historical facts and common uses (if any) of the substance. In the next section, Physical and Chemical Properties, we provide information to help the reader recognize the substance and to understand those of its properties that affect its location in, and movement through, the environment. We include information about odor, taste, color, and whether the substance is a solid, liquid, or gas under normal conditions. If the substance can be inadvertently formed or can produce some other harmful substance through chemical reactions that might occur under everyday conditions, we describe those processes.

Next, in Exposure and Distribution, we describe amounts and distribution of toxics in the environment. We describe the major sources, such as automobile exhaust and pesticides on cotton crops, and the pathways of exposure, such as breathing urban air, eating shellfish from polluted waters, and skin contact with a consumer product. For substances also produced naturally, we compare the industrial rates of production with the natural rates.

A section on Health Effects follows, which describes the symptoms and illnesses that are likely to result from various levels of exposure. We characterize the uncertainty in the health risk estimates, when appropriate, and inform the reader of any harmful effects that could result from combinations of the toxic and other substances with which it could come in contact.

Under Protection and Prevention, we focus on methods for reducing risk. If reliable information is available about antidotes or other first aid remedies that would reduce the health hazard after exposure, it is given. The main emphasis here, however, is on methods for avoiding exposure. These fall into three categories: methods for safely disposing of the substance, methods for using the substance while minimizing exposure (for example, washing fruit to remove pesticides), and methods for avoiding exposure by substituting some less harmful product or practice.

In the next section, Environmental Effects, we turn from human health to threats to other living things or the environment; effects listed here range from hazards to a household pet to risks to the entire planet. In Regulatory Status, we describe applicable governmental regulations and guidelines, and the current status of the substance (for example, "production illegal but still found in waste dumps" or "domestic use banned but exported to other countries"). Readers unfamiliar with existing pollution regulations should refer to Chapter 17 in Part I for a review of that subject.

The sections just described will provide the information sought by most people, but for those more curious about technical details, we provide additional data under Technical Information at the end of each entry in Part II. Here the scientific name is given in full if it differs from the common name. For elements, the chemical symbol is given (for example, Pb for lead) and information is provided about the decay properties of radioactive substances. Chemical formulas are provided for compounds (for example, SO_2 for sulfur dioxide). We follow this with quantitative information about typical concentrations and exposures, relations between exposure and health effects, and existing standards. This information is presented in scientific units. For readers who wish to delve into the more technical aspects of toxicology but who are unfamiliar with the relevant units, Chapter 2, section on Units Used to Describe Toxics, and Chapter 15, section on Units Used to Describe Radiation in Part I will provide some help.

Following Part II we provide a Glossary of technical terms found throughout the book and several tables deciphering abbreviations of commonly used units and abbreviations of laws and institutions. Next, an annotated list of suggested readings is provided for those wishing to read more on the various aspects of toxics. The book concludes with some important handy information: Sources for Home Testing Equipment for those seeking to measure the levels of certain pollutants to which they may be exposed, and National Hotline phone numbers for those wishing to get rapid and reliable answers to perplexing questions about toxics.

As you read Part I, "All About Toxics," you will see certain toxics set in **boldface** type. In each case, the substance is printed in boldface to alert the reader that it is listed as an entry in Part II (A Guide to Commonly Encountered Toxics), where more information can be found. Likewise, when words found in the Glossary appear in the text, they are *italicized* to alert the reader that a definition is available.

A Word on Terminology

Throughout this book, we have used the term "toxics" to refer to the hazards under discussion. This term, which is not in standard usage, is used broadly here to include chemicals, nuclear radiation, and even electromagnetic fields and noise. Most sources of information on these hazards use the term "toxic" as an adjective, as in "toxic substance." We use "toxic" as a noun because there is no other word that describes what we mean. The term "toxin" means, more narrowly, poisons produced by plants or animals; "toxic substance" suggests chemicals but not radiation. "Toxicant" is cumbersome, while "hazards" and "pollution" are, respectively, too broad and too narrow for our purposes.

Cautionary Notes

In preparing this book, we have done our best to provide the reader with the most scientifically defensible and up-to-date information about toxic substances. However, no source of information about toxic substances is complete, perfectly reliable, or permanent. The number of toxic chemicals in our environment is enormous; indeed, most toxic chemicals are not mentioned here. Our aim is a limited one—to identify and describe the most common ones. *No reader should assume that a substance is safe simply because it is not mentioned in this book.*

The data on the health risks of toxics are scanty and laden with experimental uncertainty. The technical literature is riddled with contradictions, and strong disagreement among scientists is common. The highly politicized nature of the toxics problem means that not all information available to the public is unbiased. In the light of the uncertainties resulting from incomplete information, the reader is urged to err on the side of caution when making decisions. It is for this reason that we have included in each entry in Part II information about how the reader can avoid unnecessary exposure.

Finally, we remind the reader that the material in this book dealing with disease symptoms and antidotes is not a replacement for professional and up-to-date medical advice.

Acknowledgments

Above all we thank Bill Pease and Mary Ellen Harte. Bill wrote the section on the right-to-know approach to controlling toxics and gave the entire manuscript a critical reading. His insights and suggestions for improving the text were invaluable. Mary Ellen converted our vague ideas for sketches into the illustrations used herein. She also spent many hours clarifying and enlivening our prose.

Philippe Martin was present at the birth of this project and provided many helpful suggestions about content and format. Patrick Gonzalez provided useful input for several of the entries in Part II. Paul Ehrlich made numerous constructive editorial suggestions and Anthony Nero helped us understand the nuances of many aspects of pollution.

We are grateful to Kathy Walker for a superb job of copy editing and indexing, and to Shirley Warren, who deftly managed production of the book at the University of California Press.

To Elizabeth Knoll we offer special thanks; her editorial and publishing acuity, as well as her support and enthusiasm, made working with The University of California Press a pleasure.

A final thank you goes to our spouses Mary Ellen Harte, John Holdren, Jennie Schneider, and Tony Anthony, for their unflagging encouragement, patience, and humor during the years this book was in preparation.

Cross-References to Entries by Exposure

Many readers will want to know which toxics they may be exposed to in various places or as the result of certain activities. Such information is provided in the following lists of entries from Part II, grouped by place or activity.

1. AIR POLLUTANTS (INDOOR): acrolein, asbestos, benzo[a]pyrene, carbon monoxide, chlordane, chloroform, dichlorvos, di(2-ethylhexyl)pthalate, ethylene dibromide and ethylene dichloride, extremely low frequency electromagnetic fields, formaldehyde, heptachlor, mineral fibers, napthalene, nitrogen dioxide, noise, particulate matter, radon, styrene, tetrachloroethylene, toluene, trichloroethylene, vinyl chloride, xylene.

2. AIR POLLUTANTS (OUTDOOR): acetic acid, arsenic, asbestos, benzene, benzo[a]pyrene, carbon black, carbon monoxide, CFCs, chloroform, chromium, creosote, dioxin, extremely low frequency electromagnetic fields, ethylene oxide, formaldehyde, lead, methylene chloride, nitrogen dioxide, noise, ozone, particulate matter, plutonium, radon, styrene, sulfur dioxide, tetrachloroethylene, toluene, ultraviolet light, vinyl chloride, vinylidene chloride.

3. AUTOMOBILE-RELATED ACTIVITIES: asbestos, asphalt, benzene, benzo[a]pyrene, BHT and BHA, cadmium, carbon monoxide, chloroform, ethylene dibromide and ethylene dichloride, formaldehyde, lead, nitrogen dioxide, noise, ozone, particulate matter, toluene, vinyl chloride.

4. FIRES (substances that result from the burning of insulation, plastics, fabrics, and other household products, as well as from controlled fires in the wood-stove or fireplace): benzo[a]pyrene, CFCs, cadmium, carbon monoxide, chloroform, creosote, dioxin, formaldehyde, nitrogen dioxide, particulate matter, PCBs.

5. FOOD CONTAMINANTS AND ADDITIVES: aflatoxin, alachlor, aldicarb, aldrin and dieldrin, aluminum arsenic, aspartame, azinophos-methyl, barium, benomyl, benzo[a]pyrene, beryllium, BHT and BHA, cadmium, caffeine, captan (and captafol, folpet), carbaryl, carrageenan, cesium-137, chlordane, chloroform, 2,4-D, daminozide, DDT, diazinon, di(2-ethylhexyl)-pthalate, EDB and EDC, fluoride, food colors, fosetyl Al, glyphosate, heptachlor, iodine-131, lead, lindane, malathion, mancozeb (under EBCDs), mercury, MSG, nickel, nitrates (and nitrites, nitrosamines), parathion, PCBs, pyrethrum, saccharin, selenium, strontium-90, sulfites, sulfur dioxide, 2,4,5-T, tetrachloroethylene, trichloroethylene, tritium, vinyl chloride, vinylidene chloride.

6. GARDEN AND LAWN ACTIVITIES: aldrin and dieldrin, arsenic, azinophos-methyl, benomyl, captan, carbaryl, DDT, diazinon, dioxin, glyphosate, lindane, malathion, noise, pyrethrum.

7. HOBBIES AND CRAFTS: acetic acid, acetone, benzene, cadmium, chromium, formaldehyde, dioxane, hydroquinone, methylene chloride, methyl ethyl ke-

tone, noise, tetrachloroethylene, trichloroethylene, xylene.

8. HOUSEHOLD ACTIVITIES:
   a. *Bathroom* (including cosmetics): acetic acid, acetone, ammonia, chlorine (and chloride, hydrochloric acid, hypochloric acid, and hypochlorite), fluoride, food colors, formaldehyde, hydroquinone, oxalic acid, xylene.
   b. *Kitchen* (nonfood hazards listed here, but see also number 5): benzene, carbon monoxide, extremely low frequency electromagnetic fields, formaldehyde, microwave and radio frequency radiation, nitrogen dioxide, particulate matter, radiation, noise, tetrachloroethylene.
   c. *Miscellaneous Household Products*: acetone, ammonia, barium, benzene, carbon black, dichlorvos, dioxane, di(2-ethylhexyl)phthalate, extremely low frequency electromagnetic fields, formaldehyde, laser light, methylene chloride, methyl ethyl ketone, mineral fibers, naphthalene, nickel, noise, oxalic acid, sodium hydroxide, trichloroethylene, warfarin, xylene.

9. WATER POLLUTANTS: aldicarb, aldrin and diedrin, aluminum, arsenic, barium, benzene, benzo[a]pyrene, beryllium, cadmium, captafol, chlordane, chromium, 2,4-D, DDT, diazinon, dioxin, EBDCs, fluoride, heptachlor, lead, lindane, malathion, nitrates (and nitrites and nitrosamines), parathion, selenium, 2,4,5-T, toluene, tritium.

10. SOIL CONTAMINANTS: acrolein, aldrin and dieldrin, arsenic, benzo[a]pyrene, bis(chloromethyl)ether, cadmium, cesium-137, chlordane, creosote, 2,4-D, DDT, dioxin, heptachlor, lead, lindane, PCBs and PBBs, plutonium, strontium-90, 2,4,5-T.

11. TOBACCO SMOKE: acrolein, arsenic, benzo[a]pyrene, cadmium, carbon monoxide, ethylene oxide, formaldehyde, nickel, nicotine, nitrates (and nitrites and nitrosamines), particulate matter, radon, toluene, vinyl chloride.

12. ACCIDENTAL SPILLS (for example, truck or train accidents and pipeline ruptures): ammonia, benzene, chlorine (and hydrogen chloride, hydrochloric acid, and hypochlorite).

13. WORKPLACE CONTAMINANTS:
   a. *Office*: asbestos, benzene, extremely low frequency electromagnetic fields, formaldehyde, laser light, microwave and radio frequency fields, noise, ozone, PCBs, trichloroethylene.
   b. *Agriculture, horticulture, and forestry*: alachlor, aldicarb, aldrin and dieldrin, ammonia, azinophosmethyl, benomyl, BHT and BHA, captan (and captafol and folpet), carbon tetrachloride, 2,4-D, daminozide, DDT, dicamba, EBCDs, glyphosate, heptachlor, lindane, malathion, nitrates (and nitrites and nitrosamines), noise, paraquat, parathion, sulfur dioxide, 2,4,5-T.
   c. *Services* (including schools, hospitals and doctors' offices, laboratories, gas stations, and dry cleaners; see also number 8b): acetone, asbestos, barium, benzene, bis(chloromethyl)-ether, CFCs, di(2-ethylhexyl)pthalate, ethylene dibromide (and ethylene dichloride), ethylene oxide, iodine-131, laser light, mercury, microwave and radio frequency radiation, oxalic acid, tetrachloroethylene, trichloroethylene, tritium, ultrasound, ultraviolet radiation.
   d. *Nuclear Industry*: beryllium, cesium-137, iodine-131, plutonium, radon, strontium-90, tritium.
   e. *Fossil Fuel Mining and Combustion* (including electric power plants and incinerators): acetic acid, acetone, aluminum, arsenic, benzene, benzo[a]pyrene, beryllium, cadmium, chromium, extremely low frequency

electromagnetic fields, lead, nitrogen dioxide, noise, particulate matter, sulfur dioxide.

f. *Chemical Industries* (including pesticides, plastics, rubber, cosmetics, and solvents): acetic acid, acetone, acrolein, aldicarb, aldrin and dieldrin, ammonia, arsenic, azinophos-methyl, benomyl, benzene, BHT and BHA, bis(chloromethyl)ether, carbon black, carbon tetrachloride, CFCs, chlordane, chlorine (and hydrogen chloride, hydrochloric acid, and hypochlorite), chloroform, chromium, creosote, dioxane, dioxin, di(2-ethylhexyl)phthalate, ethylene oxide, lindane, malathion, methyl ethyl ketone, methylene chloride, mercury, naphthalene, parathion, sodium hydroxide, styrene, tetrachloroethylene, toluene, trichloroethylene, vinyl chloride, vinylidene chloride, xylene.

g. *Metals Industries*: acetone, aluminum, arsenic, beryllium, carbon tetrachloride, cadmium, chromium, dioxane, lead, mercury, methyl ethyl ketone, nickel, noise, oxalic acid, particulate matter, saccharin, sulfur dioxide, tetrachloroethylene, trichloroethylene.

h. *Electronics Industries*: beryllium, cadmium, carbon tetrachloride, CFCs, lead, mercury, selenium, tetrachloroethylene.

i. *Paper and Wood Products Industries*: acetic acid, arsenic, chlorine (and hydrogen chloride, hydrochloric acid, and hypochlorite), chloroform, chromium, creosote, dioxin, formaldehyde, noise, sodium hydroxide.

j. *Textiles Industries*: acetic acid, cadmium, chromium, benzene, bis-(chloromethyl)ether, chloroform, formaldehyde, tetrachloroethylene.

14. RADIOACTIVE SUBSTANCES: cesium-137, iodine-131, plutonium, radon, strontium-90, tritium.

15. METALS (or metal-like elements): aluminum, arsenic, barium, beryllium, cadmium, chromium, lead, mercury, nickel, selenium.

16. SOLVENTS: acetic acid, acetone, acrolein, ammonia, benzene, bis(chloromethyl)ether, CFCs, carbon tetrachloride, chloroform, dioxane, ethylene glycol, formaldehyde, methylene chloride, methyl ethyl ketone, oxalic acid, tetrachloroethylene, toluene, trichloroethylene, vinyl chloride, xylene.

17. PESTICIDES: alachlor, aldicarb, aldrin and dieldrin, azinophos-methyl, benomyl, captan (and captafol and folpet), carbaryl, chlordane, creosote, 2,4-D, daminozide, diazinon, dicamba, DDT, dichlorvos, EBDCs, ethylene dibromide and ethylene dichloride, fosetyl Al, glyphosate, heptachlor, lindane, malathion, paraquat, parathion, pyrethroids, 2,4,5-T, warfarin.

18. TOXICS OF PARTICULAR ENVIRONMENTAL CONCERN: aldicarb, aldrin and dieldrin, carbaryl, carbon dioxide, CFCs, 2,4-D, DDT, EBDCs, heptachlor, lindane, nitrogen dioxide, ozone, parathion, PCBs, selenium, sulfur dioxide, 2,4,5-T, ultraviolet radiation.

PART ONE

ALL ABOUT TOXICS

FUNDAMENTALS

1 TOXICS IN PERSPECTIVE

We begin with a chapter that addresses one of the most perplexing questions concerning toxics: How much should one worry about toxic substances when there are so many other things to deal with in life? We approach this question by first exploring the meaning of risk. We highlight some of the more common confusions that arise when people talk about risk, and we try to make the reader feel more at home thinking about this easily misused notion. We then look at the changing patterns of death and disease in the United States. Here the reader will find out what the most common causes of death are and which health threats are on the rise. This information provides a useful perspective for understanding the threat of toxics.

A. Thinking about Risk

Public attitudes toward risk are varied. In response to a warning of exposure to some hazardous substance, most readers have likely heard replies such as these:

"Well, you have to die of something."

"Why should I worry, when more people get killed in car crashes than from using this chemical spray?"

"You tell me that one in a million people using that product will get cancer, but you're just telling me about odds—I'm interested in what will happen to me."

"Uncle Harry used the stuff all his life and lived to the age of 101—Why should I worry?"

"I don't want to be subject to any risk when I drink my tap water."

These quotes reflect serious and commonly encountered misunderstandings about the nature of risk. This chapter will try to clarify some of the more confusing aspects of the subject.

Risk is expressed in terms of probability, and this is what causes much of the public's confusion about risk. Risk must be expressed in terms of probability, in part because human beings are not identical and therefore do not respond in the same way to similar exposures. Even the mice used as test animals in laboratories differ from one another in their response to a given exposure. Thus, the data available from laboratory tests and from human health records will always have to be in the form of statements such as "If one million individuals drink all their water for one year from this contaminated source, then the odds are that ten of them will develop cancer as a result." The specific individuals from a group of one million who will develop cancer as a result of the contamination cannot be predicted. Nor can you even be sure that exactly ten members of the group will really develop the cancer; a hundred might or none might.

In addition, few people resemble the fictitious "average person" that scientists often refer to in expressing risk estimates. For any given hazard there are usually groups of people that are far more at risk than others. This can occur because of individual differences in age and the ways our bodies work (see Chapter 4, Section B) and because of differences in where we live and in our daily habits (which can affect the dose we receive and our response to it). Two different people can use the same product from a spray can and inhale very different levels of the toxic ingredients. Their exposures could differ because they use the spray can in places having different ventilation and because they may hold the can differently. Air pollution levels can vary widely along a single block in a polluted city, and water pollutants may not be uniformly mixed within a reservoir. At best, average levels of exposure from average everyday activities can be estimated, and even these are poorly known in many cases.

For a person who is a member of a group that is especially vulnerable to a particular hazard (or especially invulnerable), a statement about average risk is misleading. For many toxics, only the members of especially vulnerable groups need be concerned about the risk, and so throughout this book we try to characterize those who are most at risk whenever the information exists.

Even when it is understood why risk estimates are based on probability, confusion often lingers. This is illustrated by the previous quote about the greater risk of dying in a car crash than from some chemical. To understand the confusion, let's look at the dual concepts of risk and benefit. There are many situations in which we expose ourselves to some environmental hazard because we also reap some benefit in doing so. Thus, we might expose ourselves to the fumes from a paint remover to accomplish a desired goal—the removal of paint. We may live in a polluted city because it would cost us more to live elsewhere or because it is where our job is or where our friends live. Sometimes the benefit is not merely a convenience, but instead is health promoting. We add preservatives to food (which carries some risk to health) to retard the formation of molds that might pose an even greater risk.

When we compare the risk of a toxic exposure to that of other unrelated activities, we can easily be fooled into thinking that the risk of practically any exposure to a toxic is insignificant. After all, with the exception of cigarette smoking, no single activity or toxic discussed in this book causes as many deaths each year in the United States as do automobile accidents (and most cause far, far less). But this risk comparison is no reason for a car driver to continue exposure to a toxic. Rather, it is a reason for the person to ask, "Am I getting enough benefit from exposure to the toxic to make the health risk acceptable

to me?" (By the same token, we might ask ourselves whether driving is worth the risk of dying in a car crash.) By comparing each risky activity with the benefits of that activity, rather than with the risks of some unrelated activity, we can be most certain that our actions match our priorities.

Risk–benefit comparisons also help make us aware of alternative ways of deriving the same benefit. True, it is practically impossible to enjoy many of life's benefits today without exposing ourselves to the risk of car accidents. But we may be able to avoid using a toxic chemical and still get comparable benefits by using some safer alternative product. Or we might decide that the benefits of using a certain toxic simply aren't worth the risk of toxic exposure and instead find something else to do to enrich our lives.

Pursuing this theme of risk and benefit, we encounter another important subtlety: the people who benefit from a particular activity may not be the same ones who must endure the risk of harm. For example, those who benefit from a new chemical may be the consumers using it and the stockholders of the company manufacturing it, while the factory workers producing it may suffer the consequences of its toxicity. Or one group of consumers may enjoy the benefits and endure the risk, while another group may only endure the risk. The two groups may not even be alive at the same time, for the present generation may enjoy the benefit of a new chemical, while our descendants may inherit the risk. For example, some of the *nuclear wastes*[1] produced by present-day nuclear power plants remain harmful for hundreds or thousands of years and will pose a risk to our great-grandchildren long after we, the generation that enjoyed the electricity, are gone. Toxic metals (see Chapter 12) such as the **lead**[2] released into the environment

[1] Technical terms italicized throughout the book are listed in the Glossary.

[2] Toxics that are boldfaced throughout the book are listed as entries in Part II, "A Guide to Commonly Encountered Toxics."

from lead-based paints or lead additives in gasoline persist in the environment as well.

The implications of such gaps between the winners and the losers are profound. The precept "take responsibility for your own actions" is firmly implanted in our ethics, yet it is increasingly difficult to obey this in our industrial society. How far into the future should we look when we count up the people who may die of cancer because of a long-lived waste product? Will new technologies come along that will eventually permit total removal of the waste? Will a cure for cancer eventually be found? Are benefits of the product to the present generation also benefits to future ones? (For example, the use of nuclear power today leaves more oil in the ground for future generations.) These are not easy questions, yet when we evaluate the costs and benefits of a new industrial product, we must at least be aware of these issues lest we become addicts of instant technological gratification.

Further complexity surrounds the subject of risk because of the wide range of hazards associated with various activities. Some toxic substances have a high probability of harming us, but the harm is not terribly great. Perhaps we are told that temporary dizziness and a tired feeling are the worst we can expect, but we are very likely to experience these symptoms if exposed to a normal dose of the product. In contrast, suppose normal use of another product leads to a very low probability of harm, but that harm is very severe. Perhaps normal use of this second product carries the risk of developing a fatal cancer, but the probability of getting that cancer is only 1 in 100,000. Which product should we use if they both produce the same benefit?

No one can answer that question for anyone else; the choice depends on how one weighs the odds. Some people view a 1 in 100,000 chance of developing a fatal cancer as so small that it can be ignored. They would take those odds rather than accept nearly certain but temporary dizziness and fatigue.

Others, however, might reason that such a chance of a fatal cancer (that is, suffering and death) is an unacceptable risk and opt for the other product. So, risk has two dimensions: probability and magnitude. Probability tells us how likely we are to respond in a certain way to the chemical. Magnitude tells us how severe that response will be. Individuals must make up their own minds about the relative importance they attach to these two aspects of risk.

The subject of risk is also complicated by the fact that some risky activities are more subject to our control than others. It is natural to fear more those risks associated with activities that are beyond our control. For example, most people fear flying more than driving, even though, per passenger mile, the odds of dying in a car crash are greater than the odds of dying in a commercial airline accident. The perception of toxic risks is no different. Suppose that by some objective measure of risk, the odds of getting a fatal cancer from the **aflatoxin** in peanut butter (at the rate you normally eat that product) and from the aerial spraying of pesticides on agricultural fields near your home were publicized as being the same. You would probably direct more outrage and fear at the spraying. The reason is that you have some control over your peanut butter consumption—you can try shopping around for brands that are made with the best preservation techniques and you can cut down on your intake if you want to. In contrast, the spraying is out of your control. The decision to spray is imposed upon you by someone else, and you may not even know it has been made.

Some scientists and public officials argue that the regulatory process ought to deal only with the objective risks associated with various activities, not with subjective issues such as people's feeling of control over exposure. They say that each regulatory dollar should be spent to get the maximum benefit in terms of increased lifespans or other objective measures of public health. Others argue that this misses the point and that public welfare should not be measured solely in terms of objective measures such as life-span. Instead, they argue, public welfare is diminished if people are fearful because they lack control over their exposure to chemicals. Hence, regulations designed to enhance public welfare must reflect such subjective perceptions of risk. Both sides, however, can agree that in a democracy, perceptions of risk will inevitably influence regulations, and that it will be up to those who believe that the present public perceptions of risk are somehow "wrong" to work to change these perceptions.

We have seen that the notion of risk is complex and subtle, with aspects that are highly subjective and dependent on one's own perceptions. Whether you are listening to a debate over chemical hazards or are just thinking about the consequences of your own actions, it is useful to keep these lessons in mind.

B. Causes of Death and Disease

About two million people die in the United States each year: 37% from heart attacks, 22% from cancer, 7% from strokes, and the remaining 34% from a variety of afflictions listed in Table 1. The average life expectancy at birth for white women is now 79 years, for white men 72 years, for black women 74 years, and for black men 65 years. This reflects a far different picture of our overall health than that at the turn of the century. In 1900, white life expectancy in the United States was slightly less than 50 years, and black life expectancy was about 34 years. Five of the ten leading causes of death were infectious diseases, with tuberculosis, pneumonia/influenza, and diarrhea/enteritis being the top three. Today only pneumonia/influenza remains in the top ten (sixth). What accounts for this changing pattern of health and disease and how it relates to toxic substances is the subject of this section.

The most important factor in the improvement of lifespan has been the control of in-fectious diseases. Prevention of disease by improved sanitation, housing, vaccines, and nutrition, as well as treatment with antibiotics, are largely responsible for the decline in the high rate of infant and childhood mortality that marked the turn of the century. In more recent years, improved treatment for the chronic diseases of old age has also added to the average lifespan.

Cardiovascular Diseases

Cardiovascular diseases (including heart disease, stroke, and high blood pressure) are the leading cause of death, together accounting for just under half of all deaths. The underlying cause of cardiovascular disease in 85% of the cases is a progressively deteriorating condition of the arteries known as *atherosclerosis*. Atherosclerosis begins in childhood with the laying down of fatty deposits on the interior lining of the arteries. By the fourth and fifth decades of life, the deposits have grown to the point where significant narrowing of the artery has taken place. The site of accumulation begins to harden, scar tissue starts to form, and the arterial wall loses its elasticity and becomes brittle. At this point, the artery is significantly weakened and is subject to rupture, hemorrhage, or *aneurysm*. Alternatively, and especially in the case of the coronary arteries, the hardened deposit may break loose from the arterial wall and travel downstream to a narrower portion of the artery where it partially or completely blocks the flow of blood (coronary thrombosis). This is what typically happens in a heart attack.

The exact causes of atherosclerosis are not known, but various risk factors have been identified. Various nationalities of the world, such as the Japanese, have a low incidence of atherosclerosis, but when they migrate to the United States, they develop the local incidence within one generation. This points strongly to environmental or lifestyle causes. Chief among the suspected factors is the high proportion of saturated fat in the U.S. diet; also related are cigarette smoking, high blood

TABLE 1 Leading Causes of Death in the United States—1988

Rank	Cause of Death	Number of Deaths	Percent of Deaths
	All causes	2,167,999	100.0
1	Heart diseases	765,156	35.3
2	Cancer	485,048	22.4
3	Stroke	150,517	6.9
4	Accidents	97,100	4.5
	(motor vehicle	49,078	2.3)
5	Chronic obstructive lung diseases	82,853	3.8
6	Pneumonia and influenza	77,662	3.6
7	Diabetes mellitus	40,368	1.9
8	Suicide	30,407	1.4
9	All other infectious and parasitic diseases (including AIDS)	27,168	1.3
10	Chronic liver disease and cirrhosis	26,409	1.2
11	Nephritis, nephrotic syndrome, and nephrosis	22,392	1.0
12	Atherosclerosis	22,086	1.0
13	Homocide	22,032	1.0
14	Septicemia	20,925	1.0
15	Diseases of infancy	18,220	0.8
	Other and ill-defined	276,623	12.8

Source: National Center for Health Statistics. 1990. "Advance report of final mortality statistics, 1988." *Monthly Vital Statistics Report.* Vol. 39, no. 7, supplement. Hyattsville, MD: U.S. Public Health Service.

pressure, and the level of cholesterol circulating in the blood. It is unclear whether cholesterol in the diet actually determines the level of circulating blood cholesterol or whether that level is controlled by other factors. People at elevated risk for heart disease are well advised to reduce their cholesterol and fat consumption in case dietary cholesterol proves to be a controlling factor.

Regular vigorous exercise can apparently slow the atherosclerotic process by raising the proportion of so-called high-density lipoproteins (HDLs) in the blood, which actually seem to be able to scour the arteries of deposited fat. A sedentary lifestyle raises the proportion of low-density lipoproteins (LDLs), which carry cholesterol to the point of deposit. Three hours per week of vigorous exercise probably provides the maximum benefit. Moderate alcohol consumption and use of aspirin are also apparently protective against cardiovascular disease. Daily intake of aspirin is now recommended for individuals at high risk of heart disease. However, the side effects of aspirin, including the possibility of increased risk of stroke, make it unsuitable for low-risk individuals to take on a daily basis. Alcohol is associated with certain cancers (particularly among smokers) and is not recommended for the prevention of heart disease. Fish and fish oil may also protect against the disease.

The good news about cardiovascular disease is that the death rate is dropping quite rapidly. Since 1950, the number of cardiovascular deaths per 100,000 persons per year has been nearly halved (from 396 to 213). One reason for this striking decline is the identification and modification of behavior that increased the risk, leading, for example, to a reduction in dietary fat, a reduction in smoking, and an increase in exercise by many people. Another reason is improvements in medical diagnosis and treatment, including better treatment of *hypertension,* hospital coronary care units, cardio-pulmonary resuscitation (CPR), coronary by-pass surgery, and new and effective drugs. As prevention is given increased attention and as improvements in medical technology continue, we can look forward to further declines in the nation's number one killer.

Cancer

Cancer is the cause of death most people think of as associated with exposure to toxics. Currently, nearly 500,000 people die each year from cancer in the United States (nearly one in four deaths), and a million new cases are diagnosed annually. Unfortunately, in contrast to the decline in cardiovascular disease, several forms of cancer are increasing (due in large measure to cigarette smoking), leading to a rise in the overall death rate from cancer. Between 1950 and 1985 the annual incidence of reported new cancer cases rose about 1% per year (36.5% overall). The death rate from cancer rose a much smaller 0.2% per year, which partially reflects better treatment. This disparity between the incidence rate and death rate reflects better diagnosis and reporting of new cases, which makes the reported incidence rate much greater.

Most of the increase in the overall cancer rate is from lung cancer. If lung cancer is separated from the statistics, the death rate from all other cancers actually decreased by 13.3% since 1950. This overall decrease in nonrespiratory cancer deaths, however, is not uniform. It is made up of some cancers that declined markedly (such as stomach cancer) and others (such as the often fatal skin cancer melanoma) that rose, but not as much. Some of the cancers that have increased are discussed in the following sections.

The cure rate for most cancers has not improved significantly since 1950, with the important exceptions of childhood leukemia and Hodgkin's disease. The five-year survival rate (that is, the percentage of patients surviving for at least five years after a diagnosis of cancer has been made) has improved to 50%, from 39% in 1950. But much of this apparent improvement is due to earlier detection, thus lengthening the time to eventual death, rather than to more effective treatment.

The good news about cancer is that it is largely preventable. Not that all the important causes of cancer have been determined, but a comparison of the patterns of cancer among different nationalities, between migrant populations and their countries of origin, and of the changes over time within a country all show that most cancers have an environmental and/or behavioral origin. Environment and behavior in this context, however, do not only mean exposures to toxics but include all external factors over which people do or can exert control: man-made and natural toxics, viral infections, nutritional deficiencies or excesses, reproductive activities, and so on. Research on the specific causes of various cancers has begun to show that the large majority of human cancers (perhaps as much as 80 or 90%) can be avoided by suitable changes in environment or behavior.

How cancers get started is not fully understood. Several steps or stages are believed to be involved. In the first stage, called initiation, a change occurs in the genetic material (DNA) of a cell. The change can be caused by a chemical, a virus, or radiation, and it primes the cell for the next stage, called promotion. Promotion involves a second change to the genetic material that causes the cell to begin multiplying, forming a tumor. The third and final stage is called proliferation, in which some cells break away from the tumor, enter the bloodstream or lymphatic system, and colonize other tissues. This process is called metastasis, and the original tumor is referred to as being malignant. (Benign tumors do not metastasize.) Cancer becomes fatal only after metastasis has occurred. How agents alter cells to produce the various stages of cancer is not known. Some such as radiation are capable of causing both initiation and promotion (complete carcinogens) whereas others only initiate, and a second agent called a promoter must act for a tumor to form. What starts metastasis is even less well understood. There can be a long time interval between the several stages of cancer production, which is referred to as the latency period.

In our discussions of individual cancers, the currently suspected risk factors are mentioned so that individuals can take practical actions now in the hope of reducing the risk of cancer. Keep in mind, however, that only in a few cases have these risk factors been conclusively established as the most important causative agents.

Lung Cancer   Lung cancer, colon and rectal cancers, and breast cancer together account for half of all U.S. cancer deaths today. Table 2 shows the number of cancer cases, the number of deaths, and the percentage of deaths from each type for the year 1985. Lung cancer is the leading fatal cancer in both sexes, having recently overtaken breast cancer as the leading fatal cancer among women. In 1985, lung cancer caused 122,000 deaths (26.5% of all cancer deaths; 6% of deaths from all causes). The rate of new lung cancer cases among men has leveled off after rising steadily throughout this century, owing to a decrease in smoking among younger men. For women, the rate of new cases is still rising rapidly, reflecting the large increase in cigarette smoking by women since the 1950s. Lung cancer is nearly always fatal, usually within five years.

Cigarette smoking is without a doubt the major cause of lung cancer, responsible for an estimated 85% of lung cancer deaths. That tobacco smoke should cause cancer is not surprising since it contains numerous substances that, individually, are known to cause cancer, such as tars, **benzo[*a*]pyrenes, nitrosamines, arsenic,** and **cadmium**). In addition to lung cancer, cigarette smoking is implicated in many other cancers, as well as in cardiovascular diseases (see Chapter 5, Section B). If we add up the deaths from all these cancers, tobacco is responsible for about one-third of all cancer deaths.

Other known causes of lung cancer include **asbestos, radon, arsenic,** environmental tobacco smoke, and other, mainly occupational chemicals. Exactly what proportion of lung cancers among nonsmoking members of the general population is due to these substances, many of which are components of air pollution, is the subject of vigorous debate by knowledgeable experts. The U.S. Office of Technology Assessment and the EPA estimate that approximately 10% of all lung cancers are produced by environmental pollution, including naturally occurring radon gas. What everyone does agree on is that tobacco smoke multiplies the inherent risk of each of these substances, so that smokers are always at a much greater risk of dying from lung cancer than are nonsmokers exposed to similar environmental conditions. Quitting smoking (and to a lesser extent, avoiding the smoky air produced by smokers) is clearly the single most important thing one can do to avoid developing cancer.

Colon and Rectal Cancers   Colon and rectal cancers together are the second leading fatal cancers, causing 12.5% of all cancer deaths (nearly 58,000 deaths in 1985). The incidence rate has been rising gradually over the past 35 years, whereas the death rate has declined slightly. The percentage of patients surviving for five years after an initial diagnosis has improved to just over 50% from about 40% in 1950.

Dietary factors are strongly implicated as causes of colon and rectal cancers, as might be expected for cancers of the digestive tract. A high calorie intake, particularly in the form of animal fat, appears to increase the chances of these cancers; consumption of whole grains, cereals, fruits, and vegetables lessens the risk. Dietary fiber in particular appears to be protective. Stomach cancer, the leading fatal cancer in the 1930s, has declined markedly and is now responsible for only about 3% of cancer deaths. The reasons for this decline are not well understood, but may be related to the widespread use of refrigeration to preserve foods and the consequent

TABLE 2 Cancer Statistics for the United States—1985

Primary Site	Number of Estimated Cases	Number of Actual Deaths	Percentage of Cancer Deaths
All sites	910,000	461,520	100.0
Lung and bronchus	144,000	122,395	26.5
Males	98,000	83,754	
Females	46,000	38,641	
Colon and rectum	138,000	57,586	12.5
Colon	96,000	49,726	
Rectum	42,000	7,860	
Breast	119,000	40,090	8.7
Prostate gland	86,000	25,940	5.6
Pancreas		23,099	5.0
Leukemia	24,600	17,449	3.8
Non-Hodgkin's lymphoma	26,500	15,358	3.3
Stomach	24,700	13,949	3.0
Ovary	18,500	11,357	2.5
Brain and nervous system		10,265	2.2
Urinary bladder	40,000	9,785	2.1
Kidney	19,700	8,660	1.9
Esophagus		8,612	1.9
Oral and pharynx		8,290	1.8
Multiple myeloma		7,819	1.7
Uteris	37,000	5,959	1.3
Liver		5,952	1.3
Skin melanoma	22,000	5,529	1.2
Cervix	15,000	4,508	1.0
Larynx	11,500	3,501	0.8
Childhood cancers	6,000	1,840	0.4
Hodgkin's disease	6,900	1,778	0.4
Thyroid gland		957	0.2
Testis	5,000	425	0.1

Source: U.S. Department of Health and Human Services, National Institutes of Health. *1987 Annual Cancer Statistics Review*. NIH Publication No. 88–2789. Bethesda, MD: National Cancer Institute.

reduction of salting, pickling, and smoking for preservation, all of which are suspected causes of stomach cancer. The increased consumption of fresh fruits and vegetables may also have helped because of their protective effects.

Breast Cancer Breast cancer is the second leading fatal cancer among women, having just been surpassed by lung cancer. New cases are diagnosed in about 130,000 women every year; over 40,000 women die annually from the disease. The percentage of women surviving for five years after a diagnosis of breast cancer is approximately 75%. The incidence of breast cancer appears to be rising slightly, although this may be due in part to better detection and thus to more cases being reported. The causes of breast cancer are not known, but hormonal factors are strongly suspected. Factors that appear to increase the risk include no pregnancy or late age at first pregnancy, early onset of menstruation, late menopause, and a family history of breast cancer. Conversely, some protection appears to result from an early age at first childbirth, breast-feeding, late onset of menstruation and early menopause (in other words, a shorter menstrual history lessens risk, presumably by reducing the total time breast tissue is in contact with hormonal stimulus). Dietary fat consumption (particularly milk fat) correlates strongly with breast cancer, and this and other dietary factors, such as alcohol consumption, are currently receiving much study. Radiation exposure is also a risk factor.

Oral contraceptives (the "pill") for a long time were not believed to influence the development of breast cancer. The latest studies, however, are showing some linkage. At the present time, the data are difficult to interpret and further studies are under way. Experts are not recommending any change in pill use until the results of the new studies are in. One thing to keep in mind is that the dosages during the early period of pill use were much greater than the dosages prescribed today. Any cancers showing up now would be associated with these higher hormone levels in the early pills.

Other female reproductive cancers, including cancers of the cervix, uterus, and ovary, have been declining gradually among younger women, with cancer of the cervix showing a marked decline. Early diagnosis of precancerous lesions by pap smear followed by treatment is the main reason for the large decrease of cervical cancer.

Other Cancers Prostate cancer, the third leading fatal cancer among men (86,000 cases in 1985 and about 26,000 deaths), has been increasing steadily, but this, too, may reflect better detection and reporting rather than an actual increase in development of the disease. The survival rate has improved substantially so that 75% of newly diagnosed patients survive at least five years. Little is known about the causes of prostate cancer. The amount of sexual activity, the level of male hormones, the intake of dietary fat, and occupational exposures to **cadmium** have all been suggested as playing roles in development of the disease.

Leukemia and some cancers of the urinary bladder, kidney, and pancreas have all been associated with carcinogens of the workplace, and the first three, also with cigarette smoking. Cancer of the pancreas is the fourth leading fatal cancer in both sexes. Most of the current cases of cancer in this group are attributed to smoking, although there appears to be a slightly elevated risk of bladder cancer in the general population from *trihalomethanes* produced by water chlorination.

Skin cancer is by far the most common cancer, but the overwhelming majority of cases are nonfatal, easily treated, and therefore generally not reported in cancer statistics. These are the basal cell carcinomas and squamous cell carcinomas. Melanoma of the skin is the often fatal form of skin cancer, and its incidence is among the most rapidly rising of all cancers. Exposure to **ultraviolet radiation** is the main cause of melanoma. If ultraviolet radiation increases because of stratospheric ozone depletion (see Chapter 11, Section B), further increases in the incidence of fatal skin cancer are to be expected.

Toxic Substances and Cancer After reviewing the common forms of cancer and their suspected causes, we can now ask, What portion of them is due to exposure to toxics? Tobacco smoke is easily the largest single cause of all fatal human cancers, and it is composed of many toxic substances. So in one sense, a large portion of human cancers is due to toxic substances. But other than tobacco smoke, do toxic substances cause a large proportion of human cancers? The answer is unclear and vigorously debated. At one extreme, there are some experts who argue that as many as 30% of human cancers stem from exposure to toxics (including occupational exposures) other than tobacco smoke. At the other extreme are experts who claim a negligible fraction are caused by toxics. The main U.S. agencies involved in this field, including the EPA, OTA, and NIH, take the middle ground, suggesting that about 10% of cancers result from toxic exposures other than tobacco.

One important feature of the debate is that current cancer statistics only indicate past exposures. Numerous substances have been introduced in large quantities in the past 20 to 30 years whose *latency periods* (the time between exposure and effect) are only now being exceeded. Some of these materials may significantly increase future cancer rates. In the face of uncertainty about the implications of recently developed substances and the possibility that they might interact with existing carcinogens, we as a society need to carefully control the release of new chemical materials.

Other Causes of Death

Accidents are the fourth leading cause of deaths in the United States, responsible for about 100,000 fatalities, or 5% of all deaths. Motor vehicle accidents account for half of those fatalities. Other significant causes of death related to toxic substances include chronic obstructive lung diseases (fifth leading cause, 3.4% of deaths, caused by smoking, industrial exposures, and air pollution); cirrhosis of the liver (ninth leading cause, 1.3% of deaths, caused by alcohol consumption); and kidney disease (eleventh leading cause, 1% of deaths, some cases caused by exposure to toxic chemicals).

Further Reading

BAILAR, J., and WILSON, E. 1986. Progress Against Cancer? *New England Journal of Medicine* 314:1226–1232.

COHEN, LEONARD A. 1987. Diet and Cancer. *Scientific American* 257:42–48.

FEINLEIB, MANNING, and WILSON, RONALD W. 1985. Trends in Health in the United States. *Environmental Health Perspectives* 62:267–276.

TRIBE, L. H., SCHELLING, C. S., and VOSS, J., editors. 1976. *When Values Conflict: Essays on Environmental Analysis, Discourse, and Decision*. Cambridge, MA: Ballinger.

U.S. Office of Technology Assessment. 1981. *Assessment of Technologies for Determining Cancer Risks from the Environment*. Washington, D.C.

WILSON, R., and CROUCH, E. 1982. *Risk/Benefit Analysis*. Cambridge, MA: Ballinger.

2 THE LANGUAGE OF TOXICS

This chapter is for readers who want to understand the language that scientists speak when they talk quantitatively about the risk of toxics. Although most of the rest of the book is not dependent on the material here, this chapter provides a relatively painless way to understand what the numbers mean when scientists describe toxic risks. Equally important, it will help you to recognize when someone is communicating nonsensical numerical descriptions of quantities and risk of toxics in the environment, as happens more often than it should in the public media.

A. How Risk Is Described

All common measures of health risk contain several parts: a measure of pollutant exposure (including the amount of pollutant and the period over which exposure occurred), a description of the type of health damage, a description of the exposed population, and a statement expressing the odds that an individual in the exposed population will suffer the health damage. An informative statement of health risk should also tell you what the *background risk* is (that is, what proportion of the population would suffer the health damage even if they were not exposed to the pollutant). The exposed population may be smokers, asthmatics, test animals, all residents of a city, all people getting drinking water from a particular reservoir, or any other definable group. The amount of pollutant to which each individual is exposed is called the dose, and the amount of health damage is called the response. A scientific study to determine risk is sometimes called a dose–response investigation. The result of the investigation is a graph such as that shown in Figure 1, which is called a *dose–response curve* or *relation*.

Dose

A dose is usually expressed in one of three ways:

1. the amount of the substance actually in the body,

2. the amount of the material entering the body (usually in food, drinking water, or the air you breathe), or

3. the concentration in the environment.

For example, a dose can be expressed as the weight of lead in a person's bloodstream, the amount of a radioactive substance inhaled during an accidental release, or the concentration of a pesticide in a reservoir used for drinking water. If the concentration in the environment is used as a measure, the amount of time the individual has experienced that environmental concentration must be specified. Otherwise, the actual exposure to that substance would be unknown and so the risk to health could not be estimated.

It is fairly easy to relate the third example (pesticide in a reservoir) to the second one. All you need to know is the amount of tap water you drink each day from the reservoir and the concentration of the substance in the drinking water. From this, your intake of the pesticide can be estimated. It is more difficult, however, to figure out how much of a toxic substance resides in your body if all you know is how much you ingested or inhaled. The reason is that the body generally does not retain all of the ingested or inhaled pollution; some of the pollution is excreted or exhaled and some may be broken down in the body and converted to less (or more) toxic forms (see Chapter 4, Section A). Because of the difficulty in estimating amounts actually in the body, most risk estimates are couched

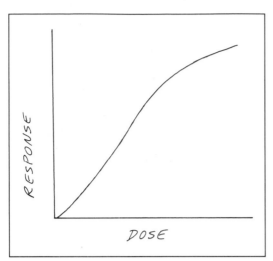

Figure 1 A dose–response relation. As the dose of a toxic substance increases, the response (for example, the severity of the effect) increases as well.

in terms of the amount of pollutant entering the body or the amount in the environment. But there are some important exceptions such as **lead**, for which direct measurement in blood provides a useful index of the amount in the body.

An additional problem arises in describing dose when it is expressed as a bodily intake. A person can ingest or inhale some specified amount of a pollutant over a short or long period of time. In many cases, the shorter the time period over which the body receives a fixed total amount of pollutant, the greater the damage will be. The reason is that the body's mechanisms for repairing the toxic damage can be overwhelmed if the uptake of the substance is sudden. Thus, ideally, a description of dose should state not only the total dose but also whether it is received over a long or short time period. The terms chronic dose and acute dose are used to describe two extreme rates of uptake. A chronic dose is one that is received over a long time interval (usually greater than a few months), and an acute dose is one received over a short interval (usually 24 hours or less).

A fourth way of describing dose exists, but is rarely used in dose–response relations.

It is the amount of pollutant coming out of a smokestack or discharge pipe. This is called the pollution emission rate. While under some circumstances this may be the easiest type of dose estimate to measure, it is difficult to relate to the actual exposure a person receives. Some of the complications that arise in trying to relate emission rate to environmental concentration and bodily intake are discussed in Chapter 9, Movement of Toxics Through the Environment.

Response

The statement of the health damage (or response) resulting from a specified dose can be couched in many different forms because there are so many different dimensions to human health and its degradation. Some of the most commonly encountered expressions of risk are listed here:

> The likelihood that a person exposed to the pollutant will, as a result of exposure, contract a particular disease sometime during his or her lifetime (or in some specified time interval, such as the year following exposure)
>
> The likelihood that the exposed person will, as a result of exposure, contract a particular disease and eventually die of it
>
> The average number of years of life that the exposed person is likely to lose as the result of the exposure
>
> The average number of days of work that a person will miss because of the exposure
>
> The decrease in some measure of performance (for example, athletic performance of schoolchildren) as a result of exposure.

Each of these five statements of response to a dose is a perfectly fine way to convey information. The one most appropriate to a particular substance and type of exposure depends on the type of damage that occurs as well as on the public's judgment about what aspect of the health damage is of concern.

When you read an estimate of the health hazard from some toxic substance that you are exposed to, the chances are that the statement of hazard will make reference to an exposure level that is not exactly the same as the one in your environment or in your body. For example, you may learn that there is a 1 in 100,000 chance that you will develop a certain type of cancer as a result of a lifetime of exposure to some specified level of a pollutant in drinking water. But in your drinking water, the level of the pollutant is twice the value specified in the risk estimate of 1 in 100,000. What should you assume is your cancer risk associated with drinking your water?

This is not an easy question, and for many substances the research has not been done to answer it. It is very tempting to speculate that if the dose is doubled, so is the response, in which case the odds of getting cancer in the situation just described would be 1 in 50,000. When the relationship between dose and response is that simple (for example, doubling the dose doubles the response), then it is called a linear dose–response relation. This relation is illustrated by the dashed line in Figure 2. For some substances, such a relation has been established, at least over some range of dose. But there is clearly one type of situation in which this cannot be true; if a certain dose results, say, in a 51% chance of dying, then doubling that dose would not result in a 102% chance. In other words, the dose–response curve has to curve over near the top end (that is, it can't be linear) for the simple reason that you can't die more than once. This is an example of a *saturation effect.* It is illustrated by the portion of the graph labeled "A."

The assumption of a linear dose–response relation can also be wrong at low doses. For example, if the body has natural repair mechanisms that fix the damage caused by low doses, then low doses may have practically no damaging effect. But at higher doses, those repair mechanisms may be overwhelmed and may not be able to keep up with the rate of damage. The part of the graph labeled "B" illustrates this *threshold effect,* so called because there is a threshold below which there is relatively little damage and above which the damage increases dramatically.

Saturation effects and threshold effects make interpretation of laboratory toxicity test results more difficult. Such tests are usually carried out at high doses so that very rare responses can be detected and so that vast numbers of test animals are not required (see Chapter 3, Section A). To determine the response at lower, more realistic doses from data on responses at higher doses, the overall shape of the dose–response curve must be known for the toxic being tested. But if the tests are only done at a few doses, it is difficult to know the overall shape of the dose–response curve. Suppose that the curve is assumed to be linear at low doses, but in fact there is a threshold effect. Then the true response at realistic low doses may be considerably less than would be deduced from the high-dose data. In other circumstances, such as when the saturation effect begins at a lower dose than assumed, it is possible to underestimate the true response at lower doses based on limited data in the saturation zone.

Confusion often occurs over the real meaning of such phrases as "the probability of your developing cancer as a result of a certain exposure to a toxic is 1%." It does not mean that out of a group of 100 people who are subjected to that exposure of the toxic, 1 and only 1 person will develop the cancer. To illustrate the true meaning of this phrase, imagine that a large number of groups of 100 people are each exposed to this same quantity of the toxic. In one of these groups, perhaps nobody will develop the cancer. In another, perhaps 4 will. If you take the average of the number of cancers from all the groups, then you have estimated that particular cancer rate. Suppose that the average is 3 per 100. Then there is a 3% chance that those exposed to the toxic will develop the cancer. But not all those cancers can be attributed to the toxic. The background risk for that type of cancer (that is, the odds that the cancer would occur if you were not exposed to the toxic) is found by looking at another collection of groups of 100 people who have not been exposed. In those

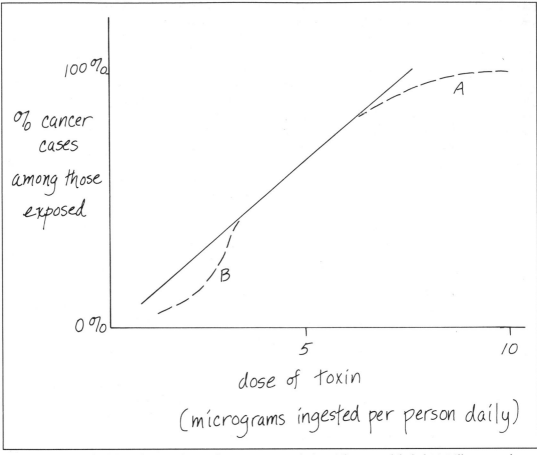

Figure 2 The dashed line shows a linear dose–response relation. The curve labeled "A" illustrates the saturation effect, and "B" shows the threshold effect.

groups, the average number of people who develop the cancer may not be 0. Suppose the average number is 2, or 2%. Then, by subtracting the background risk of 2% from the total risk of 3%, you obtain an estimate of 1% for the cancer risk attributable to the toxic.

It would be naive to take all risk estimates seriously. The information presented here is intended to show you how to interpret a statement about health risk under the assumption that the statement is correct. But not all published risk evaluations are, in fact, reliable. Many of the difficulties associated with measuring a dose–response relation are discussed in Chapter 3, Section A. Other sources of uncertainty in our knowledge of the risk of

toxics are discussed in the individual entries in Part II of this book, A Guide to Commonly Encountered Toxics.

B. Units Used to Describe Toxics

In the first part of this chapter, we explained the standard ways that risk is described. Here we acquaint the reader with the language used to characterize amounts of toxic substances in the environment. Only nonradioactive substances are discussed here because the terminology used to describe radioactivity and its effects is explained in Chapter 15, Sec-

18   ALL ABOUT TOXICS

tion E (Units Used to Describe Radiation). Units, in the sense used in this book, are simply expressions of measurements or amounts. Some familiar units are pounds, minutes, miles, dollars, miles per hour, and dollars per pound. Those used to express the amounts of pollutants in the environment are no more complicated, only less familiar. Which units are used depends on whether the substance is in water, body tissue, or air and whether the substance is a gas, liquid, or solid (such as **asbestos**). It also depends on whether the pollutant is being discharged from a source, is in the environment, or is being taken up by the body. Our discussion here highlights these distinctions.

Readers familiar with the basic ideas of scientific units may want to turn directly to the tables and lists interspersed throughout this discussion for summaries of all the relevant units and the interrelations among them.

Discharge to the Environment

The amount of pollution going into the air from a smokestack or into a stream from a factory discharge pipe is usually expressed as a rate, using some measure of pollutant weight per unit of time. For example, the emission rate of **sulfur dioxide** from a large, modern, coal-fired electric generating plant is typically several hundred tons per day. Those units (tons per day) rather than, say, ounces per year are used to avoid awkwardly large numbers (for the same reason that we express our weight in pounds, not ounces).

In the case of the routine operation of a factory, where a pollutant's discharge is fairly constant from day to day, information about the rate of release can be easily converted to an estimate of the total yearly release or total release over the factory's lifetime. In the event of an accident that suddenly releases pollution into the environment, the discharge rate is often neither constant nor accurately measured. Knowledge of the total amount that was accidentally discharged is usually more useful to the general public.

Environmental Concentrations

Does 10 tons of a pollutant in a huge reservoir pose less of a hazard than 1 ton of the same substance in a small well? It depends on how you look at it. In one very important sense, the answer is yes. The concentration of the pollutant is greater in the well water and so the amount taken into the body by someone drinking that water will be greater than if the person drank from the reservoir. However, since many more people drink from the reservoir than the well and since the total amount of pollution in the reservoir is greater than in the well water, the polluted reservoir could threaten more people.

Usually, information about amounts of toxic substances in the environment is expressed as concentrations. To augment that information, further facts are needed about how many people drink the water or breathe the air so that the total hazard to a population of people can be estimated.

Water Pollutants Concentrations of pollutants in water are most commonly expressed in terms of the weight of the pollutant divided by the volume of the water or the weight of the pollutant divided by the weight of the water. The volume of the water can be expressed in units such as pints, quarts, gallons, cubic inches, or cubic feet. These are examples of what are called British units; they are in everyday use in the United States but are not used in the scientific literature nor in most other nations. The scientific way to describe volume is by using the metric system of measurement, in which the usual units of volume are the cubic centimeter (cm^3), the liter (L), and the cubic meter (m^3). A centimeter is roughly the width of a typical thumbtack head; there are about 2.5 centimeters in an inch. So a cubic centimeter is roughly the size of a bouillon cube or a small sugar cube. A meter is 100 centimeters long— a little longer than a yard. A cubic meter of water is about twice the volume you could put in a bathtub filled to the brim. A liter is slightly larger than a quart and equals 1000 cubic centimeters. Some of the most useful relationships among these different units of length and volume are shown here.

Length
1 meter = 100 centimeters = 3.281 feet = 39.37 inches
1 kilometer = 1000 meters = 0.62 miles

Volume
1 liter = 1000 cubic centimeters = 1.057 quarts
1 cubic meter = 1000 liters = 264.2 gallons = 35.3 cubic feet

The weight of water can be given in units of ounces, pounds, or even tons, but these are also examples of British units. In the scientific or metric way to describe weight, the gram (g) is the most common unit. A pound is equivalent to about 450 grams. A gram of water has a volume of 1 cubic centimeter. The unit kilogram (kg) refers to 1000 grams, so 1 kilogram of water has a volume of 1000 cubic centimeters, or 1 liter. An even larger weight is the metric ton, sometimes spelled tonne. It equals 1000 kilograms. Here is a summary of some useful relationships among various units of weight.

Weight
1 kilogram = 1000 grams = 2.205 pounds = 35.3 ounces
1 metric tonne = 1000 kilograms = 1.102 British tons
1 pound = 16 ounces = 453.6 grams

How do we express the amount of a toxic substance in water? The customary way, for most nonradioactive water pollutants, is by weight. Because there is usually far less than 1 gram of pollutant in the volume of water you drink in a typical day, weights of pollutants are often expressed in units of thousandths, millionths, or billionths of a gram. In scientific lingo, a thousandth of a gram is a milligram (mg), a millionth of a gram is a microgram (μg), and a billionth of a gram is a nanogram (ng).

Usually the units with which a concentration is expressed are chosen so that very large or very small numbers are avoided. For example, you would not want to state the concentration of a pesticide in your drinking water in units of tons of pesticide per liter of water because the actual value would be an incredibly small number. Nor would you want to express it in units of nanograms (billionths of a gram) per cubic kilometer because the numerical value would then be incredibly large. For toxic substances such as trace metals and pesticides in water, the most often used unit for concentration is micrograms per liter (μg/L), because in that combination of units, the actual numbers are typically neither awkwardly small nor large. For example, typical drinking water has a **cadmium** concentration of a little less than 1 microgram of cadmium in a liter of water, and the EPA limits the concentration of cadmium in drinking water to 10 micrograms per liter.

There are many ways to express the same actual concentration. While it may seem unnecessary to have so many different ways to say the same thing, all of these expressions can be encountered in newspaper articles of pollution problems. It can be very useful to know how to translate one to another in the same way that it is useful for a shopper to feel equally comfortable with a label saying "25 cents each" and one saying "four for a dollar." Consider, for example, a concentration of 1 microgram per liter. It can be stated in several equivalent ways, as these three examples show:

1 microgram per liter
= 1 milligram per cubic meter (because a cubic meter contains 1000 liters and a milligram contains 1000 micrograms)
= 1 microgram per kilogram (because a liter weighs 1 kilogram, but now the concentration is expressed in terms of weight per unit of water weight rather than weight per unit of water volume)

= 1 part per billion by weight (because the toxic substance weighs one-billionth of the weight of the water it is in)

This last unit, parts per billion (abbreviated ppb), needs some explanation. A related unit is parts per million (abbreviated ppm); 1 ppm is equal to 1000 ppb. The unit parts per trillion (ppt) also arises occasionally to describe pollutants such as **dioxin**, which are found in incredibly small concentrations in water. Table 3 shows the relationships among different units of concentrations of substances in water. As an example of how to use the table, suppose you want to express the unit micrograms per liter as parts per "something." Looking across from 1 microgram in the first column and down from "1 liter," they intersect at 1 ppb.

To get an intuitive feeling for what a part per million is, think about dissolving half a bouillon cube in a bathtub full of water. The half bouillon cube weighs about half a gram, and the water in a full bathtub weighs about 500 kilograms, or half a million grams. Therefore, the concentration is 1 gram per million grams or 1 ppm. A part per billion can be thought of as roughly a drop in a medium-sized swimming pool.

We have shown how to express concentrations of pollutants in water, but the units are equally useful for any other medium. For instance, the concentration of a pesticide in milk can be expressed in just the same way as for a pesticide in water. Although it will not be exactly accurate, it can be assumed that a liter of any drinkable liquid weighs a kilogram, just like water.

Pollutants in the Human Body

Concentrations of nonradioactive pollutants in the human body are often expressed in weight per weight units. The only complication is that the whole body is not always taken as the reference. Rather, body concentrations are often based on concentrations in bone or fat or some other body component in which the pollutant tends to lodge. One important exception is blood concentrations. Quite often, pollutant concentrations in blood are given in units of weight of pollutant per volume of blood. In particular, units of micrograms (or milligrams) per 100 milliliters are most often used. A milliliter (mL) equals the volume of a cubic centimeter. With a little arithmetic, you can show that a concentration (in water) of 1 microgram per 100 milliliters is equivalent to 10 ppb.

Pollutants in Air

Air pollutants can be in any of three forms—gas, *aerosol,* or particle. Aerosols are a fine, mistlike suspension of liquid or solid. Particles, sometimes called *particulates,* are small specks of solid matter. For example, **carbon monoxide** and **sulfur dioxide** are gaseous air pollutants, a mist of pesticide spray is an aerosol, and specks of asbestos in the air are particulates. The appropriate units for describing concentrations of air pollutants depend on the form of the pollutant.

For aerosols and particulates, the customary way to refer to concentration is by weight per volume of air or number of particles per volume of air. The most commonly used weight per volume units are micrograms of pollutant per cubic meter of air ($\mu m/m^3$). A cubic meter of air at sea level weighs about 1 kilogram, and there are one billion (one thousand million) micrograms in a kilogram. Therefore, a microgram per cubic meter of air is the same, on a weight per weight basis, as a part per billion, but the latter is rarely used to describe aerosol or particulate air pollutants.

We can get an intuitive feeling for what 1 microgram per cubic meter really is by estimating the number of particles that would be inhaled with each breath or with every hour of breathing air with that concentration of particles. Relatively large particles, such as those that occur in dusty air, typically weigh up to 1 microgram, so 1 microgram per cubic meter is the same as one particle per cubic meter. With each breath, a typical individual inhales about 2 liters of air, or 1/500 of 1 cubic meter. Therefore, a concentration of

TABLE 3 Relationships Among Various Units of Concentrations of Substances in Water

Quantity of Toxic	Quantity of Water		
	1 Cubic Centimeter	1 Liter	1 Cubic Meter
1 nanogram (billionth of a gram)	1 ppb	1 ppt	1 ppq[a]
1 microgram (millionth of a gram)	1 ppm	1 ppb	1 ppt
1 milligram (thousandth of a gram)	1 ppth[b]	1 ppm	1 ppb
1 gram	—	1 ppth[b]	1 ppm

[a] ppq means parts per quadrillion.

[b] ppth means parts per thousand.

1 microgram per cubic meter of these large particles means that with every 500 breaths, a person will on the average inhale one such dust particle. Since the typical breathing rate is about 500 breaths per hour, this means that one such particle will be inhaled every hour. That represents a relatively low rate of bodily intake of dust—air that is visibly dusty probably contains several tens or hundreds of micrograms of dust per cubic meter.

Very fine particles, in contrast, such as those that are emitted with automobile exhaust, number as many as a million per microgram. For these particles, a concentration of 1 microgram per cubic meter means that about 2000 particles are inhaled with each breath (1,000,000/cubic meter × 1/500 cubic meter). Typical urban air in the United States contains about this concentration of these microscopic (invisible to the naked eye) particles.

For gaseous air pollutants, concentrations are usually expressed on a molecule per molecule basis. In a fixed volume of air, the number of pollutant gas molecules is divided by the number of air molecules to give a concentration that can be expressed in units of parts per million (ppm) or parts per billion (ppb). If one in a million air molecules is actually a molecule of some pollutant such as carbon monoxide, then the concentration of the pollutant is 1 ppm. Occasionally, however, gaseous air pollutants are expressed on a weight per weight basis. Again, the unit can be either ppm or ppb. A milligram of gaseous pollution per kilogram of air is 1 ppm. To distinguish which type of ppm is intended, the weight per weight units are often written as ppm(w) or ppb(w), where the "w" stands for weight. Similarly, the molecule per molecule units are often written as ppm(v) or ppb(v), where the "v" stands for volume. The reason that molecule per molecule units and volume per volume units are interchangeable is that a gas occupies a volume proportional to the number of gas molecules present.

Bodily Uptake

The units used to describe bodily uptake are akin to those for describing discharge to the environment. For steady exposures, such as would occur if a person drank water from a polluted reservoir, the uptake is expressed as a rate, usually in micrograms per day or year. Knowing the concentration of the pollutant in the reservoir water (say, in micrograms per liter) and the rate the person drinks water (typically about a liter per day), the uptake rate can be figured out. Sometimes doses are expressed in units such as micrograms per day per kilogram of body weight, thereby adjusting the dose to take into account the body weight. The reason for this is that if a little child and an adult each take in the same weight of pollutant, the child will be more at risk because, everything else being equal, the pollutant will be more concentrated in the child.

In the case of a sudden, accidental release of pollution that causes a brief but intense exposure, say, because a tank of toxic chemical explodes and releases a poisonous gas into the air, a public health official would be more interested in the total amount of pollutant each person takes up rather than in the amount per day. Each person's uptake might be measured in micrograms or milligrams. Sometimes it is useful to express the uptake resulting from an accidental discharge in terms of the time it would take an individual to receive the same amount of pollution during normal conditions. For example, the sudden dose received from the accident might be expressed as equal to what the individual would receive over eight accident-free years.

SOME BASIC MEDICAL ASPECTS
OF THE TOXICS PROBLEM

3 TESTING AND CLASSIFICATION OF TOXICS

How do scientists determine how harmful a substance is? How is that knowledge used to rank toxics with respect to the health threats that they pose? These two questions are the focus of this chapter. The first part discusses the scientific methods currently used to ascertain the degree to which various chemicals cause cancer. The reader will note that, despite the wealth of useful information these tests have provided, they are still imperfect. The second part of the chapter explains the major chemical classification schemes currently used by the Environmental Protection Agency (EPA) for ranking toxics.

A. Testing Toxics

Determining if a substance poses a health threat—or more accurately, at what level a substance produces a health threat (since everything becomes toxic at a high enough concentration)—is the work of environmental health scientists. Hazard assessment is approached from two main directions: the study of disease in human populations (*epidemiology*) and laboratory investigations (*toxicology*). Epidemiologists look for associations between various risk factors in a population (such as habits, living conditions, and chemical exposures) and the occurrence of disease in that population. If a strong enough association is found, those factors are usually considered to be possible causes of the disease. The link between smoking and lung cancer is a famous case. Toxicologists, in contrast, work in the laboratory on carefully controlled scientific experiments to try to understand the mechanisms of disease and the exact ways various agents cause harm. Neither approach by itself is usually enough to establish the risk associated with a specific chemical or aspect of lifestyle. Instead, both lines of evidence are used together in the evaluation of risk.

This section will describe the approaches of epidemiology and toxicology, pointing out the strengths and limitations of each. Particular attention is given to several issues that are often in the public's mind: the relevance of animal tests to humans, the application of high doses in test systems, and whether or not there is a safe level for every substance below which negligible harm is done.

Epidemiology

Epidemiologists search for statistical associations between the occurrence of disease in a population and the factors suspected of causing that disease. The groups studied might be workers exposed to varying levels of some workplace pollutant, migrants who change diets after moving to a new country, or portions of the general population that have certain habits, such as smokers. An epidemiological investigation often begins with a clinical observation, such as an unusually high occurrence of lung cancer among people who work with asbestos. Then a careful study is conducted trying to relate specific levels of the suspected cause with the rate of disease in the population. Careful attention must be paid to factors that might confuse the analysis. In the asbestos example, it might be the presence of other workplace pollutants that cause lung cancer or the degree of smoking among the workers.

When a significant relationship is found, then it is possible to estimate the risk or proportion of disease that is caused by the factor. In this way, it has been found that smokers have a ten times greater chance of developing lung cancer than do nonsmokers, that nonsmoking asbestos workers have a five times greater chance of getting lung cancer than do nonsmoking workers who are not exposed to asbestos, and that asbestos workers who smoke are fifty times more likely to develop lung cancer than workers who neither smoke nor are exposed to asbestos on the job. This last example illustrates a *synergistic* effect, in which the risk caused by two factors is greater than their sum; in contrast, some effects can simply be added.

On the basis of numerous epidemiological studies, some scientists believe that perhaps 80 to 90% of all cancers can be avoided. That is, factors within the environment, personal habits, dietary factors, and other things within the control of human decisions cause the vast majority of all cancers. Similarly, studies suggest that diet plays a part in 85% of all diseases occurring in the United States.

The enormous benefit of epidemiological methods is that the actual occurrence of real diseases in humans is studied. No questionable extrapolations from animal studies to humans are required. The full range of human susceptibility to disease is often observed (although some of the best studies are of workers who are generally much healthier than the population at large). And actual pollutants in true exposure situations are investigated.

At the same time, epidemiology has important limitations. The damage must be done to be observed, and epidemiologists can only study the consequences of past exposures— they cannot predict the results of substances newly entering the environment. Given the sometimes long time lag between exposure to a chemical and development of the disease (20 to 40 years for some *carcinogens*), epidemiological results may be a long time in coming. During that intervening period, many things can happen to confuse the association; for example, exposed people can move away and be lost from a study.

A second major problem involves separating out the contributions of two or more substances that produce the same effect. For

example, tobacco smoke, radon, and asbestos all cause lung cancer. Most people are exposed to all three to some degree. How to disentangle their respective roles is extremely difficult, particularly since good measurements of exposure are usually not available. For substances that produce lower rates of disease, the problem is even more difficult.

Another weakness is the limited sensitivity of statistical tests. Slight risks can be difficult to pinpoint. A substance that produces a 1% increase in the lung cancer rate could fail tests for being statistically significant (which means that it could be due to chance), but still be causing 1500 deaths per year. There are other technical problems, too. These include the difficulty of gathering historical exposure records for workers from businesses that are now defunct, the total lack of exposure records for other businesses, and the substantial financial and legal consequences that may result from release of the data. In spite of the limitations, epidemiology is well suited for identifying the major factors associated with disease.

Toxicology

The toxicity of compounds is determined mainly by controlled laboratory experimentation. Studies are sometimes made on human subjects if a substance is not thought to cause an irreversible effect. Components of air pollution, such as **sulfur dioxide** and **ozone**, have been used in chamber studies in which human volunteers breathe varying concentrations to measure the changes in lung performance at different levels. Certain food preservatives known as **sulfites** have been given to asthmatics to evaluate allergic reactions. For the most part, however, investigations of toxicity involve experimental animals and microorganisms.

A wide variety of experiments are possible depending on the effect in question and the time frame over which exposure takes place. Acute, subchronic, and chronic are the terms used to describe progressively longer experiments. An experiment on acute effects might be the determination of the dose that causes immediate death in 50% of the animals exposed (the LD_{50}). An experiment on subchronic effects might look for changes in blood chemistry, enzyme activities, or tissue damage over an exposure period of several months. And in chronic effects experiments, doses are administered over years or perhaps even an entire lifetime to examine such things as shortening of lifespan, cancer induction, and changes in the diseases of old age. Studies over several generations are also possible to see if exposure to a parent causes defects in the offspring. Good toxicology books, such as the two recommended at the end of this chapter, provide details on the many types of experiments that can be performed.

The object of most laboratory investigations, and one of the main benefits of them, is to find how a particular response varies with exposure, which is the *dose–response relation*. A valid dose–response curve permits prediction of effects at doses that have not been studied, including those lower doses that may be of most environmental interest. (Low-dose extrapolations do have problems, however, some of which are discussed later.) Another benefit of laboratory work is that the actual mechanisms of disease can be understood. This can lead both to prevention of disease and the development of effective treatments. A third benefit of laboratory studies, and the main reason they are required by the Toxics Substances Control Act, is that the potential hazards of compounds can be evaluated before they are released into general circulation.

Laboratory work, however, does have its limitations, which must be kept in mind when evaluating experimental results. For obvious ethical reasons, humans cannot usually be used for testing toxic substances (some exceptions were mentioned earlier). Laboratory animals, frequently mice and rats, are tested instead. It may well be asked what relevance these species have for humans. The use of nonhuman species to investigate human physiology is, of course, a long-established practice and underlies much of modern medicine. There are many similarities between other animal species and humans; what is important is choosing the correct experimental animal for any given effect. The most convincing scientific justification for using animals is that the practice works. In cancer testing, for example, all of the compounds or mixtures that have been judged by the International Agency for Research on Cancer to be carcinogenic (cancer causing) in humans have also produced cancer in at least one species of laboratory animal. Seven substances were found to be carcinogenic in animals before they were also discovered to be carcinogenic in humans. Laboratory animals can never perfectly predict human responses, but certainly in the case of cancer, positive animal results may suggest a potential human risk.

Another issue in laboratory testing is the frequent use of test dosages far greater than the concentrations to which people are ordinarily exposed. The reason for using high doses is to increase the sensitivity of the test, or in scientific terms, to avoid false negative results. A false negative result happens when a positive effect actually occurs, but the conditions of the test prevent that effect from being seen (or from being statistically significant). To understand this better, consider a typical experiment which might involve several hundred test animals. To be significant in an experiment that large, a substance would have to produce disease in 5 to 10% of the animals. If, at realistic doses, the chemical caused disease in only 1% of the animals, the result could not be distinguished from chance. Yet no one would want a substance released into the environment that caused disease in 1% of the population exposed (for the whole U.S. population that would be 2.5 million people). The high doses used increase the incidence of disease to the point where a significant result is more easily obtained.

Now the main question in this procedure is whether the high dose itself causes disease that would not occur at all at lower doses. If, for example, there are detoxification or repair processes that are overwhelmed at high doses, then low doses of the same substance might in fact be safe. This reasoning is believed to be correct for substances that do not produce cancer, and it underlies the use of safety factors in establishing permitted levels for noncarcinogens (agents that do not cause cancer). For *carcinogens*, however, it is possible that data for high doses may be valid for low doses. The uncertainties about the actual cancer mechanism make it difficult to know for sure. Even if genetic repair processes are at work in some cells, they may not exist in other cell types or may already be taxed to the limit by repairing naturally occurring genetic damage or from carcinogens now in the environment.

Safe Levels and Thresholds

Is there a safe dose for some substances, a threshold dose below which no harm is done? For noncarcinogens, the answer is thought to be yes. Virtually all chemicals act at the cellular or molecular levels to cause damage. If a large enough number of cells are damaged or killed, vital tissue may be destroyed and death or serious disorder may result. Conversely, if only a few cells are damaged, an organism may be able to repair the damage or scar it over and survive without any noticeable effect. For noncarcinogens, it is believed there is always such a point of minimal damage. The difference with carcinogens is that one change in the genetic structure of one cell may be enough to start a run-away reaction, in which that cell divides uncontrollably and spreads to other tissues. Since it may take only one "hit" to lead to cancer, no safe or threshold level would exist. Cancer caused by radiation is thought to behave this way.

For noncarcinogens, levels considered to be safe are estimated in a two-step process. The highest dose that does not cause an observable adverse effect in animal or human studies (the *No Observed Adverse Effect Level*, or *NOAEL*) is first determined. Then that level is divided by a suitable safety factor. The safety factor might be 10, 100, or 1000, depending on how closely the studies resemble the conditions of actual human exposure (for example, whether animals or humans were used in the experiment). The final number arrived at is thought to represent a safe exposure. By comparing the NOAEL to the actual environmental concentration, a margin of safety for the substance can be judged. The problem with this process is that new adverse effects may be discovered, so what might at one time seem to be a no-effect level may later be seen to be hazardous. The recognition that **lead** is far more harmful at lower concentrations than previously thought is a prime example. Safety is not guaranteed by this method.

Carcinogens are not accepted as having safe or threshold levels because a single genetic change may lead to an uncontrolled reaction. But carcinogens do differ in potency, that is, in how likely they are to produce cancer at a given dose. **Aflatoxin** B_1 is a million times more potent than **trichloroethylene**, for example. Differences in potency are not well understood, but may be related to the ease with which different chemicals gain access to the genetic material or react with it.

Mutagen Testing

Several systems have been developed to detect *mutations* of genetic material. Because cancer is thought to originate as a change in the genetic material or *DNA* of cells, materials that alter DNA (*mutagens*) may cause cancer. While not every mutation causes cancer (other diseases can result instead), a substance that is mutagenic is a suspect for causing cancer. The best known mutagen test is the Ames Salmonella test, in which a chemical is administered to a strain of *Salmonella* bacteria. Certain types of mutations can easily be seen by this method. Not all carcinogens test positive, however, so that even if the Ames test shows nothing, the chemical may still be a mutagen. And since not all mutations lead to cancer, a positive Ames test cannot be relied on to predict a cancer hazard. But what this and other microorganism tests provide is a method to screen chemicals that is relatively quick and inexpensive compared to animal experiments. With further research, we can hope that a suitable number of mutagen tests using different microorganisms can be developed that will successfully identify most carcinogens. This could both reduce the use of experimental animals in cancer testing and shorten the time over which results are obtained. Until that time, animal tests and epidemiology are the main methods used to predict the effects of toxic substances.

B. Classification of Toxics

To determine the degree and type of hazard likely to be associated with exposure to any substance, many different laboratory experiments and epidemiological studies are performed. Governmental regulatory agencies, such as the EPA, and international organizations, such as the World Health Organization (WHO) of the United Nations, evaluate the findings of such studies and, ideally, develop adequate regulations and recommendations to limit human exposure to individual toxic substances.

The EPA has developed a set of guidelines of *acute toxicity* based on the LD_{50}, defined as the dose of a substance that kills 50% of the organisms in a test (Table 4). The EPA also has a classification scheme for cancer-causing agents, which is based on an assessment of the adequacy and sufficiency of animal tests and epidemiological studies. The toxicity guidelines provide a basis for comparing the relative immediate dangers posed by different substances. For example, two closely related pesticides, **malathion** and **parathion**, produce similar immediate symptoms of poisoning in humans and other mammals, but parathion is considerably more potent than malathion, having an effect at much lower doses. Therefore, parathion would be ranked higher on the toxicity scale. Such a comparison is useful in developing appropriate regulations; use of the more toxic or dangerous pesticide is restricted to trained and certified personnel, while malathion is available for household use. In the discussions of the health effects of particular toxics in Part II of this book, the EPA's estimates (when available) of the degree of toxicity and/or the cancer-causing ability of that substance are presented.

As shown in Table 4, four categories of acute toxicity have been defined that correspond to different dose levels received through ingestion, inhalation, and skin contact. Although some substances may be uniformly toxic in small doses whether eaten, inhaled, or splashed on the skin, the toxicity level varies for many substances with the route of exposure or entry. Some toxics, for example, are particularly well absorbed from the digestive tract, but not from the lungs or through the skin. For those substances, the oral dose is the critical dose. But other substances are not readily taken up from the digestive system, but can be acutely toxic, even in very small doses, when inhaled.

The most highly toxic substances are those that cause death or severe illness in very small doses (category I). These must be labeled DANGER POISON. Somewhat less toxic chemicals (category II) are labeled WARNING, indicating that the chemical can cause death, severe illness, or other effects at dose levels slightly greater than those for category I substances. Most household cleaning products bear the word CAUTION on the label, indicating that the substance is toxic in sufficiently large doses. Consumers are advised to handle even category IV chemicals with caution, as these too can be poisonous in very large doses.

The EPA has adopted a classification system for *carcinogens* to rank the potential cancer hazard to people posed by individual chemicals (Table 5). The scheme, which is based on an assessment of the "weight of the evidence," is similar to that developed by the International Agency for Research on Can-

TABLE 4 EPA Guidelines for Acute Toxicity of Toxic Chemicals

Toxicity Category	Oral LD_{50} (mg/kg)	Dermal LD_{50} (mg/kg)	Inhalation LC_{50}	
			(mg/L dust)	(ppm vapor/gas)
I (DANGER POISON)	$\leqslant 50^a$	$\leqslant 50$	$\leqslant 2$	$\leqslant 200$
II (WARNING)	50–500	200–2000	2–20	200–2000
III (CAUTION)	500–5000	2000–20,000	20–200	2000–20,000
IV (caution)	$>5000^b$	$>20,000$	>200	$>20,000$

Toxicity Category	Eye Effect	Skin Irritation
I	Irreversible corneal opacity at 7 days	Severe irritation or damage at 72 hours
II	Corneal opacity reversible within 7 days or irritation lasting 7 days	Moderate irritation at 72 hours
III	No corneal opacity, irritation reversible within 7 days	Mild or slight irritation at 72 hours
IV	No irritation	No irritation at 72 hours

[a]The symbol $\leqslant$ means less than or equal to.

[b]The symbol $>$ means greater than.

Source: U.S. Forest Service, USDA. 1984. *Agriculture Handbook No. 633, Pesticide Background Statements. Vol 1. Herbicides.* Washington, D.C.

TABLE 5 EPA Classification System for Carcinogens

Group A. Human Carcinogen

This classification indicates that there is sufficient evidence from epidemiological studies to support a cause–effect relationship between the substance and cancer.

Group B. Probable Human Carcinogen

B_1: Substances are classified as B_1 carcinogens on the basis of sufficient evidence from animal studies and limited evidence from epidemiological studies.

B_2: Substances are classified as B_2 carcinogens on the basis of sufficient evidence from animal studies, but the epidemiological data are inadequate or nonexistent.

Group C. Possible Human Carcinogen

For this classification, there is limited evidence of carcinogenicity from animal studies and no epidemiological data.

Group D. Not Classifiable as to Human Carcinogenicity

The data from human epidemiological and animal studies are inadequate or completely lacking, so no assessment as to the substance's cancer-causing hazard is possible.

Group E. Evidence of Noncarcinogenicity for Humans

Substances in this category have tested negative in at least two adequate (as defined by the EPA) animal cancer tests in different species and in adequate epidemiological and animal studies. Classification in group E is based on available evidence; substances may prove to be carcinogenic under certain conditions.

cer. A similar system is used by the World Health Organization. The results of animal studies are assessed with respect to positive findings (cancers or noncancerous tumors), negative findings (no cancers or benign tumors), the kinds of tumors produced (lung, liver, blood, bladder, and so on), the number of tumors induced, the adequacy of test procedures, the suitability of the test organisms, and the chemical similarity to other known cancer-causing substances. Results of tests for mutagens are also considered. And where available, epidemiological data are included.

Classification of a substance as shown in Table 5 may change as new evidence, improved testing methods, or better analytical techniques become available. In the last few years alone, the ranking of several substances has changed. Generally, new regulations are made in response to such changes in carcinogen classification.

Further Reading

GORDIS, L., and LIBAUER, C. H., editors. 1988. *Epidemiology and Health Risk Assessment.* New York: Oxford University Press.

KLAASSEN, C. D., AMDUR, M. O., and DOULL, J., editors. 1986. *Casarett and Doull's Toxicology: The Basic Science of Poisons.* 3d edition. New York: Macmillan.

LOOMIS, TED A. 1978. *Essentials of Toxicology.* 3d edition. Philadelphia: Lea & Febiger.

U.S. Interagency Staff Group on Carcinogens. 1986. Chemical Carcinogens: A Review of the Science and Its Associated Principles. *Environmental Health Perspectives* 67:201–282.

4 TOXICS IN THE BODY

To understand how toxic chemicals can harm us, we need to know how they enter the body, what happens to them within, and how they exit. We also need to know how people differ in their responses to chemicals. These topics are discussed in this chapter. The most important processes that govern the movement and transformation of chemicals inside the body are explained first. Then we describe how our defense mechanisms can go awry and the sensitivities that result. Finally, we discuss the role that nutrition might play in determining our sensitivities to toxics.

A. Entry, Dose, and Exit: How Chemicals Harm the Body

When people think of human poisoning, images of someone swallowing a potion and doubling over in agony are often envisioned. In reality, chemicals can cause harm when they are breathed or spilled on the skin, as well as being swallowed, and people rarely double over in agony as a result of exposure to toxics at levels normally found in the environment. Nevertheless, toxics in the environment can and do cause severe human health problems. This section describes how chemicals enter the body, what happens to them once they are inside, and how they get out. By understanding this process, we can begin to appreciate how toxic chemicals harm us.

When a *caustic* chemical is spilled on the skin, immediate and visible damage to the skin surface is evident. Potentially more life threatening are inhaled caustic vapors that damage the lung on contact. The health consequences of this type of damage are obvious. However, internal damage caused by chemicals that make their way to the bloodstream is harder to picture.

Once a toxic substance is circulating in the bloodstream, it has access to almost all of the body's internal organs. But toxic substances are not equally damaging to all the organ systems with which they come into contact. Each organ is susceptible to damage by certain chemicals. These sensitive sites are called *target organs*. The target organ is often not the site of the chemical's highest concentration, but rather the site of highest damage potential. The amount of chemical that comes into contact with the target organs depends largely on whether the chemical is breathed in, swallowed, or spilled on the skin.

Entry Through Breathing

Inhalation through the mouth or nose is an important route of exposure to toxic substances in the workplace. Outside the workplace, it is important for certain widely distributed and common air pollutants. Gases, vapors, solid particles, and liquid *aerosols* are easily inhaled. Not all inhaled chemicals damage the lungs, however. For many industrial solvents, inhalation is a major route of exposure, but the liver or kidney is the target organ.

How much of the chemical that is actually absorbed from the lungs into the bloodstream depends on characteristics of the substance (such as particle size or how well it dissolves in body fat) and on the exposed person's breathing pattern at the time of exposure. Gases and vapors can be absorbed in the airways between the nose and lung or in the lung itself. Many water-soluble vapors become trapped in the damp walls of the tubes leading into the lung. Some of these trapped water-soluble chemicals dissolve in the dampness and are carried into the bloodstream before they ever reach the deep regions of the lung.

The lung's airways terminate at tiny air sacs called *alveoli* where waste carbon dioxide is exchanged for oxygen. Most fat-soluble vapors easily reach these deep regions of the lung and readily pass through the thin, permeable walls of the alveoli directly into the bloodstream. Because this is a rapid process, inhalation of fat-soluble toxics may pose a significant *acute* hazard to people.

Fine particles (smaller than a micron) easily reach the alveoli. Many of these inhaled particles are immediately exhaled, but some stick to the alveoli walls. Some of these pass directly into the bloodstream. Other fine particles may remain trapped forever in the aveoli, giving rise to diseases of the lung generally known as *pneumoconiosis*. Diseases resulting from specific retained fibers or particles are given unique names, such as *asbestosis* (caused by asbestos fibers) or *silicosis* (caused by fine silica dust).

Medium-sized inhaled particles ranging from barely visible to the size of a cell (a micron in diameter) can either become trapped in the airways or reach the deep lung. There are about 20 forks in the airway between the windpipe and the alveoli. This branching causes turbulence, increasing the chance that medium-sized particles will be thrown onto the moist airway walls and become trapped. The trapped particles may be absorbed in the airways or may be moved out by the normal cleansing processes in the lung and be exhaled or swallowed. Particles that do reach the inner lung can become lodged in the alveoli permanently, eventually damaging the lung.

Large, visible inhaled particles are captured by the fine hairs in the nose, where they become trapped. These are subsequently lost by blowing the nose, sneezing, or swallowing. Swallowed particles follow the path of other ingested chemicals even though the original point of entry was the nose.

The amount of air sucked into the lungs with each breath by the exposed individual and the air concentration of the toxic substance both determine the dose of toxic received from contaminated air. A person breathing hard and deep during exercise re-ceives a higher dose of chemical than a sedentary person breathing lightly, even if the air has the same concentration of toxic substance. Children breathing contaminated air receive a higher dose of chemical per pound of body weight than do similarly exposed adults because, for their size, children breathe several times more air than adults do in a given time period.

Entry Through the Mouth

Swallowed chemicals can be quickly or slowly absorbed, depending on the chemical and the state of the *gastrointestinal (GI) tract* (which depends, for example, on the time since the last meal). A few chemicals (such as ethanol) are quickly absorbed unchanged from the stomach. Other chemicals cannot be absorbed anywhere in the GI system; these pass out of the body unchanged via the feces. Chemicals that are absorbed in the GI tract pass through the liver before entering the bloodstream. Toxic substances that damage the liver are most dangerous when swallowed because they head directly to the liver. In contrast, if the same amount of liver-damaging chemical is inhaled, it is diluted in the bloodstream, and some may actually be removed by the kidney before it reaches the liver.

Whereas large doses of chemicals overwhelm the liver, sending unprocessed chemicals into the bloodstream, small doses can be rendered harmless inside the liver, or even excreted, before entering general circulation. Thus, the amount of swallowed toxic chemicals reaching the rest of the body may be smaller than the amount actually absorbed from the stomach and small intestine. In contrast, toxic chemicals entering the bloodstream via the lungs or skin are distributed full strength throughout the entire body before the liver has a chance to render them harmless.

For the most part, chemicals are absorbed slowly from the GI tract. A potentially fatal dose of toxic substance can often be removed by pumping the stomach, inducing vomiting, or giving an enema. However, these methods often cannot be used, such as when small amounts of a toxic substance are ingested everyday or when a very *caustic* agent is swallowed. These *chronic* doses must make their way out of the body naturally, either by passing through the intestines unchanged, or by being absorbed then excreted in the urine, feces, or breath. The amount of swallowed chemical absorbed from the GI tract depends mainly on how fast material passes through the stomach and intestines. The faster the chemical moves through the GI system, the less that is apt to be absorbed, meaning a lower dose is received by the liver. In general, a diet high in fiber and fluids tends to increase the amount and speed of material passing through the GI tract, thereby reducing the amount of chemical likely to be absorbed. Accidentally swallowed chemicals, however, must be removed from the stomach under medical supervision; do not eat until after such supervision is received.

Entry Through the Skin

Intact skin is an effective barrier against a wide variety of toxic substances, but it is not a complete shield. The blood supply to the skin is one of the richest in the body. If a toxic substance can penetrate the outer skin layers, it will be rapidly transported throughout the body. This is easily demonstrated by the rapid excretion of solvents through the lungs and urine after they are spilled on the skin. Contact with chemicals can also lead to a direct response by the skin ranging from burns and rashes to major allergic reactions. The term *irritant* is usually applied to chemicals that cause noninflammatory reactions such as itching or burning, as well as the more subtle effect of skin thickening. Chemicals can also cause acne-type *lesions*, hair loss, lumps and bumps, and pigmentation changes. When a chemical spilled on the skin causes inflammation of an entire limb, it usually means that the chemical was absorbed into the bloodstream and that the reaction is *systemic*, meaning that it is taken up by the whole body rather than a single organ or tissue.

The amount of chemical actually absorbed by the skin into the bloodstream depends on a variety of factors. Dry and powdered forms of toxic substance are less readily absorbed than liquids. Moist skin is ten times more permeable than dry. Oily solutions generally permit more absorption than water-based ones. Injured skin absorbs more chemical than intact skin. Drugs and other chemicals may enhance the skin's permeability. *DMSO* is an example of such a chemical because absorption of other chemicals through the skin is greatly increased when the skin has been previously exposed to DMSO.

We have seen that the way a person is exposed to a toxic chemical is important in determining the consequences of the exposure. Some chemicals are more potent when inhaled than when swallowed. Others cannot be absorbed from the gastrointestinal system, but may eventually become lodged in the lungs and cause lung cancer or other lung damage. The liver may be spared damage if the chemical is absorbed from the skin and diluted in the bloodstream before gaining access to this sensitive organ. Equally important are the processes that take place after a chemical is circulating in the bloodstream, as discussed next.

Dose to the Target Organ

Once in the bloodstream, a chemical is distributed to all the organs in the body. However, three processes limit the amount of potentially damaging chemical hitting the target organs at once. One of them—altering toxic chemicals into safe ones via *metabolism*—is discussed in the next section. The other two processes—binding toxic materials to blood proteins so they cannot cause immediate harm and removing them from circulating by storing them in other body tissue—are discussed here.

The blood is made up of a variety of different blood cells that are suspended in a watery liquid called plasma. Plasma contains a variety of salts and trace substances and a high concentration of protein. Many toxic chemicals are attracted to the plasma proteins and are capable of attaching to plasma proteins as they circulate in the bloodstream. This reduces the amount of toxic chemical free to damage the target organ, but it also prolongs the time that a toxic substance circulates in the body. Bound toxic molecules cannot harm their target organ, but eventually they become unbound and capable of doing harm. The net result is a *chronic* rather than an *acute* dose of chemical to the target organ.

In most cases this process gives the body time to break down toxic substances into harmless compounds without being poisoned. But a problem arises when a relatively harmless chemical is *bioactivated,* or rendered more toxic, when broken down by the body. Many cancer-causing chemicals fall into this category. Ideally, chemicals that need to be bioactivated before causing harm should be eliminated from the body quickly, before the body has a chance to render them harmful. Unfortunately, the body's disposal of these chemicals is often slow. Sometimes exposure to one chemical, even at nontoxic doses, can enhance the body's ability to bioactivate other chemicals. Chapter 7, Section B, gives an important example of this problem.

Another process that can reduce the amount of toxic chemicals circulating in the bloodstream or delay the time of its release is the tendency of some substances to be stored in the body tissue such as fat or bone. Some toxic substances, such as **cadmium**, can be harmful when stored in the kidneys. But most chemicals do no damage when sequestered. However, large amounts of stored chemical can be released, sometimes years after initial exposure, if the storage location is disturbed. For example, stored fat is metabolized during weight loss, and chemicals stored in the fat are released into circulation. Severe toxic effects can result if enough of this chemical is released quickly into circula-

tion. That is why it can be dangerous to lose too much weight too quickly. Fasting does cleanse the body of toxic substances, but the chemicals being removed might have caused less damage if left in place. This same phenomenon takes place at other storage locations. For instance, **lead** binds to calcium in the bones. During pregnancy, a woman's body may tap into the calcium stored in her bone mass. As the calcium is used, stored lead is released, resulting in high levels of lead in both the mother's bloodstream and that of her unborn child.

While binding to blood proteins and sequestering chemicals in body tissues are important moderators of toxicity, the most important processes for ridding the body of toxic chemicals are chemical reactions that take place within the body. The human body manufactures a wide variety of *enzymes* capable of altering the chemical structure of unwanted chemicals so that they are detoxified and/or rendered easier to excrete.

Metabolism of Toxins

Metabolism is the name given to a wide range of chemical processes that occur in the body by which nutrients and energy are derived from food and waste products are formed and prepared for elimination. Metabolism begins almost immediately after a chemical is inhaled, swallowed, or spilled on the skin.

When the original toxic chemical has been modified to a less toxic *metabolite* (the product of metabolism), it is said to be *detoxified.* But as was noted previously, harmless chemicals are sometimes bioactivated, or made more toxic, by metabolic transformations. Often it is not known whether the original chemical or its biologically activated metabolite is causing an observed toxic response. We may never know exactly how all the chemicals we absorb are metabolized nor the toxicity of the metabolites. This kind of research is extremely difficult and time consuming. Laboratory animals often metabolize chemicals differently from people, complicating the problem.

Although the metabolism of many chemicals is not well understood, a few generalizations can be made. First, much of the variation among people's susceptibility to toxic chemicals is determined by genetic variability. Some people are just born more sensitive to chemicals than are others. But it is also clear that the rate at which someone metabolizes a toxic chemical or drug also depends on that person's history of exposure to other chemicals, drugs, and diseases. It is not clear whether repeated low doses of a toxic significantly changes enzymatic action. However, following repeated or prolonged exposure to a toxic chemical or drug, some people seem to adapt by manufacturing more enzymes to process the heavier chemical load.

It is well known that people who regularly drink alcoholic beverages are able to tolerate more alcohol than nondrinkers. While some of this tolerance is due to learning how to manage inebriation, some is also due to enhanced production of an enzyme that detoxifies alcohol. But because the enzymes are not very specific, other chemicals that use the same enzymes are also metabolized faster. In some cases this is good. A chemical that is already biologically active will be detoxified and then eliminated quickly. In other cases this can lead to quick elimination of a beneficial nutrient or therapeutic drug. Even worse, the increased enzyme pool can transform biologically inactive chemicals into their bioactively toxic metabolites faster than would be the case in a nondrinker.

Exposure to high doses of a toxic chemical or therapeutic drug can also slow the production of enzymes. In some cases this can be quite dangerous. When a smaller pool of enzymes is available to detoxify a bioactive chemical or drug, the toxic substance remains in the body for a longer period of time than would be the case if a normal supply of enzyme were available. Therefore, the toxic chemical has more time in which to carry out its toxic effect.

Body Membranes

To exert a toxic effect, a chemical or its metabolite must move from the bloodstream into direct contact with the target organ. To do this, the circulating chemical passes through a variety of membranes, such as the walls of the intestines, capillary walls, or cell walls. Both the structure of the chemical and characteristics of the membrane determine how much and how easily this passage occurs.

Chemicals can pass through membranes using one of two general processes: diffusion or active transport. The process used depends on the characteristics of the chemical trying to pass through the membrane. Diffusion is a passive process. As molecules of chemical randomly strike the membrane, some pass through it. Molecules of chemical can go through the membrane from either direction. The majority of molecules move from the side of greater concentration to the side of lesser concentration. This is because more molecules are likely to strike the membrane from the more crowded side.

Molecules that dissolve readily in fat are able to pass through membranes easily. Biological membranes are primarily composed of fatty material, so fat-soluble molecules simply dissolve into the membrane when they strike it and then pass to the other side. Small water-soluble molecules diffuse by using a network of water-filled channels scattered throughout the membrane. But the channels are not very large, so if a toxic substance is composed of large water-soluble molecules, another process must be used for the chemical to get to the other side.

Active transport is used to move large water-soluble molecules across biological membranes. This special system evolved to move nutrients across biological membranes. The system works something like a shuttle bus. The molecule to be transported is first attached to a special "carrier" chemical that plays the role of the bus. The molecule is allowed on the "bus" only if its shape fits into that of the carrier. Of course, specific carriers did not evolve to transport toxic chemicals to body tissue, but many toxic substances share a family resemblance to nutrients. The number of carriers in the membrane limits the number of molecules that can be transported. This sets the stage for competition among the various molecules vying for a chance to cross the membrane. If the carriers are full of foreign molecules, they are unavailable to transport life-giving nutrients.

While membranes protect vital organs from unwanted water-soluble chemicals, no membrane can stop a fat-soluble chemical from diffusing through it. Moreover, the body does not readily get rid of fat-soluble chemicals. Every time they make it to a storage location (such as the liver, gallbladder, or small intestine) to await elimination, they are simply reabsorbed back into the bloodstream.

Some membranes are better barriers against toxics than others. The capillaries (tiny blood vessels) in the liver, for example, are "leaky" because a wide variety of chemicals must have access to liver tissue so that the liver can cleanse the blood of waste products and foreign chemicals. Likewise, the kidney is leaky to allow for the reabsorption of water. In contrast, brain capillaries are "well sealed" to protect brain cells from all but essential nutrients. This is called the *blood–brain barrier*. The placenta was once thought to be effective at keeping foreign chemicals out of the embryo and fetus, but it is proving to be leakier than first envisioned. It is not safe to assume that the placenta protects the unborn child from exposure to toxic substances.

Exit of Toxic Substances

Some chemicals leave the body the same way they came in. For instance, much of an inhaled solvent might be exhaled before crossing the alveoli membranes to enter the bloodstream. Swallowed chemicals that resist absorption are simply transported the length of the GI tract to the rectum where they will be excreted with the feces. However, once a chemical is circulating in the bloodstream, it follows a complex path before being excreted. There are three major exit routes: expired air, the urine, and the feces. Small amounts of toxic substances may also be excreted via sweat and mother's milk. Loss of toxic chemicals through exhalation is limited to those chemicals that are both fat soluble and easily vaporized, such as **acetone** or alcohol. In contrast, a wide variety of chemicals exit in the urine and feces.

Chemicals that exit in the urine are passed through the kidneys. The kidneys are the most important organs for removing toxic substances from the body. In simple terms, the job of the kidneys is to filter the blood to extract waste products. The average person filters 180 quarts (170 liters) of fluid through the kidneys each day. But nobody urinates 180 quarts of fluid each day, and the reason is that more than 99% of the filtered fluid is reabsorbed back into the bloodstream. Less than 1% is left to eventually appear in the urine or sweat. Most of this reabsorbed fluid is water, but many other substances undergo reabsorption as well, providing a pathway for chemicals filtered out by the kidneys to be reabsorbed into the bloodstream. As noted previously, fat-soluble chemicals diffuse easily through membranes and thus are easily reabsorbed, whereas water-soluble ones are not. So, fat-soluble chemicals must be metabolized into water-soluble ones before significant quantities can exit with the urine. As a practical matter, drinking plenty of water helps fat-soluble chemicals exit via the urine because a well-hydrated body reabsorbs less chemically laden water.

Toxic substances that are metabolized by the liver exit the body via the feces. Once processed by the liver, chemicals are carried in the liver's bile to the gallbladder for storage, from which they move into the small intestine. Once in the small intestine, chemicals are passed along to the large intestine where they can be excreted via the feces. This gives ample time for the fat-soluble chemicals to be reabsorbed into the bloodstream, canceling the liver's effort to remove them. Reabsorbed chemicals may be recycled more than once through the liver, usually making it out only after they have been metabolized into water-soluble compounds.

Toxic chemicals can also be secreted with sweat. The amount of toxic substances in sweat is very small. However, these substances may cause skin rash, sensitivity to sunlight, and other skin problems.

A potentially serious problem are toxics that accumulate in mother's milk. Toxic chemicals exit via mother's milk by diffusing into it. Since fat makes up about 4% of mother's milk, fat-soluble chemicals tend to accumulate in it. Compounds such as **DDT** and **PCBs** are known to accumulate in milk, making milk a major route for their excretion from nursing mothers. Metals that are chemically similar to calcium, such as **lead**, can also be found in the milk. (Remember that lead can be released from the mother's bones during pregnancy, so that lead exposure does not need to be recent to contaminate the milk.) Such contamination of mother's milk can pose a health risk to a nursing child. Not only may the child be exposed to a potentially harmful chemical, but the dose per pound of body weight is greater than if the same quantity of milk were consumed by a larger person. In addition, infants do not have mature systems for metabolizing toxic chemicals, so that a moderately harmful chemical to an adult can be life-threatening to an infant. (A good example of this is **nitrate** exposure.) In addition, when infants are exposed to cancer-causing chemicals, the tumors that may result have a good chance of showing up much earlier in life (in middle age) than for adults who are exposed. However, in spite of all these risks, the benefits of breast-feeding for baby and mother nearly always far outweigh the risks.

We have described how toxic chemicals enter and leave the body and some general ways in which they exert damage. Specific effects of individual chemicals are left to Part II of this book (A Guide to Commonly Encountered Toxics). The remainder of this chapter describes some individual responses to chemicals that are outside the normal expected range of reactions.

B. Sensitive Groups

Some people are much more sensitive to chemical exposure than others. What causes mild irritation for one person can be debilitating, even life threatening, for another. Researchers estimate that 20% of all people are at special risk from certain chemicals because of a particular sensitivity or allergy, so it is likely that you or someone you know is one of them. Here we define the terms allergy and sensitivity and describe their different biological origins to help you understand why some people react violently to chemicals while others do not.

News reports about people becoming seriously ill after eating food treated with **sulfites** illustrates how important it is to consider individual sensitivities. Until recently, sulfites were used in many restaurants to keep fresh-cut fruits and vegetables from turning brown. For most people, a little sulfite presented no risk of ill effects. But for people allergic to this chemical, it is a potentially life-threatening practice. Does this mean that everyone should avoid sulfites as if they were dangerous? Of course not. But we do owe it to people who are allergic to sulfites to provide them with the information they need to stay well. Today, products that contain sulfites are labeled, and where such labeling is impossible, their use is banned.

People often say that they are allergic to poison oak or poison ivy because they develop a rash after coming in contact with these plants. In fact, the characteristic rash is a normal reaction, in contrast to an allergic reaction, which is an abnormal response occurring only in certain susceptible individuals. Some people do show true allergic responses to poison oak or poison ivy, characterized by itchy eyes, breathing difficulties, and swelling in areas where there is no rash, but such responses are rare.

Allergic reactions generally produce symptoms that affect the whole body. They are caused by exposure to a specific chemical called an *allergen* and result when the allergen binds to a sensitized *antibody* in the bloodstream of the victim. The antibodies then become activated. The allergy symptoms are the body's response to the activated antibodies. Antibodies become sensitized as a result of previous exposures to the allergen. People prone to allergic reactions seem to inherit more allergy-producing antibodies than others. But the specific chemicals that the antibodies become sensitized to depend on the constellation of foods, pollens, dusts, and chemicals that the allergy-prone individual is exposed to during his or her lifetime.

People can be sensitive to specific chemicals without being allergic to them. Individual genetic differences, genetic abnormalities, alcoholic beverage consumption, drug regimes, age, and pregnancy cause some people to be particularly vulnerable to chemicals. Some people just *metabolize* chemicals faster than average, while others metabolize them more slowly. Some people are missing altogether the genetic information that instructs the body to make the enzymes that metabolize certain groups of chemicals, including certain drugs, industrial chemicals, and foods. Without the genetic instructions, either the enzyme is not made or it may not function properly. When a person absorbs a chemical for which there is no enzyme available to process it, that person can become quite ill. For example, many adults cannot tolerate milk because they are lacking the enzyme lactase which helps to break down the milk sugar lactose. The lactose passes unchanged into the colon, where it decomposes causing bloating, gas, and diarrhea.

There are nearly 100 conditions in which enzymes responsible for metabolizing proteins, vitamins, fats, or other chemicals are missing. In the case of drugs or toxic chemicals, missing enzymes can lead to dangerous situations. Some chemicals and drugs continue to exert their toxic effects on the body until they are metabolized and excreted. If a person cannot metabolize such a chemical, a very small amount of it may cause poisoning symptoms that normally occur only at much larger doses. And, as mentioned in the previous section, therapeutic drugs that must be metabolized to be effective will not work if no metabolic pathway exists to *bioactivate* them.

Age can also influence how sensitive a person is to toxic chemicals. The undeveloped enzyme system of an infant makes it more sensitive to chemicals than an adult. In addition, children may be more at risk than adults from developing cancer during their lifetime following exposure to cancer-causing chemicals simply because they have more time to live following exposure, and possibly because their cells are dividing more rapidly than are those of adults. Chemically induced cancers can take 20 to 30 years to develop, and their development is likely to be both a function of time and additional exposure to other environmental factors. Unfortunately, little is known about how toxic chemicals are likely to affect children. Few animal studies use rats and mice prior to adolescence, and most human studies are carried out on occupationally exposed workers. Older adults can also become more susceptible to the effects of toxics as they age. Lingering diseases, long-term drug regimes, and a reduced ability to repair damage caused by chemicals contribute to increased vulnerability.

Lifestyle can also influence a person's susceptibility to disease resulting from toxics. Smoking, excessive alcohol consumption, lack of exercise, use of medications, recreational drug use, and certain diseases can increase the discomfort or debilitating effects of some toxics. For example, smokers are five times more likely to develop lung cancer as a result of **asbestos** exposure than are nonsmokers. This is because smoking destroys *cilia*, whose rhythmic beating helps to clear inhaled asbestos fibers from the lung. Also, as described in Chapter 7, Section B, people who regularly drink alcoholic beverages are known to metabolize some chemicals faster than nondrinkers, a situation that can increase the toxicity of these chemicals. It is not known if high doses of other chemicals found in the workplace or home environment exert a similar effect. Finally, susceptibility to harm from chemicals can vary from one day to the next. As was noted in Section A of this chapter, the state of the body at the time of exposure influences how much chemical is absorbed, how much gets to the *target organ*, and how quickly it is eliminated.

A branch of health care known as clinical ecology is emerging that addresses the problems some people have living in a world of synthetic chemicals. The practice of clinical ecology is controversial. People must not be lured into believing all that they read about it. Nevertheless, insights learned during careful and controlled research by properly trained ecologists can be expected to help thousands of people (see Resources at the end of this chapter).

C. Nutrition and Susceptibility to Toxics

Since the turn of the century, people concerned about worker health have recognized that good nutrition can alleviate many of the symptoms associated with exposure to toxics. Milk was once commonly given to workers who came into contact with **lead**, in the belief that a healthy body could better defend itself against the toxic effects of lead. (Unfortunately, milk was not an appropriate food to combat lead poisoning, as will be explained.) Similarly, during World War I, a manager noticed that women factory workers exposed to chemicals suffered stomach problems more often than men. Speculating that poor nutrition might be the cause, he started a program to improve the women's nutrition. The women's stomach problems all but disappeared.

What you eat can play a crucial role in de-termining how susceptible you are to illness caused by toxic chemicals. The vitamins, minerals, fats, carbohydrates, protein, and fiber that you eat every day contribute to your overall health because these nutrients supply the raw materials needed for the body to function. Minimum requirements for most nutrients are published as the Recommended Daily Allowances (RDAs). In general, following these guidelines will protect you against diseases caused by malnutrition. But is that enough? Can vitamin supplements protect against illnesses caused by chemical exposure?

Perhaps. This section gives some examples of how nutrition can influence the toxicity of chemicals. Because interactions among vitamins, minerals, other nutrients, and toxics are complex and largely unexplored, the information presented here is incomplete. Nevertheless, enough is known about the interplay among nutrients and chemicals to convey some sense of how nutrition can influence a person's susceptibility to harm from toxics.

Lead is a ubiquitous toxic element. Children are particularly susceptible to harm following exposure to lead. There are two ways to minimize the toxic effects of lead. One way is to avoid exposure, and where possible, this is best. (The reduction of lead in gasoline was a major step in reducing exposure to this dangerous toxic; see Chapter 17 for more on this.) But good nutrition can help reduce the risk from unavoidable sources of lead. Deficiencies in dietary minerals, particularly calcium and phosphorus, but also iron, copper, and magnesium, speed the absorption of lead from the gastrointestinal system. Thus, people deficient in these minerals absorb more lead into their bloodstreams than do people who receive adequate amounts. It is also known that sugar hastens absorption of many essential nutrients, and recent research reveals that milk sugar (lactose) hastens absorption of lead as well. Thus, as hinted in the introduction, milk may not be a good source of dietary minerals when lead is known to contaminate a child's environment. Vitamins

C and E help keep the blood cells and blood-forming organs healthy, which may prevent brain damage caused by high exposures to lead. Recent research in the Soviet Union suggests that pectin, a substance found in apple skins, may also help protect blood cells from damage brought about by lead.

Interactions among nutrients and toxic chemicals are not limited to lead. The toxicity of **benzene** is also affected by nutrition. Doses of vitamin C far larger than the minimum daily requirement necessary to prevent scurvy seem to protect the body from benzene toxicity. The protective properties of vitamin C were tested in industrial workers in South Africa with positive results. Adequate amounts of complete protein in the diet also seem to help the body detoxify benzene. Selenium appears to prevent benzene from destroying the blood-forming organs in laboratory mice, but evidence confirming this effect in humans is not available. Conversely, too much fat in the diet seems to enhance benzene toxicity.

As these examples illustrate, the toxicity of some chemicals may be increased when the chemical is introduced into a poorly nourished body. While research using human subjects is inadequate to prove these interactions, a leading expert in the field, Edward Calabrese, suggests that information about the following interactions is solid enough for people to put the information to use. He suggests that:

deficiencies in vitamin A and the B vitamin pyridoxine increase the toxicity of **aflatoxin**;

deficiencies in **zinc** or the B vitamins cause an increased risk of cancer from **nitrosamines**;

a deficiency in vitamin C increases susceptibility to the toxic effects of **DDT**;

deficiencies in zinc, calcium, or vitamin C may lead to increased toxicity of the heavy metal **cadmium**;

deficiencies in vitamin E increase susceptibility to lung damage from common air pollutants such as **ozone** and **nitrogen oxides**; and

too little calcium, phosphorus, copper, magnesium, iron, vitamin C, or vitamin E may enhance the toxicity of **lead**, particularly in children.

As more research is initiated on the subject, more suggested associations such as these are likely to emerge. In the meantime, a balanced diet appears to afford some measure of protection from the harmful effects of at least some toxics.

Further Reading

CALABRESE, EDWARD J. 1980 and 1981. *Nutrition and Environmental Health: The Influence of Nutritional Status on Pollutant Toxicity and Carcinogenicity.* New York: John Wiley.

CALABRESE, EDWARD J., and DORSEY, MICHAEL W. 1984. *Healthy Living in an Unhealthy World.* New York: Simon and Schuster.

KAMRIN, M. A. 1988. *Toxicology: A Primer on Toxicology Principles and Application.* Chelsea, MI: Lewis Publishing.

KLAASSEN, C. D., AMDUR, M. O., and DOULL, J. 1986. *Casarett and Doull's Toxicology: The Basic Science of Poisons.* 3d edition. New York: Macmillan.

VANDER, A. J. 1981. *Nutrition, Stress and Toxic Chemicals: An Approach to Environment–Health Controversies.* Ann Arbor: The University of Michigan Press.

ZAMM, ALFRED V. 1980. *Why Your House May Endanger Your Health.* New York: Simon and Schuster.

Resources

American Holistic Medical Association
2727 Fairview Avenue East
Seattle, WA 98102

Referral service for clinical ecologists in local areas:
Society for Clinical Ecology
Del Stigler, M.D., Secretary
Suite 409
2005 Franklin Street
Denver, CO 80205

THE FOUR MAJOR SOURCES OF TOXIC EXPOSURE

5 TOXICS IN AIR

Air pollution poses health problems throughout the world. First we provide a general overview of the health hazards associated with air pollution, emphasizing the types of medical disorders that airborne substances can generate. Air pollution is most often associated with factories and with outdoor air. But, as discussed next, the greatest source of harmful air pollution is cigarette smoking. Moreover, as we then show, the health hazards from polluted air inside our homes are often worse than that from outdoor air, even in an industrial city.

A. Air Pollution and Health

Air pollution mainly damages the lungs and airways, although injury to other organs can happen as well. In this section, we describe the major effects of the most common pollutants in the air we breathe. Accidental release of airborne chemicals, such as **chlorine** and **ammonia**, also cause problems, but because these accidents are rare, they are not included in this chapter but left to the appropriate entry headings in Part II. Indoor air pollutants can be of even greater concern than outdoor pollutants, in part because a large proportion of our time is spent indoors. Indoor pollution is especially significant in the homes of smokers and where **radon** concentrations are high. This is discussed more in Section C of this chapter (Indoor Air Pollution).

We have divided the health effects of air pollution into four groups: short-term or *acute* respiratory effects, long-term or *chronic* respiratory effects, lung cancer, and nonrespiratory effects. Damage is said to be acute if it happens suddenly and is relatively short-lived, a few minutes to a few days. An asthmatic attack, for example, is an acute effect. Chronic effects persist over extended periods of time, generally years. Permanent respiratory loss from a decreased rate of lung growth in children and obstructive pulmonary disease (discussed later) are examples of chronic effects.

Acute Respiratory Effects

Four acute respiratory effects of air pollution are well established: (1) asthmatic attacks, (2) hyperreactive airways, (3) respiratory infections, and (4) reversible changes in lung functions. *Asthma* is a condition affecting about 10 million Americans, in which the airways suddenly narrow, obstructing the flow of air through the lungs. The narrowing is caused by spasms of the small muscles that encircle the airways and by the release of thick, excessive mucus that plugs them. An attack can be triggered by an allergic reaction to a foreign substance (either breathed or swallowed) and by a variety of other stimuli, such as respiratory infections, exercise, cold air, and emotional stress. Air pollution can bring on asthmatic attacks. In Los Angeles, attacks have been associated with **ozone** and **particulate** pollution, and in areas surrounding power plants and smelters, **sulfur dioxide** and **sulfate** particulates cause reactions. It is not known whether air pollution can actually cause asthma or whether it only triggers asthmatic attacks.

Another 20 million Americans have what are called hyperreactive airways, which are airways that constrict much more readily than average in response to foreign matter. Unlike asthma, some constriction of the airways is a normal defense mechanism to prevent inhaling noxious substances. In persons with hyperreactive airways, however, the airways respond to levels that do not bother most people. The symptoms are similar to asthma: shortness of breath, coughing, and wheezing. Sulfur dioxide, particulates, ozone, and **nitrogen oxides** are known to stimulate airway reactivity.

The incidence of respiratory infections, particularly in children, is increased by air pollution. Upper respiratory infections, such as colds, influenza, and sore throats, are associated with sulfates, sulfur dioxide, and particulates in outdoor air. Nitrogen dioxide released indoors by gas cooking stoves is associated with more frequent colds in children under the age of 10 compared with children who live in homes equipped with electric ranges. Animal studies show that concentrations of ozone and nitrogen dioxide typical of peak pollution episodes lower the resistance to bacterial infections, such as pneumonia and acute bronchitis. Air pollutants both disable the clearance mechanisms that remove viruses and bacteria from the respiratory tract and incapacitate the cells that fight the infections.

Short-term, reversible changes in lung function are also caused by air pollutants. For example, the maximum amount of air that can be inhaled or exhaled in one second is reduced in both children and healthy adults when exposed to elevated pollutant concentrations, but this returns to normal when exposure ceases. Whether such changes indicate that long-term damage is being done is not known at the present time.

Chronic Respiratory Effects

The two main chronic effects of long-term exposure to air pollutants, aside from lung cancer, are *chronic obstructive pulmonary disease (COPD)* and changes in the development and aging of the lungs. COPD is actually a group of diseases that share the common symptoms of breathlessness. Because a clear-cut diagnosis is often impossible until after death, the conditions are lumped to-

gether. The group includes chronic *bronchitis, emphysema,* and *small airway disease.* Chronic bronchitis involves the persistent secretion of excessive amounts of mucus into the airways; its leading symptom is a lasting, phlegmatic cough. Emphysema is a destruction of the walls of the air sacs (alveoli) and is indicated by breathlessness without cough. Small airway disease involves inflammation and narrowing of the smallest airways (bronchioles) and is the earliest sign of smoking-induced COPD. These diseases can appear separately or together. People with *COPD* have weakened lungs. Their long-term survival is influenced strongly by how susceptible they are to respiratory infections such as influenza and pneumonia. About 10 million people in the United States are afflicted with COPD.

The main causes of COPD are smoking; occupational exposures to such substances as coal and cotton dusts, high concentrations of sulfur dioxide, and particulates; and genetic factors. Air pollution plays a role in several ways. Some evidence suggests that a history of respiratory infections during childhood may contribute to pulmonary disease in old age, and as previously mentioned, air pollution increases childhood infections. Air pollution has also been linked to COPD in recent studies of Mormons, a group with a very low rate of smoking. The longer and greater the exposure to outdoor levels of sulfur dioxide and sulfate particulates, the more prevalent and severe the disease symptoms. Studies in laboratory animals have shown that long-term exposure to nitrogen dioxide and ozone causes destruction of alveoli walls, similar to emphysema.

Lung growth is also affected by air pollution. The lungs typically grow until the age of 20, then slowly decline in their ability to hold air with age. Slowed rates of lung growth have been observed in children ages 6 through 12 in relation to certain indoor air pollutants. The changes are greatest in homes with smokers. A smaller adult lung size means less reserve against the inevitable shrinkage of the lungs with old age and against the onset of obstructive pulmonary disease, which occurs more commonly at older ages.

Lung Cancer

Cancer of the lung is the leading fatal cancer among both men and women, responsible for over one-fourth of all cancer deaths. Smoking is the major cause of lung cancer. Air pollution causes some fraction of lung cancers, but exactly how much is in dispute. Some experts contend that air pollution causes only a few percent of all cases, while others argue that it's 20% or more. It is clear that *carcinogenic* compounds are present in indoor air and polluted outdoor urban air. Chemical analyses of air show the presence of cancer-causing by-products of burning such as **benzo-[a]-pyrenes** and **dioxins**, fibers such as **asbestos**, and metals such as **arsenic** and **cadmium**. Toxicological studies show that extracts of polluted air can produce lung tumors in mice, rats, and hamsters and can cause injury to the genetic material **DNA**. Studies in human populations have found increased cancer rates around smelters and factories, in cities compared to rural areas, and with duration of exposure to pollution.

The major question has been to what extent these materials alone have caused cancer compared with tobacco smoke. Tobacco smoke interacts *synergistically* with other carcinogens, including radon, asbestos, arsenic, and alcohol, to increase the underlying cancer risk of either material. People who are nonsmokers at death may have smoked earlier in life, and many people who have never smoked are exposed passively to tobacco smoke either on the job or at home. These and other problems blur the role of air pollutants in producing lung cancers. Nevertheless, the EPA estimates that between 5000 and 20,000 cases of lung cancer per year are caused by **radon**, with most cases occurring among smokers.

Nonrespiratory Effects

Air pollutants affect organs in the body other than the lungs. Once inhaled, pollutants can be absorbed into the bloodstream and can reach all areas of the body (see Chapter 4, Section A). Airborne **lead** has caused nervous disorders in children, including learning disabilities (decreases in IQs) and hyperactivity; kidney damage leading to high blood pressure in both children and adults; and outright poisoning. Lead levels have dropped dramatically in the last 15 years as leaded gasoline has been phased out, but deposits on the ground from years past are a lingering source of exposure.

Benzene is a cause of leukemia in rubber and chemical workers and is present in the air from refinery operations and gasoline combustion. Because the concentrations of benzene in the air are low, it is difficult to know what effect it has on the general population. Risk estimates for the Los Angeles basin suggest that benzene in outdoor air causes 100 cancer cases per year there. Various other organic solvents are associated with nervous system disorders in workers, but again, concentrations are so low that it is difficult to ascribe any particular cases to such exposures.

Carbon monoxide may play a part in the development of ischemic heart disease, in which the heart muscle does not get enough oxygen over long periods and its tissues slowly die. Similarly, the added strain on the heart and lungs caused by a lack of oxygen during peak carbon monoxide episodes (for example, when smoking cigarettes or when stuck in rush hour traffic) may trigger heart attacks. While evidence of carbon monoxide playing a widespread role in heart disease is not conclusive at the moment, most experts think it is plausible.

Summary

Air pollutants cause many health problems, ranging from the triggering of asthmatic attacks to the slow degeneration of the lungs, from cancer to brain disorders. With the notable exception of lead, air quality has not improved significantly in the last ten years, and in some instances it has gotten worse. The widespread health effects of many pollutants, such as lead, asbestos, and radon, have been generally recognized only within the last ten years, and new products and substances are constantly being introduced. Air quality must remain a top priority, both at home and in the political arena, if the quality of life is not to suffer.

B. Smoking and Health

Cigarette smoking is the single most preventable major cause of death in our society. More than one in every six deaths in the United States can be attributed to smoking, over 390,000 deaths annually. At every age, proportionately more smokers die each year than do nonsmokers. Tobacco contributes to 30% of all cancer deaths yearly, including 85% of all lung cancer deaths. Smokers overall have a 70% greater coronary heart disease death rate—the leading cause of death—compared to nonsmokers. An additional 10 million Americans suffer increased rates of various debilitating diseases caused by smoking, including *bronchitis, emphysema,* and *atherosclerosis.* Inhaling other people's smoke, or passive smoking, is now implicated in disease (particularly lung cancer) among nonsmokers.

Who Smokes and Who Doesn't: Trends in Smoking Habits

The fraction of American adults who smoked in 1987 was 29%, down from 40% in 1965. Men smokers still outnumber women smokers, but the differential has been shrinking, and among high school seniors, more girls smoke than do boys. The greatest increase in smoking has been among women aged 20 to 34. The progress made in reducing the smoking rate has been largely due to smokers quitting rather than to fewer people taking up the habit. Nearly half of all living adults who ever smoked have quit. But the most recent information about smoking among teenage boys shows that primary prevention (never smoking) is beginning to play a part in reducing the smoking rate.

Among blacks, blue-collar workers, and less educated people the smoking rate is higher than in the population as a whole. Level of education is more closely related to smoking than any other factor. The higher the level of education, the less likely someone is to be a smoker.

Smoking begins primarily during childhood and adolescence. One-fourth of high school seniors who have ever smoked had their first cigarette by sixth grade, one-half by eighth grade. For those who begin smoking before age 20, the younger they begin, the more likely they are to continue and the more likely they are to smoke heavily. These facts indicate the importance of starting smoking education campaigns at the earliest possible ages.

Diseases Caused By Smoking

Lung cancer is the disease most often identified with smoking. In 1985, smoking accounted for 87% of all lung cancer deaths. Among women, lung cancer recently overtook breast cancer as the leading fatal cancer, a direct result of the increase in female smoking over the past three decades.

Other diseases known to be caused by smoking include coronary heart disease, stroke, and peripheral vascular disease (as many cases of cardiovascular disease as lung cancer are caused by smoking); cancers of the larynx, mouth, and esophagus; *chronic obstructive pulmonary disease (COPD)*; fetal growth retardation; and low birth weight babies. Cigarette smoking is now considered to be a probable cause of unsuccessful pregnancy, increased infant mortality, and peptic ulcer disease; to be a contributing factor in cancers of the bladder, pancreas, and kidney;

and to be associated with cancer of the stomach. Tobacco smoke also interacts with various workplace substances and with alcohol to increase the risk of cancer.

There are over 4000 compounds present in tobacco smoke, many of which have been proven to be toxic or to cause cancer and mutations. A total of 43 **carcinogens** have been identified, including several **nitrosamines**, **benzo[a]pyrene**, **cadium**, **nickel**, and **zinc**. **Carbon monoxide**, **nitrogen oxides**, and **particulate matter** are some of the other toxic substances present.

Passive Smoking and Involuntary Exposure

Breathing the smoky air produced when other people smoke tobacco is called passive smoking. Practically all of the substances inhaled by smokers are present in the smoke drifting off the end of a burning cigarette or exhaled by the person smoking. Although concentrations of toxics are lower because of the dilution in the surrounding air, health effects from this smoke are now established. The EPA has recently classified passive smoke as a class A carcinogen (see Chapter 3, Section B). Lung cancer in healthy nonsmokers is the most serious outcome and has been demonstrated in families of smokers. An increase in respiratory infections and symptoms among children of smokers, increased symptoms of allergies, chronic lung conditions, and chest pains have all been reported, as well as headaches, nausea, and irritation of the eyes and nose.

Involuntary exposure to substances in tobacco smoke occurs to the developing embryos of pregnant women who smoke and to the infants of women who breast-feed and smoke. Many of the substances are able to cross the placenta and reach the fetus; other substances appear in breast milk. Some of the consequences of these exposures include stillbirth, miscarriage, premature birth, low birth weight babies, and retarded development.

C. Indoor Air Pollution

In the mid-1970s, a few scientific reports began to appear indicating that air pollution might be more hazardous in the kitchens of average U.S. homes than outdoors near a Los Angeles freeway. Since then, with the completion of many air pollution studies in homes, the problem of indoor air pollution, as it is called, is becoming clear.

Indoor Air Pollution Sources

There are five types of pollution sources in the home. These are summarized in the simplified diagram shown in Figure 3. The first to be recognized was burning fuel indoors for cooking and space heating. Natural gas, the most commonly used indoor fuel in the United States, mainly produces **nitrogen dioxide** and **carbon monoxide** along with harmless combustion products. If wood is burned in a fireplace or for cooking (as is the case in much of the world), then in addition to these two pollutants, **particulate matter** and a host of potentially hazardous hydrocarbons are produced. These hydrocarbons include the group of **benzo[a]pyrenes** that are known to be potent carcinogens. Burning coal or oil produces all of these pollutants plus **sulfur dioxide**. Because most oil-heated homes in the United States use a low-sulfur grade of oil and few houses use coal, sulfur dioxide is generally not a major problem here. However, in many other countries such as China, coal is widely used in the home and the spectrum of pollutants it produces poses a serious health threat. In developing nations where poorly vented stoves and fireplaces are common, indoor pollution from fuel burning is believed to be a major health hazard.

A second source of indoor air pollution results from synthetic, and some natural, materials used for carpeting, foam insulation, wall coverings, and furniture. Glue used in some plywood, for example, gives off **formaldehyde**. Latex carpet is a source of phenylcyclohene. **Asbestos**, used as a building mate-

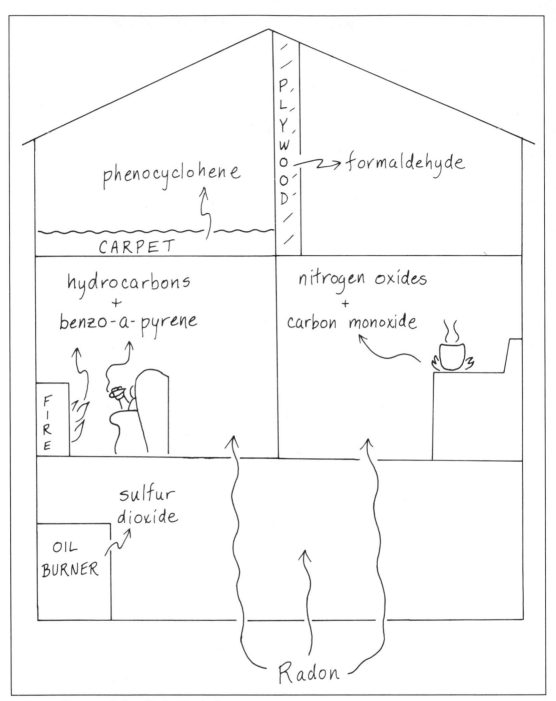

Figure 3 Sources of air pollution in the home.

rial because of its heat-resistant properties, can shed asbestos fibers into the indoor air if the material is not properly sealed. In offices, some copy machines and computer printers are a source of toxic organic substances such as **toluene**. Indeed, the air in many modern office buildings is particularly polluted because of the combination of office equipment, synthetic carpets, and poor ventilation. The phrase *sick building syndrome* has been coined to describe homes and work places where headaches and eye irritation are common as a result of poor indoor air quality. In industry, there are *Occupational Safety and Health Administration (OSHA)* regulations to protect workers against the more blatant examples of indoor air pollution generated in manufacturing. In principle, OSHA has the authority to protect office workers against sick building syndrome, but the complex nature of the pollution in sick buildings and the ambiguous nature of its health effects has resulted in very little regulatory action to date.

A third source of indoor air pollution is toxic gases leaking upward into the living area of a home from the soil beneath the house. This is the most serious of the sources in the United States, for this is the way the radioactive gas **radon** enters. Recent evidence suggests that toxic gases can probably enter houses located near chemical waste dumps this way as well, although the extent of this threat is not really known.

Many commercial products such as furniture polishes, glues, cleaning agents, cosmetics, deodorizers, pesticides, and solvents used in the home contribute to the toxicity of indoor air. (See the Cross-References at the beginning of the book for specific toxics associated with these various products.) Moreover, dry-cleaned clothes brought into the home are a source of **tetrachloroethylene.** These consumer products are the fourth source of indoor air pollution.

The fifth source is tobacco smoking. Not only is it a serious indoor air pollutant in its own right, but as was discussed in Section B of this chapter, you increase the risk of illness from other toxics such as those just discussed if you smoke or live with a smoker.

Reduction of Indoor Air Pollution

The indoor air pollution from all five sources can be reduced by increasing the ventilation in the home. Unfortunately, this strategy can be costly, for in cold weather increased ventilation means either a chillier home or higher heating bills. Also, the higher heating bills are a symptom of a host of other environmental problems such as greenhousing warming, acid rain (see Chapter 11, Sections A and C). Indeed, much of the earliest interest in indoor air pollution stemmed from concern that plugging the leaks in houses to save energy would seal in gaseous pollutants as well as warm air.

Fortunately, there are other and better ways to reduce indoor air pollution levels than to have excessive air infiltration and consequent energy waste. Cooking stoves can be vented with an exhaust fan, which increases ventilation right at the source of pollution where it's needed most. Alternatively, electric stoves can be used, although this means higher outdoor pollution levels if the electricity is produced by burning fossil fuel. Indoor pollution from space heating can be reduced, if not completely eliminated, by using properly designed, efficient furnaces or wood stoves. Pollution from synthetic materials can be reduced by avoiding their use in the home, provided they can be recognized, or by airing any suspiciously smelling new items such as plastic tableclothes until the smell goes away. New pieces of furniture, particularly sofas and easy chairs stuffed with foam, are often a much greater source of indoor air pollution than used furniture is. The reason is that by the time a foam-stuffed cushion is several years old, it will have emitted much of its formaldehyde. Reduction of indoor air pollution can thus be added to the many other reasons for recycling and prolonging the life of consumer items (see Chapter 16, Section D). Finally, sealants can be used to coat some building materials to prevent release of substances such as formaldehyde or asbestos, and indoor radon levels can be reduced by a variety of ways discussed under **radon** in Part II.

Recent studies by the National Aeronautics and Space Administration (NASA) indicate that there may be another way to at least partially reduce indoor pollution levels. NASA scientists have shown that common house plants absorb into their leaves certain polluting gases such as formaldehyde, **benzene,** and carbon monoxide (*New York Times,* July 26, 1988). It appears from these studies that some plants are better able to do this than others. Philodendrons are particularly effective at removing these gases. Other plants showing this ability are spider plants (for removing carbon monoxide), aloe veras (for formaldehyde), and gerbera daisies and chrysanthemums (for benzene). While the tests were carried out under conditions resembling airtight spacecrafts rather than ventilated homes, the results suggest that these house plants may be useful as well as ornamental.

But even after all the strategies just described have been tried, the problem of indoor air pollution will still remain in certain situations. Some houses contain construction materials that are big sources of pollution such as asbestos which cannot be removed except at enormous cost. Other houses may be located sufficiently near toxic waste dumps so that no solution short of cleaning up the dump is possible.

People concerned that they may have a serious indoor air pollution problem in their home or work place should call the appropriate hotline number listed under the heading National Hotlines (at the back of the book) to obtain information on the seriousness of their situation. If persistent headaches, eye irritation, or general malaise seem to be associated with time spent indoors at home or work, such concern is warranted.

Further Reading

AMDUR, MARY O. 1986. Air Pollutants. In *Casarett and Doull's Toxicology: The Basic Science of Poisons.* Edited by Klaassen, Curtis D., Amdur, Mary O., and Doull, John. 3d edition. New York: Macmillan.

ERIKSEN, M. P., LEMAISTRE, C. A., and NEWELL, G. R. 1988. Health Hazards of Passive Smoking. *Annual Review of Public Health* 9:47–70.

McGINNIS, J. M., SHOPLAND, D., and BROWN, C. 1987. Tobacco and Health: Trends in Smoking and Smokeless Tobacco Consumption in the United States. *Annual Review of Public Health* 8:441–467.

National Research Council. 1985. *Epidemiology and Air Pollution.* National Academy of Sciences. Washington, D.C.: National Academy Press.

NERO, A. V. 1988. Controlling Indoor Air Pollution. *Scientific American* 258(5):42–48.

TURIEL, I. 1985. *Indoor Air Quality and Human Health.* Stanford, CA: Stanford University Press.

U.S. Department of Health and Human Services. 1989. The Surgeon General's 1989 Report on Reducing the Health Consequences of Smoking: 25 Years of Progress. MMWR Supplement. *Morbidity and Mortality Weekly Report,* volume 38, number S-2.

6 TOXICS IN WATER

Clean water is a precious gift that, unfortunately, is denied to many people. In the first part of this chapter, we discuss the problems of water pollution in broad terms. The emphasis here is on hazardous substances that show up in reservoirs or that enter drinking water between the reservoir and the tap. The second section deals with a particular water pollution problem that receives relatively little publicity but is of growing importance—groundwater contamination.

A. Drinking Water and Health

Adults drink an average of 2 quarts of water per day, either directly or in other beverages. Children under the age of five consume twice as much as this in proportion to their body weights. In most of the United States, the water we drink is healthier now than it used to be, owing largely to the disinfection of drinking water beginning at the turn of the century. Nevertheless, contamination remains a problem in certain locations, and for some substances, the problem is growing worse. For some pollutants, such as **lead**, contamination is not getting worse, but scientists are discovering that injury occurs at far lower doses than previously thought.

This section discusses toxic pollutants that enter drinking water in the home, at the local water utility, and at the source. At each stage of the journey from rainwater to tap, specific pollutants tend to be added. While not the focus of this book, brief mention is also made of contamination by microorganisms since microbes have caused most of the outbreaks of waterborne disease in this country as well as most others. The section concludes with a list of measures individuals can take to reduce the risks from the water they drink.

Because all of the toxic substances mentioned here are treated in detail in Part II, only the most prominent health effects are noted here.

The Drinking Water Supply: An Overview

As most people know, water moves in a cycle on our planet. It falls to the ground as rain and snow and then runs into lakes and rivers (surface water) or percolates into the ground (groundwater). It eventually flows to the oceans where evaporation starts this hydrologic cycle over again. People take water both from the surface and from the ground to use for drinking and other purposes. For the United States as a whole, about half the population drinks surface water and the other half groundwater. But in rural areas, almost everyone uses groundwater (wells). Surface water and groundwater each tends to have its own specific kinds of problems.

Water is delivered by nearly 60,000 water utilities throughout the country to 200 million people, while approximately 40 million rely on private wells. The quality of water supplied by utilities is regulated by the EPA, although standards are set for only a few dozen of the thousands of potentially hazardous substances found in drinking water. Private wells are not regulated. Most of the population is served by large utilities, whereas rural areas are supplied by smaller systems each serving a few thousand people. As a general rule, the larger systems tend to have higher quality water because they can spread the costs of more modern facilities and maintenance over a greater number of customers.

Biological Safety of Drinking Water

Before the turn of the century, waterborne infectious diseases in the United States were rampant. Cholera and dysentery were epidemic, and as late as 1900, typhoid fever had killed as many as 25,000 people annually. With the advent of water disinfection, principally through chlorination and filtration, the occurrence of these bacterial diseases dropped dramatically. Today, the outbreaks of waterborne diseases number in the twenties per year, with only a few thousand people affected and far fewer killed. In the 1970s and 1980s, however, outbreaks have been more common than in the 1950s and 1960s, owing partly to aging water treatment plants. Also in recent years, there has been a greater occurrence of diseases caused by viruses and protozoa, organisms not effectively killed by chlorination. Although the practice of water chlorination is now being criticized for its toxic by-products, it should be remembered how important it has been in improving public health and how much for granted we take the biological safety of our drinking water.

Contaminants Added at the Source

The quality of source water varies widely, depending on the local geology, farming activities, and industrial/municipal sources of pollution. As a general rule, groundwater contains more mineral contaminants (such as **nitrates, arsenic,** and **barium**) than surface water because the water percolates through rock picking up minerals on the way. However, surface water tends to contain more biological contaminants (such as bacteria and viruses) and more natural *organic* pollution (decaying vegetable matter). Both sources can contain industrial waste of both organic and *inorganic* origins.

The latest evidence of trends in the nation's surface water quality shows a mixed picture. There have been decreases in bacterial contamination and lead pollution, the latter because of the steady elimination of lead from gasoline. But there have been increases in nitrates, chloride (**chlorine**), arsenic, and cadmium. Arsenic and **cadmium** are believed to come mainly from fossil fuel combustion because they are trace contaminants in coal and fuel oil. Nitrates come both from fossil fuel combustion (see Chapter 11, Section C) and agricultural fertilizer runoff. Nitrate pollution is a particular problem for areas east of the Mississippi River. Chloride pollution is believed to be due both to increased population growth (municipal waste and waste water) and to increased use of salt on the highways.

Groundwater quality trends are less well known. In agricultural regions, pesticide and fertilizer residues (especially nitrates) can be high. Groundwater in the vicinity of toxic waste dumps, mill tailings and coal ash piles, and other industrial storage facilities can be contaminated from leakage into underground aquifers. People served by private wells, particularly in the vicinity of potential sources of groundwater contamination, may wish to have their water tested. No federal or state agency enforces water quality standards for private wells. (See Chapter 17, Section C, for more information.)

Contaminants Added in the Distribution System

The water distribution system includes the local treatment plant and all the pipes used to bring water to the plant and move it from the plant to homes and buildings. Various contaminants can enter water from corrosion of the pipes, as additives to prevent corrosion, and as by-products of the chemicals used to disinfect and otherwise treat the water before delivery.

Corrosion of pipes can release metals such as **lead, cadmium,** iron, **zinc, nickel,** and others into the water supply. **Asbestos** can also be released by the breakdown of asbestos–cement pipe (A/C pipe), which is used in some systems. It is not known whether the asbestos released presents a significant health risk from drinking, although occupational asbestos exposure is associated with *gastrointestinal* cancers. Corrosion inhibitors are added in many supply systems to reduce the concentrations of metals and asbestos. While these substances are for the most part considered safe at the levels used, a group of inhibitors called phosphates are known to interfere with human trace metal metabolism at slightly higher concentrations.

Chlorination of drinking water for disinfection has been called the single most important public health measure ever undertaken. It has largely eliminated the occurrence of epidemic waterborne diseases in the United States common before the turn of the century. While effective against most *pathogenic* bacteria (but not against viruses and protozoa such as *Giardia*), chlorination produces toxic by-products. The most important of these are a class of organic molecules called *trihalomethanes (THMs)*, of which the best studied is **chloroform**. THMs are produced when chlorine reacts both with naturally occurring organic matter, such as decaying leaves, bark, and soil, and with industrial organic pollutants. Surface water contains more of these materials than groundwater. Approximately 80% of the population receives chlorinated water; 50% receives chlorinated surface water.

Chloroform causes cancer in rats and mice. In humans, lifetime users of chlorinated water have a higher rate of bladder cancer than users of nonchlorinated water. The effects are most plainly seen among nonsmokers. (The rate of bladder cancer in smokers is so high that it masks the relatively small effect produced by THMs.) Estimates are that chlorinated surface water may be responsible for about one-fourth of all bladder cancer cases among nonsmokers. Gastrointestinal cancers have also been associated with chlorinated surface waters in some epidemiological studies, but in other studies there has been no significant association. The National Academy of Sciences has recommended that the current federal limit for total THMs in drinking water be lowered on the basis of the latest evidence.

New methods of disinfection that may avoid or reduce some of the problems of chlorination are now in use in Europe and are being tried in the United States. These methods include using *chloramines*, **ozone**, or chlorine dioxide instead of chlorine, as well as removal of organic matter prior to chlorination. Unfortunately, at the present time the potential side effects of these alternatives are less well known than are those for chlorination. This is an area of active scientific investigation.

Fluoride and **aluminum** are two other chemicals sometimes added to drinking water prior to distribution. Fluoride is added to partially protect against dental decay (cavities), and aluminum is added in the form of "alum" (usually aluminum sulfate) to flocculate and remove organic matter that may cause odor or taste problems. The latest evidence on fluoride indicates that at the levels added to inhibit tooth decay (1 ppm), the only widespread effect is slight to moderate mottling of the teeth in a few percent of the population. There is no generally accepted evidence that fluoride causes cancer, although much higher levels than those added can cause bone disease. There is no specific hazard from the aluminum added to drinking water because most of it is removed along with the organic matter. One survey has shown, however, that in about half the systems using aluminum to treat water, the concentration in the finished water is higher than in the raw water. Aluminum causes problems for people with kidney disease, including dialysis patients and possibly a large segment of the elderly population whose kidney functioning has declined with age. Aluminum has also been associated with *Alzheimer's disease*, but there is no evidence it is a cause.

Contaminants Added in the Home

Several toxic metals are added to drinking water right in the home, the most important being lead. These metals dissolve from the service lines used to connect the city distribution system with the home, from pipes within the home, and from solder used to join copper pipes. The greatest hazards exist in older homes, where lead pipe has been used, and in homes less than five years old, which is less time than it takes for a protective scale to build up on solder joints. Since June 1988, lead has been banned from solder and other materials used in distribution systems, so the newest construction avoids most problems. Areas with soft or acidic water have the greatest risk since corrosion is most rapid under these conditions.

Lead poisoning is associated with learning impairment, reduced IQs, and hyperactivity in children; high blood pressure in adults; and underweight and premature newborns. An estimated 10 million children receive significant amounts of lead in their drinking water. Other metals that may leach or corrode from pipes include cadmium, copper, and zinc, all of which can contribute to high blood pressure, among other disorders.

Fortunately, two simple precautions can be taken to reduce metal exposures. The highest levels occur both in the first draw of water in the morning, after water has been sitting overnight in contact with pipes, and in hot water. Before water is used for drinking or cooking, the tap should be flushed for several minutes in the morning or if it has not been used for several hours. That water need not be wasted; it can be collected for watering plants. The second precaution is to use only cold water for drinking or cooking. Hot water can safely be used for washing dishes.

Ways to Improve Drinking Water Quality

There are a number of ways that you can improve the quality of the drinking water your family uses in the home.

1. Run water from the taps for several minutes every morning before using the water for drinking or cooking. (Collect the water for plants.)

2. Use only cold water for drinking or cooking. Hot water dissolves more metals from home plumbing.
3. Pay attention to warnings from your water utility company, especially if water is being used to reconstitute infant formula. These warnings often accompany monthly bills. Federal regulations require customer notification if the quality dips below standards for many substances.
4. Private well water should be analyzed if a problem is suspected.
5. If a hazard exists, bottled water may provide an acceptable substitute. Otherwise, bottled water may be no safer than tap water because it is less regulated, and in some instances it may be less safe.
6. Home purification devices can remove some contaminants, but not all. If they are not properly installed, operated, and maintained, they can actually add more substances than they remove. Home purification can only be recommended in certain situations.[1]

B. The Threat From Below: Toxics in Groundwater

Groundwater is an important source of freshwater in the United States. Half the U.S. population is served by groundwater and two-fifths of agricultural irrigation water is pumped up from the ground. Many communities depend totally on groundwater. As pressure is put on developed surface water supplies, groundwater is becoming an important source of new freshwater. Unfortunately, our untapped wells may already be polluted with **nitrates** and other industrial and agricultural chemicals.

Groundwater is water stored in pore spaces in rocks and sediments of the earth's upper crust. When rain falls or snow melts, some of the water on the earth's surface evaporates,

[1] *Consumer Reports.* 1990. Fit to Drink? Vol. 55, no. 1 (entire issue).

some is taken up by plants, and some runs over the ground into streams and lakes. The remainder seeps into pores and cracks in the underlying sediments and bedrock to become groundwater. Some groundwater emerges as surface water to supply rivers, ponds, or lakes during dry months; the rest remains in the ground. When the cracks and pores are large and well interconnected, water moves slowly through the geologic formations. A well drilled into such a rock formation will yield water fast enough to allow pumping in sufficient quantities for human use. These water-bearing rock units are called *aquifers*.

Aquifers can be contaminated by a variety of sources, including leaking septic tanks and sewers, underground gasoline tanks, landfill sites, industrial waste storage tanks, mine lagoons and tailings, oil field operations, and agricultural runoff. Bacteria, toxic chemicals, and excessive nutrients seep into the ground from such sites, following the same path of least resistance that the water takes. The pollutants tend to move down until some barrier is encountered (such as an impermeable bedrock layer) and then they spread out. In this way toxics can travel hundreds of miles before being released into a stream, lake, or well.

Aquifers can also be contaminated by saltwater. As freshwater is pumped out of an aquifer, new water flows from the surrounding area to fill vacant spaces. If the aquifer is located near the coast, the source of the new water may be the ocean. In that case, the aquifer will become contaminated, a problem known as saltwater intrusion or saltwater encroachment.

Groundwater pollution is difficult to detect and correct. Often groundwater pollution is not detected until the pollutant emerges into a well some distance from the source of pollution. In rural areas, where well water is not routinely tested for contamination, the problem can easily go unnoticed for many years. Urban areas are subject to regular municipal testing programs so a contaminated aquifer can be identified faster. But in both cases, identifying the source of pollution can be tricky. Unlike toxic spills in a river, groundwater pollutants do not follow easily identifiable paths, and they often do not mix well in the water. This makes testing difficult and often unreliable. In addition, pollutants from several sources can become mixed underground. Even if a source can be identified and the flow of toxic substance stopped, a polluted aquifer remains contaminated. The pollutant will continue to spread, becoming less concentrated as it moves away from the original source, but at the same time distributing the contamination to more people.

It is difficult, if not impossible, to reverse the effects of contamination in an aquifer. Water moves through the ground very slowly, sometimes taking days or even months to travel several hundred feet. Thus, a contaminated aquifer cannot be flushed with clean water to rinse away the contaminant. In some cases, clean-up is further restricted because the water itself lends support to the loose sediment in which it is stored. If water is pumped faster than it can be replaced, the aquifer may collapse, permanently closing the pore spaces that hold the groundwater. Even if it were possible to flush polluted water from an aquifer, the aquifer itself would remain contaminated. Many chemicals have a tendency to bind to sedimentary particles. As new freshwater replaces the removed polluted water, the bound chemicals are released, contaminating the freshwater.

An aquifer, once contaminated, can be ruined as a source of freshwater. People are only now beginning to understand the consequences of using the land as an inadvertent or deliberate recipient of waste. As such, laws are being developed to regulate the disposal of liquid wastes at landfills and in deep injection wells. The nation's six million underground storage tanks holding hazardous substances and petroleum products are also under new regulatory scrutiny. Even household septic tanks may become more strictly regulated in the years to come.

Further Reading

Concern, Inc. 1984. *Groundwater: A Community Action Guide.* Washington, D.C.

GABLER, RAYMOND, and the Editors of *Consumer Reports* Books. 1988. *Is Your Water Safe to Drink?* New York: Consumers Union.

National Academy of Sciences. 1977–1987. *Drinking Water and Health.* Vols. 1–7. Washington, D.C.: National Academy Press.

PATRICK, RUTH, FORD, EMILY, and QUARLES, JOHN. 1987. *Groundwater Contamination in the United States.* 2d edition. Philadelphia: University of Pennsylvania Press.

Water Education Foundation. 1986. *Groundwater and Toxics.* Sacramento, CA.

7 TOXICS IN FOOD

In this chapter we look at the innumerable ways in which we are exposed to toxics through eating. We first examine food additives, explaining some of the reasons why these substances are added to food, the degree to which regulations protect us from them, and some commonsense ways to reduce unnecessary exposure. Then we discuss how a particular item in many people's diet—alcohol—increases their susceptibility to other toxics to which they may be exposed. Finally, we look at what is currently a very controversial matter—the degree to which perfectly natural substances in our diet may cause more of a health risk than the generally more feared pollutants such as synthetic pesticides and other industrial chemicals.

A. Food Additives and Health

We take it for granted that our food supply is clean and wholesome. So it is often with dismay that we read that a common food additive is found to be unhealthy. Fortunately, most of the food additives in use today are not dangerous, and new ones are carefully tested before being allowed in the marketplace. Nevertheless, there are many commonly used chemical additives that are presumed safe for no other reason than that no one has complained of illness as a result of their use over the years. These are the chemicals known as *generally recognized as safe,* or *GRAS.* Once a substance is listed as GRAS, it is not subject to specific regulation. The Food and Drug Administration (FDA) requires only that "good manufacturing practice" be used for GRAS substances.

The term food additive is not very specific. It includes those chemicals intentionally added to food, contaminants from packaging material, pesticide or animal drug residues, and chemicals present in the water used to process the product. Food colors are considered separately under the Color Additives Amendment (1960) to the Food, Drug, and Cosmetics Act. Residues from new animal drugs are also considered under a separate provision of the law.

Contrary to popular belief, food additives are not a modern innovation. Salting meat was the first of many preservation techniques used over the centuries to keep meat from spoiling. But modern chemistry has provided a host of new substances that can be used to preserve food. In the early 1900s, boric acid, **formaldehyde**, **lead** salts, and salicylic acid were common but toxic food additives. In 1958, the Food Additives Amendment to the Pure Food and Drug Act was passed, which required manufacturers to do extensive testing before any new food additive could be marketed. But food additives that had been in use for a long time and those that were deemed safe by "qualified scientists" under conditions of normal use were exempt from premarket testing.

In response to the Food Additives Amendment, the FDA drew up a list of substances that were thought to be safe. The list was then included in a questionnaire that was sent to about 900 scientists. Just over one-third of those who were sent questionnaires responded, and only about 100 of the responses contained substantive comments. From this meager data, the GRAS list was finalized. It wasn't until 1969 that the FDA began to review the scientific literature to determine the safety of GRAS substances. As of mid-1987, less than 500 substances have been reviewed; 48 have GRAS affirmation pending, not because they are unsafe, but because too little is known about the chemicals to determine whether they are safe. The pending list includes such widely used additives as **caffeine, BHT** and **BHA,** mustard, gelatin, and citric acid.

The Food Additives Amendment also contains the controversial Delaney Clause, which states that "no additive shall be deemed safe if it is found to induce cancer when ingested by man or animal." The Delaney Clause defines "safe" in absolutely rigid terms. Either a chemical causes cancer or it does not. If well-conducted tests show that it causes cancer, at any amount, it must go. Period. Of course, no one wants cancer-causing chemicals added to food. But the Delaney Clause does not allow any consideration to be given to possible benefits that may be derived from using cancer-causing additives. For example, suppose that a chemical were developed that destroyed **aflatoxin** in prepared food. Now suppose that this chemical were shown to cause cancer in laboratory animals, but only using massive doses. As discussed in the aflatoxin entry in Part II of this book, very small doses of aflatoxin are capable of causing cancer in people. Thus, using this new chemical to destroy aflatoxin might be a good idea. Yet, because the new chemical causes cancer, it cannot be used, no matter how many aflatoxin-induced cancers it may prevent.

This is one of the important reasons why the Delaney Clause is so controversial. Yet it remains on the books. What member of Congress would want to be put on record as favoring the addition of cancer-causing chemicals to food? In practice, the FDA sidesteps the problem by simply ignoring potentially cancer-causing food additives that the agency determines pose an almost insignificant risk to the population eating the food. Only when members of the public believe that a risk posed by a specific additive is unacceptably high is pressure brought upon the agency to defend their decision.

Food colors must be rigorously tested before being listed as acceptable by the FDA. Only seven synthetic colors are certified to be used in food. Controversy still exists as to the cancer-causing properties of all these dyes. Yellow No. 5 is reputed to cause allergic reactions, especially among aspirin-sensitive people. Many people claim that synthetic colors are entirely unnecessary. For example, the Norwegians banned the use of all synthetic colors in 1979, and they seem unperturbed about eating gray hot dogs. Many food dyes derived from natural sources are available, but they are expensive to use, are ineffective for some applications, and do not render the bright colors that synthetic dyes do. Also, many natural food colors have not undergone toxicity testing.

Although as many as 2800 substances are used as food additives, the vast majority are used in very small quantities. Sucrose, corn syrup, dextrose, salt, black pepper, caramel, carbon dioxide, citric acid, modified starch, sodium bicarbonate, yeasts, and yellow mustard account for 95% by weight of all additives used in the United States. Of course, the average consumer is concerned about the remaining 5%. Which ones of these are actually safe to eat? There is no question that some of them are beneficial, most are harmless, and a few may cause unforeseen health problems. For example, red dye No. 3, **monosodium glutamate (MSG), sulfites,** and **nitrates** are food additives that may be potentially harmful to the population as a whole or to particularly susceptible segments of the population, especially babies and people with allergies.

With processed foods representing over half of the food consumed in the United States, concern over the health effects of food additives is not misguided. However, reliance on processed food is, in many ways, voluntary. Food additives are used because people want fast food, snack food, out-of-season food, cheap food, and food that can be stored in the pantry for long periods. And people want this food to look appetizing and have a normal texture, along with being safe to eat.

By far the best way to minimize exposure to food additives is to use fresh, unprocessed, even organically grown food whenever possible. Moreover, unprocessed food often tastes better and is nutritionally superior. Preparing fresh food may also take less effort than trying to keep up to date with the never-ending advice about which food additives to avoid, or lugging this book around the grocery store.

B. Why Alcohol and Other Chemicals Don't Mix

An estimated 10% of the U.S. population abuses alcohol. Chronic intake of alcohol (or, more technically, ethanol) is related to damage to the liver, the nervous system, the cardiovascular system, and the immune system. Regular alcohol consumption combined with smoking is also linked to cancer of the head and neck. Fetal alcohol syndrome, a set of birth defects that may affect the children of women who drink, is receiving increased attention mainly because researchers have determined that even moderate alcohol use during pregnancy is associated with adverse effects on birth weight and early childhood development. While alcohol abuse does indeed have adverse health effects and social consequences, we instead focus here on how regular alcohol consumption can alter susceptibility to the effects of other toxics.

Regular alcohol consumption, such as drinking moderately three days a week for several months or years, can lead to changes in how fast and by which pathways chemicals are broken down inside the body. In much the same way that regular exercise changes the body to accommodate more exercise, chronic exposure to ethanol causes the body to change so as to manage the heavier load. These changes are reflected in the way the body breaks down ethanol. It is broken down in the body by two sets of *enzymes* known as *alcohol dehydrogenase (ADH)* and *microsomal ethanol oxidizing system (MEOS)*. ADH is the major pathway for ethanol metabolism. This enzyme is located primarily in the liver, and there is a fixed amount of it. While a larger pool of ADH cannot be created, it can be destroyed both by abusive consumption of alcohol and possibly by toxics. When small amounts of ethanol pass through the liver, ADH is often able to process most of it. Anything in excess of the ADH capacity spills over to the MEOS.

MEOS is also located in the liver, but unlike ADH, more of it can be produced by the body on demand. A regular dose of ethanol above the small amount that can be processed by ADH stimulates one of several enzyme types that make up the MEOS until enough is created to meet the increased demand. This enzyme, however, is not very selective; it processes a wide variety of substances, including several common drugs and chemicals. Furthermore, stimulation of one enzyme type in the MEOS group stimulates the production of other chemical-metabolizing enzymes in the MEOS, thereby accelerating metabolism of a wide variety of drugs and chemicals. It is important to remember that metabolism of a chemical can make a harmless one toxic or a toxic one harmless. Consequently, people who regularly consume alcohol can be either more or less susceptible than a nondrinker to the effects of the toxics they encounter.

Increased susceptibility to a chemical may be caused by competition for existing enzyme capacity (either ADH or MEOS) or by the increased ability to *bioactivate* chemicals. For example, MEOS detoxifies *barbiturates*. However, the enzyme that detoxifies the drug is more attracted to ethanol. So, when ethanol and barbiturates are taken together, the ethanol rapidly takes over the metabolizing capacity of the MEOS. The bioactive barbiturate is left in circulation to be metabolized after competition from ethanol diminishes. For this reason, the lethal dose of barbiturate is nearly 50% lower when the drug is ingested along with ethanol.

This process also occurs when exposure to ethanol and toxics are simultaneous. **Xylene** provides an interesting example of such interaction. Xylene is attracted to fat tissue in the body. When a person is exposed to xylene, usually in an industrial setting, most of the chemical is quickly taken out of the bloodstream and is temporarily sequestered in the person's fat tissue before being metabolized. As the xylene is metabolized, it is slowly released from the fat back to the bloodstream. In this way a constant concentration of xylene is maintained in the bloodstream until all of it is removed from fat stores. Ethanol is metabolized by the same enzyme that xylene is, but again, the enzyme is more attracted to the ethanol. So, when a person exposed to xylene during the day consumes an alcoholic beverage during the evening, the xylene suddenly has no metabolic pathway available for detoxification. Indeed, blood levels of xylene have been found to double when ethanol is ingested several hours after the initial exposure to xylene. Such an increase can result in toxic symptoms due to xylene poisoning.

In contrast, those who use alcohol regularly are less susceptible to the effects of chemicals metabolized by the MEOS at times when there is no ethanol in their bodies. This is because a larger pool of enzyme is available to detoxify the drugs and chemicals than would be present in the nondrinker. However, chronic alcohol intake can increase a person's susceptibility to harm from chemicals that are nontoxic when ingested or inhaled but which are toxic when bioactivated. For example, it has been observed that alcoholics display a greatly increased susceptibility to **carbon tetrachloride** poisoning. This is because alcoholics tend to have a much greater pool of enzymes available to change the carbon tetrachloride into its toxic *metabolite*.

These examples illustrate how regular alcohol consumption can influence an individual's susceptibility to toxics. The destruction, stimulation, or inhibition of enzymes often play a crucial role in determining individual suceptibility to harm following chemical exposure.

C. Food and Cancer: How Much Is Nature to Blame?

Pesticides and other chemical contaminants found in our environment have come under heavy fire from scientists and public interest groups because of the threat they may pose to our health. In recent years, a counterargument has been made with increasing vigor. It states, in a nutshell, that the threat of cancer from synthetic chemicals in our environment has been greatly exaggerated and that many foods contain larger amounts of natural cancer-causing substances than those for which the chemical industries are responsible.

The strongest proponent of this argument is biochemist Bruce Ames, who developed the *Ames test* for screening cancer-causing substances by detecting substances that cause mutations in bacteria (see Chapter 3, Section A). To clarify his reasoning, it is useful to consider three categories of potentially cancer-causing ingredients in our food and water:

1. Pollutants: These include pesticide *residues* in food and a variety of trace metals and other chemical pollutants found in drinking water. They appear in our environment not because people want them there, but because they are the by-products of human activities.
2. Additives: These include substances such as **nitrates**, for food preservation, or **chlorine**, for water treatment. They are deliberately added to our food and water for some beneficial purpose.
3. Nature's toxics: These include numerous natural ingredients of foods. Some are an inevitable part of the food or are produced by growing plants when they are stressed by insects or fungi. Others are produced by molds that can contaminate foods (such as **aflatoxin** produced by the mold *Aspergillus flavus*), and still others are produced when foods are cooked, fermented, or become rancid.

Ames argues that the threat from categories 1 and 2 has been greatly exaggerated and that much money is wasted and fear unnecessarily generated because of the governmental, scientific, and media attention given to toxics in those categories. He goes on to state that the hazards of category 3 exceed those of the first two. In particular, he argues that the amount of natural pesticides in foods such as mushrooms, many herbs and spices, celery, potatoes, lima beans, and many other fruits and vegetables far exceeds the amount of pesticide we receive because of synthetic pesticide use. While the cancer-causing potential of most of them has not been adequately tested, he asserts that natural pesticides are so much more abundant in the average diet that they pose a greater threat to us than do synthetic pesticides. Furthermore, to put the issue of pesticides in perspective, Ames concludes that the threat from all such pesticides, natural or synthetic, is insignificant to the health of the general public in comparison to the threat from smoking, alcohol, dietary fat, and nondietary hazards.

It ought not be a surprise that some fruits, nuts, and vegetables contain natural chemicals that are poisonous to at least some animals that can eat those foods. Such chemicals act as the plants' defenses against being eaten. Just as natural selection has led to the evolution of quills on porcupines and shells on turtles, it has led to chemical defenses for plants. Often, the chemical defense is so noxious to some animals that they avoid eating it altogether, but Ames' evidence indicates that perfectly tasty foods can be hazardous as well.

There is little doubt among most scientists that the cancer threat to human health from smoking greatly exceeds that from chemicals in categories 1 and 2. More controversial are Ames' conclusion that we concern ourselves needlessly with chemical pollutants and additives and his conclusion about the relative health threat from nature's pesticides versus those manufactured industrially. There have been numerous criticisms of his writings, the more compelling of which are listed here.

1. Estimates of the cancer-causing potential of most of the chemicals in all three categories are very uncertain. Relatively few natural pesticides in foods have been tested to determine how potent they are as causes of cancer, and for those that have been tested, there are large uncertainties in interpreting the results (for reasons discussed in Chapter 3, Section A). Given those uncertainties, critics argue, it is inappropriate to conclude that fears of synthetic chemical pollutants and additives are groundless. A "better safe than sorry" philosophy would warrant that we at least maintain our present level of concern over these substances.

2. Ames exaggerates the amounts of moldy foods and other cancer-causing natural ingredients in the typical human diet. For example, Ames' critics charge that he assumes ten or more times as much mushrooms and basil in the average diet than is realistic; both of these foods contain potentially toxic natural chemicals and are important to Ames' argument. Moreover, he may be underestimating the amount of synthetic pesticides in the average diet because the two pesticides he primarily used to derive his dose estimates were **DDT** and **ethylene dibromide (EDB)**, both of which have been banned in the United States. Synthetic pesticides in widespread use today are likely to be more abundant in the diet than these two substances.

3. People can choose which foods they eat, whereas they often have no choice about what contaminates the air they breathe and the water they drink. Hence, the risk from nature's toxics in the diet and the risk from pollution differ in an important, albeit subjective, way. Also, the people that benefit from pollution are often not the same as those who suffer the risk, whereas the risks and benefits associated with diet both occur to the same individual. Thus, ethically these two situations are quite different. (See Chapter 1, Section A, for more discussion of these issues.)

4. Whatever the risk from nature's toxics in our diet really is and regardless of whether it exceeds that from chemical pollutants, we have to eat, but we don't have to pollute our environment as carelessly as we now do. Such pollution does threaten health. Therefore, we can and should take strong actions now to reduce pollution.

5. Ames' assessment of the relative risk of diet and chemical pollutants is based solely on cancer risk. Chemicals in our environment (in all three categories) pose numerous other health threats besides cancer, including liver damage, reproductive and lung impairment, damage to the nervous system, and weakening of the body's natural immune system. (Such risks, along with that of cancer, are discussed for individual toxics in the entries in Part II.) Statements about the priority that the government should give to any of the three categories of toxics should be based on knowledge of all health risks, not just that of cancer. While in the scientific literature, Ames carefully specifies that his arguments pertain only to the cancer risk, the public media reporting on his results often fail to qualify the argument. As a result, the public is led to believe that Ames is saying that nature's pesticides are more of a total health threat than are industrial pesticides.

6. Ames' arguments pertain only to human health and ignore the threat of pollution to the other living organisms with which we share this planet. Examples of major ecological damage from pesticides such as DDT or from acid rain should convince us that we jeopardize other forms of life when we pollute the environment. Chemical pollutants can also alter our climate (see Chapter 11, Section A) and the stratospheric ozone layer that protects us from **ultraviolet radiation** (see Chapter 11, Section B), thereby threatening life. To many scientists, these are reason enough for the current level of concern over chemical pollutants.

Ames' evidence that the cancer threat from chemical pollutants and additives is insignificant compared to that from nature's toxics may or may not stand the test of time. Nevertheless, he has performed a useful service by pointing out that "natural" does not necessarily mean "healthy." As we have done throughout this book, we urge the reader to err on the side of caution in all such issues. In this case, caution would dictate making all reasonable attempts to minimize exposure to those chemical contaminants in the environment that appear to pose a serious health risk. It would also dictate that reasonable care be taken to minimize consumption of moldy foods and other food items that may pose a health risk. Readers wanting to learn more about which foods Ames believes contain relatively large amounts of natural pesticides are urged to refer to Ames' writings listed under Further Reading.

Further Reading

AMES, B. N. 1983. Dietary Carcinogens and Anticarcinogens. *Science* 221:1256–1264.

AMES, B. N., MAGAW, R., and GOLD, L. S. 1987. Ranking Possible Carcinogen Hazards. *Science* 236:271–280.

EPSTEIN, S. S. 1984. *Science* 224: 664.

———. S. S. 1979. *The Politics of Cancer*. New York: Anchor.

GARRO, A. J., and LIEBER, C. S. 1990. Alcohol and Cancer. *Annual Review of Pharmacology and Toxicology* 30:219–249.

JACOBSON, MICHAEL F. 1978. *Eaters Digest: The Consumer Fact Book of Food Additives*. Garden City, N.Y.: Doubleday and Company, Inc.

LIEBER, CHARLES S. 1988. Metabolic Effects of Ethanol and Its Interaction with Other Drugs, Hepatotoxic Agents, Vitamins, and Carcinogens: A 1988 Update. *Seminars in Liver Disease* 8 (1):47–68.

PERERA, F., and BUFFETTA, P. 1988. Perspectives on Comparing Risks of Environmental Carcinogens. *Journal of the National Cancer Institute* 80:1282–1293.

8 TOXICS IN CONSUMER PRODUCTS

Everyday household products contribute measurably to our daily exposure to toxic chemicals. Such products as new carpeting, art and craft supplies, and cleaning fluids emit toxics into the air. Many of these hazards are hidden; there may be no labels for the consumer to read to learn of a possible hazard. Other products may be safe to use, but during their manufacture or following disposal, toxic chemicals are released into the air and water. It is just as important to recognize this environmental hazard as it is to recognize the more personal hazard associated with using a product that emits a toxic chemical. This chapter describes some of the hidden hazards and provides a simple introduction to some of the environmental issues that consumers need to consider when choosing alternative products.

A. Inert Ingredients

In the world of product labeling, the word "inert" can be as misleading as the words "lite" or "natural" on food packaging. There are well over 1000 inert ingredients added to pesticides, cleaning products, and home improvement products to make them sprayable, spreadable, sticky, slippery, or less concentrated. While these inert components are not active in the sense that they do not, in and of themselves, kill the intended pests, color a wall, or remove dirt, many are chemically and biologically active. In other words, inert ingredients may be toxic or may cause environmental problems. Of the 1200 "inert" substances known to the EPA to be used in pesticide products, over 100 are of toxicological concern, including phenol, **tetrachloroethylene**, **methylene chloride**, and **carbon tetrachloride**. Inert ingredients are also used in industrial and consumer products. **Methylene chloride**, **xylene**, **methyl ethyl ketone**, **acetone**, and tetrachloroethylene have been reported to be used as inert ingredients in products ranging from furniture and shoe polish to carpet cleaners.

Even though their use is widespread, it is often difficult to find out exactly which inert ingredients are used in particular products. This is because manufacturers select the inert ingredients based on the prices and availability of suitable chemicals during the time that a batch of the product is being made. Thus, one batch of product may contain a different inert base than another batch manufactured two months later.

Inert ingredients have received little regulatory scrutiny because regulations have traditionally focused on the active ingredients. Inert ingredients used in pesticides, for instance, are exempt from tolerance requirements, which specify how much of a residue from a pesticide product may be left on food. The EPA has recently required manufacturers of pesticides to relabel products to identify the presence of 50 selected highly toxic inert ingredients. The EPA is also encouraging pesticide manufacturers to substitute less toxic inert ingredients for the more toxic ones whenever possible.

Inert ingredients in consumer products have received almost no attention. Although they are usually nontoxic substances such as water, this is not always the case. People who suffer allergic or other abnormal reactions while using a consumer product should contact their doctor. While treating a patient, a doctor may be able to persuade a company to divulge the types of chemicals used as inert ingredients for a particular product. It helps to bring the product in its original container to the doctor's office. Unfortunately, identifying the inert ingredients used in common products when no adverse reactions are reported is next to impossible.

B. Hobbies and Crafts

What could be more pleasurable than whiling away the hours on a special project in the basement shop or creating a beautiful wall hanging out of wax and dye in the kitchen? Who thinks, at these times, of the toxic hazards associated with art and craft supplies? Yet, art and craft materials can be dangerous to your health—even life threatening. Many art and craft materials are laden with pigments containing heavy metals and with dangerous solvents. Some processes emit toxic gases into the air, while others bathe the craftsperson with intense **ultraviolet radiation**. Here we briefly outline the more common hazards associated with art supplies. At the end of the chapter, we also provide references and telephone numbers to help people who use art and craft supplies assess the risks associated with their own particular situation.

Heavy metals such as **lead, cadmium**, and **chromium** are commonly found in art and crafts supplies. Lead is used in some ceramic glazes and in stained glass materials. Cadmium is used in silver solders, fluxes, and ceramic glazes. **Arsenic**, cadmium, chromium, cobalt, lead, manganese, and **zinc** are all used as pigments in paint, dyes, and ceramic glazes. Many other substances in addition to heavy metal are also common. **Toluene, xylene, methylene chloride**, petroleum distillates, glycol ethers, alcohols, ketones, and even **benzene** are some of the solvents used in oil- and solvent-based paints, markers, finishes, and coatings. **Formaldehyde** is used as a preservative in many acrylic paints, fabric finishes, and photographic products. **Hydroquinone** is used in photographic developing chemicals. **Asbestos** insulates kilns and contaminates talc and soapstone. Kilns emit gases such as carbon dioxide, **sulfur dioxide**, formaldehyde, fluorine, **chlorine**, lead, and cad-

mium during use. **Ultraviolet radiation** exposures in the arts come from such sources as arc welding, carbon arcs, photo printmaking, printing, and dyeline copying.

This is just the tip of the iceberg! There are literally hundreds of art and craft products on the market, many that contain toxics. These can be breathed, swallowed, or absorbed through the skin of unsuspecting users. Although professional artists and craftspeople, art teachers, and art students face the greatest dangers because they are constantly exposed to these products, they tend to be better informed about the risks. They are more likely to take measures to protect themselves than people who dabble and schoolchildren and the elderly using materials at the community center.

People who use art and craft materials should take the time to learn which harmful chemicals they may be using and take measures to avoid exposure. This is not as difficult a task as it was just a few years ago. In 1988, a bill was passed that requires the U.S. Product Safety Commission to regulate the labeling of art and craft materials for health hazards. The new law stipulates that young children, the elderly, and disabled people must be taken into consideration when labeling a product.

Unfortunately, since art and craft materials have a long shelf life, it may be years before all the products in the marketplace are properly labeled. In the meantime, look for products that bear the AP or CP seal. These can be safely used by small children, with certain exceptions. For example, metal enamels, ceramic glazes, and clays that contain talc may bear the seal, but should not be used by small children.

Experts suggest that hobbyists follow these guidelines.

1. Work in a well-ventilated area. An open window may not provide adequate ventilation. An exhaust fan that vents to the outside often provides sufficient ventilation, but consult an expert before instal-

ling one. Avoid working in a closed basement or garage.
2. Substitute nontoxic materials for the toxic ones whenever possible.
3. Avoid the use of aerosols, dry powders, or other forms of products that are difficult to apply precisely.
4. Don't eat, drink, or smoke in your workrooms when using hazardous materials.
5. Don't leave open containers of art and craft supplies around the room, and clean up spills quickly. Keep your work area clean.

Several books have been written for the amateur as well as the professional artist on the hazards of art supplies. Also, several organizations are available to help people use art and craft materials safely. (See the Further Reading list and Resources list at the end of the chapter.)

C. Some Product Comparisons

Whenever we buy, use, or clean products, we assume a pollution burden. It cannot be avoided. Hazardous waste results from the production of common products such as polyester fabric, acrylic sweaters, kitchen appliances, and plastic milk jugs. Table 6 lists some of the common products we use and the hazardous wastes they create, many of which are discussed throughout this book.

The products listed in Table 6 are common and may even be necessary for people to live comfortably. Nevertheless, it is possible for people to minimize their pollution burden with some knowledge, some smart shopping, and some advance planning. We are not attempting here to answer all questions that may arise, but we do present some of the issues that a consumer could consider when trying to choose among alternative products. Our analysis here is not definitive, but rather is intended to encourage people to think about the criteria for making environmentally sound consumer choices.

Paper Versus Plastic

Perhaps the most common question asked of grocery shoppers these days is "paper or plastic?" The bag with the lowest pollution burden may not be the paper one, as is commonly assumed. The pulp and paper industry is one of the top five polluters in the United States. When compared by weight, plastic is produced with less toxic waste. But this fact doesn't tell the whole story. In general, the toxic waste produced during the manufacture of paper is caustic. It may burn on contact and can even destroy a population of fish exposed to it. However, most of the toxic waste resulting from paper manufacturing does not cause cancer or other long-term human health effects.

In contrast, some of the waste associated with plastics manufacture is persistent in the environment and tends to cause cancer and other long-term health problems in exposed people and wildlife. In addition, when plastic is burned, the smoke tends to be more hazardous to health than is the smoke that results from burning paper.

The argument based on the amount of pollution released per pound of material also does not take into account how the bags are reused or what happens to them following their disposal. It can be argued that the bag likely to be reused most often is the better choice. If the paper sack is recycled, the choice of paper may come out slightly ahead. Unfortunately, the brown paper that grocery sacks are made of is of poor quality so that there is little demand for used grocery sacks. Once the sacks make it to the dump, there is little difference between them. Paper can last a remarkably long time in a municipal dump. However, if the local dump is located in a coastal area, the paper comes out way ahead. Paper falls apart quickly should it make its way to the water, whereas the plastic persists and becomes a hazard to marine life. Fortunately, the issue can be avoided entirely by choosing an alternative, which in this case is a canvas or string mesh shopping bag that can

TABLE 6 Everyday Products and the Hazardous Wastes They Generate

Product	Hazardous Wastes
Plastics	Organic **chlorine** compounds and *solvents*
Pesticides	Organic chlorine and organic phosphate compounds
Drugs	Organic solvents and residues, and heavy metals (**mercury** and **zinc** are common)
Paints	Heavy metals, pigments, solvents, and organic residues
Oil and gasoline	Phenol, **benzene**, and other organic compounds; **lead**, **ammonia**, salt, acids, and caustic liquids
Metals	**Lead**, **mercury**, **zinc**, **fluoride**, cyanide, acid and alkaline cleaners, solvents, pigments, plating salts, oils, and phenol
Leather	**Chromium** and organic solvents
Textiles	Heavy metals, dyes, organic chlorine compounds, and solvents

be carried to the store and reused hundreds of times before it wears out.

This discussion shows that in choosing among alternative products, the following questions should be asked:

1. How often will the product be reused before being discarded? Favor the one that will be reused.
2. Can it be recycled? Favor the one that can.
3. How toxic are the wastes produced or released during manufacture or disposal?
4. Is there a better alternative?

How does the paper versus plastic comparison look for that morning take-out cup of coffee? Insulated plastic cups are made using **styrene** puffed with **CFCs** or pentane. Cups puffed with CFCs should be avoided, since the release of CFCs destroys stratospheric ozone (see Chapter 11, Section B). Otherwise, the plastic cup may carry less of a pollution burden, partly because fewer raw materials and less energy are necessary to manufacture it. Many plastic cups can also be recycled, whereas the coatings and glues used to make paper cups interfere with recycling. Both cups share the disadvantage that they are single-use products. As an alternative to disposable cups, bring a reusable ceramic mug to the coffee shop every morning. The factors involved in the choice between plastic versus paper are shown in Figure 4.

Disposable Versus Cotton Diapers

Disposable diapers are big business in the United States. Whereas they were once used only during travel, more than 80% of the diaper crowd now wears disposable diapers exclusively. These paper and plastic products have revolutionized the old job of changing diapers. If the toxic waste question is just considered per diaper, then cotton and disposable diapers carry similar pollution burdens (see Chapter 14, Section E). However, the average baby will go through over 170 disposable diapers for every cotton diaper that is purchased and reused. The manufacture of enough disposable diapers to meet the needs of a typical child uses more raw materials and creates more manufacturing waste than does the manufacture of enough cotton diapers. Cotton diapers do use more energy and water, and contribute more effluent to sewage treatment plants than do disposable diapers. Nevertheless, the amount of waste associated with the manufacture, use, and disposal of disposable diapers so overwhelms that of using cotton diapers that cotton diapers clearly come out ahead from an environmental perspective. In addition, disposable diapers add human waste to municipal dumps that were not designed to manage such wastes in a healthful way. As such, some scientists fear that local groundwater may be-

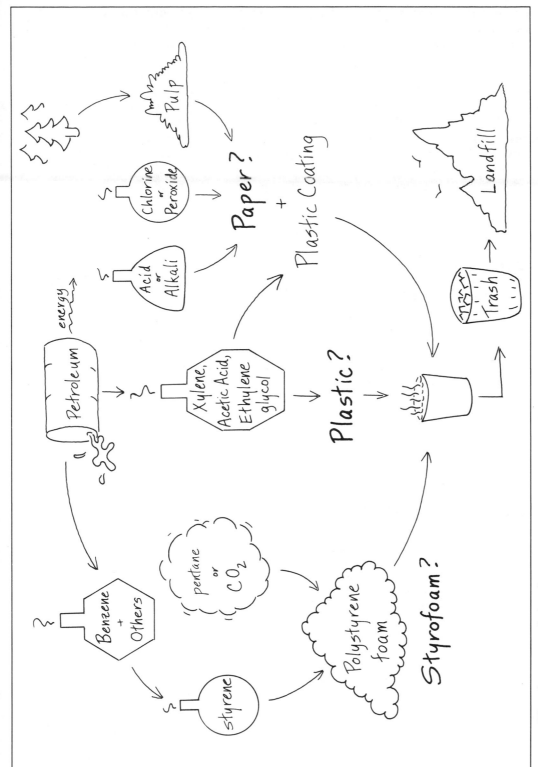

Figure 4 The take-out cup choice: foam versus paper.

come contaminated with bacteria, viruses, and other *pathogens*. These microorganisms also threaten the health of people who work at landfills, and they are able to persist long after the dump is closed, making future use of dump sites risky. Used disposable diapers also take up a great deal of space at already crowded municipal landfills. There is a consensus among people who manage municipal dumps that disposable diapers are a growing problem.

While disposable diaper manufacturers are experimenting with recycling used disposable diapers, diaper recycling is not yet being practiced commercially. Under certain circumstances, it may be necessary or vastly more convenient to use disposables. For example, if cleaning facilities are unavailable or it is impossible to store used diapers for later pick-up, disposables may be appropriate. Figure 5 presents the factors involved in the choice between disposable and cotton diapers.

Whenever products are purchased, consumers who want to minimize their pollution burden should work through similar thought processes. Fortunately, the information that allows consumers the opportunity to make a choice is becoming more available.

Further Reading

Earthworks Press. 1989. *50 Things You Can Do To Help Save the Earth*. Berkeley, CA.

HOCKING, MARTIN B. "Paper versus Polystyrene: A Complex Choice." *Science* 251:504–505.

McCANN, MICHAEL. 1985. *Health Hazards Manual for Artists*. New York: Lyons Burford.

ROSSOL, MONONA. 1990. *The Artists' Complete Health and Safety Guide*. New York: Allworth Press.

Resources

Center for Safety in the Arts, Inc.
   5 Beekman Street
   New York, New York 10038
A clearinghouse for information about dangers found in the visual and performing arts. They answer questions about specific products and publish datasheets, pamphlets, and books on several dozen subjects. These are available at many art supply stores or directly from the Center. In addition, they publish a newsletter called *Art Hazards News* ten times a year.

Arts, Crafts, and Theater Safety
   181 Thompson Street, Number 23
   New York, New York 10012
   (212) 777-0062
This group will answer questions about the hazards of art materials by telephone.

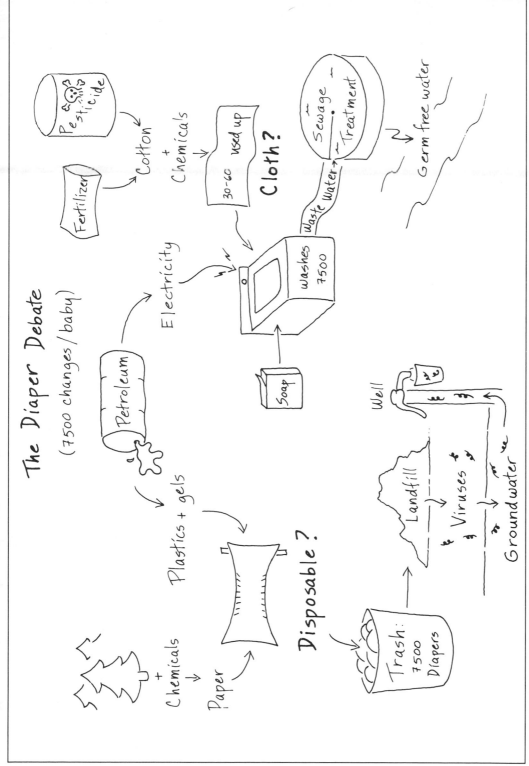

Figure 5 Disposable versus cotton diapers: some of the factors involved in choosing between these two types.

TOXICS AND THE ENVIRONMENT

9 MOVEMENT OF TOXICS THROUGH THE ENVIRONMENT

The journey a pollutant takes from its source to our bodies can be simple or complex. If a can of paint thinner is opened in an unventilated room, the fumes will probably not undergo any chemical changes as they travel the short distance from can to nose. Everyday experience tells us the relationship between the way we hold the can and how much of a noseful of the fumes we will get. In contrast, if a factory belches out gaseous pollutants in a city 50 miles upwind, the pathway through the atmosphere by which the pollution travels is relatively complex. Chemical reactions in the atmosphere are likely to change the composition of the gases as they travel with the wind, and the amount of the pollution that reaches us will depend on a host of weather conditions. In such situations, everyday experience may not provide us with the insights we need to predict human exposures.

In this chapter, we describe the major chemical and physical processes that influence the character and movement of pollutants between their sources and our bodies. The emphasis will be on the role played by the three physical media—air, water, and soil. Pollutants can also be transported and transformed in living tissue; some discussion of this living arena will be found here, but further discussion can be found in Chapters 4 and 10.

A. Air

The atmosphere is the point of entry to the environment for many pollutants such as chemical vapors from industry and exhaust gases from cars. Within the atmosphere, numerous chemical processes occur that can change the form and toxicity of air pollutants. Some of these pollutants are gases, some are in the form of a suspension of small liquid or solid particles (called *aerosol*, or *particulates* if they are solids only) and some are dissolved in cloud vapor or raindrops. Pollutants reach our bodies from the atmosphere either directly by inhalation and skin contact or indirectly in food or water after the pollutant has fallen from the atmosphere to the land or water.

Atmospheric Inversions

There are days within a city when the pollution level is low and others when it is high, even if all factories and other sources in the city spew out pollutants at a constant rate. Two atmospheric conditions contribute to the buildup of air pollutants in a city. One is straightforward—the stronger the winds sweeping across the city, the lower the pollution levels (assuming that there are no major upwind pollution sources that could be swept into the city by those winds).

The second factor—the vertical structure of the atmosphere—requires some explanation. At most times in most places, the atmosphere gets steadily colder with greater altitude. Under generally prevailing conditions, the temperature at ground level is 6.5°C warmer than it is 1 kilometer above (or 19°F warmer than it is 1 mile above). Since warm air is less dense than cold air and rises relative to it, the warmer air at the surface is continually rising. This would tend to cool the surface and eliminate the temperature difference were it not for the fact that the sun provides warmth to replenish the heat lost by the upwelling warm air. From the viewpoint of city inhabitants, this upwelling is a blessing because it removes polluted air at the earth's surface, thus serving as a natural air ventilation system.

However, if for some reason the temperature at the surface becomes cooler than it is higher up, then the denser, cooler air near the surface cannot get enough lift to rise. In this case, an *atmospheric inversion* occurs and the upwelling stops. Without upwelling, any pollutants injected into the atmosphere at the surface from chimneys and tailpipes build up in the air near the surface where people breathe.

In Los Angeles, atmospheric inversions are common and often result in severe smog episodes. Here the inversions occur because of cool ocean air that blows in near ground level, cooling the lower atmosphere relative to the air above. Inversions can also occur following a cloudless night because, while a cloud layer traps surface heat, a clear sky permits the surface to radiate its heat away to space quite effectively. In cities surrounded by mountains at high elevations, inversions are frequent in winter when cold air slides down the surrounding slopes and squats over the city. Inversions can also occur when high-altitude dust or light-absorbing pollutants absorb sunlight and cause the upper atmosphere to heat up. Aerosol formed from **sulfur dioxide** is an example of such a light-absorbing material.

The two conditions that remove pollution from a city—horizontal winds and upwelling—are connected. During times of inversions, winds are less likely to sweep pollutants across and out of a city. This is because the cooler air that is trapped at ground level in an inversion is denser and therefore more resistant to movement in both the horizontal and vertical directions.

Downwind Transport

If a serious accident occurs at a chemical factory or a nuclear power plant, people living downwind have good reason to be concerned that they might be exposed to dangerous levels of airborne toxic substances. A moving mass of pollution, whether resulting from an accident or the smaller, continuous output from a properly functioning industrial facility, is called a *plume*. What determines the path and shape of a plume? Obviously the direction of the wind is the major determinant, but it is not the whole story. As anyone who has watched the smoke pouring from a chimney knows, a plume spreads out as it travels downwind. So, even if you don't live directly downwind, you can be subject to a substantial dose. A plume spreads out as it travels downwind for several reasons.

First, winds near ground level are rarely from a single direction over distances greater than 20 to 30 miles. When a weather report states that the winds are from the northwest, this means only that the average direction is from the northwest; they may vary substantially from this at any given time. Careful observation of smokestack plumes indicates that they usually follow a zig-zag course immediately downwind of the source. Moreover, usually within 50 miles from a source, a plume will veer off to one side in an arc. For example, the trails of plumes from coal-burning industries in the lower Ohio River valley and in the middle and sourthern Atlantic states are generally sweeping clockwise arcs that begin to move toward the north or northwest and then sweep eastward. They eventually bring a substantial amount of pollution into the northeastern United States and southeastern Canada, where some of that pollution contributes to the problem of acid rain (see Chapter 11, Section C).

Another reason why plumes spread out is that, even at one location, wind direction can shift suddenly. For example, following the nuclear power plant accident at Chernobyl in the Soviet Union, the initial plume of airborne *radioactive isotopes* (mainly **iodine-131** and **cesium-137**) took a generally northwesterly course toward northeastern Europe and Scandinavia. But within a few days, a shift in winds in central Europe brought another plume of radiation on a southeasterly course toward Italy and southern France. Shortly thereafter, the winds shifted again, and subsequent emissions from Chernobyl took off on an easterly path across Asia and the Pacific Ocean and over to the western coast of North America.

Even when the wind is perfectly steady in direction, plumes spread horizontally and vertically because of diffusion and atmospheric turbulence. Diffusion is the same process that causes gases or smoke particles from a cigarette that are released in a still room to spread out slowly to all parts of the room. Turbulence is the choppy motion of a fluid (such as air or water) that results in random stirring. Under conditions of steady wind direction and an average wind speed of 10 miles per hour (which is typical of lower atmospheric winds), diffusion and turbulence can cause a spread of as much as 20 miles to either side of the centerline in a plume by the time it has traveled several hundred miles from a source. And even if the source is a tall smokestack, such as the quarter-mile-high stacks on the coal-fired power plants in the mid-western United States (installed to reduce local ground level air pollution), the plumes may touch the ground downwind because of these processes. The extent to which diffusion and turbulence spread a plume depends considerably on weather conditions. If substantial upwelling is occurring in the lower atmosphere (for reasons described in the previous section), a plume will rise as it moves downwind. Because the weather conditions that give rise to strong upwelling usually also produce turbulence, these two processes occur together and result in plumes that both touch ground at their bottom edge and, as a whole, rise and spread as they move downwind. In an inversion, a plume is prevented from rising and reaching the swifter winds often found aloft, so it moves downwind more slowly. Under these conditions, the flow is trapped, and horizontal spread occurs mainly because of diffusion.

Deposition of Atmospheric Pollutants

Suppose that a hypothetical accident occurs upwind of you and you are standing on the ground while the plume of pollution passes overhead. The dose of pollution you receive will depend on two factors: the distance from the ground to the lower edge of the plume and the rate of deposition of material straight downward out of the plume. The altitude of the bottom of the plume is determined by those same factors that govern the spreading of the plume—turbulence, diffusion, and upwelling. Strong upwelling will cause the plume as a whole to rise as it moves downwind, while strong turbulence will cause the plume to spread downward as well as sideways and upward.

Atmospheric pollution will also fall from a plume under gravity. This may occur as individual particles of the toxic material fall to the ground or as the material is contained in falling raindrops (or snowflakes). The former process is called *dry deposition* and the latter process is called *rainout* or *wet deposition*. The speed with which isolated particles of pollution fall from the atmosphere depends on particle size and weight. Some solid particles of pollution are smaller than tiny bacteria (that is, they are smaller than 1 *micron* in diameter, which is about 40-millionths of an inch) and may never fall to the ground because atmospheric turbulence keeps them suspended. These small particles are individually invisible, but in large numbers they block sunlight, creating the hazy conditions observed over many industrial areas of the world. They remain in the atmosphere for weeks or months until they are washed out in rain or until many of them join together to make larger particles that are pulled to the ground by gravity.

Sooty particles, such as those that blacken window ledges and laundry hung outdoors in cities, are typically tens to hundreds of microns across and usually remain in the atmosphere for at most a few hours or days.

Raindrops and even snowflakes generally fall much faster than particles of pollution, so deposition in rain is usually the way most atmospheric pollution reaches the ground. Thus, if a toxic plume is passing overhead, the greatest danger you face occurs if it is raining or snowing. In the aftermath of the Chernobyl accident, rainout was the major process that led to higher than normal radiation exposures for those living downwind under the plume.

Atmospheric Chemistry

Over the industrialized regions of the world, the atmosphere is a complex mixture of chemical pollutants in gaseous, solid, and aerosol form. The fate of atmospheric pollution is governed not only by the physical movements just described, but also by a host of chemical reactions that occur in the atmosphere. These chemical reactions can dramatically change the toxicity of the pollution by producing new chemicals from combinations of existing ones.

The formation of acid rain is one example. Sulfuric acid and nitric acid, the two acids that make up acid rain, are formed in the atmosphere from the gaseous pollutants **sulfur dioxide** and **nitrogen oxides** that are emitted when coal or oil is burned. The formation of these acids in the atmosphere occurs during a chemical reaction called *oxidation*. Oxidation reactions are complex and can occur through several different processes.

Within the atmosphere are chemicals called *oxidants* that cause oxidation by readily transferring oxygen to sulfur dioxide and nitrogen oxides. An example of an oxidant in the atmosphere is hydrogen peroxide, the familiar chemical used to bleach hair and reduce infection in cuts (by oxidizing and thus killing oxygen-sensitive microbes that inhabit many wounds). Another important oxidant in the lower atmosphere is **ozone**. (It should be noted here that ozone in the lower atmosphere acts as a pollutant while the upper atmospheric ozone layer acts as an important protective barrier to incoming *ultraviolet radiation*.)

Oxidants are produced in the atmosphere when sunlight triggers what are known as *photochemical reactions*. These reactions are particularly important during mid-day in polluted urban areas that receive abundant sunshine, such as Los Angeles.

Very small soot particles produced from burning coal and oil can also cause oxidation. These particles are *catalysts*, which means that they stimulate the reaction, but are not consumed in the process and are therefore available to react again and again.

In addition to acid-forming atmospheric oxidation processes, other types of atmospheric chemical reactions can also affect toxicity. For example, a wide variety of reac- can destroy the upper atmospheric ozone layer, exposing us to higher doses of **ultraviolet radiation**. This is the source of concern about ozone depletion in the upper atmosphere, a topic discussed further in Chapter 11, Section B.

The chemical reactions that form smog are also important to the creation of toxic pollutants in the air. *Smog* is the name used to describe the mixture of air pollutants first investigated in Los Angeles, but which is also found in numerous other cities with heavy automobile traffic. Smog consists of organic and inorganic chemicals that form when nitrogen oxides and *hydrocarbons* emitted by automobiles react in the presence of sunlight through photochemical reactions. The major components of smog produced from these ingredients are ozone and a class of organic chemicals called aldehydes, of which **formaldehyde** is a common example in smoggy air. As smog levels build up in an urban atmosphere during the daytime, the ozone produced from the initial reactions then reacts with the aldehydes and nitrogen oxides to produce a particularly hazardous group of chemicals known as *peroxyacetyl nitrates* or *PAN* (see discussion of PAN toxicity under the ozone entry in Part II).

We have seen that the atmosphere is a

medium for both the transport and chemical transformation of pollutants. Substances that leave the atmosphere often end up in water. As we show in the next section, water is a medium with similar capabilities to transport and transform toxics.

B. Water

The collection of all the waters on earth is called the *hydrosphere.* Within the hydrosphere, water continually recycles as rain and snow fall, as streams flow to lakes and oceans, and as seawater and freshwater evaporate to form clouds that create more rain. Because many pollutants dissolve in water, the movement of water through the hydrosphere results in the movement of toxic substances. Water can dilute pollution as well as convey it. Water is also a superb medium for speeding up chemical reactions among dissolved substances, making the hydrosphere a kind of chemical reactor that can change the toxicity of many substances.

Flow and Mixing

Suppose you draw drinking water from one edge of a lake while pollution is being dumped in along the far shore. How concerned should you be about exposure to toxics? Clearly it is preferable to draw water from a large lake than from a small one, if pollution is entering both at the same rate, because the larger lake will dilute the chemical more. But other less obvious factors should also govern your level of concern, as listed here.

1. Does the pollutant dissolve in water (as acids do) or float on the surface (as many petroleum products do)? If it either dissolves or floats, then it might reach the site where you withdraw water. If it does neither, it will *precipitate,* that is, settle to the bottom of the lake near its point of entry, which is often the case with trace metal pollution. However, this does not

mean that the chemical poses no risk to you, as discussed later.

2. Does the pollutant turn to vapor quickly? Just as some pollutants sink to the bottom, others readily escape into the atmosphere. Such substances are called *volatile.* Included among this group are many organic toxics such as **benzene** and **toluene.** Volatile substances may not pose a water pollution problem, but they become air pollutants when they leave the water. In some cases, volatile substances in domestic water supplies may pass from water to air when you take a shower, resulting in indoor air pollution in the bathroom (see Chapter 5, Section C).

3. How well flushed is the lake? A lake is well flushed if its water is replenished often with new water from incoming streams and if it is drained by an outlet stream. In such a lake, pollution levels are less likely to build up to hazardous levels. Of course, flushing does not eliminate the pollution hazard; the people downstream are receiving the pollution flushed from the lake.

4. How well stirred is the lake? Shallow lakes are usually well stirred because wind keeps the waters mixed. In such lakes, pollutants will spread and become uniformly mixed within a few hours or days of a sudden pollution spill at one point. In contrast, deep lakes often have a well-stirred upper layer mixed by the wind and an unmixed deeper layer (Fig. 6). Such lakes are called stratified (meaning layered). Lake stratification is particularly common in summer when the top 10 feet or so of a lake warms in the sun and floats above the colder, deeper water. In this case, a pollutant dumped in the well-stirred upper layer will mix rapidly throughout that layer, but the deep water will remain relatively free of the substance for weeks or months. Any pollution discharged to the deep layer will mix very slowly. However, even stratified lakes generally become completely mixed periodically. This often happens in the autumn when the surface waters cool, be-

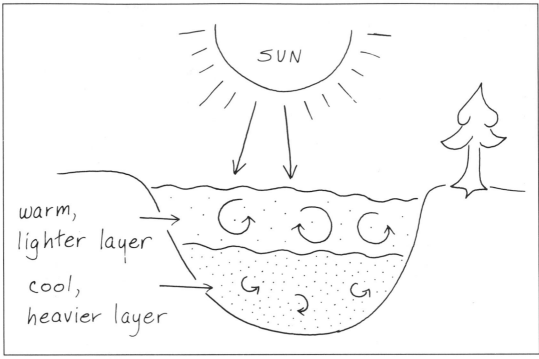

Figure 6 The two layers of water that often occur in lakes.

come more dense, and begin to sink. When this occurs, pollutant levels that had built up in the upper layer will be diluted as they mix with the deep waters.

5. Are the lake's fish contaminated with the pollutant? Drinking water from the lake is not the only way to receive a hazardous level of the pollutant. It might be taken up by aquatic plants and small animals and passed on through the food chain to fish and then to fish eaters (including people). This can happen whether the substance dissolves or settles to the lake bottom. As a chemical moves in this manner from one living organism to another, it can build up in concentration in a process called *bioconcentration* (discussed in more detail in Chapter 10, Section A).

These same considerations also apply to other types of water. For bays and other marine waters from which fish and other food sources are obtained, volatility, solubility, flushing, mixing rates, and bioconcentration are all factors to be considered when assessing the hazards of pollution. Pollution can be conveyed vast distances in seawater just as it can in the atmosphere. For example, tars from heavy crude oil are found on beaches worldwide. They are the result of oil spills from accidents involving tankers or offshore drilling rigs and from routine discharges at rigs and at locations where oil is loaded or unloaded from ships.

The basic issues surrounding toxics in groundwater are the same as for surface water, although here there are some added complications (see Chapter 6, Section B). Little is known about the underground flow of water, the sizes of *aquifers*, the chemical composition of groundwater, and the places where groundwater comes to the surface. Moreover, it is difficult to get samples of groundwater that are typical of the whole aquifer to test for chemical concentrations. Hence, estimates of the amount of toxic substances from dump sites that will enter groundwater are often inaccurate, as are predictions of where groundwater pollution will eventually show up in wells and reservoirs.

Chemical Processes in Water

Water molecules are very effective at pulling apart other molecules and leaving them in paired but separate pieces. This process is called ionization, and the pieces are called ions. An ion has an electrical charge; one member of the pair has a positive charge and the other a negative charge. Ions are also very reactive, so the positive ion from one pair can combine with the negative ion from a different chemical's pair to make yet a third substance. In this way, a toxic substance can become something that is more or less toxic, more or less dissolvable, more or less volatile, and more or less able to bioconcentrate.

The rates at which various chemical processes occur in water depend upon water temperature, with warmer water generally causing reactions to go faster. The types of organisms in the water can also affect the chemical reactions. For example, mercury pollution in water can occur when the mercury is in its *inorganic* form, but certain aquatic microorganisms can convert inorganic mercury to the more hazardous methyl mercury.

Two other major controlling factors influencing the rates of reactions and the types of possible end-products are oxygen levels and the acidity of the water. For example, toxic metals (see Chapter 12) can occur in different molecular forms characterized by varying proportions of oxygen in the molecules. Generally, the less oxygen combined with the metal and the more acid in the water, the more dissolvable the metal. Dissolved metals are more likely to be taken up by plants and ingested by animals. So the higher the acid level in the water (from acid rain) and the lower the oxygen level (from decomposing sewage in the water), the more likely it is that toxic metals will pose a biological threat. The solubility of nutrients such as phosphorus (essential for the growth of green plankton which provide the food for aquatic animals) is also generally increased by raising acid levels or lowering oxygen levels.

In summary, water, like air, is a medium in which pollutants are transported and chemically transformed. Prior to their entrance into our bodies, some pollutants pass through one additional medium—soil.

C. Soil

Since air pollutants are generally emitted over land, it is understandable that many toxics leave the atmosphere by falling to the ground and entering the soil. Here the pollutants may be transformed chemically by the organisms that inhabit soil. For example, ammonia gas in the atmosphere is quite soluble in water. Upon dissolving in rainwater and reaching the soil, ammonia can be transformed by soil microorganisms to nitrate, which, like ammonia, is a plant nutrient. It may also be transformed by microorganisms to nitrite, which is more toxic than either of the other two forms.

Whether or not pollutants in the soil are chemically transformed, they (or the products they are transformed to) will eventually meet one of four fates. First, they may be taken up by plants growing in the soil (and possibly be ingested by people or other organisms). For example, the trace metal selenium sometimes found in soil downwind of oil-burning industries is readily taken up by many leafy green plants that we eat as vegetables. A second possibility is that soil pollutants will be flushed out by rain into water bodies. For example, many pesticides pass from agricultural fields to streams and lakes in this way. A third possibility is that the soil pollutant is sufficiently volatile that it passes into the atmosphere. DDT is an example of such a pollutant. It *co-distills* with evaporating water from the soil surface, and once in the atmosphere, it can travel great distances.

Finally, some soil pollutants, particularly certain toxic metals (see Chapter 12), reside virtually forever in the soil because they are neither volatile, soluble, nor accessible to plants.

pollutants can tavel a tortuous path and undergo many changes from their source to your body. Figure 7 summarizes the most important processes we have discussed in this chapter.

Summary

From this introduction to the three physical media—air, water, and soil—it is clear that

Further Reading

Environmental Protection Agency. 1985. *National Air Quality and Emission Trends Report, 1983*. Report EPA-450/4-84-029. Washington, D.C.

GARRELS, R. M., MACKENZIE, F. T., and HUNT, C. 1982. *Chemical Cycles and the Global Environment*. 2d edition. Los Altos, CA: William Kaufmann.

GRAEDEL, T. E., and CRUTZEN, P. J. 1989. The Changing Atmosphere. *Scientific American* 261(3):58–68.

LA RIVIERE, J. W. M. 1989. Threats to the World's Waters. *Scientific American* 261(3):80–94.

WILSON, J., ed. 1984. *The Fate of Toxics in Surface and Ground Waters: The Proceedings of the Second National Water Conference*. Philadelphia Academy of Natural Sciences.

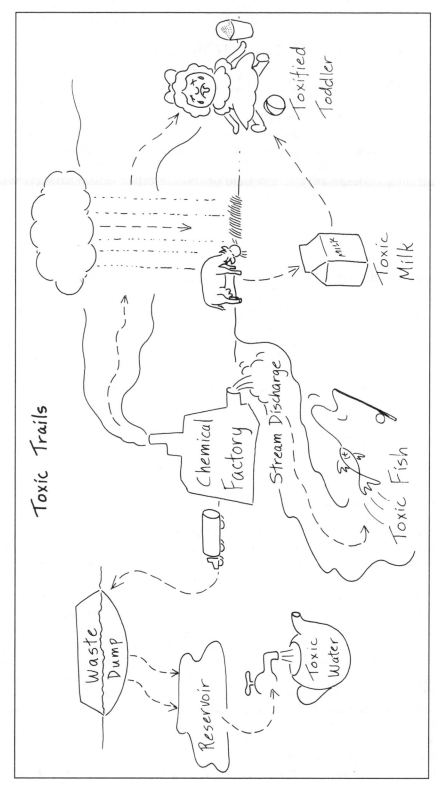

Figure 7 Some of the important pathways by which toxics can reach our bodies.

10 TOXICS IN THE BIOSPHERE

This chapter reminds us that we do not poison just our own species when we release toxics into the environment. First, we deal with an unfortunately widespread phenomenon—the buildup of the concentration of certain toxics in ecological food chains. Not only does this pose a threat to wildlife, but it can also seriously harm people that eat the animals that have concentrated those substances in their bodies. We then review our incomplete knowledge of how wild plants and animals respond to toxics and discuss the relatively new field of science called ecotoxicology, which seeks to further our understanding of these responses.

A. How Toxic Concentrations Build Up in Animals

If an animal eats food containing a toxic substance day after day, under certain circumstances that substance will concentrate in the animal to a higher level than in the food. This phenomenon, called *biomagnification* (or bioconcentration), can lead to dangerous levels of toxic substances in the food we eat. What are the circumstances under which biomagnification will occur, and how severe is this problem?

An animal grows by metabolizing some of the food it eats into new body tissue. Even an animal that is not actually growing larger uses some of its food to replace worn-out tissue. Typically, only 1 to 10% of the food eaten by an animal is retained for these purposes; the remainder is used in the body as a source of energy or is excreted. If the toxic substance in the food is retained at a higher rate than the food itself, then the concentration of the toxic substance in the animal will gradually increase.

Some toxic substances are readily excreted by animals (see Chapter 4), and in those instances the substance will not bioconcentrate. Substances usually bioconcentrate when they are stored in certain tissues or organs of the body. **DDT**, for example, bioconcentrates because it lodges in body fat. Although only a small portion of the food eaten by an animal

is retained, a large fraction of ingested DDT is. Hence, the concentration of DDT in the body gradually increases.

The tendency for a toxic substance to be retained in some part of the body is usually a property of the substance. Certain characteristics of the animal also determine the extent of bioconcentration. The more inefficient an animal is in turning its food into new tissue, the more it has to eat to grow. If both an efficient and an inefficient animal eat the same food containing the same level of toxic substance, for every new pound of weight put on, the inefficient animal will ingest more of the toxic substance. If the two animals retain the toxic substance equally, the inefficient one will have a higher concentration in its body.

Now suppose that an animal that has bioconcentrated a toxic substance is itself food for some other animal. Then the concentration of the substance in the second animal can reach an even higher level through the same process. A third animal eating the second can bioconcentrate still more, and so on. A sequence of animals organized according to who eats whom is called a *food chain* (Fig. 8). The farther up the food chain an animal is, the more likely it is to have a high level of bioconcentrated toxic substances in its tissues.

At the base of every food chain are plants, which get their nourishment from air, sun-

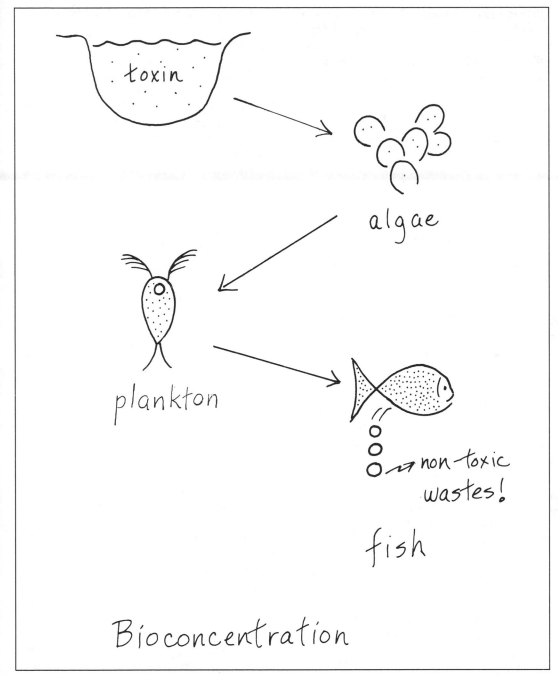

Figure 8 In this food chain, a toxic substance becomes increasingly bioconcentrated as it passes from the water to algae to plankton and finally to fish. Bioconcentration occurs if the toxic substance is preferentially retained in the organism rather than excreted. If people eat the toxified fish, the substance may concentrate still further in them.

light, and raw chemicals in the soil or water in which they grow. The amount of toxic substance that moves through the food chain will be determined in part by how much of the substance resides in the soil or water, for that is where the process of bioconcentration begins. All else being equal, the higher the concentration of the toxic substance in the soil and water environment, the more that will be taken up by plants and passed from the plants to the plant-eating animals, and then on to the meat eaters.

Many examples of bioconcentration exist in nature. The case of DDT is a well-documented example. Bald eagles, white pelicans, peregrine falcons, and other predatory birds that eat substantial amounts of fish were found in the 1960s to be dying out in the United States as a result of reproductive failure brought on by excess DDT in their tissues. Although these birds did not feed on the farmlands where DDT was used, these predators were at the end of a long food chain along which DDT bioconcentrated. Rain runoff carried DDT away from the farms to the natural ecosystems where they hunted.

Another example of bioconcentration occurred in the Arctic. Nuclear weapons testing in the atmosphere during the 1950s and early 1960s led to the fallout of **cesium-137** onto the tundra. Lichens soaked up some of the radioactive substance and passed it on to the caribou that graze on the lichens. Eskimos eating caribou meat were found to have roughly twice the concentration of cesium-137 than in the caribou, and the caribou had over two times that in the lichens.

A final example of bioconcentration is one involving a great human tragedy. During the 1970s, Japanese villagers in the fishing village of Minimata were seriously poisoned by **mercury** that had been discharged from a nearby chemical factory. The mercury had bioconcentrated in fish and then in villagers eating those fish. The result was approximately 50 agonizing deaths and over several thousand cases of severe and permanent nervous disorders.

B. Ecological Effects of Toxics

This book is concerned primarily with the effects of toxic substances on people. Indeed, nearly all the media attention on toxics focuses on the human dimension of the problem. In only a few cases, such as with acid rain or the banning of **DDT** in the United States, are the effects of toxic substances on wild plants and animals of greater immediate interest than their effects on people. Yet, in numerous cases, nature can be harmed by the same toxics that threaten us.

Ecological Versus Human Risk

While human self-centeredness places the risk to us in front row center, it is important to realize that the quality of human existence depends upon the numerous benefits we derive from healthy natural ecosystems. For example, forests purify our air, reduce the risk of flooding, and moderate our climate; wild insects pollinate many of our crops; tropical plants are the source of many modern medicines; and strains of wild seeds have been the basis of agricultural productivity and will continue to sustain food production as we seek new crop strains from nature that can cope with the changing future climate (see Chapter 11, Section A). Thus, there are good reasons why the branch of science called ecotoxicology, which seeks to understand the ecological effects of toxics, is of great relevance to the well-being of humanity. This section discusses some of the differences between the study of human health effects and ecological effects of toxics and describes a few of the current questions that concern ecotoxicologists.

Human beings are far more sensitive than other living organisms to some kinds of toxic substances. Radiation is a good example, for it generally takes at least ten times the dose of radiation (measured in terms of amount of radiation absorbed per unit body weight) to do the same damage to most animals or plants as it does to people (see Chapter 15). Thus, if people are protected from dangerous radiation levels by the enforcement of appropriate regulations, then other creatures are likely to be protected as well. This is true not only because of the great sensitivity of humans to radiation, but also because they are more likely to receive high doses of it than are wild plants and animals.

For many kinds of toxic substances, however, people are far less sensitive than other organisms. This fact has been exploited by the use of especially sensitive organisms as early warning systems. A famous example is the former use by miners of caged canaries, which are more sensitive than miners to poisonous gases trapped in mine shafts. If the miners saw the canary die, they knew they should exit the mine. Many pesticides are far more lethal to insects (or, as with DDT, to birds of prey) than to people. And concentrations of certain trace metals such as **aluminum** or **selenium** that can kill fish or birds are only slightly toxic to people. Thus, the relative sensitivity of people and other creatures justifies our self-centered approach only for some classes of toxic substances such as radioactive isotopes.

Another reason why we are often more concerned with human toxicity than with that of wild species relates to human individuality. We are concerned with each individual in the human population. When we evaluate risk, we try to determine how many individual people will die or suffer illness. In contrast, with a species of wild animal or plant, our concern is less with the health or survival of each individual organism than it is with the survival of the species. We may also be concerned about the *gene pool*, the local population, or an economically valuable collection of individuals within the species (such as harvestable trees). Hence, we have an Endangered Species Act in the United States, but not an endangered organism act. Only when a species is nearly extinct, or when we protect certain special animals such as whales or song birds, do we protect individual organisms. The basis for this distinction between concern for individuals and concern for groups is rooted in human ethics.

The implications of this ethical distinction in toxic substances policy are significant. The discharge of toxic waste from an industrial facility usually does not threaten an entire species of plant or animal because the range of most species is much larger than the area affected by a factory's emissions (even though many individuals from many species may die as a result of the discharge). An exception occurs when a pollutant is discharged in the vicinity of a species found only in a small geographical area. But even if the species is widely distributed, a policy of only protecting species can lead to serious damage. Most species are composed of many distinct populations, which are collections of individuals from within a species that live and reproduce together. Because populations are often genetically unique, loss of a population can be nearly as irreversible as loss of a species. Unfortunately, the Endangered Species Act does not protect populations, and thus toxic discharges can eliminate rare and valuable genes from a species' gene pool.

Goals of Ecotoxicology

The general considerations just discussed provide insight into the importance and challenge of ecotoxicology. This science has several major goals. One is to identify organisms that are useful early warning indicators—such as the canary in the mine—so that we can determine when we are beginning to overload our environment with toxic substances. Such indicators may warn us of either a human or an ecological hazard. For example, certain species of salamanders have proven to be very sensitive to acid rain, leading some researchers to suspect that their demise is a warning of impending widespread damage to forests. Closer to this book's focus, certain species of organisms have been identified as being particularly useful indicators of human health risk from contaminated water. In some cases, the indicator is a species that thrives in polluted waters, such as *Escherichia coli,* a *coliform bacteria* often found in waters contaminated with sewage. In other cases, the disappearance of an animal or plant population that could not tolerate the polluted conditions indicates an impending problem. This was the case in the Kesterson Wildlife Refuge in California's San Joaquin Valley, where high **selenium** concentrations first became apparent when fish and waterfowl began to succumb to this toxic metal.

A second goal of ecotoxicology is to understand when a species or genetically distinct population is threatened by a toxic substance. This is tougher than it may seem, for we don't always know how much stress a population can absorb before it will become extinct. Here, ecotoxicology combines forces with the newly developing science of conservation biology in this important investigation.

A third and most challenging goal is to understand how damage to one species might affect the entire ecosystem of which it is a part. An ecosystem is more than just a collection of species sharing space and preying upon one another. Through the interactions of its parts, an ecosystem performs functions that could not be accomplished by its individual parts. These functions include the cycling and storage of nutrients, the efficient exploitation of the sun's energy, the prevention of soil erosion, and the maintenance of favorable local climatic conditions. These functions are not only necessary for the ecosystem to thrive, but they also provide many benefits to humanity, as previously mentioned. When individual species or populations within the ecosystem are threatened, so may be the integrity of the entire ecosystem. And to that threat, our species must take heed because the very quality of our lives depends upon the maintenance of those ecosystems.

Further Reading

LEVIN, S. A., HARWELL, M. A., KELLEY, J. R., and KIMBALL, K. D. 1989. *Ecotoxicology: Problems and Approaches.* New York: Springer–Verlag.
WOODWELL, G. M. 1967. Toxic Substances and Ecological Cycles. *Scientific American* 216(3):24–31.

11 THREE GLOBAL ENVIRONMENTAL HAZARDS OF POLLUTANTS

Most of the concern over pollution, both in this book and in the public media, is focused on the health threat to individuals from direct exposure to hazardous substances. Generally, the nearer you are to such pollution sources, the greater your risk. Some pollutants, however, pose an entirely different type of threat. They can do harm thousands of miles from where they are discharged into the environment, and the harm they cause is not due to their direct toxicity to individuals, but rather to their ability to disrupt atmospheric chemistry, climate, and ecosystems. We discuss here three such problems—the greenhouse effect, stratospheric ozone depletion, and acid rain—explaining the current hazards and the options for preventing these problems from becoming even worse in the future. The success of the solutions we present all depends on political leadership and individual responsibility working hand-in-hand. But there is one crucial condition that must also be met if these (and indeed, all other problems associated with pollution) are to be solved—a halt to the growth of the human population. For if the population continues to increase, so will the amount of toxic wastes and the threats to our well-being that those toxics pose.

A. The Greenhouse Effect

Within 50 years, there is a good chance that our planet will be warmer than it has been at any time in the past 100,000 years. The reason is that we are loading the atmosphere with gases that trap heat (Fig. 9). This is called the greenhouse effect (although the reason a real greenhouse heats up is different).

The gas most responsible for this change in climate is carbon dioxide, which is released to the atmosphere from the burning of coal, oil, and natural gas. Another source of carbon dioxide is the clearing of vast areas of forests, particularly in the tropics. When felled trees rot or are burned, the carbon contained in the trees is released to the atmosphere as carbon dioxide. Unless a similar amount of living plants replace the lost forest, the level of carbon dioxide in the atmosphere rises. Other gases released to the atmosphere from industrial and agricultural activities, such as methane, nitrous oxide, and chlorofluorocarbons (CFCs), also trap heat and contribute to the greenhouse effect. All of these gases are called greenhouse gases.

Even before the industrial revolution and the beginning of coal burning, the atmosphere contained natural greenhouse gases such as water vapor and carbon dioxide. But today the levels are higher, and by the middle of the next century, with the expected continued emission of greenhouse gases, their levels are expected to be high enough to warm the planet by an average of 2° to 5°C (about 4° to 9°F). In some regions, such as the Arctic, the predicted warming is likely to be considerably higher than average, while in the tropics, the amount of warming will be less than average.

Along with a rise in temperature, changes in rainfall will most likely occur, with increases seen in some regions and decreases in others. Unfortunately, it is difficult to predict exactly where it will become wetter and where it will become drier. Because temperatures, and therefore evaporation, will increase and rainfall rates will change, it is likely that soil moisture levels will change, which is of extreme importance to farmers. Moreover, river flow rates and reservoir levels, which determine water supply for agricultural, industrial, and domestic use, will be altered. In regions where snowmelt is a

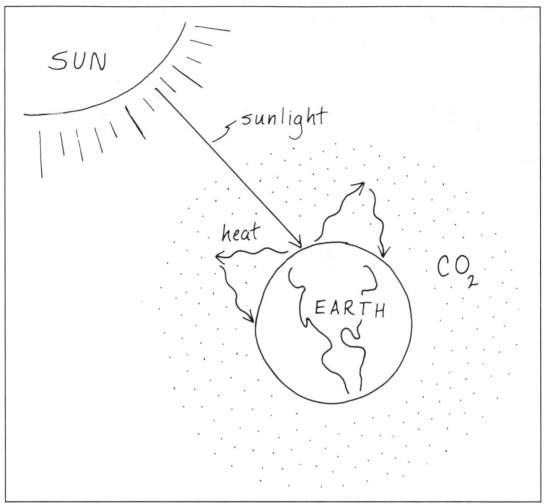

Figure 9 The greenhouse effect. Gases such as carbon dioxide, methane, nitrous oxide, and chlorofluorocarbons absorb heat radiated outward from the earth's surface and reradiate it back to the surface, thereby warming it.

major source of water supply, it is likely that water scarcity will become more of a problem in late summer because snowmelt will occur earlier in the spring. But for the most part, we cannot predict exactly how regional climates will change or how this will affect water supply in any particular region. Summer heat waves will be more severe and late summer frosts will be less likely. Melting of glacial ice, and perhaps even the Antarctic icecap, will increase, contributing to a rise in sea level of possibly 1 or 2 feet within 50 years and maybe 3 or 4 feet within 100 years.

Why should we believe the prediction that the planet will warm? After all, meteorologists are not always right about next weekend's weather, and surely it is easier to make a reliable prediction about tomorrow than about next century. In fact, there are several reasons for placing confidence in the predictions about the greenhouse effect.

1. It is possible that the predicted warming has already begun. During the past 100 years, the average temperature of the planet, as measured at sites all over the

globe, has increased about 0.6°C (1.1°F). Although we cannot be sure that this is due to the slow but steady buildup of greenhouse gases, no other explanation matches the facts as well. During this 100-year period of warming, sea level has also risen by several inches, which would be expected as a result of the warming.

2. When the mathematical models used to predict the greenhouse effect on earth are applied to Mars and Venus, which have different levels of greenhouse gases in their atmospheres, predictions for the average temperatures of those planets are remarkably accurate.

3. Throughout the geological history of our planet, periods of high temperature generally coincided with periods of high atmospheric carbon dioxide. It is possible, however, that warmer temperatures of the past were not induced by elevated levels of carbon dioxide, but rather that the high temperatures caused carbon dioxide levels to rise. Hence, it is difficult to know how much weight to give this argument.

4. The earth's atmosphere contains natural levels of greenhouse gases, without which our climate would be inhospitably cold. The models used to predict the impending global warming reliably explain the warming effect of these natural levels of greenhouse gases.

5. In defense of meteorologists, a prediction of next weekend's weather in your hometown requires much more detailed and unavailable information than does predicting the average global climate of the next century and is therefore less reliable.

The implications of the greenhouse effect for human life are profound. Some coastal cities and lands may be flooded by rising seas. Inhabitants of cities that presently have just barely tolerable summer heat waves are likely to experience health-threatening heat episodes in the next century. Water supplies may be increased in some areas and reduced in others, but no one can predict with great certainty just where these increases and decreases

will occur. The same holds for agricultural productivity—some nations or regions may be able to increase food production, while others will face declines in yields.

Adapting food production to the changing climate may not be easy. Some people have spoken blithely of moving the corn-growing region of the United States north several hundred miles to where the eventual greenhouse climate will resemble that of Kansas. Some have suggested that sugar cane could then be grown in the present corn belt. But temperature is not the only factor influencing what can be grown where. While the temperature in Kansas may be ideal for sugar cane, the amount of rainfall may be unsuitable. Because the changes in rainfall are so uncertain, no one can predict how successfully crops will grow in the future climate, even if farmers are flexible about which crops they grow.

The world's forests are likely to be stressed by greenhouse warming as well. Of course, in the past natural changes in climate have occurred and forests seem to have survived. Indeed, trees have adapted over the thousands of years since the last ice age to a changing climate. From the last ice age to the present, the planet has warmed by about the same amount as is expected during the next 100 years. Because the pace of future warming greatly exceeds that since the last ice age, it is far less likely that forests will be able to adapt. Difficult as it may be for corn farming to move north, it is even more unlikely that our commercial forests will move northward to keep pace with the changing climate. Coming at a time when many forests already appear to be under stress from air pollution, the damage is likely to be heightened.

In short, major changes can be expected for the entire planet and its inhabitants. Even with further advances in our ability to model and predict the climate, a good deal of uncertainty will remain. Thus, we need to plan for an uncertain future. Because of the enormous risks, it is vital that we do not forget that the greenhouse effect is of our own doing and is therefore partially within our power to prevent. There is no practical way to reverse the warming that may have already occurred or to prevent some additional warming, but by making wise choices, we can reduce the amount of greenhouse gases we add to the atmosphere and thereby reduce the severity of the coming greenhouse effect. Some of the actions we can take are listed here.

1. Stop deforestation, particularly in the tropics where every year an area the size of Pennsylvania is stripped of trees, and accelerate efforts to reforest denuded areas of the planet.
2. Increase the efficiency with which we use coal, oil, and gas. In the United State we could enjoy our current standard of living by using only half as much energy as we now do if we made use of available technologies for saving energy in transportation, industry, home heating, and appliances. By doing this, we would produce carbon dioxide at half the rate we now do.
3. Develop new energy sources to replace coal, oil, and gas. From the standpoint of environmental safety, solar energy is most promising, but research is needed to make it as cheap to use as existing fuels.

While it is best to reduce the size of the impending climatic change as much as possible by these preventive actions, it is also sensible to plan how to adapt to some change. Currently, our seed stocks used for agriculture are adapted to the present climate. But they lack genetic variety and thus are not likely to be well adapted to a different and uncertain future climate. It would be prudent of all nations to begin now to select and store seed stocks for strains of crops that are suited for a wide variety of climate conditions, including more frequent and prolonged droughts. Also, water conservation should be encouraged in agriculture, the home, and industry. Implementation of all these measures, including the three preventive steps just listed, make good sense even if no threat of greenhouse warming existed because they would improve the quality of our environment and in many cases lead to cost savings for the public.

B. Stratospheric Ozone Depletion

Ozone is both a hazard and a benefit to people. As an *oxidant,* ozone contributes to the formation of acid rain and can be a health hazard in urban air where levels tend to be high (see Chapter 9, Section A). But ozone occurring in a layer high above the earth, in a region of the atmosphere called the stratosphere, is a lifesaver. There it absorbs **ultraviolet radiation** from the sun, preventing that radiation from striking living creatures at the earth's surface (Fig. 10). Were it not for the protective ozone layer in the upper atmosphere, ultraviolet radiation would cause many more cases of skin cancer, including the often fatal form *melanoma*. Ironically, human activities are causing ozone levels to increase in the urban air we breathe, where ozone is a threat, and to decrease in the stratosphere, where ozone is a blessing. Our concern in this section is with its decrease in the stratosphere. (See the **ozone** entry in Part II for a discussion of ozone as an air pollutant.)

Recent measurements in the stratosphere over the Antarctic have revealed a temporary decrease each year in the normal ozone levels there. Scientists have described this as a "hole" in the Antarctic ozone layer. The hole has been occurring each year between September and November when one-third or more of the ozone disappears over central Antarctica. Since it was first observed, the hole has grown in area, and toward the end of the 1980s, it extended northward beyond the Antarctic circle. In 1987, more evidence for ozone decline was announced, this time over much of the Northern Hemisphere. Analysis of satellite data has indicated a decline of about 2 or 3% in the ozone of the northern stratosphere during the past decade.

In the United States, it is estimated that

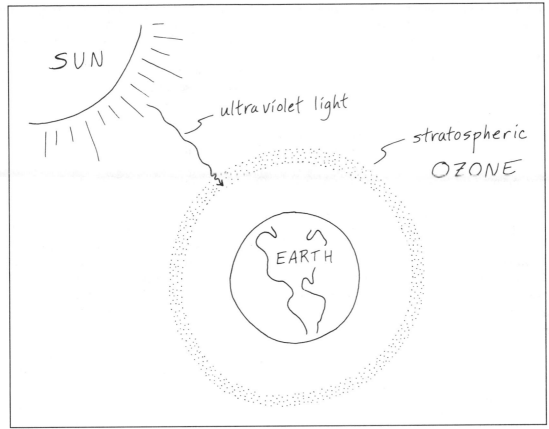

Figure 10 The earth's protective ozone layer. Stratospheric ozone absorbs ultraviolet radiation, thereby preventing it from striking the surface where it would be harmful to life.

a 2% decline in stratospheric ozone will result in about 25,000 to 50,000 additional cases of skin cancer each year (out of a total of about 500,000 new cases diagnosed annually). Nearly all these cases are treatable, but the annual incidence of melanoma is expected to increase by about 1000 for every 2% decrease in stratospheric ozone. Melanoma is a more serious cancer that can be caused by ultraviolet radiation and that is presently fatal in about one-fourth of all cases. Other species are also at risk, although the specific damage to other animals and plants from ultraviolet radiation is poorly understood. Recently, special concern has been voiced about the risk to oceanic plankton.

Scientists have intensively studied the cause of the decline in stratospheric ozone. The evidence points convincingly toward a particular group of atmospheric pollutants called **chlorofluorocarbons** (abbreviated **CFCs**) as the culprit. In the atmosphere, the **chlorine** atoms in CFCs are split off and form molecules of chlorine oxide, a gas that reacts with and destroys ozone molecules. This gas increases in concentration in the south polar stratosphere just prior to the opening of the ozone hole there. In late 1988, scientists announced that chlorine oxide was also building up in the stratosphere above the north polar region, thus generating concern that an ozone hole may begin to form there as well.

Chlorofluorocarbons have many applications for human use, such as refrigerants in automobile air conditioners, foaming agents to create insulated packing material, cleansers in the electronics industry, and propellants in spray cans (this last use has been virtually eliminated in the United States, but is still in common practice elsewhere).

In all these applications, the CFCs are eventually released as pollutants to the lower atmosphere, from whence they travel to the stratosphere. It appears that the only way to slow and eventually stop the further loss of stratospheric ozone is to stop releasing these pollutants into the atmosphere. In practice, this means to discontinue their use and find substitutes for all essential uses. Realizing this, scientists and government representatives from most of the industrialized nations of the world met in 1987 to develop an international treaty limiting the production of CFCs. In September 1987, an agreement was reached in Montreal that has now been approved by nearly all participating governments, including the United States, which is the leading manufacturer of these chemicals. The terms of the agreement are as follows:

1. The participating nations will hold annual CFC production constant at 1986 levels starting in 1989. The only exception is the Soviet Union, which will hold CFC levels constant in 1990 levels starting in 1990.
2. Then, starting in 1993, the nations will decrease annual production by 20% from the 1986 levels; starting in 1998, production will decrease by 50% from the 1986 levels (1990 level for the Soviet Union).
3. Developing nations with an annual CFC production rate of less than 0.3 kilograms per person can delay compliance with the above points for ten years.

In early 1989, the European nations and the United States met again to discuss a timetable for the complete elimination of CFC use by the turn of the century. It appears that this is one environmental problem that many of the world's leaders are truly taking seriously.

The Montreal agreement is noteworthy not only because it deals constructively with the particularly serious hazard of ozone depletion, but also because it sets an example for multinational cooperation on global environmental problems. With this successful track record, the nations of the world now have a working model of how to attack other global environmental threats, including greenhouse warming, acid rain, deforestation, and soil erosion.

C. Acid Rain

Over large regions of North America and Eurasia, the rain is polluted with acid. This pollution mainly comes from the burning of coal and oil, which leads to the emission of tens of millions of tons of **sulfur dioxide** and **nitrogen oxides** from smokestacks and tailpipes each year. These gases convert to sulfuric and nitric acids in the atmosphere and then fall to earth in rain and snow and as dry acid particles (Fig. 11). Often the acids fall to the earth many hundreds of miles away from where the original gases were emitted. Hence, one nation's pollution can fall as acid in another nation.

The acid levels in rain and other waters such as lakes and streams are measured on a pH scale (Fig. 12). This scale may seem confusing because high acid levels correspond to low values of pH. Also, on the pH scale, a change of one unit of pH, say from 5 to 4, is a factor of ten increase in acid concentration. Figure 12 shows a pH scale with some values indicated to characterize some aspects of the acid rain problem.

In some regions, acids are so strongly concentrated in the rain and snow that they can increase the acid in lakes to levels that kill certain types of plants and animals. Populations of trout and salamanders in many lakes of eastern North America and Scandinavia have been wiped out as a result. It is also possible that forests are being destroyed by acid rain. A phenomenon called "forest dieback," characterized by the death of large parts of a forest over thousands of square miles, was first observed in West Germany. Forest dieback is spreading rapidly and threatens the

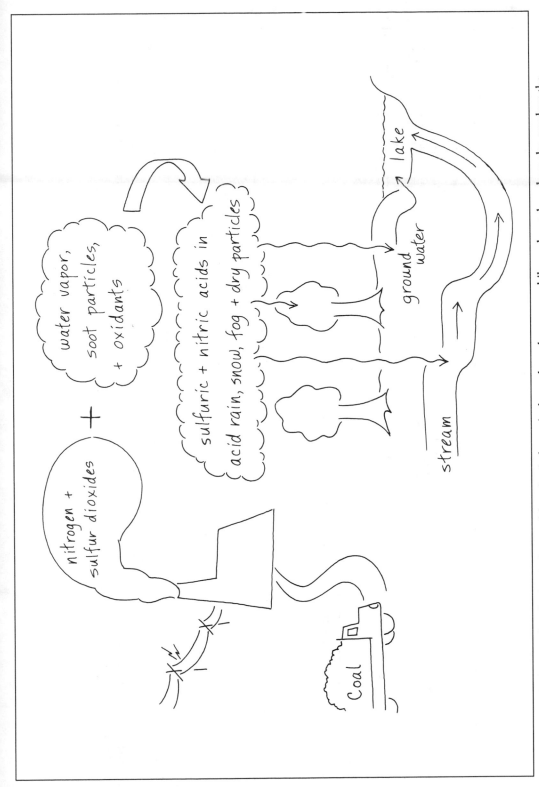

Figure 11 The formation of acid rain. Only a coal-burning industry is shown here, but automobiles and metal smelters also produce the gases that form acids.

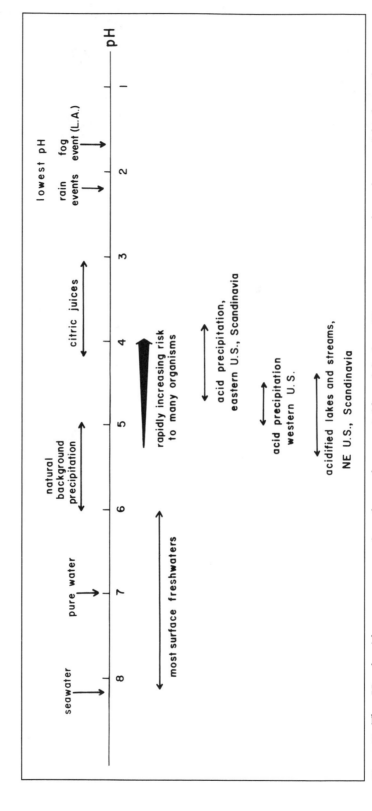

Figure 12 The pH scale with some representative values and ranges. Acid precipitation pH ranges correspond to volume-weighted annual averages of weekly precipitation samples.

economic as well as aesthetic value of much of Germany's revered forests. It is also occurring in eastern Europe and to a lesser extent in the eastern United States. Acid rain is strongly suspected as contributing to forest dieback, but the exact way in which the trees are being killed is not understood.

Does acid rain pose a direct threat to human health? You can drink a solution of sulfuric or nitric acid as strong as typical acid rain and not suffer. And it won't burn your skin. But inhalation of acid fogs and *aerosols* does appear to affect the human respiratory tract, increasing the incidence of bronchitis and interfering with the ability of the lungs to cleanse themselves. The effects on people already suffering from asthma are particularly worrisome. For these reasons, a science advisory panel to the EPA recently recommended that acid aerosol levels in the atmosphere should be regulated under the Clean Air Act (see Chapter 17, Section B).

There is another more speculative way that acid rain could cause illness. Acidified waters, such as those found in lakes and streams in the Adirondack Mountains of the United States and in Scandinavian mountains, often have highly elevated concentrations of **aluminum** and to a lesser extent **lead** and other toxic metals (see Chapter 12). The reason is that acid rain dissolves these metals from soils and flushes them into the water. In some regions, aluminum concentrations reach several hundred parts per billion, which is toxic to some species of fish. It is not known if human health is adversely affected by long-term exposure to these levels of metals found in acidified drinking water. People drinking reservoir water supplied by mountain streams in acidified regions need not worry; reservoirs are not acidic enough to dissolve the metals. Perhaps the greatest risk is from eating fish that have high levels of toxic metals due to *bioconcentration* (see Chapter 10, Section A), although even this risk is purely speculative at present.

Present evidence suggests that food crops are not at risk from acid rain because their soils generally contain a large stock of chemicals that neutralize acids. Damage to materials such as rubber, synthetic fabrics, paint coatings, and the marble of our statuary is a more serious problem. The annual cost of this damage just in the United States is estimated to be as much as several billion dollars each year. The aesthetic loss from damage to outdoor sculptures and historic building facades throughout the world is inestimable.

What can be done about the acid rain problem? Solutions have been proposed that range from absurd to useful but politically difficult to enact. An absurd solution is to genetically engineer fish and other acid-sensitive organisms to be more tolerant of acid. (Will we also engineer our own genes so that we become tolerant of high toxic metal levels that bioconcentrate in the fish we eat from acidified lakes?) Slightly less absurd is the proposal to add acid-neutralizing chemicals to the thousands of threatened or acidified lakes. The cost of providing such chemical protection to these lakes is estimated to be roughly the same as the cost of cleaning up the major polluters that cause the problem. And this would still leave vast areas of threatened forest soils unprotected. Limiting such protection to lakes would be a costly way to solve only a small part of the problem.

Far more sensible would be to use a similar chemical approach to remove the acid-forming gases in the smokestacks of the most offensive industries. This technique is called "scrubbing." Other solutions involve cleaning up our industries by switching to coals and oils that contain less sulfur or by switching to completely different forms of energy (such as solar or nuclear) that do not produce acid-forming pollutants. The 1990 revisions to the Clean Air Act mandate that such solutions will be gradually adopted to reduce sulfuric acid levels and, to a lesser extent, nitric acid in precipitation. For more specifics, see the entries on **nitrogen oxides** and **sulfur dioxide**.

Another approach to reducing the acidity of rain is use energy more efficiently so that we could derive our present level of benefits from less energy, that is, without burning so much coal, oil, and gas. This means making automobiles that get more miles per gallon, encouraging the use of mass transit, more efficient refrigerators and other appliances, and designing or renovating our homes and commercial buildings so they are more energy efficient. Such solutions would not only reduce the problem of acid rain, but would also reduce the severity of potential greenhouse warming, save the consumer money, and reduce our dependence on foreign fuels.

Further Reading

Environmental Protection Agency. 1984. *The Acidic Deposition Phenomenon and Its Effects.* Washington, D.C.

GRAEDEL, T. E., and CRUTZEN, P. J. 1989. The Changing Atmosphere. *Scientific American* 261(3):58–68.

HOUGHTON, R. A., and WOODWELL, G. M. 1989. Global Climatic Change. *Scientific American.* 260(4):36–44.

FOUR SPECIAL GROUPS OF TOXICS

12 TOXIC METALS

Trace metals, heavy metals, and toxic metals are terms usually used interchangeably to describe a group of metallic elements, many of which are hazardous if taken into the body. This chapter will present an introduction to metals: what they are, where they come from, how people are exposed to them, and some of their health effects. At the end, there is a brief list of ways to reduce exposure to metals. Because many of the metals mentioned here are treated as individual entries in Part II, most of the detail is spared. General features are illustrated by specific examples, the details of which can be found elsewhere.

A. Significance and Sources of Toxic Metals

The term "trace metals" refers to metals that are present either in the environment or in the human body in very low concentrations, such as copper, iron, and zinc. Heavy metals are those trace metals whose densities are at least five times greater than water, such as cadmium, lead, and mercury. Toxic metals are all those metals whose concentrations in the environment are now considered to be harmful, at least to some people in some places. All of the metal entries in Part II of this book are examples of toxic metals.

Metals have many properties that make them both interesting to study and important to human health. For example, some metals are essential for good health, and their deficiency can lead to disease. Not enough iron, for example, causes anemia. At the same time, metals that are necessary for good health in small amounts can become toxic if ingested in large doses. Molybdenum is required for certain *enzymes* to function properly, but too much can lead to gout. Finally, some metals, such as lead, have no known functions in the body and any internal exposure may be harmful. Another important property of metals is that they never degrade. Unlike many *organic* pollutants that break down with exposure to sunlight or heat, metals persist. They can be buried in landfills or washed into sediments, but they never disappear entirely and always remain a threat to be remobilized in the future.

Metals were present in the earth from its very beginning several billion years ago. They are found in nearly all rock types, but are concentrated in ores throughout the world, depending on the geological history of the region. They are brought to the surface naturally by erosion and volcanic activity and are washed in streams and eventually deposited with sediments in rivers, lakes, and oceans. There they are imbedded in sedimentary rocks, which are eventually uplifted to start the cycle again. Human actions have greatly altered the natural cycle of metals, and in many instances, contributions from humans are much greater than those from natural sources.

Some of the ways people mobilize metals are obvious, and others are quite subtle. Burning coal and oil releases vast quantities of metals to the air because they are natural contaminants of the fuel. Prior to the 1970s, lead was intentionally added to gasoline to prevent engine knock, and cars became the greatest source of lead to the environment. Ore refining, trash burning, and cement production are other important sources of airborne metals. Discarded products that contain metals are buried in dumps along with the metal-containing ash from coal and trash burning. These landfills often leak metals into underground water supplies.

Some of the subtle ways of adding metals

to the environment are through the use of fertilizers and *pesticides* and through acid rain. **Arsenic** has long been a component of pesticides, and though its use is now declining, permanent contamination of many orchards and croplands has occurred. Cadmium is a trace contaminant of phosphate fertilizers and is slowly but steadily building up in agricultural soils. This may become the most important source of cadmium exposure in the future. Acid rain, caused largely by the burning of fuels, dissolves **aluminum** from surface rocks and soil and washes it into lakes and streams. Along with the acid, aluminum contributes to the fish kills of the Northeast and Canada.

Once mobile in the environment, metals find countless ways into the body through drinking water, food, and breathable air. Water sitting overnight in household plumbing can leach lead and cadmium out of pipes and solder joints to appear in the first draw for morning coffee. Organisms such as bacteria can take a harmless form of mercury and turn it into harmful methyl mercury, a form that is absorbed and concentrated by fish and then eaten by people. Metals released into the air waft down on food crops, working their way into the diet. Food processing exposes food to contact with metal equipment. Autos, refineries, smelters, and power plants pump lead, arsenic, cadmium, **nickel**, and a host of other substances into the air. Often people find themselves watching this process from nearby freeways stuck in rush-hour traffic, breathing these dangerous compounds all the while. And tobacco smoke containing cadmium, arsenic, zinc, **chromium**, nickel, **selenium**, and lead is inhaled both by smokers and nearby nonsmokers. These are just some of the many examples of exposure routes into the body detailed throughout this book.

B. Human Health Effects

Metals exert their effects in many ways, but usually within body cells. Some disrupt chemical reactions, others block the absorption of essential nutrients, while still others change the shapes of vital chemical compounds, rendering them useless. Some metals bind to nutrients in the stomach, preventing their absorption into the body. The outcome of these actions depends on the specific metal and body organ involved.

Acute poisoning by metals is not something most members of the public experience. Workers exposed to metals on the job may suffer lung damage, skin reactions, and gastrointestinal symptoms from brief contact with high concentrations. Lead poisoning in children, a far too common occurrence, can lead to convulsions, brain damage, or death. Occasionally, metals can be introduced to foods through the dissolution of metallic containers by acidic foods. The symptoms are typical of food poisoning: vomiting and diarrhea, usually developing several hours later in all who ate the meal.

Chronic poisoning from long-term exposure to low levels of metals is of more concern than acute effects. Some metals accumulate in the body over time, reaching toxic concentrations after years of exposure. Cadmium, for example, builds up in the kidneys and after many years can cause kidney disease. Lead, methyl mercury, and organic tin compounds slowly cause brain degeneration. Arsenic can damage the peripheral nervous system, leading to tingling sensations, pain, and eventual loss of muscular control in the extremities. Years of exposure to metal dusts cause scar tissue to form in the lungs (*pulmonary fibrosis*), along with progressive difficulties in breathing. Damage to the liver, kidney, and skin can also be caused by persistent exposure to various metals, such as chromium, selenium, cadmium, nickel, and arsenic.

Cancer is another type of chronic effect. Arsenic, **beryllium**, cadmium, chromium, and nickel dust can cause lung cancer. Arsenic can probably also cause skin cancer if swallowed. Other metals and metal-containing compounds are suspected causes of cancer, but the data are not yet sufficient for proof.

Mutations are changes in the genetic material that can lead to cancer and various illnesses or to genetic damage in later generations (such as mental illness or physical handicaps) if mutations occur in reproductive cells of the ovaries or testes. Lead, cadmium, chromium, selenium, nickel, and arsenic have produced mutations in laboratory tests of human and other cells, but no specific genetic disease other than cancer has been definitively linked to metal exposure.

A final group of effects occur in the developing embryo and newborn child. These stages of human development are particularly vulnerable because key nervous system structures are being formed and rapid cell division is occurring throughout the body at a time when the genetic material is relatively unprotected. Exposure to methyl mercury or lead at this time can cause gross deformities in development, including incorrect placement of brain structures, severe cerebral palsy, blindness, and poor or nonexistent language development. Lead exposure in children has been linked to low IQs.

There are several commonsense ways to reduce exposure to metals and related pollutants.

1. Tobacco smoke is a source of many metals. Eliminate tobacco smoke by personally quitting and by having nonquitters smoke outdoors.
2. Industries such as refineries, chemical plants, cement manufacturers, power plants, and smelters release large quantities of metals into our atmosphere and water. Spend as little time as possible in the immediate vicinity of such sources. In particular, do not let children use playgrounds downwind of these factories. Small chrome-plating shops are found throughout cities and should be avoided on a regular basis.
3. Cars emit metals, particularly lead from older vehicles burning leaded gasoline. Children should avoid playgrounds near heavily traveled streets and freeways.
4. Dirt and dust often contain metal particulates. Wash hands and make sure that children wash their hands before eating.
5. Water left overnight in pipes tends to accumulate metals from the plumbing. Run the water for several minutes in the morning from all taps from which water is consumed. (The water can be collected in pitchers for watering plants.)
6. Hot water dissolves more metals than cold water. Always use cold water for cooking.
7. Pay attention to public notices of contamination. Public water suppliers are required in many instances to notify consumers if levels of contaminants in drinking water exceed permitted allowances. Occasionally, food is contaminated as well.

Further Reading

FRIBERG, L., NORDBERG, G. F., and VOUK, V. B. 1986. *Handbook on the Toxicology of Metals.* Amsterdam and New York: Elsevier.

GOYER, R. A. 1986. Toxic Effects of Metals. In *Casarett and Doull's Toxicology: The Basic Science of Poisons.* 3d edition. Edited by Klaassen, C. D., Amdur, M. O., and Doull, J. New York: Macmillan. Pp. 582–635.

13 PETROCHEMICALS

As noted throughout this book, modern technological societies depend, to a large extent, on the chemical industry. Ultimately, chemicals are used in the production of virtually all consumer and industrial goods—food, medicine, cosmetics, lumber, appliances, fuels, plastics, electronic equipment, textiles, paper, and many other products. While most of us probably think of paints and pesticides as chemicals, the relationship between chemicals and certain finished products such as computers may seem obscure. But consider that all of the parts—the plastic housing and keyboard, the microchips, the wiring, the glass-covered screen, and the cathode ray tube or liquid crystal display—all are end-products of chemical manufacturing. And the underpinnings of the chemical industry are fossil fuels, specifically petroleum and natural gas, and to a lesser extent, coal. While the major proportion of fossil fuels are burned to provide energy for power plants and automobiles, roughly 10% of the petroleum and natural gas we use is funneled into chemical production.

In this chapter, we briefly describe the petrochemical industry, including the raw materials, the intermediate chemicals, and the end-products (Fig. 13). To illustrate some of the problems associated with this industry, we focus on one group of very widely distributed chemicals: solvents.

A. Sources and Products

Such everyday products as toys and detergents start out as raw materials, which are turned into intermediary process chemicals. These, in turn, undergo a variety of reactions to produce the desired chemical products, which may be end-products in themselves, such as paints or cleaning fluids, or which may be used in the manufacture of other goods.

Raw Materials

While some raw materials used in chemical production are obtained by mining naturally occurring metal and mineral deposits in the earth, most of the chemicals in use are derived chiefly from petroleum and natural gas; hence, the chemical industry is commonly referred to as the petrochemical industry and the products are called petrochemicals. Prior to the 1940s, the petrochemical industry was essentially nonexistent. Basic industrial

chemicals were obtained from the distillation of agricultural products, such as molasses, and the processing of coal tar. Following World War II, new and improved methods for obtaining basic chemicals from petroleum and natural gas were developed, resulting in the rapid growth of the petrochemical industry. In 1950, for example, about 2 million tons of basic chemicals were produced; by 1986, production had risen to nearly 100 million tons.

Today, while some products are still derived from processing cellulose and coal tar, more than 90% (by weight) of *organic* chemicals are petrochemicals. Moreover, a substantial fraction of *inorganic* chemicals, such as **ammonia** and sulfur, are produced from petroleum and natural gas. Prior to the 1930s, ammonia was produced from hydrogen gas generated during coke (processed coal) production. About half of the sulfur currently produced is recovered from refineries that produce natural gas and oil containing hydrogen sulfide. The rest is extracted directly from sulfur mines.

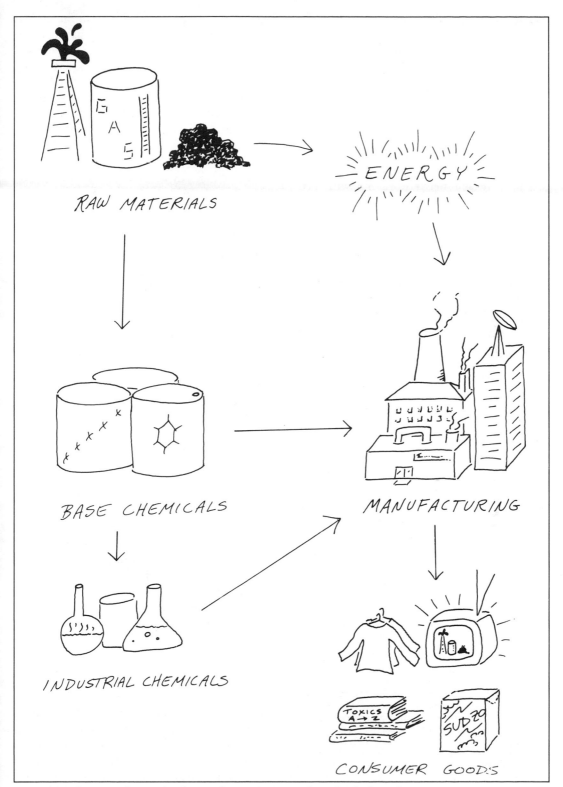

RAW MATERIALS

ENERGY

BASE CHEMICALS

MANUFACTURING

INDUSTRIAL CHEMICALS

CONSUMER GOODS

Figure 13 The petrochemical industry: from raw materials to finished products.

The Chemicals

Chemical compounds can be distinguished into two groups by the presence (or absence) of carbon. Organic compounds, often called *hydrocarbons,* basically are made up of carbon atoms usually in combination with hydrogen.[1] Inorganic substances, on the other hand, are not based on carbon. Examples of inorganic and organic substances are given in Table 7.

Ethylene and **benzene**, along with propylene, butylenes, **toluene**, and **xylene**, are important base organic chemicals that supply manufacturing industries or are converted to other chemical products, such as industrial solvents or plastics. **Hydrochloric** and sulfuric acids, major inorganic chemicals, are used extensively as reactants in industrial processes, but are not incorporated into the final product. In contrast, certain metals and *halogens,* such as chlorine and bromine, are critical constituents of the finished organic products, as in *organochlorine* pesticides. (As discussed elsewhere in this book, the addition of halogens to organic products poses risks to human health and the environment. For example, see Chapters 11 and 14 and individual entries in Part II.)

The Chemicals and Allied Products Industry (as the chemical industry is classified by the U.S. Department of Commerce) produces about 500 million tons of chemicals in eight product categories: industrial inorganic chemicals; synthetic resins and plastics; soaps, toiletries, and detergents; paints and coatings; drugs; industrial organic chemicals; agricultural chemicals; and miscellaneous chemicals.

Production of these chemicals is big business. Chemical manufacturing is the fourth largest manufacturing industry in the United States exceeded (in dollars) only by the food, transportation equipment, and petroleum and coal products (fuels) industries. Of the roughly $2 trillion ($2000 billion) worth of manufactured goods produced and shipped in the United States annually, chemical products account for about 10% of the total, about $206 billion in 1986.

Most of us would agree that our washing machines, allergy remedies, easy-care fabrics, paperback books—all products made possible by the petrochemical industry—have made life easier or better for us. Unfortunately, dirty air, contaminated drinking water wells, oil-covered beaches and birds, and other evidence of pollution have become familiar accompaniments to the petroleum and chemical industries. Chemical products enter the environment as a result of intentional introductions, as in the case of pesticides; incidental or routine releases, as in gaseous emissions and solid and liquid effluents; and accidental spills, such as the oil spill from the Exxon supertanker *Valdez.*

In the following essay, we discuss some of the problems associated with one group of chemical products. *Solvents* are a common group of chemicals used in nearly every human activity, from heavy industrial settings to the home workshop. Certain of these chemicals have been found as contaminants in well water, particularly in areas with heavy concentrations of electronics or computer industries. Some are airborne pollutants and, as such, can be widely distributed. Because solvents are so common and widely dispersed, nearly everyone is exposed at some time to these substances, which cause a variety of adverse health effects.

B. Solvents

Solvents are a group of chemicals that have many varied uses in industry and the home. The word "solvent" is generally defined as a liquid used to dissolve other substances, a definition that includes water as a solvent.

[1] Because of the way that carbon atoms (the backbone of organic compounds) can link to other carbon, simple to very complex arrangements are possible; some carbon-to-carbon linkages form chainlike structures. These are called *aliphatic compounds.* Other organic compounds, in which the carbons are tightly linked to form a ringlike structure, are called *aromatics.* Various chemical constituents, such as nitrogen, oxygen, chlorine, and sulfur, are attached to the backbone structure to form the vast array of organic compounds, ranging from alcohols to proteins.

TABLE 7 Examples of Chemical Compounds

Inorganic	Organic
Acids 　Hydrochloric acid 　Sulfuric acid Bases 　Sodium hydroxide 　Ammonium hydroxide Metals 　Aluminum 　Chromium Salts 　Sodium chloride (table salt)	Aliphatic 　Ethylene 　Acetic acid (vinegar) 　Methylene chloride 　Formaldehyde Aromatic 　Benzene 　DDT 　PCBs

Here we restrict its meaning to a group of organic compounds (*hydrocarbons*) that are used to dissolve other hydrocarbons such as tars, waxes, oils, and other petrochemicals. Because solvents evaporate quickly and leave almost no residue they are used to wash dust from precision electronic and machined parts. Solvents are also used to thin paints and glues, dry-clean fabrics, and extract oils and waxes from impure materials. They are also used in many household products and drugs.

Types of Solvents

The variety of solvents available to industry and the household is large. Hundreds of individual solvents are used to make over 30,000 proprietary blends that have become widely known by their trade names, such as Chlorox (**chlorine** bleach), Freon (**CFC**), and Arctic (methyl chloride or chloromethane). The most common solvents fall into five general categories. These are the alcohols (such as methanol and isopropyl alcohol), the ketones (such as **methyl ethyl ketone** and **acetone**), the aliphatic ("chain") hydrocarbons (such as hexane), the aromatic ("ring") hydrocarbons (such as **benzene, toluene,** and **xylene**), and finally the halogenated hydrocarbons (such as **trichloroethylene, methylene chloride,** and **CFCs**). Other less commonly used groups of organic solvents are glycol ethers and acetates.

Most solvents are hazardous: some are flammable, others explode easily, some are corrosive, and most are toxic. In general, the solvents that contain *halogens* (chlorine, fluorine, bromine, and iodine) are less apt to catch fire, explode, or corrode tanks and pipelines than nonhalogenated organic solvents. The most commonly used halogenated solvents are the chlorinated ones. Unfortunately, chlorinated solvents, like most other halogenated solvents, are toxic. Nevertheless, demand for chlorinated solvents in 1987 was 1.5 billion pounds. Only 1% is reused or recycled, whereas about 94% is eventually released into the environment, mostly into the air. The rest is incorporated into various products such as polyvinyl chloride plastic, CFCs, and plastic food wrap. Nearly all of the demand for chlorinated solvents is filled by only four chemicals: methylene chloride, **trichloroethane,** trichloroethylene, and **tetrachloroethylene**. These four chemicals are either used directly, or they are further processed to yield more specialized solvents, plastics, and pharmaceuticals.

Demand for chlorinated solvents is dropping due to increased recycling, technological changes, and substitution with less toxic water-based solvents. Nevertheless, chlorinated solvents will continue to be used in large quantities for years to come. These solvents are used during the manufacture of a huge variety of everyday products, and it takes time to find less toxic substitute chemicals and integrate them into industrial processes. Chlorinated solvents are also used by a myriad of small- and medium-sized businesses, which are often difficult to incorporate into recycling programs. Finally, chlorinated solvents are relatively inexpensive for industries to buy, and many of the costs associated with cleaning up contamination by chlorinated solvents is not borne directly by the users of the chemicals. Thus, industries have no economic incentive for finding ways to reduce the use of these solvents.

Human Health and Environmental Effects

Human health effects due to exposure to solvents can include damage to the skin, liver, blood, central nervous system, and sometimes the lungs and kidneys. Some solvents are irritants, while others are capable of causing cancer. Since solvents generally evaporate easily at room temperature, most solvent exposure results from breathing vapors. But leaks in underground storage tanks, surface impoundments, and accidental spills have exposed significant numbers of people to solvents via groundwater.

Solvents can also be absorbed into the body upon skin contact, although this is a minor exposure route for most people. Solvents spilled on the skin strip skin cells of vital oils and fats, causing red, cracked, or scaly skin. Once exposure stops, the skin usually heals itself. Some solvents are *allergens* and cause allergic *dermatitis* among sensitive people, even if they do not actually touch the solvent.

Inhaling solvent vapors, even for very short periods, can lead to lung and throat irritation, *pulmonary edema,* dizziness, lightheadedness, blurred vision, nervousness, sleepiness or insomnia, nausea, vomiting, disorientation, confusion, irregular heartbeat, and even unconsciousness and death. Many of these symptoms pass quickly when exposure stops. Some symptoms of acute exposure cannot be felt immediately. Certain chlorinated solvents, for instance, cause delayed lung, liver, and kidney damage. Chemicals that do not cause an immediate display of symptoms of overexposure are said to have poor warning ability because dangerous concentrations cannot be detected by overexposed people.

Repeated exposure to some solvents can lead to chronic bronchitis, permanent liver and kidney damage, and permanent neurological problems. Solvents can affect the body's ability to manufacture blood, while some can damage the immune system. Many commonly encountered chlorinated solvents, including benzene, trichloroethylene, tetrachloroethylene, and methylene chloride, are suspected of causing cancer. Some solvents cause, or are suspected of causing, birth defects. For example, glycol ethers have recently been found to cause birth defects and reproductive problems among test animals. Most solvents readily pass from maternal to fetal blood, thus exposing unborn children to potentially toxic compounds.

People concerned about solvent exposure should learn the composition, scientific names, toxicity, and degree of hazard associated with all solvents they use. *Material Safety Data Sheets (MSDS)* containing this information should be readily available to people exposed to solvents at the workplace. Unfortunately, the precise chemical composition of proprietary solvent mixtures may not be available, and the toxicity information presented on the MSDS may be incomplete or confusing. Should this be the case, contact your local department of health or the Occupational Safety and Health Administration (OSHA).

Consumers may have a more difficult time finding information about the toxic hazards associated with architectural coatings (house paint), art and craft materials, and cleaning supplies can be difficult. Consumer product labels are not presently required to list specific solvent ingredients. The so-called *inert* ingredients are solvents that are subject to lax regulation. California's right-to-know regulation is an attempt to inform consumers about the presence of chemicals in products that cause cancer or birth defects. But the law's effectiveness has not been demonstrated because not all consumer products are labeled clearly. Also, cancer and birth defects are a small subset of the potential problems associated with solvents in consumer products. A report issued by the California State Department of Health Services states that over 60 different solvents are commonly used in consumer products. The most common solvents found in consumer products are ethanol, isopropyl alcohol, kerosene, propylene glycol, isobutane, butane, and propane, none of which are highly toxic or are known to cause cancer or birth defects, but about 250 tons per day of these materials are released into California's air every year.

Some of these commonly released solvents cause serious environmental problems when released into urban air. Many volatile solvents contribute to the formation of urban ozone, while others, including CFCs, trichloroethane, and **carbon tetrachloride**, contribute to stratospheric ozone depletion. Chlorinated solvents are often persistent in soil and water, leading to the environmental problems associated with *bioconcentration* and groundwater pollution. Sometimes solvents released into the environment mix with other chemicals or degrade to form more toxic products. For example, trichloroethane degrades in soil to form the more toxic chemical **vinyl chloride**.

Until products are clearly labeled, allowing people to make informed choices, consumers are urged to buy water-based products whenever they are available and effective. When water-based products are not available, learn the names of the solvents used in various product formulations and try to choose the ones that are the least toxic to people or the environment.

Further Reading

ANDREWS, LARRY, and SNYDER, ROBERT. 1986. Toxic Effects of Solvents and Vapors. In *Casarett and Doull's Toxicology: The Basic Science of Poisons*. 3d edition. Klaassen, C. D., Amdur, M. O., and Doull, J., eds. New York: Macmillan.

LAVE, LESTER B., and UPTON, ARTHUR C., eds. 1987. *Toxic Chemicals, Health, and the Environment*. Baltimore: The Johns Hopkins University Press.

14 PESTICIDES

Enormous quantities of pesticides are used globally in the production of food, fiber, and lumber; in the management of public lands; and in the control of disease-carrying insects and common household and garden pests. In the last 40 years, people have become increasingly reliant on chemicals to control unwanted insects, weeds, molds, and rodents. Recent scientific findings regarding the safety of many of the pesticides in use have begun to suggest the need for a reevaluation of our current practices with the intent to develop a more rational policy. Also, growing evidence shows that safer, alternative methods of pest control are available that can be effective and economically profitable.

A. Overview

Each year about 2.6 billion pounds of *pesticides* are consumed in the United States. Although the amount of pesticides produced and used is a relatively small percentage of all synthetic organic chemicals, pesticides are of particular concern because they are by definition toxic chemicals (the word "pesticide" literally means "pest killer"). They are specifically intended to kill insects (*insecticides*), plants (*herbicides*), molds and mildews (*fungicides*), rats and mice (*rodenticides*), mites and ticks (*acaricides*), bacteria (*bactericides*), birds (*avicides*), roundworms (*nematicides*), and even coyotes—whatever people have deemed to be pests. Moreover, they are intentionally introduced into the environment.

In the United States, agriculture accounts for more than 90% of our domestic pesticide consumption. The remaining fraction—a hefty 260 millon pounds or so annually—is used to control fungi and other pests in a great variety of products including paints, dentures, shampoos, disposable diapers, mattresses, paper, flea powders, hair wigs, carpets, and contact lenses. Pesticides are used to control algae in lakes and swimming pools and to prevent damage from termites and fungi (dry rot) in wooden structures; they are sprayed on golf courses, lawns, playing fields, and pastures.

Because of their extensive use and the manner in which they are applied, pesticides are found everywhere—in our drinking water, our food, our air, and our soils. In short, pesticides are a part of our everyday life.

Plants are the basic food source for the world's rapidly growing human population. Today more than five billion people worldwide compete for food with many thousands of major plant pests, including as many as 100,000 species of plant *pathogens* (disease-causing agents), more than 10,000 species of voracious insects, 1000 species of crop-destroying roundworms, and 1800 species of economically important weeds. Many more thousands of species are minor agricultural pests that have the potential to become serious pests. Consequently, agriculture may be hard-pressed to keep pace with the demands of an exploding and hungry human population.

Historically, people and pests have had a long association, and the use of chemicals to rid ourselves of pests is not new. The early Romans, for example, sterilized the soil using salt brines and ashes. Water extracts of tobacco plants (**nicotine**) have been effectively used to kill sucking insects for over 300 years. Extracts of chrysanthemum flowers (**pyrethrum**) have been used as insecticides in Asia at least since 1800 and probably longer. Inorganic compounds containing sulfur, copper, mercury, and **arsenic** were used extensively as insecticides, herbicides, or fungicides in the first half of this century.

Following World War II, there was a burgeoning of the synthetic organic chemical industry. An entirely new array of apparently superior, inexpensive pesticides, suitable for application over vast acreages, became readily and widely available. Chemically unlike traditional pesticides, the synthetic organic pesticides have largely replaced the inorganic and botanical or naturally occurring compounds. These so-called miracle chemicals promised to eliminate hunger and disease and improve the quality of life for the world's population. Indeed, over a short period of time, these pesticides have changed the nature of the association between people and pests.

Consider the magnitude of the changes. In the last 40 years or so throughout most of the world, we have made a rapid shift from merely slapping mosquitoes (although this certainly is not a dead art) to treating entire lakes, marshes, swamps, and other mosquito breeding grounds with chemical insecticides. Many farmers throughout the world have switched from manual or mechanical weeding of a few acres to aerial spraying of herbicides over hundreds or even thousands of acres of agricultural fields.

As the scale of operations has vastly expanded in terms of more crops, more acreage, and more frequent applications, the volume of pesticides used has increased dramatically. Just since 1960, the total amount of pesticides produced has doubled (with peak usage in 1975 and 1980), as can be seen in the graph of Figure 14. In the late 1940s, about 50 million pounds of pesticides were used annually in the United States. Now about 50 times as much is being used. During just the last 25 years, there has been roughly a doubling in pesticide consumption in the United States alone. Pesticides are applied so routinely and extensively that, to many, pest control is now synonymous with chemical control.

Interestingly, the overall increase in pesticide usage has been accompanied by a shift in usage pattern among the principal categories of pesticides. While fungicide production and use have remained approximately constant since 1960, herbicide use has increased. Insecticide use, in contrast, peaked in the late 1970s and has subsequently returned to 1960 levels.

Soaring pesticide use is tied to the development and extensive cultivation of high-yield grains and a correspondingly large increase in the use of chemical fertilizers. But since 1945, a 10-fold increase in insecticide use and a 100-fold increase in herbicide use has been accompanied by only a bit more than a doubling in wheat, rice, and corn output. Despite massive chemical pest control efforts, about one-third of the world's food crops are lost to pests. Spiraling pesticide inputs and persistent agricultural losses clearly indicate that there are limits to the effectiveness of massive pesticide applications.

Nevertheless, the benefits of pesticides for all manner of uses from large-scale food production to small-scale home gardening and the control of household pests are widely touted. But perhaps the most important applications are those associated with public health. Here again, however, there are signs that the trend toward greater and greater reliance on chemical pest control is of limited usefulness. For example, until as recently as 1955, about 100 million people throughout the world were infected with malaria, a debilitating and often fatal disease. With the introduction of DDT to control the disease-carrying mosquitoes, the number of human deaths has been significantly cut—from an estimated 6 million in 1939 to 2.5 million in the 1970s. Furthermore, in some parts of the world, the disease had been virtually eliminated, at least until strains of mosquitoes appeared with natural resistance to the effects of the pesticide (see Section D of this chapter). The resistant mosquitoes evolved as a result of both direct exposure to high levels of DDT, sprayed in mosquito-infested areas, and indirect exposure when significant concentrations of DDT were carried by the wind

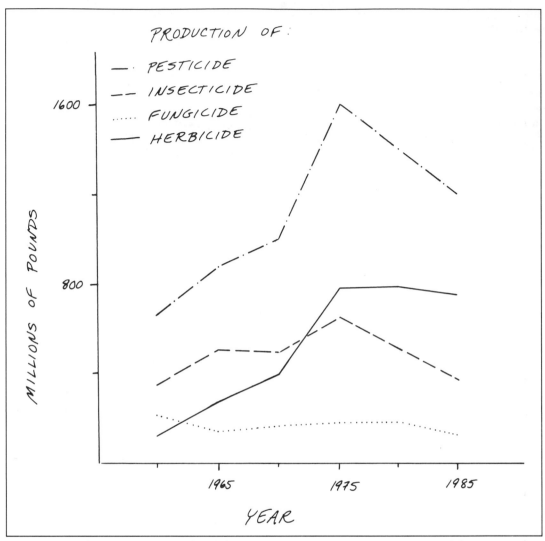

Figure 14 Synthetic organic pesticide production, 1960 to 1985. (From U.S. Bureau of the Census. 1989. *Statistical Abstract of the United States: 1989.* 109th edition. Washington, D.C.: USGPO.)

(aerial drift) following spraying of agricultural fields.

In 1962 Rachel Carson called attention, in her book *Silent Spring,* to the potential hazards associated with excessive reliance on synthetic pesticides. Her warnings, which primarily concerned chlorinated hydrocarbons such as DDT, were applied more generally to synthetic organic compounds and provided the initial impetus for much of the environmental legislation enacted in the 1970s. Nearly three decades after the publica-

tion of *Silent Spring,* we are now beginning to understand fully the nature of the chemicals we use in such great abundance and to recognize the social and environmental costs imposed by that usage. Among the costs are an estimated 45,000 (possibly as many as 300,000) acute accidental human poisonings a year in the United States alone, the exposure of a large segment of the population to pesticide residues in food, persistent crop losses despite increasing pesticide inputs, the development of pesticide resistance in pest species, and adverse (sometimes devastating) effects on beneficial and nonpest species.

What accounts for these problems? Are they significant? What choices do we have? Answers to these questions are complex and related to the chemistry of the synthetic compounds, the biological properties of the pests, the ecological relationships among pests and beneficial species, and the changing perceptions of costs and benefits. This chapter is intended to acquaint the reader with some of the basic chemical and functional relationships among pesticides, the major social and environmental problems and issues associated with pesticide use, and the current ideas about alternatives to existing pesticide practices.

B. Classification and Patterns of Use

Pesticides are chemically and functionally very diverse. There are more than 600 different *active ingredients* (the actual substance that kills) registered for use in the United States. These are combined with various other ingredients, such as other pesticides, *synergists,* and *inert ingredients,* into about 40,000 pesticide products. These range from widely available moth crystals, snail baits, and flea and tick collars for pets to highly restricted pesticides for use only by trained and properly equipped personnel. Some pesticides are toxic to a wide variety of species and kinds of organisms; these are called *broad spectrum* agents. A broad spectrum herbicide might be used, for example, to kill all of the shrubs, weeds, and grasses at a construction site. In contrast, other pesticides are highly specific or *selective,* effective against a narrowly defined group of organisms such as moths and butterflies.

Insecticides, herbicides, fungicides, and so on are available in various usable forms such as liquid sprays, wettable powders, dusts, and granules. The products are designed for specific application methods: aerial or ground spraying onto the plant leaves, spraying or dusting onto the soil surface, or injecting directly into the plant or soil around the roots.

In theory, the method of application is designed to deliver the pesticide in the most effective or readily usable form for its mode of action. Some pesticides act on contact with the intended victim or target organism, as it is called. *Contact* (or *knockdown*) pesticides are rapidly effective, capable, for instance, of killing houseflies on the wing. In contrast, the slower acting *systemic* insecticides and herbicides are applied to plants, which are themselves either the target pest or serve as food for a pest insect species. The systemics are absorbed by the roots (when applied to the soil) or leaves (when applied to the foliage) of the plant and moved to other tissues. Systemic herbicides interfere with normal plant functions. Systemic insecticides, in contrast, poison plant-eating insects after being absorbed from the stomach following ingestion of the food plant. While systemic insecticides generally do not harm the plant, their effectiveness depends on systemwide transport and accumulation in those parts of the plant—the fruits, nuts, seeds, and leaves—that not only insects but, ultimately, people eat (see Section D).

Various schemes have been devised for classifying pesticides. Here, they are first classified on the basis of their primary function or use—as insecticides, fungicides, herbicides, and so on. Then, within each functional class, the substances are grouped according to their chemical and structural similarities or relationships. This arrangement permits discussion of common properties of the substances, such as the way they kill the target species; their effect on nontarget species, including people; and their behavior in the environment.

Insecticides and Acaricides

About 13% of U.S. crops are lost before harvest to insects. Additional losses occur during harvest and storage. Today, insecticides and the related *acaricides* account for about

35% of all agricultural pesticide use. Outside the agricultural market, however, insecticides are the predominant pesticide.

Most of the insecticides currently in use are synthetic organic compounds, but some, the botanicals, are produced naturally by plants. By design, some of the synthetics are chemically and functionally very similar to the botanicals. Although the array of insecticides available is chemically very diverse, the most widely used fall into one of four major groups: the *organochlorines*, the *organophosphates*, the *carbamates*, and the botanicals and related synthetic compounds. Gaining in popularity are the microbial insecticides.

Organochlorine or chlorinated hydrocarbon[1] insecticides are part of a broader class of halogenated hydrocarbons, which includes the well-known, troublesome **polychlorinated biphenyls (PCBs)** and **dioxin**. As a group, the organochlorine insecticides are *neurotoxins* that stimulate the nervous system of both insects and mammals, causing tremors and convulsions. But the symptoms of poisoning caused by **DDT** (and its analogs) differ slightly from those caused by other organochlorine insecticides (see individual entries in Part II).

Chlorinated hydrocarbons have been used extensively since their development in the 1940s and 1950s. Although highly effective and inexpensive, use of most organochlorines has been banned or severely restricted throughout much of the industrialized world on environmental grounds. DDT and certain other chlorinated hydrocarbons, such as **lindane, aldrin/dieldrin,** and **heptachlor,** have gained widespread notoriety because of their

persistence in the environment, their tendency to accumulate in the tissues of living organisms, and their adverse effect on non-target species. These compounds are very stable chemically, that is, they are not readily broken down in the environment or in animal or plant tissues. In fact, they remain unchanged in soil and water for decades, ready to be absorbed or ingested by organisms. Through the process of *bioconcentration*, they accumulate in plant and animal tissues and can endanger animals high in the *food chain*. Certain other organochlorines, such as methoxychlor, chlorobenzilate, and uncontaminated dicofol (which is often contaminated with DDT during manufacture), are slightly less persistent in the environment. Toxaphene, although relatively persistent in soil, air, and water and highly toxic to fish, is metabolized and excreted fairly readily by mammals and little is stored in tissues.

A second class of insecticides, the organophosphates (OPs),[2] have been in use for several decades; the first OP insecticide was introduced in 1946, just two years after DDT. The OPs are generally the most *acutely toxic* pesticides to vertebrate animals, such as fish, birds, lizards, and mammals. In fact OP insecticides have been associated with more human poisonings than any other pesticide. Although they are closely related to some of the most potent nerve gases developed for use as chemical weapons, the OPs range in toxicity from that of nerve gases to that of table salt.

To a large extent, the chemically unstable OPs have replaced the persistent organochlorines, particularly in products available to consumers. Unlike DDT and many other organochlorines, the OPs break down rapidly in the environment and do not have a tendency to accumulate in tissues.

The OPs interfere with the normal function of the nervous system in a complex way that ultimately affects the respiratory and cir-

---

[1] Organochlorine compounds contain carbon, hydrogen, and chlorine; some also contain oxygen and less often sulfur. There are basically two kinds of chlorinated hydrocarbons: those that form ringlike structures ◯ and those that exist in chainlike forms ∿∿∿. In the first category are some of the earliest developed, most widely used, and most notorious synthetic organic pesticides such as **DDT, chlordane,** and Kepone. The chainlike compounds are generally used as *fumigants* and *nematicides.*

[2] Structurally the OPs are very diverse, forming various ring or chain shapes, and contain some combination of phosphorus, carbon, hydrogen, oxygen, and often sulfur.

culatory systems, causing muscular twitching and paralysis. Basically, the OPs block the activity of *cholinesterase,* an *enzyme* that plays a crucial role in the transmission of nerve signals. Each signal is carried from one nerve fiber to another by a chemical transmitter that must be broken down after the signal is relayed to make ready for new messages. Normally, cholinesterase breaks down the transmitter, thus keeping the circuits clear. When the action of the enzyme is hindered, as occurs when an organophosphate insecticide becomes bound to the enzyme, the chemical accumulates at the junction of nerve fibers. As a result, certain target organs, such as the heart, are subjected to continuous stimulation, which may cause muscular twitching, paralysis, or death, depending on dosage and treatment. Because the bond between the organophosphate and the enzyme is relatively strong, the inhibitory effects are very slowly reversed and may persist for as long as a week.

Additionally, some OPs induce other neurotoxic effects that resemble the effects of alcoholism, diabetes, or various prescription drugs. Other organic phosphorous compounds have the ability to enhance the toxicity of related insecticides by blocking the body's detoxifying mechanisms. This is called *potentiation.* There is some concern that OP insecticides may potentiate pharmaceuticals, other kinds of pesticides, and even the solvents or other substances in pesticide products. It has been shown, however, that some chlorinated hydrocarbon insecticides interfere with the toxic effect of the OPs probably because they stimulate a major detoxification system.

Carbamates,[3] a third class of insecticides, are among the most widely used pesticides in the world. The U.S. consumption of carbamates in 1982 was estimated to be roughly 26 million pounds a year, equal to about 50%

[3] Carbamate compounds, like other complex organic pesticides, vary greatly in structure, but all contain nitrogen, carbon, hydrogen, and oxygen in varying amounts and configurations.

of total global use. Most of the 50 or so carbamates have been in commercial use since the 1950s. Not all carbamates have insecticidal activity; some act principally as *herbicides* or *fungicides.*

Like the organophosphates, insecticidal carbamates inhibit certain enzymes, particularly cholinesterase, and they may enhance the effects of other toxics. Unlike the OPs, however, there is a relatively quick recovery time following carbamate poisoning. Moreover, carbamates do not mimic the effects of alcoholism, diabetes, or certain drugs. Carbamates undergo essentially the same breakdown processes in plants, insects, and mammals. Generally the resulting breakdown products are less toxic than the parent compounds, but there are exceptions; some are more persistent and considerably more toxic. Carbamates are rapidly excreted in mammals and do not *bioconcentrate.* They do, however, bioconcentrate in fish.

Despite a long history of use, little information exists on carbamates from animal studies or human data on long-term toxicity, including its cancer-causing ability, ability to cause DNA changes, tendency to cause birth defects, and such reproductive effects as increased spontaneous abortions, decreased fertility, and decreased survival of the young. It is known, however, that in the presence of **nitrates**, carbamates can be converted to **nitrosamines**, which are carcinogenic. Studies indicate that these substances could form in the mammalian stomach. Other tests show that many carbamates appear to be associated with liver and kidney impairment and/or degeneration.

Few carbamates have been classified according to their degree of acute toxicity to people, but some are highly toxic to various nontarget organisms. Honeybees, for example, are extremely sensitive to insecticidal carbamates. Many aquatic invertebrates are also very susceptible to poisoning by specific carbamates.

In the environment, the fate of the carbamates is a function of their chemical properties and the physical conditions they encounter. Under aqueous conditions, they are rapidly decomposed by sunlight. Because they do not dissolve very readily in water, carbamates do not leach or diffuse much in soils. Soil acidity (pH) plays a role in the breakdown of some carbamates. For example, carbofuran, linked to the death of about two million birds in and around Chesapeake Bay, has a *half-life* of about one year in neutral or *acid* soils (with a *pH* less than 7.0), but degrades rapidly in *alkaline* soils.

Another major group of insecticides, the botanicals, is composed of a diverse array of compounds produced naturally by plants, which kill or deter plant-eating insects. Differing in origin, chemical structure, stability, and specific toxic effect, the botanicals have evolved over millions of years in response to direct attack by herbivores. These naturally occurring plant products are highly effective insecticides and some (such as **nicotine**, rotenone, **pyrethrum** extracts, camphor, and even turpentine) have been used by human beings for this purpose for the past few hundred years. Use of botanical insecticides peaked in the mid-1960s and had declined by the mid-1980s. They are generally impractical for use in large-scale farming operations because they are relatively expensive, but they continue to be used by householders and alternative gardeners, especially pyrethrum extracts (see Section F).

Several synthetic **pyrethroids** (structurally very similar to the naturally occurring pyrethrum extracts) have been developed recently and are used extensively in agriculture. Unlike pyrethrum extracts, synthetic pyrethroids, such as **permethrin** and fenvalerate, resist chemical and photochemical degradation and are highly effective at low rates of application. In fact, about 1 pound of a synthetic pyrethroid is generally as effective as 10 pounds of a carbamate or organophosphate insecticide.

A new variety of insecticide, the microbials, may prove far more effective than the various chemicals so widely used today. Microbial insecticides constitute a diverse array of microorganisms, including bacteria, viruses, fungi, and protozoans, that are fairly selective in their action. Of the microbials, the most commonly used at present is a species of bacterium, *Bacillus thuringiensis*, that is selectively effective against moths and butterflies.

Finally, *fumigants,* a special group of simple, volatile compounds that exist as gases at temperatures greater than 40°F, are used to kill insects in several stages of development in soils and in confined spaces, such as warehouses, grain elevators, greenhouses, and food packages. (Fumigants are not only insecticides; they are used also to kill plant seeds, roundworms, and certain microorganisms in soils and enclosed structures.) Fumigants readily penetrate the skin and membranes that line the human respiratory and *gastrointestinal tracts.* Moreover, they can penetrate the conventional rubber and plastic of protective clothing and are not efficiently filtered by ordinary respirators. Most fumigants, including methyl bromide and **naphthalene**, act as narcotics, that is, they induce sleep or unconsciousness. Some, notably **ethylene dibromide** (**EDB**) and hydrogen cyanide, are not simply narcotic; they are also highly toxic to humans.

Herbicides

Weeds, unwanted plant species that compete with cultivated plants for nutrients, light, and water, destroy roughly the same proportion of crops as do insects, roughly 10 to 15% in the United States. As previously noted, herbicide production and use has increased enormously in the last 25 years, overtaking and exceeding insecticide use. More than 60% of the pesticides used in agriculture are herbicides. Nearly all agricultural land planted with corn, soybeans, cotton, peanuts, and rice in the United States is treated with at least one herbicide. But herbicide use is not limited to farming. Of the millions of pounds of herbicides used annually in the United States, a substantial amount is used to clear weeds from public lands, railroad embankments, roadsides, irrigation canals, power lines, golf courses, and backyard gardens.

The organic herbicides[4] are a chemically diverse group, which includes not only the well-known **2,4-D** and **2,4,5-T**, but also atrazine, **dicamba, paraquat,** and linuron. Because herbicides do not fall into a few tidy groupings, few generalizations can be made regarding their mode of action, environmental fate, or effects on nontarget species. Thus, the reader should refer to their individual entries in Part II. Herbicides vary in selectivity, persistence in tissues and the environment, and ability to be absorbed by plants.

Herbicides are applied by a variety of methods and at varying times during a plant's growing cycle, depending on the desired effect. Some are applied over relatively large areas, either in bands along crop rows or over entire cropland areas. Other applications are on a smaller scale as spot treatments or directed spraying on selected targets. Timing of applications depends on the chemical used, the crop species, the weed species, and the climate, among other things. Herbicides are used prior to planting, after planting but shortly before the crop or weeds emerge, or after the plants have begun to grow.

Fungicides

Traditionally, fungi (molds and mildews) have been classified by biologists as plants. More recent schemes, however, treat them as a distinct and separate group of organisms. Along with bacteria, fungi decompose organic material, be it cloth, paint, cardboard, bread, or living plants. Fungi are parasites on living organisms, deriving nutrients by penetrating the host's tissues. This characteristic makes controlling them without injuring the living plant a bit tricky.

Some 80 million pounds of fungicides are applied annually in the United States to prevent fungal destruction of such crops as pota-

toes, apples, peanuts, tomatoes, and plums. Most of the 150 or so fungicides in use function only on the surface that has been treated, necessitating repeated applications to new plant growth. Recently, however, several new and effective *systemic* fungicides have been developed, eliminating the need for frequent spraying and reducing the possibility of environmental contamination.

The most widely used organic fungicides, developed mostly in the 1930s and 1940s, fall into just a few chemical groups. The first group includes **captan, captafol,** and **folpet.** Structurally quite similar to the drug thalidomide, which has been found to cause extensive birth defects, this group has been well studied. To date, there is no evidence that captan, captafol, or folpet cause birth defects or other reproductive problems, but recent data suggest other potential chronic effects (see entry in Part II).

Carbamate derivatives, another major group of fungicides, include the comparatively new and successful systemic fungicide **benomyl** and the most widely used fungicides in the world, namely, **mancozeb, maneb, metiram,** and **zineb.** Known collectively as the ethylenebisdithiocarbamates or **EBDCs,** more than 30 million pounds of these four structurally and chemically similar compounds are used in the United States alone. Generally of low acute toxicity, the EBDCs are contaminated with and are readily degraded to ethylene thiourea (ETU), a substance that has been implicated as a cause of cancer, mutations, and birth defects, as well as being a specific toxin to the thyroid gland. As a result, the EBDCs are undergoing a *Special Review* by the EPA. Other fungicides chemically related to the EBDCs do not break down to ETU, but like other carbamates, they can potentially form nitrosocarbamate compounds in the stomach of humans and other mammals. Unlike the insecticidal carbamate derivatives, the fungicidal carbamates do not inhibit cholinesterase, the enzyme involved in the transmission of nerve signals.

[4] Most of the herbicides discussed here are based on a carbon–hydrogen ring structure to which oxygen, nitrogen, chlorine, or sulfur have been added.

Several fungicides, such as chlorothalonil, pentachlorophenol, and hexachlorobenzene, can be loosely classified as **benzene** ring derivatives. Pentachlorophenol is used not only as a fungicide, but also as a wood preservative against termites and as an herbicide.

C. Human Health Concerns

All of us are unavoidably and routinely exposed to a smorgasbord of pesticides in the air we breathe, the water we drink, the foods we eat, and even the consumer products we buy. Pesticides are lodged in tissues of people living in even very remote places throughout the world. As a result of environmental contamination, the concentration of certain pesticides in human breast milk has at certain times in some areas exceeded the *tolerance* level for milk (which is the maximum amount of pesticide residue legally permitted by the EPA). Around the country, many drinking water wells—the primary source of water for about half of the nation's population—have been closed as a result of pesticide contamination. Recent surveys show that a substantial fraction of both our domestically grown and imported fruits and vegetables reach the market with detectable levels of pesticide residues. As many as 4.0 to 4.5 million agricultural workers (including farmers, pesticide mixers and applicators, and field hands) are exposed to relatively high levels. The U.S. Department of Health, Education, and Welfare has estimated that more than 350,000 workers are potentially exposed to pesticides in chemical plants where the active ingredients are manufactured or the pesticides formulated.

Recently, media attention, public interest, and legislative discussion—even action—have focused on the issue of exposure to pesticides. Is there cause for concern about pesticides in our food and water or about occupational exposures? To address that question, we examine a number of incidents and problems associated with worker, community, and consumer exposure to pesticides.

Human Exposure

That workers engaged in the manufacture of pesticides can be and have been exposed to dangerously high levels of the materials is a matter of record. And the consequences of excessive exposure have been documented. Over a 14-month period in the mid-1970s, for example, dozens of factory workers from a plant producing the pesticide Kepone (technically known as chlordecone) were treated for a severe disorder of the nervous system. Called the "shakes" by the workers, this ailment eventually was tied to the pesticide and the grossly negligent working conditions under which it was produced. In 1976, the EPA cancelled the registration of Kepone following the 1975 shutdown of the manufacturing plant in Hopewell, Virginia. This decision was made only after a drawn-out series of investigations revealing that workers were exposed to high levels of Kepone, which was known to be very toxic (the manufacturers had possessed numerous studies disclosing neurologic and adverse reproductive effects). Workers were not required to wear respirators or protective clothing and, in fact, did not (workers stated that they had even handled the material with bare hands). Safety equipment installed in the plant was evidently either inoperable or inadequate; casual on-site inspections revealed heavy coatings of white powder everywhere. Also, waste water from the plant had contaminated both the local municipal sewage plant and, as a consequence, the James River, resulting in the closure of the important commercial fishing and shellfishing industries there.

Despite numerous complaints about illness and safety and reports that dozens of workers had been hospitalized, the Occupational Safety and Health Administration failed to respond meaningfully. Moreover, very little follow-up has been done on the long-term effects on the workers, although animal studies have indicated that Kepone causes liver abnormalities, possibly including liver cancer, as well as reproductive impairment. A court case on environmental contamination by Kepone, however, did result in record penalties under the Clean Water Act.

A similar situation in California resulted in the 1977 cancellation of the EPA registration of the soil fumigant dibromochloropropane (DBCP). Although DBCP was considered to be a possible human carcinogen, production and use were stopped only after the compound was linked to sterility in male factory workers. By that time, it was too late to prevent widespread exposure. Thousands of pounds of the pesticide had been used since 1955 to kill root-eating worms and had percolated into groundwater systems. At last count, more than 2000 wells in California's San Joaquin Valley had detectable levels of DBCP. Of course, DBCP is not the only pesticide found in the groundwater of agricultural communities. A 1985 report to the California State Assembly pointed out that 36 different pesticides have been detected in the groundwater of six agricultural counties.

The causal link between exposure to pesticides and community-wide, chronic, or long-term health effects has not been established, but suggestive evidence exists. In several farming communities in California's Central Valley, unusual clusters of childhood cancers have been reported. That is, the number of cases of specific cancers in the communities appears to be higher than would normally be expected. The cancer victims shared a common factor; most of their fathers had worked in treated fields before the child's conception. To date, however, no link has been established between intensive pesticide use and the apparent high incidence of certain cancers, but neither the greater than normal number of cases nor the occurrence of particular kinds of cancer has been explained. While investigations into these cases continue, studies of other agricultural areas have found evidence of greater than expected incidences of stomach cancer, cancer of the lymphatic system, and certain birth defects.

Incidents such as the Kepone and DBCP cases have made both industry and the government aware that lax safety standards and regulatory efforts are economically and socially costly. But the lessons learned have not been translated into comprehensive protection for agricultural workers or for the communities in which they live.

It is far more difficult to develop and enforce occupational standards for farmworkers than for people engaged in pesticide manufacturing, in part because of the difficulty in accurately assessing the amount of exposure. Unlike the manufacturing process, which concentrates the chemicals in a relatively confined space, agricultural use disperses pesticides widely and unpredictably. In the United States, approximately 65% of all pesticides are applied by aerial spraying, a large fraction of which may drift one-fourth mile or more from the target site.

Moreover, we do not have accurate estimates of the number of people exposed and affected, largely because so many farmworkers are seasonal or migrant workers and we simply do not keep track of them. Some authorities suggest that more than 300,000 farmworkers in the United States may have symptoms of pesticide-related illness. Most of the cases go unreported because even many of the acute symptoms, such as dizziness and vomiting, are relatively nonspecific and cannot be readily distinguished from those caused by other illnesses. Furthermore, many farmworkers, particularly field hands, do not know that they are entitled to medical care. And an unknown number are illegal workers who are unlikely to seek help in any case.

Most instances of reported and estimated pesticide-related illnesses are based on acute exposure, in which symptoms show up shortly after direct contact with the chemical or its *metabolite* (breakdown product). Even more uncertain is the number of people who may suffer chronic or long-term effects, ranging from cancer to sterility to liver damage.

There are significant regional differences in the amount of exposure and the compounds to which workers are exposed. About 30% of the country's field hands are employed in California, Texas, and Washington—three states that rely heavily on *restricted pesticides,* that is, those available only to certified personnel. In contrast, only about 10% of all fieldworkers work in the grainbelt, where they are exposed primarily to less toxic chemicals. Different climatic conditions contribute to regional variations in exposure. For instance, atmospheric inversions and heavy ground fog can reduce the rate at which pesticide vapors are diluted and carried away in the atmosphere. Consequently, entire communities can be exposed to unusually high concentrations of airborne pesticides. In California's San Joaquin Valley, heavy ground fog commonly blankets the area during the winter. In one incident, an entire town had to be evacuated when an atmospheric inversion trapped pesticide vapors.

Farmworkers are exposed to pesticides in a variety of ways. Like industrial workers, farmers and laborers who actually mix and apply pesticides may come into direct contact with high concentrations of the chemicals. According to EPA regulations, private and commercial pesticide applicators must be trained and certified. Inappropriate pesticide use is illegal and can result in penalties, but monitoring and enforcement are haphazard. While there are regulations for particular pesticides requiring the use of protective clothing and special equipment (such as long-sleeved shirts, long pants, boots, gloves, masks or respirators, and enclosed cabs), compliance is inconsistent. In 1982, nearly 200 cases of pesticide poisoning were reported in California among all farmworkers, including applicators. The number is a significant reduction from the 1975 level of more than 300 cases, suggesting an increased use of effective protective measures. When fieldworkers alone are considered, however, a different picture emerges. The number of reported poisoning cases increased between 1975 and 1982, probably largely as a result of increased awareness among field hands that medical treatment was available. Most authorities agree that the actual number of fieldworker poisonings is vastly underreported. Even so, it is claimed that the highest rate of occupationally related illness (7 per 1000 full-time workers per year in California) occurs among field hands.

It is the field hands who reenter fields to prune, pick, and weed soon after pesticide treatment and are thereby often exposed to dangerously high levels of residues. Neither the EPA nor OSHA have adequately addressed the issue of reentry into treated fields. At issue are several concerns: (1) the rate of breakdown of pesticides, (2) the breakdown products themselves, and (3) the effectiveness of protective gear. Both EPA and OSHA have proposed specific reentry waiting periods or intervals for individual pesticides to allow them to degrade sufficiently. Unfortunately, growers have not been happy with extended reentry periods, and the shorter periods that have been adopted by EPA appear to be based more on convenience than on safety. California, the nation's largest agricultural producer, has developed substantially longer reentry intervals than those recommended by the federal government, as shown in the comparison of federal and California reentry intervals in Table 8.

Standardized reentry periods for specific pesticides may be inadequate, in any case, because pesticides break down at varying rates, depending on ambient moisture, rainfall, temperature, and humidity. In the hot, dry California climate, for instance, residues remain on the plant surfaces longer than they do in the Southeast, where frequent precipitation washes the residues from the leaves. In addition, some breakdown products are considerably more toxic than the parent compounds, such as **parathion**.

Farmers may legally permit early reentry to fields (that is, after intervals shorter than those specified in Table 8) as long as the field hands are provided with protective clothing. In this respect and, more generally, in permitting the continued use of extremely toxic compounds at all, EPA policy relies on the

TABLE 8 A Comparison of Reentry Intervals: California versus Federal Regulations

| Pesticide | California | | | Federal |
	Citrus	Peaches	Grapes	All crops
Parathion	30 days[a]	21 days	21 days	48 hours
Azinophos-methyl	30 days	14 days	21 days	24 hours
Chlorobenzilate	14 days	—	—	None
Diazinon	5 days	5 days	5 days	None
Methomyl	2 days	2 days	2 days	None
Malathion	1 day	1 day	1 day	None
Endosulfon	48 hours on all crops			None

[a]The interval varies depending on the application rate; at the highest rate, the interval is 60 days.
Source: Adapted from Wasserstram, R. F. and Wiles, R. 1985. *Field Duty. U.S. Farmworkers and Pesticide Safety.* Washington, D.C.: World Resources Institute. Study 3.

efficacy (and consistent use) of protective clothing. Few studies, however, have shown that such clothing is actually effective.[5] Studies do show that pesticides have differing abilities to penetrate fabrics. For some pesticides, extending the reentry period, taking into account regional differences in breakdown times, and requiring protective outerwear no doubt suffice, but some pesticides, like parathion, appear to cause illness in direct proportion to the amount used.

Some regulations to protect fieldworkers apparently have been completely disregarded. There are, for example, reported cases of field hands being exposed during spray operations, either directly or from aerial drift from adjacent fields. Even more horrifying are stories of migrant workers and their families who actually live in or near treated fields and who obtain their drinking, bathing, and cooking water from contaminated irrigation canals or use discarded pesticide containers to hold water.

[5]A recent study comparing the protective properties of commonly used clothing fabrics found that cotton and cotton/polyester blends afford considerably better protection (that is, they allow less pesticide to penetrate from the surface) than 100% nylon, acrylic, or polyester fabrics. None of the common apparel fabrics, however, repelled pesticides nearly as well as the moisture-resistant protective clothing, such as 100% olefin, made for agricultural pesticide applicators.

Consumer Safety

During the summer of 1985, about 1000 people were poisoned after eating watermelons that contained residues of the *systemic* insecticide **aldicarb**. Although it is not and was not registered for use on watermelons, aldicarb was the most frequently detected pesticide on the fruit during that year. Similarly, illegal residues of **heptachlor** have been detected in the milk of dairy cows in Hawaii, Arkansas, Oklahoma, and Missouri. The insecticide turned up in the milk after the cows had been fed fodder containing residues. In Hawaii, a considerable amount of the contaminated milk was consumed before the problem was discovered and the milk recalled. Several long-term studies to monitor babies exposed to heptachlor have been initiated because the insecticide was found in the breast milk of nursing mothers.

Poisoning and contamination incidents, recent studies, and scientific reports have served to focus public attention on the issue of pesticide residues in or on food. A recent survey conducted by the Natural Resources Defense Council (NRDC), covering foods sampled by the federal Food and Drug Administration (FDA) and the California Department of Food and Agriculture (CDFA) between 1982 and 1985, revealed a high frequency of pesticide residues on both domestic and imported produce. Nationwide, about

48% of the produce tested (domestic and imported combined) contained detectable residues. In contrast, only 14% of the samples of California-grown fruits and vegetables had residues. In all, 110 pesticides were detected. Of the 25 pesticides that were found most frequently, 9 are listed as (probable or possible) human carcinogens by the EPA. They are acephate, **captan**, chlorothalonil, **DDT**, **dieldrin**, **folpet**, methomyl, **parathion**, and **permethrin**.

Furthermore, the number of residues found is undoubtedly lower than the number of residues that exist because routine tests employed by both the FDA and California testing laboratories can detect only about half of the pesticides registered for use on any given crop. For example, of the nearly 90 different pesticides registered for use on potatoes, roughly half cannot be detected by the FDA's routine testing methods. Even so, one-fifth of the potatoes sampled contained residues of one or more of 38 different pesticides. More than 110 pesticides are permitted on apples, although, again, standard tests can detect only half of them. The NRDC report revealed that 43 different pesticides were found on apples and about one-third of the apples sampled contained residues. Potatoes and apples are important constituents of the American diet: the average consumer eats about 54 pounds of potatoes and 22 pounds of apples a year.

Among the residues that are not detected using routine analytical methods are several that have been associated with long-term adverse health effects. The list includes **alachlor, benomyl, daminozide** (Alar), and the **EBDCs**. Benomyl, for instance, is a systemic fungicide that is mutagenic in animal tests and is listed as a possible human carcinogen by the EPA. Nevertheless, it is used on 43 food crops. Moreover, evidence shows that it becomes concentrated in certain processed foods as a result of the processing. Consequently, residues of the pesticide are found in higher levels in fruit juices and dried fruits than in fresh fruit.

Pesticide residues are distributed unevenly among food crops. Corn, for example, contains few residues and those only infrequently. In contrast, certain crops for which there are high cosmetic standards, such as peaches, pears, and strawberries, frequently have many different residues. High cosmetic standards necessitate pesticide use to produce perfect-looking, blemish-free fruits and vegetables, even though the blemishes do not affect the taste or nutritional value of the food.

A Congressional report released in 1982 pointed out that most of the 600 pesticides currently in use were registered prior to 1984 under considerably less stringent standards than those that newer pesticides must meet. The report also found that 85% of registered pesticides have not been adequately tested for *carcinogenicity,* that more than 90% have not had sufficient testing for *mutagenicity,* and that there is too little information regarding the possibility of birth defects for 60 to 70% of the pesticides on the market. Similarly, a study by the National Academy of Sciences was unable to assess fully the health effects of about 90% of the pesticides it examined because so much pertinent information was missing.

Despite such glaring gaps in the data, EPA policy permits a pesticide to be sold if it judges that the product is not likely to cause more than "one additional case of cancer in the lifetime of 1,000,000 people." According to a recent report by the National Academy of Sciences, the dietary *oncogenic* (tumor-producing) risk for 23 of 28 commonly used pesticides exceeds this operational cancer standard. These risk estimates, it should be noted, are considered to be conservative, meaning that the cancer risk is not likely to be higher and may be as low as zero.

At the heart of the food safety issue is the question of whether existing *tolerances* (maximum allowable residue levels) are reasonable. For pesticides that do not appear to cause either benign or cancerous tumors, the EPA calculates an *acceptable daily intake (ADI)* on the basis of the *no observed effect level (NOEL)* in test animals, which often is information supplied by the pesticide manufacturer. Dividing the NOEL by a safety factor, usually 100, yields the ADI, a level of dietary exposure deemed generally safe. The ADI is compared with another estimate, the theoretical maximum residue contribution (TMRC). The TMRC is calculated for each food item in which a given pesticide could be found. The EPA effectively overestimates exposure by assuming that the pesticide in question is used on all crops for which a tolerance exists and that pesticide residues are present at the maximum level permitted on all food items. If the TMRC is smaller than the ADI, the tolerance is approved. Tolerances for compounds that have been found to produce tumors are determined differently. EPA instead uses quantitative risk assessment models.

These procedures have a number of problems, even beyond the obvious one that relevant health and safety tests have not yet been performed for most pesticides. First, because the Federal Insecticide, Fungicide, and Rodenticide Act (FIFRA) permits the EPA to consider benefits when registering a pesticide, tolerances have been established for many carcinogenic pesticides on raw agricultural commodities even though there may be no "safe" level (see Chapter 1, Section A). Until recently, the EPA declined to issue tolerances for processed foods because the Delaney Clause of the Federal Food, Drug, and Cosmetic Act (FFDCA) specifically prohibits cancer-causing additives on or in processed food (see Chapter 17, Section D). This policy has been changed; in effect, the EPA has abandoned the Delaney Clause and now applies a cancer risk exception of 1 in 1,000,000 uniformly.

Many of the tolerances set for raw agricultural commodities were established on the basis of outdated assumptions about the average American diet. Eating habits have changed considerably over the last 20 to 30 years. We eat much more fresh produce—26 pounds more per year on the average—than just 10 years ago. There has been a shift to formerly exotic or less available foods such as artichokes, nectarines, zucchini, and mushrooms. Also, food tolerances generally do not take into account differences in diet and relative intake between adults and children (children eat proportionally more of fewer foods and more food per unit body weight), which suggests that children are less well protected.

Tolerances are rarely revised even when new data become available. No tolerances for *inert ingredients* have been established, although several, including **benzene** and **carbon tetrachloride**, are known carcinogens. These inert ingredients occur in pesticide products and may well show up as residues on food. Nor are there tolerances for certain breakdown products, many of which are hazardous to human health. Finally, the limits set for exposure to pesticides through food do not take into account additional exposure through nonfood sources, such as manufactured goods.

As already mentioned, many residues escape detection because the FDA testing methods are inadequate. What is found is alarming enough. Mevinphos, an acutely toxic organophosphate that is supposed to break down in one or two days (thus, in theory, would not be detectable by the time the produce reached the market), was the most frequently detected residue on lettuce, according to the NRDC survey. Despite being banned in 1972, **DDT** was the most frequently found residue on carrots. The DDT residue in or on root crops may be a result of *persistence* in the soils. Another possible explanation is that DDT is a contaminant of two widely used pesticides, dicofol and chlorobenzilate. Also, DDT continues to be used in other countries and shows up on imported foods.

In fact, there is no doubt that unwanted and unwarranted pesticides turn up on imported foods. In a comparison of imported and domestic produce, the NRDC report showed that nearly two-thirds of the imported produce sampled contained detectable pesticide residues (Table 9). What Table 9 does not reveal is that many of the residues on imported foods, such as DDT, are illegal (banned, restricted, or never registered) in the United States. Many of these, such as DBCP and **2,4,5-T**, continued to be

TABLE 9 Comparison of Pesticide Residues Found on Domestic versus Imported Produce

Sample	Number of Samples	Number with Residues	Percentage with Residues
Domestic	11,729	4,450	38
Imported	7,686	4,922	64
Total	19,415	9,372	48

manufactured here and shipped abroad long after domestic use was curtailed. The Government Accounting Office estimates that 25% or more of the pesticides exported from the United States cannot be used domestically. The so-called circle of poison is complete when those residues return here on luxury crops such as coffee, cocoa, and pineapples (and out-of-season melons, tomatoes, and grapes) produced chiefly in developing countries.

While agricultural working conditions in the United States need improvement, conditions in developing countries are even more lamentable. To produce luxury export crops for our tables, Third World workers are exposed to excessively high levels of particularly dangerous chemicals, in many cases without even minimal protection. Warning labels and directions for handling, mixing, applying, and storing pesticides are often written in English, a language that laborers and fieldworkers in other countries are unlikely to know.

Legislative efforts to change our pesticide export policy, to address the issue of residues on foods, and to speed up the process of testing older pesticides have gained increasing attention and momentum. To promote needed legislative changes, the consumer can become better informed about the issues (see the reading list at the end of this chapter) and can follow-up by encouraging state and federal action. Lifestyle can reduce exposure to pesticide residues, as well. The following suggestions can be particularly helpful.

Wash, peel, or trim fresh produce; many pesticides can be removed or reduced in this way.

Grow fruits and vegetables at home.

Buy certified organically grown produce; it is increasingly available and even large chain supermarkets are responding to demand.

Buy fruits and vegetables in season and select domestically grown produce.

If pesticides are used at home, the precautions and instructions on the label should be heeded. Since the major route of pesticide poisoning is through the skin, it is particularly important to cover up when handling pesticides. Many product labels suggest that consumers wear gloves and protective clothing. They do not, however, specify the type of clothing or gloves that are most effective. As previously mentioned, cotton and cotton/polyester blend fabrics do a reasonably good job of preventing pesticides from reaching the skin. Cloth and leather gloves, however, can easily become wet and absorb pesticides. (Commercial applicators use gloves of neoprene or some other impermeable material for most purposes, but only natural rubber provides an adequate barrier to organophosphates.) Just as cloth or leather gloves can become soaked with pesticides, so can canvas or leather shoes; rubber boots thus provide better protection. Because so many pesticides cause eye irritation and can be absorbed into the body through the eye, goggles or other eye covering should be worn.

D. Environmental and Economic Constraints

Just as it is clear that pesticides pose health risks, evidence is growing that there are undesirable ecological and economic consequences of their ever-increasing use. Widespread distribution of pesticides, harmful effects on non-target species, and unwanted and unanticipated effects on the pests themselves are the end results of an excessive reliance on chemical pest control that cannot be sustained.

Today, pesticides are widely distributed in the environment. Why? The answer lies in our methods of application and in natural processes. Of the tremendous quantity of pesticides used domestically in agriculture, only a small fraction actually reaches the intended target, be it the Colorado potato beetle decimating the potato crop, the morning glory running rampant in the corn field, or the powdery mildew dusting the leaves of the peach trees. Washed from the leaves and soil by rain or carried by the wind, pesticides disperse to adjacent fields, streams, lakes, pastures, and woodlands. Pesticides travel through soils to underground water systems. They have been found in drinking water wells from Maine to Texas to California and throughout the world. Residues contaminate the sediments of our major rivers, and some, ultimately, are deposited in the sea.

Pesticide residues are taken up from soil and water by pest and nonpest species alike. The *persistent* substances that can be transferred through the *food chain,* such as the *organochlorines,* evidently reside in all living organisms. Residues have been found in the tissues of seals and penguins in Antarctica, in fishes from coral reefs and the deep ocean, and in human breast milk throughout the world. **DDT,** for example, continues to be found in human fat tissue at readily detectable levels, although those levels have declined steadily since use of the insecticide was banned in the United States in 1972.

There is plenty of evidence that the more toxic but less persistent pesticides, such as the *organophosphates* and *carbamates,* can have harmful effects not only on pests but also on nontarget species, including humans, cows, fishes, birds, plants, soil microorganisms, and beneficial insects. In fact there have been numerous incidents of unintentional poisonings of wildlife, including fishes, waterfowl,

and mammals, as a result of improper spraying, inadvertent spills, or inappropriate choice of pesticide. Typically such incidents, although unfortunate, have relatively limited impact; the effects are commonly localized and of short duration, and affected populations normally can recover following a single exposure.

But some exposures do have more severe effects. For example, each year in the United States thousands of honeybee colonies are killed inadvertently by pesticides. It has been estimated that roughly 11% of California's honeybee colonies are lost each year to pesticides. Dozens of agricultural crops, including orchard fruits and alfalfa, depend on pollination by honeybees. Because the bees are particularly susceptible to certain carbamates, efforts are being made to restrict carbamate use and to rely on other less harmful pesticides.

Ecological Constraints

Today's agriculture appears locked into a system that is utterly dependent on chemical pest control, but signs of problems are becoming increasingly apparent. Despite increasing volume and greater diversity of chemicals, agricultural returns are declining. Although worldwide agricultural yields have doubled since 1950 as a result of new agricultural practices (including use of high-yield grains and massive chemical inputs), we are getting less yield per unit effort. In the period from 1945 to 1984, losses to insects nearly doubled from 7 to 13% and losses to weeds increased from 8 to 12%, all while pesticide inputs soared. Why?

Basically, pesticides have become less effective as a result of several biological consequences of repeated, heavy doses of pesticides. These include *resurgence* or rebound of the primary pest species following an initial suppression of numbers; *secondary outbreaks* of other, previously minor pests; the promotion to pest status of previous nonpest species; and the development of pesticide *resis-*

tance (the ability of a pest to withstand the effects of a pesticide).

To understand these responses to pesticide use, it is necessary to know a bit about the underlying ecology and biology of pest species. In a natural ecosystem, say a meadow, many kinds of organisms, such as grasses, wildflowers, aphids, spiders, worms, soil bacteria, lichens, birds, and field mice, are interdependent. They interact with each other in a variety of ways, the sum of which maintains the health and vitality of the meadow. Although the number of individuals of each species changes over time (days, months, or years), the populations generally remain within certain bounds, held in check by the availability of food and habitat, by the presence of natural enemies and competitors, and by environmental factors such as temperature and rainfall.

Characteristically, pest species are able to adapt readily to a variety of living conditions and to produce many offspring rapidly. That's why they are such effective pests. Aphids, for example, can produce a new generation each week during the period in which they reproduce (Fig. 15). A termite queen can produce as many as 150 million eggs during her several year lifespan. Such tremendous reproductive capabilities coupled with the ability to survive under less than ideal conditions make pest species able to recover easily from setbacks and quick to take over, which is why they are so difficult to eliminate.

Prevailing agricultural systems differ from natural systems in several important ways that tend to upset the balance of organisms. Throughout much of the country, soybeans, cotton, apples, and most other crops are grown as single, intentionally uniform crops, or *monocultures*, on large plots of land. For plant-feeding insects, monocultures present a lavish and inviting banquet of readily available and tasty food. And compared to a grassy meadow studded with a variety of bushes and trees, there are fewer nesting or hiding places for natural enemies and fewer alternative food sources for competitors. Moreover, if not for the intensive human intervention in the form of plowing and spraying, the fields and orchards would be overrun by numerous other plant species and a variety of animals would move in.

What happens when a farmer intervenes with pesticides? Certainly, the pest is killed in large numbers, but as previously mentioned, so are many other species—including the predators and parasites that normally keep the pest population relatively small. In fact, it is not uncommon for nontarget species to be more severely affected than the pest; sometimes nonpest species are more sensitive to certain pesticides, as honeybees are to carbamate insecticides. And even if they are not directly affected by the pesticide, the loss of their primary food source can cause predators or parasites to starve or move away.

When a cornfield or an apple orchard is sprayed, many of the pests are killed, but not all of them. Even when spraying can be likened to saturation bombing, some fraction of the population escapes by chance or because they are genetically resistant to the effects of the poison. With astonishing swiftness, the survivors are able to build up the population to high levels, sometimes far greater than the original, and with particular ease, because their natural enemies either have disappeared or there are too few left to be effective. This is resurgence of the primary pest.

Another consequence of the loss of predators, parasites, or competitors due to pesticide use, is that other species, especially insects and fungi, erupt. Secondary outbreaks involve species that normally would be considered minor pests at worst. Typically, the secondary pests coexist with the target species, but do far less damage to the crops because their numbers are so few. Their population size is kept low by natural controls. But human intervention alters the normal relationships, and in some cases, a new pest not only erupts, but takes center stage, as has occurred with the cotton bollworm (see Section E, this chapter).

Typically, in response to the resurgence of

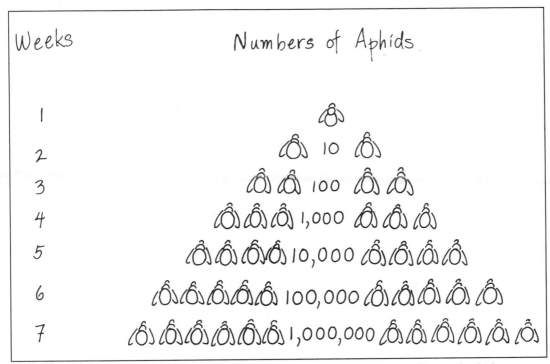

Figure 15 Aphid reproduction. A single female aphid can establish a large population of aphids very quickly. If each daughter produces 10 daughters each generation, then there will be 1,000,000 in just 6 weeks. Imagine the numbers if each female produced 100 daughters instead of 10.

the original target species and/or a secondary outbreak, the farmer sprays again, which leads to further suppression of remaining or returning natural enemies, permitting another cycle of increase and so on. The farmer is caught on the pesticide treadmill.

Because the resurgent and outbreak populations are produced mostly by pesticide-resistant individuals, the natural (genetic) capacity for resistance is passed on to succeeding generations. This is a form of natural selection, the same principle applied by plant and animal breeders, such as the dairy farmer who chooses to breed those cows that produce the most milk in an effort to develop a highly productive herd. The more intense the selection effort or pressure, the more quickly a particular characteristic can be established. Very simply, the more choosy the breeder, the more quickly will the proportion of high-milk producers in the herd be increased. So, too, increasing pesticide exposure pushes the pest population toward pesticide resistance.

The ability of highly adaptable, fast-breeding pests to resist the effects of pesticides is a growing problem. The number of resistant species has increased dramatically in response to modern pesticides (Fig. 16). As shown in the figure, nearly 450 insect and mite species have become resistant to one or more insecticides or acaricides. Similarly, about 150 resistant fungi and other agents that cause plant disease have been identified. Weeds have also developed resistance, with approximately 50 resistant species found so far. Some pests, such as houseflies, mosquitoes, cotton boll-worms, cattle ticks, and spider mites, are not susceptible to the effects of any of the pesticides to which they have been extensively exposed.

Both resurgence and secondary outbreaks have resulted in substantial agricultural losses. A 1970 California study found that 24 of the major insect and mite pest species had become pests as a result of resurgence or secondary outbreaks. Moreover, 21 of those

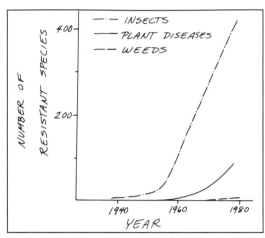

Figure 16 Resistance to pesticides is increasing among all pest species. (Adapted from Wasserman, R. F., and Wiles, R. 1985. *Field Duty: U.S. Farmworkers and Pesticide Safety.* Washington, D.C.: World Resources Institute.)

species were found to be resistant to the preferred insecticides. Especially distressing is the development of DDT resistance among malaria-carrying mosquitoes in Asia, Africa, and Latin America and the subsequent resurgence of the disease—once thought to be nearly eradicated. DDT resistance, a significant factor in the resurgence, was hastened by excessive agricultural spraying with DDT, which drifted into mosquito-breeding areas. Other pesticides, such as some of the organophosphates, are effective against the mosquitoes, but pose health and environmental problems of their own.

The development of resistance is no real surprise to biologists. After all, while plants have been evolving poisonous and other nasty compounds to discourage insect feeding, the vast majority of plant-eating insects have been evolving detoxification mechanisms, out of necessity. For millions of years, both the plant chemicals and the insects' mechanisms to deal with them have been undergoing small modifications. It is evidently not a big leap for many pest species to detoxify synthetic pesticides. Moreover, resistance to one class of pesticides often conveys resistance to another, very different class. For example, at

least ten species of DDT-resistant mosquitoes are resistant to one organophosphate (**malathion**), and another four species are resistant to at least one carbamate.

Economic Constraints

Maintenance of current patterns of pesticide use is becoming increasingly costly in monetary terms, too. It has been estimated that decimation of honeybee colonies and the consequent loss of pollination has cost California farmers and beekeepers millions of dollars each year. Generally, it is very difficult to assess the costs and benefits of pesticide use in economic terms. The perspective held by many scientists is that if all the costs of pesticide use could be taken into account, including all harmful effects on human health, the environment, and agriculture, the costs would outweigh the benefits. In practical terms, the easy, inexpensive chemicals have already been developed. The next generation of pesticides will have to be more highly selective for a particular pest organism to reduce the potential for harm to nontarget species. But as selectivity increases, so does the likelihood of resistance. Thus, the life expectancy of new pesticides is likely to be reduced.

A case in point is the focus in the last several years on the development of *systemic* fungicides. From an environmental point of view, they are preferable because application is more directed, the total dosage is lower, and the number of treatments required is less. Unfortunately, their greater specificity has already demonstrated a greater tendency to generate resistance. Moreover, while the fungicide market is important, it is small and cannot sustain the ever-increasing costs of developing new products to circumvent fungicide resistance.

More stringent government regulations that impose rigorous testing of new pesticides for long-term human health and environmental problems make the development of new pesticides more expensive. These costs are ultimately reflected in higher food prices.

E. Cotton: A Case Study

Throughout the world, cotton is a major cash crop; in some countries it is the main export item. Because of its economic importance, vast acreages are devoted to cotton production. This, plus the fact that domestication and selective breeding of cotton have resulted in strains of cotton plants that have lost some of their natural defenses against a variety of insect pests, make cotton highly vulnerable to insect attack. Cotton hosts at least half a dozen major pest species, including the pink bollworm, the cotton bollworm, the lygus bug or fleahopper, the boll weevil, the cotton aphid, and the tobacco budworm. Consequently, in many parts of the United States and other regions of the world, cotton is the major recipient of pesticide overload, accounting for roughly one-half of the volume of all insecticides applied.

In cotton-growing regions around the world—Central and South America, Egypt, Mexico, the southwestern United States, and Australia—a pattern of ecological backlash and economic setbacks has repeated itself over and over again as a result of excessive insecticide use. The combined effect of pesticide resistance, high mortality among natural enemies, secondary outbreaks, and resurgence are particularly well illustrated by the Peruvian experience.

In the coastal Canete Valley of Peru, cotton growers controlled pest species reasonably well until the late 1940s. They used inorganic and botanical insecticides, such as calcium arsenate and nicotine sulfate, both of which have a relatively small impact on the pests' natural enemies. With the introduction of the *organochlorines*, including **DDT**, **lindane**, endrin, and toxaphene, huge increases in cotton yields initially occurred. Following the dubious principle that if a little is good, then more is better, farmers blanketed the cotton-growing region with pesticides, increasing both the volume used and the frequency of application. The initial success story was short-lived.

By 1952, only a few years after the synthetic organic pesticides were introduced, the cotton aphid had become resistant to benzene hexachloride. Following in quick succession, toxaphene's effectiveness against the tobacco budworm was markedly reduced. By the mid-1950s, the boll weevil population had reached extremely high levels, predators and parasites of the pests had been killed or weakened, new pest species had appeared, and there was resurgence of the cotton bollworm, which had become resistant to DDT. To deal with the organochlorine resistance and multiple outbreaks, farmers switched to organophosphate insecticides and reduced the interval between sprayings from one or two weeks to three days. Nevertheless, cotton yields dropped to levels far below those obtained before the introduction of the organochlorines. Economic disaster ensued and prompted the establishment of an *Integrated Pest Management (IPM)* program, which proved to be a major success (see Section F).

Similar events have occurred in the United States. In California, for example, efforts to wipe out the lygus bug backfired, and instead, a variety of insect predators were killed, thereby causing massive outbreaks of the cotton bollworm and other moth caterpillars. Ironically, studies indicate that the lygus bug probably does little real damage to cotton crops since it generally feeds on surplus flower buds, that is, those that would not open anyway. The bollworm, however, is a serious cotton pest; the pink bollworm, for example, can easily destroy half of the crop or more. Efforts to control the pink bollworm with insecticides have succeeded in causing a secondary outbreak of the tobacco budworm, a cotton pest that is resistant to a variety of conventional insecticides and normally is held in check by an array of predators and parasites. Also, secondary outbreaks have occurred on noncotton crops in adjacent fields. Aphids and the beet armyworm, for example, have caused extensive damage to sugar beets and alfalfa. The pink bollworm problem is compounded by the feeding habit of this pest; it lives and feeds inside the closed cotton fruit, making it relatively inaccessible to insecticides.

It has been amply demonstrated, however, that the bollworm can be effectively controlled by some combination of IPM methods, as discussed in the next section. Spraying for the lygus bug only when and where needed reduces the amount of pesticides used, thereby minimizing the impact on its natural enemies. Planting early maturing cotton strains, harvesting early, and promptly destroying the residues deprives the bollworm of food and hiding places when it needs them most. Another approach involves the release of sterile adult male bollworms (moths) to reduce the reproductive success of the natural population.

F. Alternatives to Conventional Pest Control

The treadmill of conventional pesticide practice, with its continuously increasing requirements for synthetic pesticides and its constantly decreasing effectiveness, is fortunately not the only option available. Scientific data and practical experience show us that there are ecologically acceptable and economically feasible alternatives.

One of the best alternatives is *Integrated Pest Management (IPM)*. As the name implies, IPM is a carefully planned strategy that integrates a variety of pest control methods. It relies on a complementary mix of tactics, including biological control, modifications of agricultural practices, regulatory actions, and if needed, the selective use of both synthetic organic chemicals and naturally occurring pesticides. Although still in its early stages of development, IPM has gained wide acceptance and has proven effective in agricultural, forestry, and municipal applications. It has

reduced the use of the most hazardous pesticides by as much as 70% in some crops, with no losses in crop quantity or quality. Several California cities have had enormous success with IPM programs designed to maintain healthy shade trees along city streets. They have essentially eliminated the use of synthetic pesticides and have saved money at the same time. The Office of Technology Assessment has estimated that fully implemented IPM programs for major crops in the United States could reduce pesticide use overall by as much as 75%, while cutting losses to pests by about 50% and reducing costs as well.

Organic growers, however, entirely shun the use of any synthetic pesticides and growth regulators, as well as synthetic fertilizers and livestock feed additives. Instead, organic growers, including farmers and nursery growers, use a combination of naturally occurring pesticides (which are not without health risks; see **pyrethrum**) and the nonchemical methods that have been incorporated into IPM programs. Commercial organic farming has been practiced for years on a relatively small scale, but in the last few years, growing public concern with health and fitness has spurred expansion of the market for organically grown produce and animal products. In California, for example, several major supermarket chains routinely carry some certified organically grown produce. IPM programs are frequently employed as a transitional phase when growers switch from conventional, pesticide-laden agriculture to fully organic practices free of any synthetic chemicals.

Alternative pest control systems, whether IPM or organic, are based on sound ecological principles. An effective IPM program, for example, combines an understanding of the characteristics of the particular crop to be protected, the biology of the pest species in question, the local climatic conditions, and the presence or absence of the pest's natural enemies with careful monitoring of the levels of primary and secondary pest species. The important distinction between organic and

IPM methods is that the farmer using IPM may resort to synthetic pesticides when pest species reach some critical level, if other methods are considered inadequate or inappropriate at that point in the crop's development and the pest's life cycle. In either case, there are no cookbook strategies. Tactics to control a pest are geared to the particular problem at hand. Thus, alternative methods require more careful planning and attention than the conventional spraying by the calendar. As with conventional pest control, no method is completely free of risks or problems. The risks associated with alternative methods, however, are not only substantially different than those of the conventional approaches, but also less hazardous to human health and the environment.

Biological or Biorational Control

Biological or biorational control is a catchall category encompassing multiple approaches that exploit certain biological properties of pest or plant. Much biological control emphasizes the central role of natural enemies—predators, parasites, and disease-causing agents or pathogens—in controlling pests. Another approach involves genetic or reproductive manipulations of insect populations or plant chemistry. Finally, naturally occurring chemicals, such as those that regulate plant or insect growth, as well as synthetic analogs of these compounds, have great potential in biorational control.

Natural Enemies or Biological Control Agents

In nature, populations of most species of organisms are controlled or limited in size, in part, by natural enemies—predators, parasites, or competitors. Thus, pest species can also be held in check by their natural enemies. Both organic and IPM growers successfully control pests of citrus, corn, alfalfa, apples, olives, and so on by encouraging the pest's natural control agents. For this approach to work, it is necessary to provide nesting sites, hiding places, and alternative food sources for beneficial species. Where synthetic pesticides are used, as in the IPM programs, the method of application, the particular pesticide used, and the timing of the treatments are carefully designed to have a minimal impact on biological control organisms. Once established and left undisturbed, populations of natural enemies often can check excessive growth of pest species.

Many of the major pests are introduced species. They become pests as a result of arriving in an environment free of their natural controls. To correct the balance and contain such pests, specific natural enemies can be intentionally introduced. This is an effective tactic that has a long track record. For example, populations of the introduced European cabbage butterfly were contained following the importation in 1884 of a parasitic wasp that selectively lays its eggs in the developing caterpillars of this butterfly. At about this same time, a parasitic fly and a predatory beetle were imported from Australia to deal with the inadvertently introduced cottony cushion scale, which was decimating the California citrus industry. By 1890, two years after its importation, the ladybird beetle had been so completely successful that the cottony cushion scale was relegated to nonpest status—until the late 1940s when growers began using DDT against other pests. The ladybird bettle proved susceptible to DDT; the scale insect, however, was not. It caused severe economic damage to the citrus industry until DDT spraying was stopped and biological control was reestablished.

The ability of insects and other plant-eating pests to devastate a crop, a forest, or a backyard garden has been exploited to control a diverse array of weedy species. The garden plant lantana became a pest in Hawaii after its introduction, overrunning and crowding out native plants. Introduction of a lantana-loving moth has checked its destructive progress. Similarly, the association between insects and plant *pathogens* has been turned to our advantage. In Australia, a cactus introduced from North America as an ornamental became a tremendous pest, spreading rapidly through the arid regions of the continent. The introduction of a moth that transmits a disease-causing bacterium to the cactus while feeding on it has helped halt the spread of the pest plant. Various beetles, flies, and wasps also have all been used with good results in weed control efforts.

Microbial pesticides as a group show great promise as biological control agents. These are viruses and bacteria that infect the target pests (plants or animals) and cause disease. Most microbials are quite selective, infecting only one species or a limited number of closely related species. Although microbial pesticides are in an early stage of development, several are commercially available and widely used. The most well-established microbial pesticide is the insecticidal bacterium *Bacillus thuringiensis,* which is used against moth and butterfly pests of crops and forests.

Genetic and Reproductive Manipulations

Biological control through genetic manipulations has proven highly successful. One approach is to use insects for their own self-destruction by taking advantage of their mating behavior. Laboratory-reared sterile or genetically inferior individuals of the pest species are released into the population in sufficiently large numbers to result in a preponderance of sterile matings or the production of offspring unable to survive or compete for mates. The screwworm, for example, a major pest of livestock in several regions of the United States, has been controlled by an aggressive program involving the release of sterile males.

Another kind of genetic manipulation is the selective breeding of strains of plants that resist attack by particular insects or diseases. Conventional selective breeding, as done to obtain a higher yield in many crop species, has resulted in some losses of natural defense mechanisms. This increases the need to "breed back" the defensive compounds. Development of resistant varieties has economic as well as ecological merit. It has been esti-

mated, for instance, that Canadian and U.S. wheat farmers save hundreds of millions of dollars annually by growing strains of wheat that are resistant to two species of highly destructive flies. There are, however, drawbacks to restoring natural defensive compounds; many, such as solanine, are quite toxic to humans as well as to pests.

Behavior and Growth Control Regulators

Additional biorational methods use a diversity of naturally occurring compounds (or their synthetic analogs) to affect the behavior or growth of insects or plants. Insect pheromones, for example, are highly selective hormone-like substances that affect behavior by eliciting specific responses (sex attraction, alarm, or aggregation) in other members of the same species. Pheromones are commonly used in IPM programs to monitor population levels by luring insects to traps. They are also used successfully to disrupt mating in the cotton pest, the pink bollworm. Insect growth regulators (IGRs), such as *juvenile hormone,* disrupt the insect's life cycle by interfering with normal developmental processes.

An assorted group of naturally occurring or synthetic compounds that affect plant growth and development called plant-growth regulators are technically considered to be pesticides and are used by both alternative and conventional pest control operations. These compounds act variously to stimulate or inhibit growth; to regulate development, flowering, or fruit ripening; to prevent sprouting in stored potatoes and onions; to prolong dormancy in fruit trees; and to stimulate root development.

Control Using Mechanical and Cultivation Techniques

Among the simplest approaches to alternative pest control are those involving modification of agricultural practices to make the environment less favorable to the pests. Cultural and mechanical farming practices that effectively discourage or destroy pests include increasing crop diversity (to increase natural enemies or provide other food for pests), rotating crops (to prevent pest buildup on a single crop), changing planting and harvesting times (to avoid periods of pest buildup), disposing of crop residues (to remove overwintering sites for some pests), tilling after harvest (to kill weeds and insects outright), and flooding of fields (to drown insects and weeds).

One particularly good example of this approach is the control of the lygus bug, an especially destructive pest of cotton, alfalfa, beans, and other major crops. In California, two methods of control have been developed on the basis of ecological studies to determine the preferred food plants, the dispersal patterns into the agricultural area, and the pest's life cycle requirements. In the spring, the lygus bug develops on wild plants in the areas surrounding the cultivated fields. As those plants dry up, the insect moves to alfalfa fields. Although cotton is not a preferred food plant, the bug is then forced to switch to cotton when the alfalfa is harvested. Both control methods exploit the lygus bug's preference for alfalfa rather than cotton and permit survival of natural enemies. The first method is used to protect cotton and is called trap planting. Alfalfa is interplanted in strips among the cotton crop, and the lygus bug preferentially stays on the alfalfa. Similarly, the lygus bug's predators and parasites stay with their preferred food source. The other method is used to protect alfalfa and is a modification of alfalfa harvesting practices done to avoid totally depleting the lygus bug's preferred food. Only half of the alfalfa is harvested at a time, in strips, so that the bug has no incentive to move onto the cotton. Since in this case the alfalfa is grown for feed, proper timing of alfalfa cutting in relation to the insect's development cycle is critical. The farmer, not wanting to lose the alfalfa harvest to pests, cuts before the bug's population reaches destructive levels.

Simple physical or mechanical methods have proven to be successful alternatives to fumigating stored grains after harvest. Lowering oxygen levels, increasing the level of carbon dioxide in storage facilities, or irradiating stored foods effectively kill a variety of pests (see Chapter 15, Section H). Simply stirring the grain abrades or crushes many species of pests, thus reducing their numbers.

Regulatory Control

In the United States, a large fraction of our agricultural losses are due to introduced species, which are the targets of most of the pesticides used. The first line of defense and the most rational way of avoiding pest problems is by preventing the original entry of pest species. To achieve this, federal laws restrict the importation of plants, plant products, animals, and animal products. Customs checks, quarantines at points of entry to the United States, agricultural inspection of imported foods, plants, and animals, and fumigation of airplanes on certain international flights are intended to prevent the accidental introduction of unwanted plants, animals, and diseases. While some pests have been controlled by the deliberate introduction of imported enemies, sometimes these enemies can become pests themselves, as discussed in more detail later. To prevent mistakes of this kind, there are regulations governing the introduction of exotic species for pest control. The U.S. Department of Agriculture is responsible for evaluating the safety of imported species, while the safety of introducing microbial pesticides into the environment is regulated by the EPA.

Agricultural states such as California, Arizona, and Hawaii that have favorable growing conditions for a wide variety of organisms have very stringent restrictions concerning interstate movement of potential pest species. Unfortunately, agricultural inspections at points of entry are not adequate in the detection of all pests, such as gypsy moth eggs and pupae that "hitchhike" attached to the underside of a car or infestations in commercially imported fruits and vegetables. Both the gypsy moth, a voracious, indiscriminate plant-eating pest on the East coast, and the highly destructive Mediterranean fruit fly have been accidently introduced into California many times, prompting great alarm about threats to California agriculture and the initiation of massive chemical treatment programs. Similarly, flying insects and windborne plant seeds are not stopped by international and state borders. To deal with that problem, a number of cooperative efforts have been established to control the numbers and distribution of pests on a regional basis.

Chemical Control

The use of chemical pesticides to control pests has been discussed extensively in terms of effectiveness and potential hazards. Given current conventional practices, it is unlikely that there will be an overnight shift to nonchemical or limited chemical control. Reduced dependence on chemicals, however, is not only possible, it is desirable. Toward that goal, the criteria that have been established by IPM programs for the sensible use of synthetic pesticides can be applied.

IPM criteria focus on the choice of chemicals to be used, the timing of application, and the method of delivering the pesticide. In general, the materials chosen should be short-lived in the environment and as selective in action as possible. *Broad spectrum pesticides* do far more damage to beneficial populations than do selective ones. The timing and placement of treatments is critical. Ideally, pesticide application should coincide with the most vulnerable stage in the pest's life cycle. Treatment should be done only when monitoring shows that predator and parasite populations are too low to suppress pests effectively. If the goal is to reduce the number of pests, not wipe out the pest, the amount of pesticide needed is considerably less. The method of application is also important and, like the pesticide, should be as selective as possible. For example, direct injection into the soil or plant is preferable to broadcast spraying or misting. Many situations permit effective control with just spot treatments to the affected plant or a small group of plants. Adoption of these criteria can effectively limit human exposure and environmental contamination.

Problems of Alternative Methods

Although biological and cultural control methods are less likely to cause harmful effects on human health and the environment than pesticides, they are not entirely free of problems or risks. For example, organisms introduced to control a particular pest may themselves become pests or cause secondary outbreaks. Consider the Indian mongoose. Imported to Jamaica to control sugarcane rats, it reduced the population of the target pest, but with devastating side effects. Tree rats, able to evade the mongoose and freed of competiton from the sugarcane rats, damaged crops and decimated populations of native birds and small mammals. Elsewhere, the mongoose became a carrier of rabies. An introduced species may interfere or directly compete with other beneficial species, as in the case of a parasitic wasp introduced into California to control the black scale (also a newcomer). The wasp parasitized not only the intended target, but also another species of parasitic wasp, which was an enemy of the black scale.

Some additional problems and risks are associated with the development and deployment of pest-resistant plants. First, many of the compounds that deter pests are often toxic to humans and domestic animals. Potatoes, for example, contain several poisons known as alkaloids, which are not only effective against the potato blight disease but also have killed people. Some plant compounds, while deterring certain pests, actually enhance the attractiveness of the plant to other species. Furthermore, beneficial organisms can be adversely affected by defensive chemicals. Honeybees and other nectar-feeding insects have been poisoned by high concentrations of naturally produced toxic compounds in nectar. Finally, selective breeding for resistance is tricky, time-consuming, and of limited usefulness. Most efforts focus on genetically enhancing the production of a single compound. Wild plants, however, are more resistant to herbivore attack because they generally produce several different compounds. Insects and other pests can more readily develop the ability to detoxify a single compound than several.

While relatively simple, cultural and mechanical pest control must be employed with care and under appropriate circumstances. For example, interplanting can make harvesting more difficult. But more important, selecting the right combination of plant species is crucial. Some mixed crop cultures support not only more predators and parasites, but also a greater number of pest species. Tillage, the mechanical plowing of a field after harvest, is a time-honored and effective method of controlling weeds, insects, and pathogens. It can, however, substantially increase soil erosion, which is a major problem in the United States and elsewhere. Controlled irrigation or flooding of fields works well to drown certain insects and weeds, but it is not appropriate in arid regions or during periods of drought. Moreover, flooding can lead to accumulation of salts in the soil and other soil problems, such as **selenium** contamination.

Pest Control for Home and Garden

Many of the pest control measures used in IPM programs and by organic growers can be readily applied around the home. Beneficial organisms should be recognized and encouraged (Fig. 17). A great variety of predatory insects and parasites can be ordered by the gardener through mail-order houses. A list has been compiled by the Connecticut Agricultural Experiment Station and is shown in Table 10.

In addition to biological control, there are many other techniques for dealing with house and garden pests. Indoor and outdoor plants can be washed free of pests by spraying with plain water or a mixture of pure soap and water, if hand picking is too difficult. More intractable pests can be sprayed with tobacco, hot pepper, or garlic water, using the following recipes.

Recipes for Pest Control in the Home and Garden

TOBACCO WATER:
Steep 1 large handful tobacco in 4 quarts of warm water for 24 hours, dilute and spray.
Caution: Handle with care; this solution is poisonous to humans and domestic animals (see **nicotine**).

HOT PEPPER SOLUTION:
Blend 2 or 3 very hot peppers, ½ onion, and 1 clove of garlic in water; boil, then let steep for 2 days; strain.
Comment: This mix can be frozen for later use.

GARLIC SOLUTION:
Combine 2 Tbs garlic juice (not powder), 1 tsp rubbing alcohol, and 1 oz diatomaceous earth in 4 qt water.
Comment: This solution can also be frozen for later use.

SOAP SOLUTION:
Mix 2 Tbs liquid soap in 1 qt water or 1½ to 2 oz dry soap in 1 qt water.
Comment: Use only pure soap because detergents will harm plants.

When necessary, **pyrethrum** dust, diatomaceous earth, and insecticidal soaps are generally considered safe for the home garden. Weeds can be suppressed either by mulching with organic material, such as grass clippings, redwood bark, or plastic, or by weeding. Indoor pests, such as ants, cockroaches, and moths, can be controlled using a variety of common nontoxic household products rather than conventional pesticides.

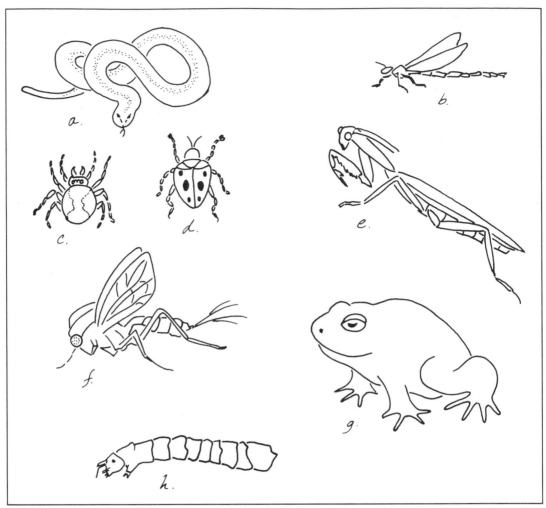

Figure 17 Beneficial species that may live in your backyard. a. garter snake, b. damselfly, c. spider, d. lady bird beetle, e. praying mantis, f. wasp, g. frog, h. larval beetle.

Controlling Household Pests

ANTS:

Squeeze lemon juice at point of entry, leave the peel.

Other effective barriers are chalk, damp coffee grounds, bone meal, charcoal dust, and cayenne pepper.

COCKROACHES:

Plug cracks along baseboard, wall shelves, and cupboards, and around pipes, sinks, and bathtub fixtures, then dust with borax. Trap insects by greasing the inner neck of a bottle baited with raw potato or stale beer.

FLIES:

Trap them on sticky flypaper (nonpesticidal), which can be made at home using honey and yellow paper.

MOTHS:

Keep clothes clean and well aired; use camphor for storage. Trap them using 1 part molasses to 2 parts vinegar placed in a yellow container.

TABLE 10 Common Garden Pests and Their Common Biological Control Agents

Pest	Biological Control Agent
Pests controlled by nonselective predators:	
Aphids	Ladybird beetles (ladybugs)
Mealybugs	Ladybird beetles (ladybugs)
Scales	Praying mantids
Thrips	Green lacewings
Pests controlled by specific predators or parasites:	
Moth eggs	Parasitic wasp (*Trichogramma*)
Whitefly (greenhouse)	Parasitoid (*Encarsia formosa*)
Spider mites	Predatory mites
Root maggot	Predatory roundworms

SILVERFISH:

Trap them with a mixture of 1 part molasses to 2 parts vinegar and set traps near holes and cracks; repel them with borax dusted along baseboards and cupboard cracks.

STORED FOOD PESTS (moths and weevils):

Put dry food that is to be stored in a warm oven at 70° for 1 hour or freeze for 2 or 3 days, then store in airtight containers.

Summary

Alternative agricultural practices have been proven to be socially, ecologically, and economically sound. But because effective control requires careful planning, thorough monitoring of the pest–plant complex, and diligence, it is more labor intensive than the conventional approach and may appear less economically attractive in the short-term than reliance on chemical pesticides. Nevertheless, as costs to society and the environment resulting from misuse of pesticides are increasingly recognized and as costs to pesticide manufacturers increase in their search for better pesticides, it is likely that alternative pest control methods, particularly IPM, will become the new conventional approach. The use of IPM will also be speeded up as evidence of the effectiveness of alternative methods become more widely apparent. Just as the farmer has an increasing set of choices to control pests, householders also have a range of relatively simple and inexpensive options available.

Further Reading

CARSON, R. 1962. *Silent Spring*. Greenwich, CT: Fawcett Publications.

CAWCUTT, L., and WATSON, C. 1984. *Pesticides: The New Plague*. Collingwood, Australia: Friends of the Earth.

EHRLICH, P. R. 1986. *The Machinery of Nature*. New York: Simon and Schuster.

HAYES, W. J. 1982. *Pesticides Studied in Man*. Baltimore, MD: Williams and Wilkins.

KIPLING, E. F. 1979. *The Basic Principles of Insect Population Suppression and Management*. Washington, D.C.: USDA/USGPO.

MOTT, L., and SNYDER, K. 1987. *Pesticide Alert*. San Francisco: Sierra Club Books.

National Academy of Sciences. 1987. *Regulating Pesticides in Food: The Delaney Paradox*. Washington, D.C.: National Academy Press.

National Research Council. 1989. *Alternative Agriculture*. Washington, D.C.: National Academy Press.

Natural Resources Defense Council. 1989. *Intolerable Risk*. Washington, D.C.: NRDC.

Pesticide Handling: A Safety Handbook. 1987. Ottawa, Canada: Canadian Government Publishing Centre.

U.S. Department of Agriculture. 1978. *Biological Agents for Pest Control.* Washington, D.C.: USGPO.

U.S. Department of Agriculture. 1982. *Report and Recommendations on Organic Farming.* Washington, D.C.: USDA.

U.S. Department of Health, Education, and Welfare. 1978. *Occupational Exposure During the Manufacture and Formulation of Pesticides.* Washington, D.C.: USGPO.

VAN DEN BOSCH, R. 1978. *The Pesticide Conspiracy.* New York: Doubleday and Co.

WARE, G. W. 1978. *The Pesticide Book.* San Francisco: W. H. Freeman and Co.

WASSERMAN, R. F., and WILES, R. 1985. *Field Duty: U.S. Farmworkers and Pesticide Safety.* Washington, D.C.: World Resources Institute.

WEIR, D., and SHAPIRO, M. 1981. *Circle of Poison.* San Francisco: Institute for Food and Development Policy.

15 RADIATION

To many people, *radioactivity* is a mysterious and ominous subject. An attitude of "leave it to the experts" prevails, with all the accompanying social harm that can arise from such a neglect of responsibility by the public. The unfamiliarity of the lingo has much to do with this attitude. The basic units with which we describe non-radioactive toxic substances are familiar to everyone. For example, for lead in drinking water, we use ordinary units of weight, or for asbestos in the air, we use the number of particles inhaled with each breath. Weight and number are concepts ingrained in us since childhood, and there is little mystery associated with them. In contrast, the language used to describe quantities of radiation in the environment—replete with curies, rems, and half-lives—seems foreign.

In this chapter, we demystify the topic of radiation by explaining the terminology. We also describe the unique nature of radiation and discuss some of the risks associated with old and new applications of nuclear technology. The readings listed at the end of the chapter provide a more in-depth discussion of many of the topics discussed here.

A. The Nature of Radioactivity

Just as a cake is made up of flour, eggs, and other ingredients, all the objects around us, from eggs to stars, are made of one or more types of basic matter called *elements*. Each of the elements of matter, such as oxygen, calcium, phosphorus, lead, and uranium, is symbolized by one or two letters. For example, O stands for oxygen, Ca for calcium, P for phosphorus, Pb for lead, U for uranium, and so on for each element. A total of 92 different elements occur in nature, and 13 additional ones have been created in the laboratory.

Elements are made up of atoms, and each atom in turn is composed of tiny particles called *electrons* orbiting around a central *nucleus*. The nucleus is also made up of tiny particles called *protons* and *neutrons* that are arranged in a tight cluster. Each element is unique, differing from all others by the number of protons in the nucleus of its atoms. For example, a hydrogen atom has 1 proton in its nucleus, an oxygen atom has 8, and a lead atom has 82. However, the exact number of neutrons in the atomic nucleus of any given element may vary. For instance, all lead

atoms have 82 protons and most have 126 neutrons, but some have 122, 128, or some other number of neutrons. These different forms of an atom, with the same number of protons but a different number of neutrons, are called *isotopes*. The total number of protons and neutrons in the nucleus of an isotope is called the *atomic weight* of that isotope; the number of protons in the nucleus is called the *atomic number*. For example, in Figure 18, carbon is shown to have an atomic weight of 12 and an atomic number of 6.

The notation used to label isotopes requires explanation. Consider the example of the isotope uranium-238. The number 238 refers to the total number of protons plus neutrons in the isotope, that is, the atomic weight. Since all uranium isotope atoms have 92 protons in the nucleus (remember, the number of protons defines the element), the number of neutrons is 238 minus 92, or 146. Another way to name isotopes is to use the element symbol preceded by its atomic weight as a superscript. Thus, uranium-238 is ^{238}U, which is pronounced the same way as the spelled-out version. (Uranium-238 is not the isotope of the uranium in fuel for nuclear

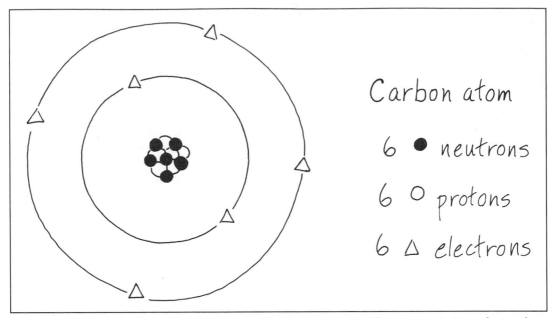

Figure 18 A schematic view of a carbon atom, which has 6 protons and 6 neutrons in its nucleus and 6 electrons in orbit about the nucleus.

weapons and power plants; that is uranium-235; see Section D, this chapter.)

The different isotopes of an element are similar chemically, which means that they react with other chemicals in the same way. But they differ slightly in weight and in another important way—some isotopes are stable while others are unstable. Stability means that they remain the same forever. Unstable isotopes, in contrast, change their form and turn into other isotopes. An isotope that is unstable is called *radioactive*. When a radioactive isotope decays to some other isotope, the latter isotope is called the *decay product* or *daughter* of the former. In the process of changing form or *decaying*, radioactive isotopes shoot out particles. These moving particles are what is called *radiation*. The concern over radioactive substances is that the radiation they produce can cause biological damage when it enters living tissue.

The three main types of radiation particles are designated by the terms *beta rays*, *alpha rays*, and *gamma rays*. The term ray was used historically to describe radiation when it was first discovered, but it is a useful term to re-

tain because it conveys the correct notion that the particles of radiation possess both particle-like and wave-like characteristics. Beta (pronounced "bay-tuh") rays are electrons. Alpha ("al-fa") rays are the nuclei of helium atoms, and each alpha particle has two protons and two neutrons. Gamma rays are like ordinary light in some respects, but each gamma particle contains much more energy than do the particles that compose visible light. (The nature of gamma rays and their relationship to light and to X-rays are discussed in Section B.)

A batch of radioactive atoms will decrease in number over time. This should be no surprise because the atoms are changing their form (or decaying) and becoming other isotopes. But what may be a surprise is that the decrease is very regular—it follows a consistent pattern. Consider the radioactive isotope lead-210. After 22 years, half of the original lead atoms remain. The other half no longer exists in their original form; they have decayed. After another 22 years, half of the remaining half have again decayed, leaving one-fourth of the original batch of atoms.

And after every 22 years that follow, the number remaining will be reduced in half again and again.

For that particular lead isotope, 22 years is the length of its *half-life*. The half-life is the time it takes for half of the batch of atoms to decay. Only a very small fraction of the atoms in the batch will remain after many half-lives have elapsed. Every radioactive isotope has a different half-life. The half-life of some isotopes is incredibly short. For instance, there is an isotope of the element polonium with a half-life of less than a thousandth of a second. For other isotopes, the half-life is very long; the uranium isotope ^{238}U, for example, has a half-life of 4.5 billion years!

Not all radiation is produced by radioactive isotope decay. For example, beta rays can be produced by heating certain types of nonradioactive metals. This is how the radiation is produced that forms the image on a television screen or computer monitor. Some of the radiation produced in nuclear reactors also does not originate from radioactive isotopes. X-ray machines used in dentistry and cyclotrons and other types of "atom smashers" used in science and medicine produce radiation without radioactive isotopes, and the sun's intense radiation is also not produced by such isotopes (see the next section).

B. The Electromagnetic Spectrum

Early in this century it was discovered that light had a dual nature. It could be thought of as a wave and it could also be thought of as a stream of particles. These particles were given the name photons. Each different color of light is composed of photons of different energy. They have no mass and they invariably travel at a very high speed, simply defined as the speed of light. Photons of blue light, for example, differ from those of red light in one very important way—photon for photon, they carry more energy. The visible spectrum of light, ranging from violet to red, can be thought of as a spectrum of photons, with the most energetic ones at the violet end and the least energetic ones at the red end.

Light also has wave-like characteristics. A wave is characterized by a wavelength, which is the distance from the crest of one wave to the crest of the next. Violet light has a wavelength of about 20 millionths of an inch; the wavelength of red light is almost twice as long.

The spectrum of photon energies actually goes well below the red and well above the violet. **Ultraviolet radiation**, while not visible to the human eye, is made up of photons more energetic than those in the visible part of the spectrum. The wavelength of ultraviolet light is shorter than that of violet light. Infrared light, however, is made up of photons less energetic than those in the visible realm, and its wavelength is longer than that of red light. Above the ultraviolet spectrum, there are even more energetic photons called X-rays, well known for their diagnostic and therapeutic applications in medicine. More energetic than X-rays are photons called *gamma rays* (discussed in the first section), which are sometimes emitted in the decay of radioactive isotopes. Ultraviolet light, X-rays, and gamma rays can all inflict biological damage. But even ordinary visible light can be harmful to health if it is sufficiently intense (see **laser light** entry in Part II).

At the other end of the spectrum where energies are below that of infrared light, there are, in order of decreasing energy (and increasing wavelength), photons associated with microwaves, television waves, and radiowaves. This range of the electromagnetic spectrum is called **extremely low frequency electromagnetic fields** (the health risks of which are discussed under its entry in Part II). The *frequency* of a wave is the number of waves per second that pass by a certain point. The relationship between wavelength and frequency is simple: wavelength multiplied by frequency equals the speed of light, which is the same for all these forms of electromagnetic energy. Hence, the long-wavelength part of the spectrum is low frequency, and the short-wavelength end is high frequency.

All of these forms of energy, from radiowaves through visible light to gamma rays, make up what is called the *electromagnetic spectrum*. Exposure to parts of the electromagnetic spectrum can result in health damage if the energy of the radiation is sufficiently high.

C. How Radiation Affects Us

Radioactive isotopes differ from one another in ways that determine how harmful they are. They can have different half-lives, they can emit different forms of radiation, and the radiation they emit can have different energies. In addition, various isotopes can differ in three other important respects. First, isotopes can be either gases, liquid, or solids. Second, isotopes of different elements can differ from one another in the way they interact chemically with various substances in the body. Third, radioactive isotopes differ in the type of daughter isotopes they produce when they decay. Some radioactive isotopes produce daughters that are themselves harmful, while others produce harmless nonradioactive daughters. All of these characteristics influence the degree and type of damage that the isotope can cause. To understand this, let's first look at the way in which radiation damages biological tissue.

When a particle of radiation penetrates the human body and passes through and out the other side without interacting with bodily tissue, no damage is inflicted. It is when the particles deposit some of their energy in tissue that damage could occur. When a ball rolls across a lawn, the grass slowly stops the ball. Each impacted blade of grass bends in the path of the ball, taking from the ball some of its energy of motion. Some of the blades may even bend and break as a result of the impact. The grass is slightly damaged as a result, even if some of the broken blades recover.

Much the same thing happens with radiation in biological tissue. The individual molecules in tissue absorb some of the energy of the passing radiation. Some of the energy is absorbed in a way that is like the grass bending—the molecules just roll with the punch, so to speak. In other cases, however, a molecular bond is snapped or a molecule returns to a different shape after absorbing the energy of the radiation. If those molecules happen to be a part of some sensitive piece of the biological machinery, such as a *DNA* molecule, then damage can result. (DNA is the chemical that carries the genetic information in all plants and animals.) For example, a gene may *mutate* or an organ may become cancerous. Some of the molecular damage that occurs, however, is naturally repaired by the body before the organism as a whole suffers.

The various particles of radiation differ in the way they plow through tissue. If beta rays and alpha rays both start out with the same energy at the same place, both will lose energy uniformly over their paths through tissue, but the beta rays will travel farther into the tissue than the alpha rays. Because these two types of radiation tend to lose roughly the same amount of energy in each collision with a molecule, the total number of impacted molecules will be about the same in both cases. This number will depend on the initial energy of the particles, but not on the type of particle. The type of particle mainly influences the concentration of impacted molecules. Particles of radiation that spread their damage over a shorter path, such as alpha rays, will leave behind a trail of damaged molecules that are closer together.

Alpha rays are particularly dangerous under some circumstances because of this characteristic. If an alpha particle source, such as a speck of plutonium-239, lodges in the thin layer of tissue lining the lung, the alpha particles will concentrate their damage in this thin but highly sensitive tissue. Lung cancer is a likely result. In contrast, if a beta ray emitter is lodged in the same tissue, only a small fraction of the damage would be to molecules in that sensitive tissue.

The relative hazard of these two types of radiation is reversed, however, if the radioactive isotope producing the radiation is outside the body. Since alpha particles typically cannot even pass through skin, it is unlikely that vital internal tissues will be damaged, although skin cancer can result. Beta particles, in contrast, can penetrate the skin, and thus a beta emitter outside the body can damage vital internal organs. Thus, the type of particle emitted by an isotope affects the health risk. The energy of the emitted particle is also important. The greater that energy, the greater the number of damaged molecules and, therefore, the greater the odds that a cancer or mutation will develop.

The half-life of an isotope also affects its potential for damage. An isotope with a long half-life, say, hundreds or thousands of years, will not decay very fast, and so large quantities of it are required to produce substantial radiation in the short run. However, it will linger in the environment for a long time, subjecting future generations to its radiation. Isotopes that have short half-lives (seconds or minutes) probably will not travel from their source to a person's body before they have substantially decayed. Their radiation will probably be emitted harmlessly into the surroundings where the short-lived isotope was produced (such as in a nuclear reactor). An exception occurs, however, if the isotope is produced in the body as a decay product, or daughter, of some other radioactive isotope. This can happen, for example, with the radioactive gas **radon**, which can decay through several intermediate steps to a polonium isotope with a half-life of less than one-thousandth of a second. It emits an energetic alpha particle that can cause severe lung damage.

Although there are important exceptions (such as the polonium isotope that results from radon decay), isotopes with half-lives of intermediate length generally pose the greatest risk to human health because they linger long enough to travel from the source to a person, but decay fast enough so that a substantial portion of the radioactive atoms decay within a human lifetime.

The previous examples of radon and polonium illustrate the importance of the physical state of the isotope. Because radioactive radon is a gas, it can readily enter houses. Because some of its decay products are gases or can attach readily to fine *particulates*, they can easily enter deep inside the lung to cause damage. Isotopes that form solids differ in the degree to which they are soluble in water; those that are more soluble can generally be more readily ingested by animals.

The strength and type of chemical bonds that the isotope forms and the ability of the body to excrete the isotope (see Chapter 10, Section A) also affects the risk it poses. An isotope of iodine, iodine-131, follows the more common and beneficial isotope iodine-127 in its pathways through the human body. The thyroid gland, where iodine accumulates, can become cancerous as a result of the radiation from this unstable isotope. Strontium is chemically similar to calcium and hence lodges in bone tissue. The radioactive isotopes of this element can cause leukemia, a cancer of the bone marrow where white blood cells are produced. The element cesium is chemically very similar to sodium and potassium, substances found throughout the body, and hence the radioactive isotope cesium-137 is generally not localized in one particular organ.

D. Nuclear Fission and Nuclear Fusion

A famous isotope of uranium is uranium-235, which is used as the explosive material in an atomic bomb. Why is this isotope used for bombs? The reason is that it rapidly splits apart when struck by neutrons, a process called *fission*. When the isotope splits apart, it produces two isotopes that together have slightly less mass than the parent uranium. It is because of this small difference in mass that energy is released. Einstein's famous formula $E = mc^2$ correctly predicts how much energy is released in a fission process. In this formula, m is the small mass difference between the parent and the products. Because c, the speed of light, is a very large number, the energy released, E, is enormous.

The two isotopes produced in the fission process are called *fission fragments*, labeled 1 and 2 in Figure 19. In addition, the fission process results in the production of a variety of particles of radiation. Included in these particles are neutrons, which can initiate yet additional fission events. This chain of events—fission events producing neutrons that cause further fission events—happens very fast, leading to the enormous explosive force of the nuclear fission weapons. (Note that nuclear is pronounced "new-klee-er," not "new-cue-ler.") The fission process need not be explosive, however; it can be controlled by keeping most of the neutrons from causing additional fission events. This is what occurs in a properly functioning nuclear power plant, where the fission events occur slowly and steadily over time, producing heat that generates steam to drive an electricity-producing turbine.

Fission produces harmful radiation in two ways. First, particles of radiation are directly produced in the fission process. This process is not the one previously described as radioactivity, and the concept of half-life does not apply to it. In a fission event, this direct radiation emerges instantly. The second source of fission radiation comes about because the fission fragments are unstable (or radioactive) isotopes. Some of the most hazardous fission fragments are iodine-131, strontium-90, and cesium-137. These isotopes have half-lives of 8 days, 28 years, and 30 years, respectively. Thus, when a nuclear weapon explodes or a serious accident occurs at a nuclear power plant, the radiation from these fission fragments lasts over a long time period and can cause health damage long after the explosion or accident.

Fission powers nuclear reactors and atom bombs, but it is not the energy source of the more powerful hydrogen bombs. A process called *fusion* is responsible for powering this second type of weapon. Fusion is also the source of energy that keeps the sun glowing. In the future it may provide energy to generate electricity at an acceptable cost and with much less risk to human health and the environment than conventional nuclear fission power plants. Nuclear fusion, as the name suggests, is the joining together (or fusing) of two nuclei to form a heavier one. This is not possible for most elements except by using an enormous amount of energy. For certain very light elements, however, such as deuterium (an isotope of hydrogen) and lithium, the nuclei can be joined and energy can be produced in the process. Again, $E = mc^2$ describes the source of energy: the sum of the masses of lithium and deuterium is slightly greater than the mass of the nucleus produced when they coalesce, and this difference in mass multiplied by the speed of light squared (c^2) is the amount of energy released.

When fusion reactions occur rapidly and uncontrollably, they can produce the great explosive power of the fusion weapons or hydrogen bombs. For commercial applications, however, it is necessary to control and contain the reaction so that a "slow burn" occurs. There are great technical difficulties in doing this in the laboratory, and the technology probably will not be available for electricity generation in this century.

E. Units Used to Describe Radiation

The effect of radiation in biological tissue is both physical and biological. The physical effect is the dumping of energy in the body. This is measured in units that physicists use to describe energy. The biological effect is measured in units relating to disease and death.

A deposit of energy from radiation in tissue (or for that matter, in any type of sub-

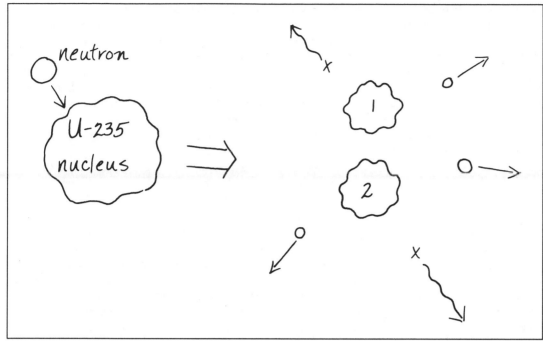

Figure 19 The nuclear fission process. A neutron hits a ^{235}U nucleus, causing it to split into two fission fragments, labeled 1 and 2. Various particles of radiation are also produced, some of which are neutrons that can initiate additional fission processes if other ^{235}U atoms are nearby.

stance) is measured with two units: *grays* and *sieverts*. A gray is defined in terms of the amount of energy absorbed in a given weight of body tissue. Specifically, an object is said to receive 1 gray (abbreviated Gy) of radiation when every gram of that object has deposited in it (from the passing radiation) exactly 10,000 ergs of energy. An erg of energy is a very small amount, roughly the energy in the motion of a large crawling beetle. One milligray is one-thousandth of a gray. The gray unit was recently introduced into scientific nomenclature to replace an older unit called the *rad*; 1 gray equals 100 rads.

The phrase "a 0.05 gray dose to the liver" means that the liver has absorbed enough radiation to deposit 500 ergs of energy in every gram of the liver. The actual distribution of the absorbed energy in the liver is not described by that phrase, however. Certain parts of the liver absorbed more and some less, so that on the average, 500 ergs was absorbed by each gram of liver tissue. The

phrase "a whole body dose of 1 gray" means that, on the average, every gram of tissue in the body has absorbed 10,000 ergs.

The concept of 10,000 ergs of energy being deposited in each gram of a human body is hard to grasp. One way to think of it is to imagine that all the energy is in the form of heat. If 10,000 ergs of heat were deposited in every gram of a person's body, it would increase body temperature by less than one-thousandth of a degree. This would hardly be noticed. Yet, as discussed in Section G (this chapter), a whole body radiation dose of 1 gray can cause serious injury. The reason is that a relatively small amount of nuclear radiation energy, unlike the same amount of heat energy, can damage vital molecules in the body.

The sievert (abbreviated Sv) is a unit very much like the gray except that it takes into account (in a crude way) the biological damage that might result from the absorbed energy. You will recall that beta, alpha, and gamma rays deposit their energy within living tissue in different ways (see Section C). For that reason, absorption of 100 ergs from alpha rays within the body is more harmful than absorption of the same energy from beta rays. In other words, if a person receives a certain number of grays from beta rays, the biological damage is probably less than if the dose results from alpha rays. The number of sieverts received equals the number of grays times a so-called *quality factor*. The quality factor takes into account the relative biological hazard of the different types of particles. For betas and gammas, the sievert dose equals the gray dose; in other words, the quality factor for betas and gammas is 1. For alpha particles, a dose of 1 gray equals 20 sieverts; in other words, the quality factor for alpha particles is 20. This means that a 20-gray beta dose is, in terms of biological damage, equal to a 1-gray dose from alpha particles. For protons and neutrons, the quality factor is 10.

Just as the old unit rad was replaced by the new unit gray, so the older unit rem was recently replaced by the sievert. The sievert is related to the rem in the same way that the gray is related to the rad: 1 sievert equals 100 rem.

The units used for radiation can be summarized as follows:

1 gray (Gy) = 100 rad
  (10,000 ergs absorbed per gram)
1 sievert (Sv) = 100 rem
Dose in sieverts equals dose in grays times:
  1 for betas and gammas
  10 for protons and neutrons
  20 for alphas

The units of gray and sievert are used to describe a dose—they refer to the amount of energy deposited in the body when a beam of radiation is absorbed there. They do not tell us anything, however, about the amount of radiation in the environment (to which we may or may not be exposed). For the purpose of describing an amount of radioactive material, the mass of the material is not as interesting to us as is the rate at which radiation is being emitted by it. This rate is called *activity*; to describe it, the unit of *becquerel* (abbreviated Bq) is most often used. To understand the unit becquerel, consider a certain amount of radioactive material. Every second, some number of atoms of that material will decay into another material. One becquerel of radioactive material is the amount of that material in which every second, one atom decays.

There are some subtleties about the becquerel. Consider a piece of radioactive strontium-90, with a half-life of 28 years. Suppose that at the present time, this amount is known to be a 10-billion becquerel source. In other words, 10 billion nuclei in this piece are decaying each second. In 28 years, half of the strontium-90 in this piece of material will have decayed, leaving only half as much of it as was initially present. Therefore, only half as many atoms will be decaying each second as compared to today. It will then be a 5-billion becquerel source. Thus, activity is not an unchanging characteristic of a piece of radioactive material; as the material decays, the number of becquerels left decreases. The number of becquerels in a short-lived isotope decreases very fast, while the change in the number of becquerels in a long-lived isotope can be so slow as to be undetectable over a human lifetime.

The unit of becquerel has replaced an older unit called the *curie* (abbreviated Ci). One curie of radioactive material is equal to 37 billion becquerels. There is a historical reason for the peculiar number 37 billion in this relationship: it is the number of nuclei that decay per second in 1 gram of radium, the radioactive element that was first intensively studied by Marie Curie (hence the name).

It is also useful to have a unit of radiation that expresses the total dose to an entire population. For example, following the 1986 accident at the Chernobyl nuclear power plant in the Soviet Union, scientists estimated that the dose to the entire world population was in the range of 800,000 to 2,000,000 person-sieverts. The unit *person-sievert* is simply the product of the number of people exposed times the average dose, in sieverts, to each person. Equally useful for describing the health consequences of an accident or even of the routine operation of a nuclear facility is the unit of *person-sievert per becquerel*. The becquerels referred to here are the becquerels of radiation released to the environment. So this unit expresses the potency of the radioactive isotopes that are released—how much of these isotopes will come in contact with people and how much radiation the people will receive as a result. The release of radioactive isotopes far from human habitation will generally not produce as many person-sieverts per becquerel as will the same amount released near a city.

F. Background Exposure and Radiation Standards

When an accident occurs involving the release of radioactive materials, public officials and industry spokespersons often describe the estimated radiation dose to people in relative terms. The usual yardstick against which the accidental exposure is compared is the *background level,* or sometimes the *natural background level,* of radiation. For example, following the nuclear power plant accident at Chernobyl in the Soviet Union, it was announced that people living in Scandinavia might receive a 20% increase in radiation dose above their background exposure during the subsequent year. First, let's look at what is meant by natural background level.

The natural background level is the amount of a substance that would be in the environment if there were no people on the planet to produce it. It describes nature's contribution. The natural background dose is thus the rate at which a person would breathe, eat, or otherwise uptake that substance if it existed at the natural background level. By comparing an accidental dose from human activity to the natural background dose, we are putting the hazard resulting

from the accidental dose into perspective. If the former is very small compared to the latter, we can be assured that however many people die from the man-made dose, far more are dying anyway from the natural dose of the same substance. How reassuring this is to the affected population is a matter that can only be decided personally by each individual.

The natural background dose of radiation to the general public is estimated to be 3 millisieverts (300 millirem) per year (see the previous section for an explanation of these units). Table 11 shows the various contributing factors that make up this natural background. (Note that we are including **radon** and its *daughters* as natural background even though our exposure to radon largely occurs because we live in houses rather than outdoors.)

The values given in Table 11 are averages for the entire U.S. population. The cosmic radiation dose to people living at high elevations is higher than that shown. For example, in the mile-high city of Denver, Colorado, the cosmic radiation dose is about 0.6 millisieverts per year. The indoor radon daughter dose varies tremendously from one location or house to another (as discussed in the entry for radon in Part II). Also, the radon dose estimate is the average for both smokers and nonsmokers; for smokers it averages about 3 or 4 millisieverts per year, but for nonsmokers, only about 0.4 or 0.6 (because smoke particles increase the time that radon daughters spend in the lungs). Thus, while the sources listed in Table 11 are presented as natural sources, it is clear that we have some influence over the magnitude of the dose we receive from them.

Even in the absence of accidents at nuclear facilities, we are exposed to other sources of radiation besides those listed in Table 11. These nonnatural (that is, *anthropogenic*) sources that result from human use of radiation are given in Table 12 for the U.S. population. As for the natural sources, these figures represent averages, and there is con-

TABLE 11 The Main Sources of Natural Background Radiation in the United States

Natural Radiation Source	Whole Body Annual Dose (millisieverts/year)
Cosmic radiation	0.3
Carbon-14 in the atmosphere	0.01
Isotopes in the earth's crust that decay externally to the body	0.3
Radon and its *daughters*	2.0
Potassium-40 and other isotopes decaying in the body	0.4

TABLE 12 The Major Anthropogenic Sources of Radiation to the U.S. Public

Anthropogenic Sources	Whole Body Annual Dose (millisieverts/year)
Diagnostic X-rays	
dental	0.03
medical	0.35
Therapeutic radiation	0.14
Fallout from past atmospheric testing of nuclear weapons (estimate for 1988)	0.01
Television receivers	0.005
Airline travel (additional cosmic radiation dose)	0.005
Nuclear energy (routine operation)	0.0005

TABLE 13 Current U.S. Regulations for Permissible Radiation Doses

Individual of Concern	Maximum Dose to Individual Permitted (millisieverts/year)	
Workers in nuclear or medical industries	50	(5 rem)
Each individual in the population	5	(0.5 rem)
Average of U.S. population	1.7	(0.17 rem)

siderable variation within the public in the actual dose received. A cancer patient undergoing radiation treatment will receive in one year many times the therapeutic dose listed in Table 12. A frequent flyer will get many times the average airline travel dose.

Together the natural and nonnatural background doses make up the background radiation dose. It is approximately 3.6 millisieverts per person per year in the United States. How many deaths from cancer can be attributed to our exposure to this background radiation? The following section answers that question after first describing the nature of the evidence upon which our understanding of the potency of radiation is based.

The U.S. Nuclear Regulatory Commis-

sion is currently responsible for setting and enforcing radiation protection standards in the United States. The current regulation for permissible doses, exclusive of radiation from naturally occurring sources and for medical diagnosis or treatment, are shown in Table 13.

G. Estimating the Risk of Radiation

Most of our information about the risk of getting cancer or other illness from exposure to radiation comes from studying the initial survivors of the nuclear explosions at Hiroshima and Nagasaki in 1945. Different parts of those cities received different radiation doses, and people living in the different locales exhibited different chances of later developing cancers. From this, it has been possible to estimate the relationship between radiation dose and cancer risk.

For very high doses delivered rapidly (so-called *acute doses*), the effects of radiation are apparent shortly after exposure and the symptoms are quite obvious. Hence, we know with a good deal of certainty what large doses do to us. Information from Hiroshima and Nagasaki, along with scattered lessons learned from accidents in the nuclear industry in the United States, have provided a general picture of the short-term health effects of large, sudden, whole body doses, which is shown in Table 14.

But what about the long-term risk of developing cancer from lower doses of radiation? Here we are concerned with doses so low that no short-term symptoms of radiation exposure are necessarily noticeable. From data on Japanese who survived the initial radiation exposure and the other immediate consequences of the two bombs, a relationship between dose of radiation and risk of cancer has been determined. The relationship appears to be a simple one: the chances of developing most cancers from radiation are directly proportional to the dose of radiation received. This sort of relationship between dose and damage is called a *linear dose–response relation* (discussed in more detail in Chapter 2, Section A). An alternative assumption, called the *threshold effect*, holds that below some threshold level of radiation, the risk is inconsequential because at low levels of exposure, the body can repair the biological damage as fast as it is created. Leukemia is one type of cancer whose induction may be described better by a threshold relation than a linear relation.

A specific relationship between dose and cancer risk has been derived from the Japanese data. If 100,000 people each receive a one-time dose of 100 millisieverts (10 rem) of radiation, then on average, about 800 of those

people will die of cancer as a result of this additional exposure. From this use of the data, the cancer risk from the typical background level of radiation can be roughly estimated. To do this, the **radon** dose must be treated separately from the other sources of background radiation because of the special nature of *alpha particle* damage to the lung. Moreover, it must be taken into consideration that a given dose of radiation spread out over every year of a person's life could be less harmful than if it is administered in one dose. The result is that the dose (3.6 millisieverts) from both natural and *anthropogenic* sources of radiation received by the typical U.S. citizen each year causes roughly 10,000 to 20,000 cancer deaths in the United States annually. Since each year about 500,000 people in the United States die of cancer, background radiation may be responsible for about 2 to 4% of the total cancer deaths in the United States.

Previous estimates of the risk of low-level radiation based on the Japanese data had given a lower cancer risk than that just quoted. However, it came to light that the radiation dose received by the Japanese had been less than previously estimated. Thus, less radiation was actually needed to produce a cancer than previously thought. Also, medical studies began to reveal that as the Japanese victims grew older, an unexpectedly higher death rate occurred. For these reasons, the dose–response relation was reevaluated, yielding the results just given. A reevaluation of radiation protection regulations is now in progress; a tightening of the regulations on permitted radiation exposures to the general public and to workers in the radiation industries may result.

H. Food Irradiation

About one-third of all the food produced each year in the United States is discarded because of spoilage. Moreover, if spoiled food is eaten, it not only has an unpleasant taste, but it can also cause illness such as salmonella

TABLE 14 The Short-Term Health Effects of Large Radiation Exposures

Acute Dose (millisieverts)	Short-Term Symptoms	Comments
1000–3000	Vomiting, malaise, fatigue, and loss of appetite	Antibiotic treatment necessary; recovery from short-term effects likely
3000–6000	Above symptoms plus hemorrhaging, infection, hair loss, and sterility	Blood transfusion and bone marrow transplant needed; recovery likely in roughly 50% of cases
More than 6000	Above symptoms plus damage to central nervous system and total incapacitation	Death nearly certain

poisoning. By properly exposing foods to radiation, shelf life can be greatly prolonged and many of the risks of eating spoiled foods can be reduced. Moreover, the risks of using *fumigants* and chemical preservatives can be avoided. Several nations, such as South Africa and the Netherlands, are already making considerable commercial use of food irradiation technology. Paving the way for future use of this technology in the United States, the Food and Drug Administration (FDA) in 1986 authorized commercial use of food irradiation for fresh fruits and vegetables, herbs and spices, and pork.

Just as nuclear power has met with persistent public opposition in the United States, plans to allow widespread commercial use of food irradiation are also likely to meet with resistance. Already, several citizens groups have voiced concern, and a debate over the safety of the technology is under way.

One misconception is that irradiated food would become radioactive, but this should not be a real concern. To kill the microbes that cause spoilage, *gamma rays* from a radioactive *isotope* are aimed at the food. Under proper use of the technology, the radioactive isotopes, most commonly cobalt-60 or **cesium-137**, do not come in contact with the food. Moreover, the gamma rays from those isotopes lack the energy to create radioactive isotopes in the food. It would take the deliberate action of a saboteur to implant the isotopes in the food, and there already exist much easier ways for saboteurs to carry out such a goal.

Of greater concern is the inevitable increase in the transport and handling of radioactive substances, increasing the opportunity for an accidental spill. Workers in the food irradiation industry will be at the greatest risk from this, although a potential threat to the general public is posed by the possibility of rail, air, or highway accidents involving vehicles carrying radioactive materials. One of the isotopes that can be used for food irradiation, cesium-137, is a by-product of nuclear power plants so, at least in one sense, its use in the food irradiation industry would not create a new isotope management problem. Using that isotope as a gamma ray source for food irradiation is a way of making use of an otherwise useless waste product. However, extracting the cesium-137 from nuclear power plant wastes requires a process called "fuel reprocessing" in which the nuclear wastes are sorted into useful components. This process presents risks to the workers involved and also provides one more step in the nuclear fuel cycle at which terrorists could obtain dangerous nuclear materials.

While the direct risk of radioactivity from a growing food irradiation industry in the United States will be relatively small, other concerns have arisen. One possibility centers on potentially harmful nonradioactive chemicals that may be created when food is irradiated. These chemicals are called *radiolytic products* and include a group known as unique radiolytic products, or URPs, which are found only in radiated substances. Insufficient scientific information exists at present to evaluate the health risk posed by URPs, but it is around this issue that much of the present debate about the safety of food irradiation revolves.

Various other risks exist that are not directly related to the radiation hazard. Consumers may find that some irradiated foods have unfamiliar or unpleasant textures or tastes. Moreover, some foods will suffer a loss in nutrient content as a result of irradiation. Some irradiated foods could appear unspoiled because the microbes that create visual symptoms of rot have been killed, but they may actually harbor a dangerous organism that was relatively resistant to radiation. In such a case, it would be better for the consumer to be able to recognize by its appearance that the food was spoiled.

Finally, increasing use of food irradiation is likely to have consequences throughout the various stages of food production and distribution. The price of food should change only slightly, as it typically costs only a few cents a pound to irradiate foods, and there will be cost savings because more food will be available. But the growing, harvesting, storing, transporting, and packaging of foods are likely to be affected in ways difficult to foresee. As an example, it is possible that food irradiation will result in a decrease in the use of pesticides on the farm as well as a decrease in the use of preservatives in packaged foods. As the discussions on preservatives and pesticides in this book have made clear (see Chapters 7 and 14), this will have a positive impact on our health.

This discussion suggests that many issues should be considered openly before embarking on a major commitment to food irradiation. Both pros and cons exist. As the history of nuclear power in the United States teaches, clear and credible lines of governmental authority and responsibility will have to be established for the hazards to be effectively regulated. Radiated foods should be labeled as such in the market so that consumers can avoid them if they so choose. Most important, full and truthful communication among governmental agencies, industry, and the public is essential if the welfare of the public is to be best served by this new food-processing technology.

I. Nuclear War

No single human act could result in as much toxicity as the waging of a nuclear war. Nuclear weapons kill by a variety of means. Immediately following the detonation of a nuclear weapon, *X-rays* and intense heat are produced that are sufficient to kill practically everyone within about a mile radius (depending on the size of the weapon and the hilliness of the terrain). The heat produces a pressure wave called a "blast" that can topple buildings and turn a city into rubble.

Two types of radiation are produced by the detonation of a nuclear bomb: prompt and delayed. Prompt radiation consists of the particles released by the nuclear reactions that power the weapon and of X-rays that irradiated air molecules produce almost instantaneously. Delayed radiation is mainly due to the radioactive decay of *fission fragments* (see Section D, this chapter), which will remain in the environment for many years. They are dispersed great distances from the detonation site and will slowly emit particles of radiation.

In addition to the direct lethal effects from heat, blast, and radiation, which can totally destroy a city, there are a variety of indirect ways in which nuclear war can kill. Fires produced by the heat of the weapons, particularly in urban areas, will produce massive amounts of pyrotoxins (harmful chemicals produced when plastics and other substances are burned) that may blow out to the suburbs and pose a hazard to those that escape the direct effects of the weapons.

The ozone layer (see Chapter 11, Section B) will be severely damaged in the aftermath of nuclear war by **nitrogen oxides** produced from the fires. This will expose people over much of the planet to harmful **ultraviolet radiation**.

It has also been theorized that the urban

fires and forest fires ignited in a major nuclear war would seriously alter the earth's climate for a period of many months following the war. The reason is that the fires would produce enough sooty smoke to block much of the sunlight, leading to a dark and cold climate popularly known as "nuclear winter." Like the effect of ozone depletion, this climate alteration would not be limited to the region where the bombs fall, but would most likely extend over much of the inhabited planet. The cold, dark conditions would make it difficult or impossible for many nations to grow food, leading to the possibility of mass starvation among those who survived the other hideous effects of nuclear war.

Further Reading

EISENBUD, M. 1984. *Environmental Radioactivity.* 3d edition. New York: Academic Press.

Office of Technology Assessment. 1984. *Nuclear Power in an Age of Uncertainty.* Washington, D.C.: OTA.

Royal Swedish Academy of Sciences. 1982. *Nuclear War: The Aftermath.* A special issue of the journal *Ambio.* Vol. XI, nos. 2 and 3.

Union of Concerned Scientists. 1975. *The Nuclear Fuel Cycle: A Survey of the Public Health, Environmental, and National Security Effects of Nuclear Power.* Revised edition. Cambridge, MA: MIT Press.

MANAGING TOXICS

16 THE WASTE CRISIS: SOURCES AND SOLUTIONS

In the last few years, Americans have been deluged with television and newspaper stories and photos of toxic waste dumps, overflowing landfills, contaminated drinking water wells, closed swimming beaches, and improperly stored radioactive wastes at U.S. government nuclear weapons facilities—all indicators of the waste crisis. The images are graphic and, in many cases, close to home. In response to the waste problem, industry, the public, and the government are beginning to develop long-term, sustainable solutions and a comprehensive policy. In this chapter, we examine the problem from the perspective of its sources, the current disposal and treatment methods, and its long-term solutions, which involve changes in attitudes and specific measures to reduce the ever-increasing flow of toxic waste.

A. Overview of the Waste Crisis

From East Africa to Germany, from Chinese villages to New York City, people produce a variety of wastes—the inevitable end-product of human activity. Highly technological societies, such as ours and those in Europe and Japan, are responsible for both a staggering array and excessively large amounts of waste. Here in the United States, when something is emptied, breaks, falls apart, or becomes worn, it is likely to end up in the garbage pile, contributing to the growing mound of municipal garbage (Fig. 20). The refuse, including disposable diapers, food wastes, plastic bags, styrofoam cups, broken toys, paint thinner, plant prunings, scrap lumber, bed springs, pickle jars, worn carpet, old appliances, aluminum and tin cans, cleaning compounds, and paper, is a manifestation of what has been called the disposable economy.

In contrast, in much of Africa, for example, an empty Coca-Cola bottle is so valuable that curb-side vendors keep careful track of each bottle dispensed, insist that each is returned, and have been known to chase a busload of tourists to take possession of one missing bottle. Similarly, throughout much of the world (and here in days past), broken objects are not casually discarded, but are mended and restored to usefulness or cannibalized and used for parts.

Not too long ago, about 1960, the average U.S. citizen disposed of roughly 2.5 pounds of garbage each day. Today, 30 years later, the average per capita disposal rate is about 3.5 pounds per day—twice the amount produced by the average European. Our output totals about 160 million tons or more than 300 billion pounds of unwanted stuff a year. The increase in per capita garbage, along with the greater number of people (65 million more) producing garbage than in 1960, the lack of places to dump our junk, and the toxic or otherwise hazardous nature of much of our garbage, all adds up to what has been aptly termed the waste crisis. The syringes, dressings, and other medical wastes that washed up on East Coast beaches during the summer of 1988; the closure of sport and commercial fisheries due to **PCB** contamination; dead marine birds and mammals choked by plastic six-pack beverage can yokes; aluminum beer cans littering the landscape; **dioxin**-laden rivers and sediments from pulp and paper mills; abandoned, uninhabitable homes at Love Canal in Niagara Falls, New York; and leaking, rusty barrels full of unknown chemicals—all these are signs of the times, graphic and disturbing symbols of the waste crisis.

Pollution control regulations, established to limit the volume and impact of airborne wastes and sewage and industrial effluents,

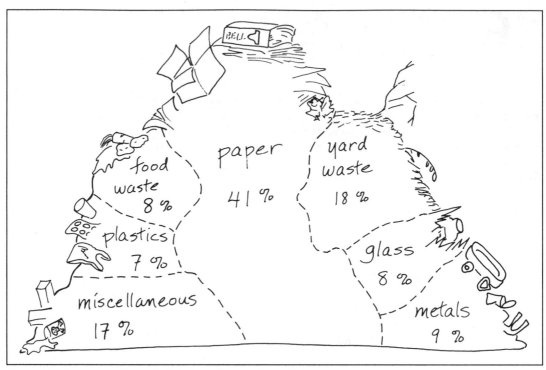

Figure 20 Anatomy of a typical garbage dump—by weight.

have succeeded to a certain extent in reducing the burden of wastes dispersed in the nation's air and water (see Chapter 17). The technology, the know-how, and the legal and economic incentives exist (although they may not be fully employed) to prevent continued use of our air and water as dumping grounds for wastes. We have been slower to react to the ever-increasing loads of solid wastes, those that typically get buried or burned. Consequently, both the volume and diversity of solid wastes are overburdening our capacity to protect human health and the natural environment.

Solid waste is defined by the Resource Conservation and Recovery Act (RCRA) as garbage, refuse, sludge, or any other discarded material resulting from industrial, commercial, mining, agricultural, or community activities. It broadly applies to nearly all types of waste in most forms—solid, semisolid, liquid, or contained gaseous. Furthermore, hazardous wastes, the by-products of

industrial activity, are distinguished from nonhazardous wastes on the basis of toxicity, flammability, corrosiveness, or reactivity. Hazardous wastes are further defined by RCRA, the primary law governing hazardous wastes, as materials that can cause death or contribute significantly to fatal, irreversible, or incapacitating diseases. The law specifies additional criteria of quantity, concentration, and physical, chemical, or infectious properties that pose a serious threat to human health and the environment when "improperly treated, stored, transported, disposed of, or otherwise managed." The overall objective is to ensure that hazardous wastes are managed in an environmentally sound manner (see Chapter 17).

Typically, the refuse produced by households, small businesses (including small manufacturers), and local governments has been considered to be nonhazardous or of sufficiently small volume as to pose no hazard and thus has been disposed of in municipal facilities. But, as discussed later, the view that such material can be excluded from more stringent regulation is currently being reevaluated. Municipal refuse, however, accounts for just a small fraction of the estimated six billion tons of all wastes (including sewage, dredged material, and industrial wastes) produced annually by our society. Moreover, much of what constitutes municipal garbage, such as plastic soft drink containers and paper packaging material, are commercial end-products whose manufacture inevitably yields wastes, many of them toxic.

In a 1983 report, the Congressional Budget Office estimated that the chemical, metal, petroleum, rubber and plastics, wood preserving, and other industries generated nearly 300 million tons of hazardous waste each year. A 1987 EPA survey estimated that more than 11 million tons of toxic wastes (a subset of hazardous wastes) were being discharged into the nation's water, air, and soil. The chemical manufacturing industry, which produces about a billion tons of chemicals a year, accounted for more than half of the toxic wastes generated; paper manufacturing and primary metal production (smelters and steel mills) together accounted for nearly 25% of the total. In addition to the nonhazardous and hazardous wastes, there are radioactive wastes from nuclear power plants, weapons production facilities, and research and medical institutions that require very careful handling, storage, and disposal.

Conventional approaches to dealing with the wastes generated by our industrialized society do not differ much from the methods employed by our early ancestors. Most wastes are disposed of by being dumped or buried on land or dumped into streams, lakes, or oceans. The rest is incinerated. Serious drawbacks to dumping or burning have become increasingly apparent, leading municipalities, industries, and government facilities to seek sensible long-term solutions dictated by necessity, public concern, and more stringent government regulations.

More than a decade ago, the EPA concluded that waste reduction at the source is the best long-term solution to the waste problem, followed by recycling as the second best, then incineration, and finally, disposal by burying. Unfortunately, EPA's conclusions have not had a significant impact on the way our society deals with its wastes. While some communities across the country are trying to reduce the amount of garbage, for example, by banning disposable diapers and plastic food packaging and by opening municipal recycling centers, the volume of waste continues to grow, the hazards remain unabated, and we persist in burying or burning our junk. In the following two sections, we describe what we currently do with nonhazardous, hazardous, and radioactive wastes. We then conclude with a section on alternative approaches to reducing waste at its source.

B. Waste Disposal

Most wastes are disposed of on land, either in landfills, waste piles, underground injection wells, or surface impoundments (Fig. 21). Each type of waste—nonhazardous, hazardous, and radioactive—is dealt with in a different way.

Municipal Nonhazardous Wastes

About 80 to 90% of municipal wastes end up in landfills. One problem confronting municipalities is the rapid disappearance of adequate disposal sites. It has been estimated that of the 6500 operating municipal landfills, from one-third to one-half will close in the next few years, having exhausted their capacity. In the last few years, U.S. and foreign newspapers, magazines, and television news programs have featured one story after another about the lack of available disposal sites. Perhaps one of the more memorable stories was the saga of the garbage barge that wandered at sea for seven weeks, looking for a place to unload its burden of trash from Islip, New York. The circumstances were

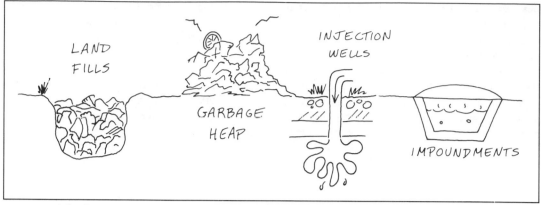

Figure 21 The four options commonly used to dispose of wastes on land.

not unusual; the city's dump was overflowing, so an alternative site was sought. Six states and three countries, themselves undoubtedly feeling the pinch of diminishing disposal sites, rejected the cargo, forcing the barge to return to New York.

As the value of land and the demand for new building sites both increase, the availability of new suitable disposal sites decreases. This, in turn, leads to an increase in the cost of disposal. As a result, some municipalities have found it cheaper and politically more popular (at home) to export their garbage rather than open new facilities or enlarge existing sites. Many heavily populated states typically rely on out-of-state disposal, trucking municipal wastes to landfill sites in less populated areas. Furthermore, many industrial countries now routinely export their wastes, both nonhazardous and hazardous, to less developed nations. More and more, though, local residents here and abroad are refusing to accept someone else's garbage.

Hazardous Wastes

Typically, reference to hazardous wastes or waste sites conjures images of pits full of noxious, foul-looking, deadly chemicals of industrial origin or perhaps reminds us of the buried time-bomb of industrial chemicals discovered at Love Canal in Niagara Falls, New York. Love Canal, a national symbol of

the hazardous waste problem, was the first mismanaged hazardous waste site to be recognized, but certainly not the last. Since 1980, when nationwide cleanup of such sites began, more and more sites requiring priority cleanup have been identified each year. As of 1989, more than 1000 priority sites had been listed by the EPA. Moreover, it has been estimated by the EPA, the Office of Technology Assessment, and the Government Accounting Office that many thousands more uncontrolled hazardous waste sites remain to be found.

Since the discovery of Love Canal, the problems of groundwater, surface water, and soil contamination, threatened species, and human illness, all of which arise from uncontrolled dump sites, have become all to familiar. Yet, while cleanup of already identified priority waste sites goes on and while additional sites requiring massive cleanup efforts are identified each year, we continue to generate and carelessly dispose of large amounts of hazardous wastes, despite regulations intended to prevent future problems. Under RCRA, EPA regulates the management (transport, treatment, storage, and disposal) of large-volume hazardous, chiefly industrial, wastes from cradle to grave. The central problem concerning the disposal of hazardous wastes is the prevention of environmental contamination, particularly groundwater contamination. Unfortunately, the adequacy of past and present disposal methods and sites is doubtful.

The Congressional Budget Office estimates that about 96% of industrial wastes, the major source of hazardous wastes, is disposed of on-site, that is, at the production site. There is some concern that on-site disposal may be less stringently managed and more difficult to monitor and enforce than off-site commercial facilities. One advantage of on-site management, however, is the reduction of risks associated with transportation of hazardous material.

About 70% of hazardous wastes are disposed of on land, but the distribution differs from that of municipal wastes. According to the EPA, only 5% of land-disposed hazardous material goes to landfills. Roughly 60% of it is injected into underground wells, about 35% is dumped into surface impoundments, and slightly less than 1% ends up in waste piles. Certain kinds of wastes, such as halogenated solvents and sludges, **PCBs**, liquid pesticides, and metal-containing liquids are prohibited from land disposal, but must undergo some kind of treatment (see Section C).

Regulations specify features of design, construction, and containment ability for disposal sites, but the EPA acknowledges that existing techniques will probably not prevent eventual environmental contamination. For example, hazardous waste landfills must have double liners and leachate collection systems, but most landfills, even those operating in compliance with the regulations, are likely to leak. Moreover, an unknown number of hazardous waste landfills that do not meet the specified standards are in operation. Despite acknowledged problems with long-term containment of untreated hazardous wastes, less than 5% of the wastes are chemically or physically stabilized to reduce the chance of migration to groundwater. Similarly, although regulations require liners in surface impoundments, many are unlined. Consequently, it is estimated that 90% of existing surface impoundments pose a potential threat to groundwater. Furthermore, the caps or coverings over both surface impoundments and landfills can (and do) break down, allowing surface runoff of wastes.

Deep well injection, the most popular technique, provides large capacity and is relatively inexpensive. It involves drilling of disposal passages and pumping wastes into underground geologic formations—such as salt caverns and even aquifers. Amendments to RCRA in 1984, however, specifically prohibit the pumping of hazardous wastes into underground drinking water sources. Nevertheless, because of the possibility of undetected cracks and fissures in underground caverns, the potential for migration into groundwater supplies exists. Despite the threat to groundwater, it is likely that injection wells will continue to be used as other land-based methods are phased out.

A major problem, only now becoming widely recognized, is that municipal wastes, not just industrial wastes, contribute substantially to the problems of hazardous wastes. Municipal garbage consists of a mix that includes hazardous and potentially hazardous material. Pesticides, oil-based paints, solvents, waste motor oil, and used car batteries are just a few of the unquestionably hazardous materials that ultimately end up in the local dump, if not simply poured down the drain. Unfortunately, most people are unaware of or unconcerned about the hazards stowed in the garage or basement, hazardous materials that, at cleanup time, are hauled off to the dump along with the tree prunings and broken aluminum garden chair. Most municipal landfills are not designed to monitor, regulate, and contain the flow of hazardous materials, so the stuff is buried and forgotten—until contaminants are detected in groundwater or in nearby surface waters.

Reliable estimates of the amounts of such hazardous materials that end up in ordinary landfills are hard to come by, but it is a good guess that a substantial quantity is dumped. It has been estimated that as much as 100,000 pounds of **DDT** is sitting around on shelves in homes just in the Seattle, Washington, area.

The EPA estimates that of the roughly 200 million gallons of used motor oil extracted at home, only about 15% is taken to collection centers. In the early 1980s, about 90% of old car batteries were recycled. By 1987, only 60% were being recycled, thanks to a drop in the price of **lead**. Moreover, hazardous wastes from certain kinds of small businesses (those generating less than 220 pounds per month), such as printing, gardening, dry cleaning, electrical repair, woodworking, and painting, are excluded from federal regulations governing the disposal of hazardous and toxic substances. Consequently, such wastes are commonly hauled to municipal disposal sites.

Radioactive Wastes

The material produced in nuclear reactors is called *radioactive waste*. The two main sources of this waste in the United States, the manufacture of nuclear weapons and commercial nuclear power plants, have handled their wastes differently. To make nuclear bombs, **plutonium** is required. It is made and then extracted from the fuel of military production reactors, leaving a large quantity of a highly radioactive liquid called high-level waste. This waste contains such *isotopes* as radioactive **strontium-90**, **iodine-131**, and **cesium-137**, among others. Nuclear power plant fuel, by contrast, is replaced about once a year and the highly radioactive spent fuel rods are temporarily stored at the power plant to cool down in large pools of water. Spent commercial fuel is also called high-level waste, but it still contains plutonium and uranium that could be removed and reused for further power generation, a technology called reprocessing. For a combination of economic and health reasons and, more important, because the plutonium separated from power plant fuel could be stolen and used by terrorists (or other countries) to make nuclear weapons, reprocessing has never taken place with commercial nuclear fuel.

The long-range plan is for all nuclear waste to be stored in permanent waste repositories.

But since a plan for permanent waste disposal has not yet been agreed upon, spent fuel rods are piling up at power plants around the United States, and liquid military waste has been stored for decades longer than anticipated at military production sites. Unfortunately, leaks involving hundreds of thousands of gallons of high-level waste have occurred at temporary storage sites at Hanford, Washington, and Savannah River, Georgia.

Several ideas for permanent storage have been discussed over the past few decades. Schemes to rocket the wastes to outer space, to dump them under the Antarctic ice cap, or to deposit them in the ocean can be readily dismissed on economic and/or environmental grounds. The best ideas proposed to date are either to bury the radioactive wastes in deep salt deposits or bedrock, or to keep them in massive concrete and steel vaults at the earth's surface. Germany uses abandoned salt mines for disposal of their nuclear wastes. Such mines are considered to be good places to store these wastes because the presence of undissolved salt indicates that water does not flow through the site and thus the wastes are not likely to get transported into water supplies. Some salt mines that were originally thought to be disposal sites, however, have subsequently been found to occasionally contain water. Hence, the debate persists over the wisdom of this disposal method.

A major stumbling block to implementation of these ideas is that local governing bodies have been reluctant to accept the wastes in their areas of jurisdiction, including those states where nuclear power supplies a significant fraction of the electricity. Like the famous barge of garbage from New York City, which no one was willing to accept, radioactive wastes have generated a strong NIMBY ("not in my backyard") response. Apparently, the public is not convinced that deep burial (the federal government's chosen method of disposal) is as safe as the government says it is.

Nuclear wastes are often considered to be more of a burden on future generations than are ordinary wastes, such as municipal garbage and sewage, because nuclear wastes can remain a hazard for a very long time (see the discussion of *half-life* in Chapter 15, Section B). Indeed, nearly one-tenth of the original radioactivity in typical nonreuseable nuclear waste from a power plant will still remain after 100 years. Since some of the radioactive constituents have a half-life of several hundreds of thousands of years, a radiation hazard will exist far longer into the future than humanity could conceivably plan for. In some ways, the situation is not so different from some of the more conventional types of waste. Toxic metals have an infinite half-life, meaning that they last forever (see Chapter 12). When wastes containing toxic metals, such as **cadmium** or **mercury**, are dumped into the oceans or contaminate soils, their threat to the ecosystem and to human health lingers on indefinitely.

The nuclear industry has pointed to the relatively small volume of nuclear wastes from a typical nuclear power plant (compared, say, to the volume of municipal wastes from a city served by the power plant) as an argument that nuclear wastes pose a relatively minor problem. In one sense, this is a valid point; the sheer volume of ordinary wastes makes transport and disposal more of a problem. But in another sense, it is misleading, for the toxicity in nuclear waste repositories is extremely concentrated and thus a small leak or spill poses more of a threat.

One significant difference between nuclear wastes and ordinary wastes is that nuclear wastes can be used by terrorists or by nations seeking the material to make a nuclear weapon. At reprocessing plants where the reusable materials are separated from the true wastes, the possibility exists that such groups could steal the reusable materials after separation (this would be virtually impossible before separation because of the intense radiation of the useless wastes). To many scientists concerned with these issues, this connection between nuclear wastes and international security is a far greater threat to humanity than the risk of radiation from permanently stored nuclear wastes.

Ocean Dumping

In the last decade or so, as land disposal of wastes has become more expensive (or undesirable), advocates of ocean disposal and ocean incineration have become increasingly vocal.

The open oceans and coastal marine areas have served as dumping grounds for all manner of wastes—raw and treated sewage, industrial effluents, low-level radioactive wastes, sewage sludge, municipal garbage, dredge spoils, and drilling wastes from offshore gas and oil operations. Wastes enter the marine environment directly through pipelines or by being dumped from barges, or indirectly as a result of discharge into rivers, which eventually carry their loads to the sea. Federal regulations, developed over the last two decades to curtail indiscriminate dumping into the marine environment, allow the EPA to issue disposal permits. In theory, then, substances are subject to regulation as pollutants in accordance with either the Clean Water Act or the Marine Protection, Research, and Sanctuaries Act. Specific provisions have been developed to regulate the kinds and amounts of materials disposed of in the oceans, such as low-level radioactive wastes, and the locations of permissible disposal sites, such as near shore versus deep ocean sites.

Until recently, most wastes have not been dumped into the open oceans (100 or more miles from shore), but have been routinely discharged, directly or indirectly, into near shore coastal waters and estuaries. These are biologically and commercially important areas that serve as the feeding and nursery grounds for a substantial portion of commercial fish and shellfish species. Approximately 80% of marine-disposed dredged material and nearly all sewage have been dumped in estuaries and along the coast.

Estimates exist for the amounts of sludge, sewage, industrial effluents, industrial wastes, and dredge material that have been dumped directly into the seas, but the extent to which these various wastes have been contaminated with hazardous substances is uncertain. Most of the nearly 200 tons of dredge spoil that is disposed of in the oceans is thought to be nonhazardous. But dredge spoil and sewage sludge, dumped into the New York Bight (until recently, an approved dump site just 12 miles off the New York–New Jersey coast) contained **PCBs** and various toxic metals, including **cadmium**, **lead**, and **mercury**.

Similarly, while there are reasonably good estimates of the toxic load in industrial effluents discharged into rivers, it is difficult to estimate what proportion of the hazardous substances actually gets transported to coastal marine areas. About 6.4 trillion gallons of industrial wastes containing some 400 million pounds of toxic metals and another 170 million pounds of toxic organic chemicals are discharged into the nation's rivers. How much of that ends up in the marine environment is unknown; how much is retained in freshwater sediments is also generally undetermined. But some proportion of the contaminated sediments, such as those from navigable waters, become the dredged material that is ultimately dumped into the ocean.

As pressure has increased to use the oceans as dumping grounds, it has become apparent to the public and to Congress that more stringent laws regarding ocean disposal of wastes are needed to protect human health, marine species, and the marine environment. Changes in RCRA in 1984 that apply to land-based disposal and modification of the laws governing ocean dumping have forced waste generators to consider alternatives to previously cheap land-based and ocean disposal that have resulted in pollution. Consequently, there has been a shift toward increased reliance on incineration and the development of waste-processing technologies, both of which reduce the volume of wastes and/or change the nature of the waste.

C. Waste Processing

Before waste is disposed, there are numerous opportunities to alter its form, reduce its bulk, and recycle its components. Incineration, for example, is often thought of as waste disposal, but it is only a step in that direction, for the end-products of burning must themselves be disposed of. Because of its controversial aspects and great public interest, a separate discussion of incineration follows.

There are fundamentally three approaches to processing waste: physical treatment, chemical treatment, and biological treatment. Physical treatment includes compaction, separation, distillation (boiling off various components), and evaporation. Each of these methods tends to reduce the volume of waste. A separation stage allows recyclable materials to be recovered. Chemical treatment can be neutralization of *acidic* or *alkaline* materials, precipitation of dissolved substances out of solution, and chemical dechlorination. Incineration is actually a form of chemical treatment since burning is the chemical reaction of oxygen with combustible materials. The third approach is biological treatment, or allowing microorganisms to consume, alter, and detoxify waste. This is what is done in secondary treatment of human sewage.

Incineration

Perhaps the most controversial technique of waste processing is burning. As landfills increasingly approach their limits, communities are searching for ways to reduce the volume of waste they must dispose of. One such method is mass incineration in which municipal solid waste is fed directly and continuously into combusters. Many of the new plants produce electrical power as a by-product. Currently, more than 100 garbage-burning plants exist in the United States, more than three-fourths of which are waste-to-energy facilities, and many more are planned. However, as new plants are proposed, community opposition to them rises, usually on the basis of potential health and environmental effects.

Incineration changes the form of the waste, reduces its volume and weight, but does not destroy many of its hazardous components.

In fact, burning releases many harmful substances that were once fairly safely embedded in solid material. Two new forms of waste are produced: gaseous emissions and solid residues. Gases exit from the smokestacks of the incinerators, with or without special treatment. Solid residues include both the ash that falls through the grates of the combustion chamber (bottom ash) and the fly ash that rises up the smokestack. As regulations require more of the air emissions to be cleaned up, more of the hazardous waste ends up in the bottom ash.

The most important toxic products of incineration are **dioxin**, furan, and toxic metals. They are found in both the gaseous emissions and the solid residues. Quantitatively, the most significant components are the metals **lead**, **cadmium**, arsenic, **mercury**, **selenium**, and **beryllium**. Other identified metals include **nickel**, **aluminum**, **zinc**, copper, and manganese. Many of these metals cause cancer and produce diseases of the nervous system, kidneys, liver, blood, and other organs. Dioxin and furan are potent causes of cancer and other illnesses.

When trash is burned, the physical or chemical form of metals can be changed, often making them more hazardous. For example, mercury is turned into a gas, which is then difficult to trap and is released into the air. Many metals end up on very small particles that more easily escape filtering devices or become more dispersible by wind or rain from ash piles when they are collected. The smaller particles are more easily and deeply inhaled into the lungs or swallowed, making their intrinsic hazard greater both for people and animals. The **chlorine** that is a widespread ingredient in modern plastics creates metal chlorides when burned, which are more easily dissolved in water than the original metal product and become more mobile in the environment as a result. Even treatments to reduce the hazard of some of the gases make the metals problem worse. Lead, for example, dissolves more readily in water after acid gases have been treated with lime to neutralize them. Recent research has shown that the lead

and cadmium that dissolve out of ash piles attain levels that are legally defined as hazardous waste, thus requiring special disposal, despite the fact that virtually all ash is buried in sanitary landfills along with unburned municipal trash.

Other criticisms of incineration revolve around cost and whether a commitment to burning reduces the incentive for recycling. Many environmentalists believe there is a place for incineration in the mix of waste-processing options, but only after all reasonable attempts have been made to separate potentially hazardous products from the waste prior to burning and only if gaseous emissions are properly controlled and solid residues properly buried.

New Hazardous Waste-Processing Technologies

Engineers are continually at work devising new methods to treat toxic wastes in an attempt to eliminate or render them less harmful. As government policy makes it more difficult and expensive to dispose of hazardous materials, the financial incentive to develop treatment processes increases. Some of the creative directions being pursued involve solar energy and plasma torches.

At the U.S. government's Solar Energy Research Institute in Colorado and Sandia National Laboratory in New Mexico, solar technologies are being used to destroy toxic chemicals in industrial waste and in polluted groundwater. Contaminated water containing a *catalyst* is pumped through tubes in solar collectors that focus the sun's ultraviolet energy on the waste water mixture. In one pass through the collector, one-third of the contaminants are converted to harmless products; in several passes, 90% are destroyed. In another technique, the sun's heat is focused on collectors containing organic chemicals in a special chamber with a catalyst. At temperatures approaching 1000°C, the organics are converted to carbon monoxide and hydrogen, which can then be made to react to produce methanol for fuel. A third process focuses light at an intensity of 300 suns on a quartz vessel containing **dioxin**. The sunlight quickly breaks down 99.9999% of the dioxin into relatively harmless compounds.

Westinghouse Electric Company is developing a "plasma torch" that generates temperatures up to 5500°C (10,000°F). The torch, which resembles an arc welder, can be used to blast difficult organic chemicals, such as **PCB** transformer fluids, into harmless gases that can be vented or used as fuels. The torch is small enough to be truck mounted and brought to the waste site so hazardous materials do not have to be transported. The destruction is so complete that Westinghouse is considering using it to destroy old chemical warfare weapons.

These examples demonstrate the possibilities for dealing successfully with toxic wastes. Nevertheless, not producing toxic compounds in the first place is the surest way to minimize toxic hazards.

D. Recycling and Other Approaches to Source Reduction

Our society is hooked on manufactured chemical products. Like a smoker faced with the option of either quitting smoking or learning to cope with the prospect of getting lung cancer, we can either reduce our dependency on toxics or we can "manage" toxics. In the preceding two sections we discussed ways to manage toxics through disposal and waste processing. But there is a growing sentiment in the United States that the best approach to the hazard of toxics is to greatly reduce our use of them. A *Los Angeles Times* editorial of April 11, 1988, put it bluntly: "The best way to avoid toxic waste is to make fewer toxics in the first place. If more time were spent figuring out how to do with less, less time would be wasted searching for dump sites to dispose of waste."

Quitting toxics will require imagination and restraint on the part of both industry, by reducing toxics used in manufacturing, and

the public, by reducing consumption. In this section, we discuss how both these groups can reduce or eliminate the use of toxics. Although this may involve a slight change in lifestyle, what is more important is a change in attitudes. Industries can reduce their use of toxics by improving manufacturing techniques. Consumers can do it simply by consuming less. Reducing consumption can be achieved in a variety of ways, including conservation, recycling, and finding substitute products for those containing or producing toxics.

Industrial Options

The traditional view of industry as some sort of gigantic machine that eats raw materials and spits out finished products is starting to be replaced by a more comprehensive picture, that of an industrial ecosystem. Whereas the former view simply emphasized productivity, the latter now emphasizes efficient recycling of resources to achieve that productivity. Industries have already started to figure out how to reduce their dependence on the many toxic substances used in the manufacture of goods that in themselves may or may not be hazardous. Many segregate toxic and nontoxic wastes, a first step toward recycling toxics, or at least permitting them to be disposed of separately in designated toxic waste sites.

Industrial recycling is already established and growing in several major industries, although weak points along the recycling pathway still hinder the process. In producing the plastic polyvinyl chloride (PVC), the toxic ingredient **vinyl chloride** is tightly controlled. It may be converted to the product, recovered for further use, or broken down into harmless by-products. Almost all in-house scrap PVC is recycled at factories making PVC products. Because PVC is so widely used, however, collection and recovery of it is difficult once it enters the marketplace.

Two industrial processes that illustrate the benefits and opportunities of recycling have recently been developed. A way has been found to use discarded auto tires to produce a wide range of new products, including gaskets, exercise mats, storage bins, railroad crossing pads, and new tires. The system is in use in Minnesota, Massachusetts, and Michigan. It uses no water, so it produces no effluents; it has no smokestack because it produces no air pollutants. There are two billion tires in official waste tire dumps, with another 240 million discarded each year in the United States alone. The process is economical, costing half as much as virgin rubber, and it produces a product cheaper than plastic.

In the second example, a Swiss company has developed a process to use unsorted plastic wastes to make durable goods, such as fence posts and vine stakes. It was previously thought that different plastics were not compatible because of their different compositions. This inhibited the recycling of plastics because of the need to sort and separate different kinds. But this process shows that some useful products can be made from mixed plastic waste. The main disadvantage is that the recycled plastic is not of uniform strength, so it cannot be used to provide structural strength in construction products. Nevertheless, these two examples show how industrial innovation can provide environmental benefits as well as profitable business opportunities.

Some industries have developed ways to make use of the toxic waste of other industries. For example, certain chemicals used in the process of refining oil cannot be reused by the refinery, but they can be sold to chemical or cement manufacturers for their subsequent use. In the absence of such interindustry recycling, the wastes would have been disposed of in hazardous landfill sites or other disposal sites.

There are other ways that industries can reduce environmental releases of toxics besides recycling. The California Public Interest Research Group (CALPIRG), a nonprofit organization dedicated to environmental quality and consumer welfare, has documented three different pioneering approaches that several industries have taken:

Finding nontoxic substitutes for toxics,
Redesigning production methods to eliminate the need for toxics, and
Making production more efficient so as to reduce toxics use.

For example, some paper-processing companies have substituted relatively harmless bleaches for toxic **chlorine** bleaching agents, and other industries, such as Christmas wrapping paper producers, have substituted water-based solvents for more toxic organic solvents. To avoid altogether the use of toxic cleansing solvents, other industries have redesigned their production systems so that cleaning is accomplished by rotating metal brushes or plastic beads propelled at high speed. To make more efficient use of toxics, some industries have plugged up leaks in pipes conveying toxics, have used evaporation barriers to prevent unnecessary loss to the atmosphere, or have removed defective product components from the production line before toxic solvents are wasted on them. Many dry cleaning businesses are using machines that recycle the cleansing solvents.

All of these industrial strategies still lead to the production of the same consumer goods that were being made before. Their purpose is to reduce the volume of toxics that industry is discharging to the environment and to which it is exposing its own workers. But an equally great opportunity for source reduction is available to each consumer. There are three major ways for us to consume fewer toxics: conservation of energy, recycling, and purchasing less toxic substitutes.

Consumer Options

Conservation of Energy Conservation of energy is one of the easiest ways to reduce the amount of toxics in the environment because conventional methods of producing energy create a host of hazardous substances (including **sulfur dioxide, nitrogen oxide,** carbon dioxide, and **carbon monoxide**). One can conserve energy not only by turning off lights, televisions, and other appliances when not in use, but also by minimizing the need for them. When buying new cars or appliances, make use of consumer organizations and magazines to find out which ones are most energy efficient and invest in them. Some appliances, such as refrigerators, are now labeled with efficiency ratings. There are some incredible advances on the market now, such as 15-watt light bulbs that produce as much light as standard 75-watt bulbs and last longer.

Recycling   It is increasingly common to find recycling centers in local communities. These centers recycle paper, glass, tin, aluminum, and even plastics. Many communities now also have recycling programs mandated by the local government in which residents are provided with color-coded containers for sorting recyclable materials. Pickups for the various materials occur on specific days. Often, more than half of a family's garbage can be recycled in this way. If your community does not have such a program, lobby for one!

Many thrift shops have a home pickup service for people who do not have time to drop off used items. When you need a product, first check out local yard sales, estate sales, flea markets, consignment and thrift shops, and personal newspaper ads for used items on sale. Not only are the savings and diversity usually tremendous, but nearly new or untouched products can often be found this way. It is amazing how easy it is to ignore these reusable resources when we are continually presented with advertisements and promotions of seemingly plentiful new goods. One word of caution is necessary, however. Be alert to the sale of products that may have already been banned because of toxics problems or other safety reasons, such as unsafe toys and fire-resistant pajamas contaminated with **TRIS.**

The case of paper illustrates the tremendous benefits of recycling and the successes that can be achieved. Production of paper produces a considerable amount of air and water pollution, destroys vast acreages of forest, contributes to soil erosion and siltation of streams, and threatens wildlife habitats. Moreover, paper and cardboard are the largest single component of municipal waste (about half the volume and two-fifths of the weight), thus contributing greatly to the problem of inadequate disposal sites. Nearly all used paper can be recycled. If it cannot be used for fine quality stationary, it can be turned into nursery pots, insulation, or the poorer quality paper used for newspapers. Each ton of paper recycled saves 17 average-sized trees, along with 25 barrels of oil and 7000 gallons of water used in manufacturing, and 3 cubic yards of landfill space. Recycling just one edition of the Sunday *New York Times* would save nearly 100,000 trees. The public has shown that recycling paper works. Many towns now provide scheduled curbside collection of used paper, and public cooperation has been great. Indeed, the effort has been so successful that the next step is to increase the demand for recycled paper products. Here, too, the actions of the consumer are essential—ask for and buy recycled paper products when the opportunity exists.

Purchasing Less Toxic Substitutes for Toxic Products   While energy conservation and recycling can really help reduce the use of toxics, finding less toxic substitutes for toxic consumer goods is a more direct way to stop the toxics flow. For example, some garden pesticides such as **pyrethrum** and some food preservatives such as **acetic acid** are less toxic than others, and certain power lawn mowers and wood stoves pollute less than others. Other good candidates for substitution are plastic and styrofoam; the manufacture of both require toxics. And neither is biodegradable: the so-called biodegradable plastics that have recently been developed will merely break down into tiny pieces, not chemically degrade into other usable substances. Use paper or other degradable substitutes when possible, especially when dealing with packaging materials, where the use of plastics has exploded within the past few years. (Popped corn, a great substitute for styrofoam pellets, is increasingly used in commercial packing applications.)

To reduce personal consumption of packaging, buy concentrates and in large sizes or bulk. One European company, for example, sells fabric softener concentrates in small pouches that consumers pour into a bottle they already have and add water. Avoid products sold with excessive packaging. If consumers write to companies selling over-packaged products and explain why they are not buying them, manufacturers will eventually get the point and change their ways. Maximize the reuse of plastics and styrofoam when their use is necessary. The styrofoam that an appliance came packed in, for example, can be broken up and reused to pack other items for shipping.

Under the entries in Part II, the subhead Protection and Prevention provides numerous suggestions for how consumers can reduce their exposure to specific toxics by either switching to alternative products or being more careful in their use of products containing toxics. But a thorough product comparison for all major consumer goods is beyond the scope of this book, so in most cases, the consumer will have to rely on a careful reading of the ingredients on products. We hope that with reference to the entries in Part II, the information in ingredients lists can be better evaluated. In some instances, the best choice is far from obvious.

Often the best way to reduce dependence on toxics is simply to avoid altogether the activity that requires toxics. For example, is it really necessary to use a gasoline-powered lawn mower? Rather than shopping around for the least polluting power mower, consider switching altogether to a manual mower. Mowing the lawn with a manual mower avoids exposure to the fumes from a power mower and is a good form of aerobic exercise (so it won't be necessary to drive to an expensive aerobics class!). Going one step further, is it really necessary to have a manicured lawn? By replacing some of it with a vegetable garden, food can be grown that contains no pesticides. Just as some cities try to reduce their pollution problems by encouraging light industries over the more polluting heavy industries, try to choose recreational or other activities that involve lower material consumption and to minimize consumption when participating in activities that consume materials. Walking or bicycling rather than driving on short trips and carpooling rather than driving alone save energy and reduce the quantity of toxics in the environment.

Summary

Reducing the need for toxics by any of the methods just described is a very important step for an individual to make. A decision by an individual consumer not to use a particular toxic substance (or a product whose manufacture requires use of toxic substances) not only reduces the health threat to that person, but also sends a message to industry that the toxic product is not wanted. In the long run, this will entice industries to place more emphasis on making products that are less toxic. And when no nontoxic substitutes are available, it will entice industries to invent them. In our economy, individual consumer actions can add up to a very potent force. It is senseless to wait until others take the lead; it is in both the self-interest of the consumer and in the interests of the wider society that individuals act now rather than later.

Other ways of reducing toxics involve attitudes that are not new, but seem to have been forgotten in recent decades. When buying a product, avoid the disposable versions and look for ones that will last longest and/or are readily recyclable or *biodegradable*. Before throwing out a broken product, first try to repair it to a reasonably usable state—even if it costs nearly as much as a new one, you are saving both the resources to go into producing a new one and junking the old one! Stick to simple versions of products, avoiding the "frills" since these often involve extra substances that are sometimes toxic. (A good example is printed or colored toilet paper, which in most cases uses slowly biodegradable ink.) Not only does the simpler product lead to lower levels of toxics in the environment, but it saves the consumer money as well. Likewise, reupholstering a drab-looking sofa or easy chair rather than buying a new one reduces the amount of indoor air pollution in the home (because new sofas and easy chairs usually contain a foam filling that is a source of **formaldehyde**) and costs less as well.

Lest this discussion mislead, it must be pointed out that decisions to use a substitute product or to substitute one type of activity for another can backfire. A substitute chemical may seem safer only because less is known about it. The choice of walking rather than driving to a destination, while laudable from the perspective of reducing pollution emissions and providing good exercise, may expose that person to far more air pollution from the cars of all the people who have not made the switch. How can risk be minimized, given the large number of factors that have to be considered? No easy answer to that question exists. Risk is a complex and subtle concept, as we showed in Chapter 1. The most people can do is to be well informed and act on the basis of the best available information. In that way people will not be at the mercy of commercial interests who care chiefly about their own profit and not necessarily the public's well-being. Like the survival of democracy, the protection of individual health and safety is ultimately dependent on a citizenry that follows its own educated instincts.

Further Reading

BECK, M., HAGER, M., KING, P., HUTCHINSON, S., ROBINS, K., and GORDON, J. 1989. Buried Alive. *Newsweek* November 27.

COLBURN, T. E., DAVIDSON, A., GREEN, S. N., HODGE, R. A., JACKSON, C. I., and LIROFF, R. A. 1990. *The Great Lakes Great Legacy?* Washington, D.C.: The Conservation Foundation.

Concern, Inc. 1989. *Household Waste: Issues and Opportunities.* Washington, D.C.

Congressional Budget Office. 1985. *Hazardous Waste Management: Recent Changes and Policy Alternatives.* Washington, D.C.: U.S. Government Printing Office.

DENISON, R. A., and RUSTON, J. 1990. *Recycling and Incineration: Evaluating the Choices.* Environmental Defense Fund. Washington, D.C.: Island Press.

DENISON, R. A., and SILBERGELD, E. K. 1988. Risks of Municipal Solid Waste Incineration: An Environmental Perspective. *Risk Analysis* 8(3):343–355.

DOYLE, J. K. 1989. *The Wastoid Handbook.* Dallas, TX: Leadership America.

FROSCH, R. A., and GALLOPOULOS, N. E. 1989. Strategies for Manufacturing. *Scientific American* 261(3):144–152.

HAYES, D. 1978. *Repairs, Reuse, Recycling—First Steps Toward a Sustainable Society.* Worldwatch Paper 23. Washington, D.C.: Worldwatch Institute.

Office of Technology Assessment. 1986. *Serious Reduction of Hazardous Wastes.* Washington, D.C.: U.S. Government Printing Office.

Office of Technology Assessment. 1987. *Wastes in the Marine Environment.* Washington, D.C.: U.S. Government Printing Office.

17 REGULATING TOXICS

The number of toxic or potentially harmful substances that we use or come in contact with everyday is staggering. Over the last two decades, Congress has enacted a great variety of laws in recognition of the need to identify the culprits, to understand their potential effects, and to limit human exposure to such substances. Although most of the principal laws share the broad goal of protecting human health and the environment, each has one or more specific mandates: to protect air quality, to protect water quality, to enhance public health and safety, or to improve waste management. Several new bills, proposed to fill in some gaps in the regulatory blanket, are currently before Congress. While a review such as this is bound to be partially out of date soon after it is written, we briefly describe some of these proposed laws pending in Congress that we believe are likely to have a significant effect on the future regulation of toxics. A final section discusses a novel approach to regulating toxics recently implemented in California, namely, Proposition 65.

A. The Regulations: An Overview

In the United States there are more than two dozen statutes or laws whose purpose, at least in part, is to protect people and the environment from the potentially harmful effects of toxic or hazardous substances. Most of the more far-reaching environmental legislation was enacted in the 1970s when it became clear that unexpected costs, as well as benefits, were associated with the nation's tremendous industrial productivity and that these costs—human health problems and environmental deterioration—had to be addressed. By regulating every phase in the life cycle of toxic substances from extraction, production, and marketing, to transportation, consumption, storage, and disposal, the laws limit our exposure to potentially harmful materials.

The major federal regulations governing toxic or hazardous substances are briefly described in Table 15. As shown, most of the laws have been amended one or more times; in some cases, the specific titles of amendments are given. Many laws were originally written or amended with explicit expiration dates, which are also indicated in the table. Once a law expires, it must be rewritten and reenacted, that is, reauthorized. Reauthorization of some expired regulations has proven to be a difficult and protracted exercise, often involving several years; reauthorization of certain pieces of legislation is pending, as noted.

For many of these statutes, Congress writes broad goals into the legislation, leaving it to the overseeing agency, usually the EPA, to write detailed guidelines and regulations. The EPA assumes the primary burden of regulating toxic chemicals and is empowered to set standards for toxics in the air and in surface and underground water (drinking water specifically), to monitor air and water quality, to test and register new pesticides, to test and reregister in-use pesticides, and to evaluate data on the roughly 1000 new chemicals introduced annually. But because many of the laws are vague, the EPA has considerable latitude in interpretation and implementation.

Taken as a whole, the laws have been likened to an incomplete crazy quilt, with large areas of overlap, mismatches, and glaring omissions. Since they were first enacted, the laws have been frequently reevaluated and amended (patched up) to take into account

TABLE 15 The Major Federal Legislation Focusing on Toxic Substances

Statute	Date Enacted, Amended, Expired, or Reauthorized	Mandate
Atomic Energy Act	1954	To regulate utilization, storage, distribution, and disposal of radioactive materials
Clean Air Act (CAA)	1970	To "protect and enhance the quality of the nation's air resources . . . to promote the public health and welfare"
Amended	1977	
Expired	1981	
Reauthorized	1990	
Clean Water Act (CWA)	1972	To "restore and maintain the chemical, physical, and biological integrity of the nation's waters"
Amended	1977	
Expired	1982	
Reauthorized	1987	
Coastal Zone Management Act	1976	To preserve, protect, and enhance coastal zones
Comprehensive Environmental Response, Compensation, and Liability Act (CERCLA) (the Superfund)	1980	To clean up hazardous waste sites and spills
Expired	1985	
Reauthorized as Superfund Amendments and Re-authorization Act (SARA)	1986	Establishes new cleanup standards for hazardous waste sites, emphasizes permanent cleanup, and regulates underground storage tanks (with SDWA and HSWA)
Consumer Product Safety Act	1972	To protect consumer from hazardous products that pose an "unreasonable risk" of injury or illness
Amended	1976, 1978	
Emergency Planning and Community Right-to-Know Act (EPCRA) (also known as Title III of SARA)	1986	Provides tools for improved management of industrial toxic chemicals; requires annual Toxics Release Inventory by industries
Federal Food, Drug, and Cosmetic Act (FFDCA)	1938	To protect consumer food, drugs, and cosmetics
Food additives amendment	1958	
Color additives amendment	1960	
DES proviso amendment	1962	
New animal drugs amendment	1968	
Federal Insecticide, Fungicide, and Rodenticide Act (FIFRA)	1947	Originally written to protect farmers from dangerous and ineffective pesticides
Amended	1972	Requires the registration of pesticides on
	1975	the basis of test data; no registration
	1978	permitted if "unreasonable adverse risk
Expired	1984	to environment" disclosed
Partially reauthorized	1988	Major issues not included
Federal Meat Inspection Act	1967	To regulate food and feed, color additives, and pesticide residues in meat, poultry and eggs
Poultry Products Inspection Act	1957	
Egg Products Inspection Act	1970	

TABLE 15 The Major Federal Legislation Focusing on Toxic Substances (continued)

Statute	Date Enacted, Amended, Expired, or Reauthorized	Mandate
Federal Land Policy and Management Act	1976	To protect public lands, specifically regulating mining
Federal Mine Safety and Health Act	1977	To regulate toxic substances in coal and other mines
Hazardous Liquid Pipeline Safety Act	1979	To regulate pipeline transportation (and incidental storage)
Hazardous Materials Transportation Act	1974	To protect against risks associated with transport of hazardous materials
Amended	1975, 1976	
Expired	1986	
Lead-Based Paint Poisoning Prevention Act	1973	To regulate use of lead paint in toys and furniture, and in cooking, drinking, and eating utensils
Amended	1976	
Low-Level Radioactive Waste Policy Act	1980	To regulate disposal of wastes, e.g., clothing, paper, sludges, and equipment, contaminated with small amounts of radioactivity
Marine Protection, Research, and Sanctuaries Act (MPRSA)	1972	To regulate the transport and dumping of wastes in open ocean and coastal marine waters
Amended several times		
Expired	1982	
Reauthorized (part)	1988, pending	
National Environment Policy Act (NEPA)	1969	To establish policy to prevent damage to environment and to promote human health and welfare
Noise Control Act	1976	To protect against noise levels that jeopardize health or welfare
Occupational Safety and Health Act (OSHA)	1970	To ensure so far as possible safe and healthful working conditions for every working man and woman
Poison Prevention Act	1970	To protect children from injury or illness by requiring special packaging of household substances
Ports and Waterways Safety Act	1972	To regulate shipment of toxics and petroleum products by water
Dangerous Cargo Act	1952	
Public Health Service Act	1944	To regulate biological products
Resource Conservation and Recovery Act (RCRA)	1976	To protect health and environment by conservation of resources and "cradle-to-grave" management of hazardous wastes
Amended	1980	
Hazardous and Solid Waste Amendment (HSWA)	1984	Bans land disposal of certain toxic chemicals, unless treated
Reauthorization	Pending	

Statute	Date Enacted, Amended, Expired, or Reauthorized	Mandate

Safe Drinking Water Act (SDWA)
  Amended
  Expired
  Reauthorized
	1974
	1977
	1982
	1986
		To ensure minimum standards for public water supplies; regulates contaminant levels in public water supplies

Surface Mining Control Act	1977	To protect society and the environment from pollution problems of surface coal mining

Toxic Substances Control Act (TSCA)
  Expired
  Reauthorization
	1976
	
	1983
	No action
		To regulate toxic substances (other than alcohol, tobacco, radioactive materials, food, drugs, food additives, and pesticides); the intent is to minimize toxic hazards of industrial chemicals

Asbestos School Hazard Abatement Act	1984	Amendment to TSCA to help defray the costs of inspection, management, and removal of asbestos in schools
Asbestos Hazard Emergency Response Act Amended	1986 1988	To strengthen EPA regulations of asbestos and set deadlines for school response Extends deadlines for school inspections and asbestos removal plans
Uranium Mill Tailings Act	1978	To control hazards to public from tailings sites

the most obvious problems, weaknesses, and gaps in the original statutes. Many of the amendments have been stopgap measures to deal only with the most glaring problems. But there have also been significant mid-course corrections, notably the 1977 amendments to the Clean Water Act. Most of the laws need extensive and fundamental reworking, which is more appropriately done at the time a law expires and is being prepared for reauthorization or renewal.

Unfortunately, the reauthorization process is neither an easy one nor a quick one. Many of the laws are allowed to expire and remain in limbo for years, while Congress debates the specific goals and provisions of renewed legislation. Proposals for renewed legislation, in the form of bills, often become mired in Congressional committees because of overlapping jurisdiction, opposing interests, and a persistent failure to reach

agreement. Despite expiration, existing laws do not become inactive if, as is usually the case, Congress votes for emergency funding to maintain basic programs. But the much needed strengthening of the regulations is stalled, sometimes indefinitely.

Ten of the statutes, which are particularly broad in scope, form the legislative backbone of toxics regulation in the United States. In this chapter, the goals and effectiveness of these major laws are described. Problems of implementation, loopholes, and inadequate coverage and funding are noted. These problems, coupled with new and better scientific information on the risks posed by toxics, have led to a general agreement among federal and state legislators, representatives of the various chemical industries, environmentalists, scientists, and informed members of the public that most of the laws are imperfect and need a major overhaul.

B. Protection of Air Quality

Several laws are involved, directly or indirectly, with the protection of air quality. Indirectly, the Toxic Substances Control Act (TSCA), the Comprehensive Environmental Response, Compensation, and Liability Act (CERCLA), and the Resource Conservation and Recovery Act (RCRA) all play significant roles in promoting and maintaining clean air. Because of differing mandates, however, these are discussed elsewhere; TSCA more broadly concerns public health and safety, and CERCLA and RCRA focus more specifically on waste management. The primary law directly concerned with air quality is the Clean Air Act.

Clean Air Act (CAA)

Enacted in 1970, the Clean Air Act is the major law intended to protect and enhance the nation's air quality. With it, Congress required the EPA to establish National Ambient Air Quality Standards (NAAQS) for air pollutants characterized by wide dispersal and emission by many sources, such as cars. These *primary air quality standards* define the level of air quality to be achieved and maintained nationwide for six conventional pollutants: **sulfur dioxide, carbon monoxide, nitrogen oxide, ozone, particulate matter**, and **lead**. Both human health and environmental effects are taken into account in setting the standards. In addition, the EPA is required to identify locally distributed *hazardous air pollutants* for which it intends to establish national emission or performance standards (allowable limits) because exposure to them could "result in an increase in mortality" or serious illness; such as cancer, damage to the reproductive or nervous systems, and other chronic or acute health effects. Although hundreds of potentially hazardous air pollutants exist and may ultimately be regulated, to date only eight hazardous air pollutants have been listed: **mercury, beryllium, asbestos, vinyl chloride, benzene**, *radioactive* substances, coke oven emissions, and inorganic **arsenic**. Emission standards have been set for all but certain coke oven emissions.

The primary goal of the original legislation—the establishment and attainment of air quality standards—has proven difficult to achieve. Key elements of a 1977 amendment to the CAA authorize the EPA to

1. impose penalties (including bans on certain types of construction and withholding of federal funds for highway construction and sewage treatment facilities) on communities that fail to meet air quality standards,

2. tighten emission limits on new stationary sources of air pollutants,

3. require areas that have not attained the standards for **ozone** and **carbon monoxide** to retrofit controls, and

4. establish motor vehicle inspection and maintenance programs.

There have been some positive results of the CAA. Most significant has been the dramatic decrease in ambient air concentrations of **lead** in the United States as a result of steady reductions in the content of lead in gasoline beginning in the 1970s. It has been estimated that about 86% of the 250,000 tons of lead released globally to the air each year is from automobile emissions. In 1985, the EPA ordered refiners to remove 90% of the lead in gasoline by the end of the year. The agency initially went further than expected by proposing a total ban on lead by 1988, seven years sooner than previously proposed, but it has subsequently backed off on this. The new move was prompted by two studies that linked only slightly elevated levels of lead with high blood pressure, particularly in white males. Projections suggested that the reduction in lead could prevent 1.8 million cases of high blood pressure and reduce the number of heart attacks by 5000 and strokes by 1000 in 1986. Furthermore, the EPA estimates that removal of 90% of the lead in the air will prevent lead-linked disease in 172,000 children. The action was supported by a cost–benefit analysis indicating that consumers will save $914 million on engine maintenance, $187 million on fuel economy, and $600 million in health costs of toxic effects on children.

Until recently there was a steady improvement in air quality around the country, with the primary standards being met in most areas. Overall, there have been substantial (20%) reductions in emissions of particulates, sulfur dioxide, and carbon monoxide over the last decade. But, these successes have been accompanied by an increase in nitrogen oxide emissions. Also, more than 100 areas nationwide have ozone and carbon monoxide levels in excess of the standards for part of the time. Not surprisingly, most of these areas are metropolitan, but some, such as Acadia National Park in Maine, are rural. The EPA has estimated that as many as 100 million people live in the affected areas. Compounding the concerns with occasional high levels is new scientific information indicating that low levels over an extended period of time also pose a health threat.

It has been pointed out by a number of experts that even with additional pollution controls and stiff penalties, it could take many years for the most heavily polluted areas, namely, Los Angeles, Houston, and the Connecticut–New York corridor, to meet the standards. They suggest that drastic measures, including shutting down industrial plants, rationing gas, and restricting automobile use, would speed up compliance. To set an example and hasten compliance, the EPA issued a ban on the construction of facilities in Los Angeles that cause air pollution (those that emit more than 100 tons of pollutants a year). Unfortunately, a construction ban does not address a major source of ozone and carbon monoxide—the automobile. Los Angeles, however, seems to regard the need to improve air quality seriously. The city recently proposed an air quality plan that would require substantial changes in life-style habits that contribute to air pollution. For example, one idea in the plan is to eventually ban all gasoline-fueled vehicles and to redesign the city to reduce reliance on the automobile.

Failure to meet air quality standards is just one problem that Congress has grappled with in the decade-long effort to reauthorize the Clean Air Act, which expired in 1981. One of the most controversial issues in the renewal struggle was acid rain (see Chapter 11, Section C). Despite the improved technologies and restrictions on emissions imposed on power plants, industrial facilities, and automobiles by the law, we still produce roughly 20 million tons each of sulfur dioxide (down from a previous high of 26 million tons) and nitrogen oxides a year, both of which are implicated in the problem of acid rain. Agreeing in principle that the emissions levels of oxides of sulfur and nitrogen must be lowered, Congress had difficulty determining an acceptable level of emissions and a satisfactory method of achieving those levels.

On November 5, 1990, President Bush signed the new Clean Air Act Amendments that

1. tighten pollution control requirements in cities that have not attained the National Ambient Air Quality Standards,

2. require 40% reductions in acid-rain causing emissions of SO_2,

3. list nearly 200 hazardous air pollutants and mandate control technologies for all major sources of air toxics,

4. require more stringent auto emission standards, cleaner gasoline, and the introduction of clean-fueled vehicles in the nation's most polluted cities, and

5. specify a phase-out schedule for the production of chemicals that contribute to the depletion of the stratospheric ozone layer.

Implementing the new law will not be cheap. The yearly price tag is expected to be about $25 billion. The savings in human health costs and environmental damage are incalculable.

C. Protection of Water Quality

The integrity and quality of the nation's rivers, lakes, drinking water, groundwater, and coastal marine waters are addressed by a set of laws. The Clean Water Act (CWA) and the Safe Drinking Water Act (SDWA) are the principal laws governing freshwater systems. The Marine Protection, Research, and Sanctuaries Act (MPRSA); the Comprehensive Environmental Response, Compensation, and Liability Act (CERCLA); and the Resource Conservation and Recovery Act (RCRA) protect water chiefly by regulating the introduction of pollutants into the marine environment, freshwaters, and certain groundwater supplies. As yet, no single statute exists expressly to prevent contamination of groundwater, other than drinking water supplies (see Section F, this chapter).

Clean Water Act (CWA)

The primary law protecting the "chemical, physical, and biological integrity of the nation's waters" is the Federal Water Pollution Control Act, more popularly known as the Clean Water Act (CWA), which was enacted in 1972. Intended to regain or maintain fishable and swimmable water quality, the CWA requires the EPA to set and revise water quality *criteria* based on the most recent scientific information. (The criteria are not rules; they are a compilation of data about pollutants that can be used to formulate enforceable standards or regulations. The EPA issues the criteria, and the states adopt water quality standards, which consist of a designated beneficial use limit and a supporting numerical concentration limit.) Three classes of pollutants are covered by the law: conventional pollutants such as *Escherichia coli, a coliform bacterium* present in sewage; nonconventional pollutants such as **ammonia**, nitrogen, and phosphorus; and toxics. Originally the principal focus was the regulation of potentially polluting discharges from fixed, localized sources (point sources) such as municipal sewage treatment facilities and industrial plants.

The 1972 Clean Water Act established two mechanisms to achieve the clean water goal. First, point source dischargers are required to treat wastes to specified minimum levels using the best available technology in compliance with the quality standards of the receiving water. Second, to help municipal dischargers meet requirements, Congress provided federal financial assistance for construction of sewage facilities. A major amendment in 1977 provided additional funds for construction of sewage treatment plants, established a program to encourage innovative and alternative wastewater treatment, emphasized the control of toxic pollutants, and imposed new compliance dates for conventional, priority, and other toxic pollutants. Amendments enacted in 1981 reduced federal assistance, putting an increased burden on the states.

Measured in terms of conventional pollutants, some of the nation's surface waters have improved since the implementation of water pollution legislation designed to control point source discharges. Coliform bacteria counts and dissolved solids have been reduced, while oxygen levels have increased sufficiently to permit the reestablishment of plants and animals that had died out in many polluted lakes and streams. According to the 1982 National Water Quality Inventory, about two-thirds of the states responding to a survey indicated overall positive trends in water quality. The effectiveness of the CWA, however, has been mixed. Nationwide, there has been improvement in about 13% of the rivers and streams that have been assessed and degradation in about 3%. In contrast, only about 3% of the assessed lakes have improved, while about 14% have degraded. Water quality in the vast majority of fresh surface waters has remained unchanged.

Application of the technology-based controls required by CWA has resulted in reduced pollution loads, although the population has grown and industrial discharge has substantially increased. Certainly, the amount of municipal and industrial wastes undergoing *secondary* and *tertiary treatment* (intended to deal with organic chemicals and heavy metals) has increased. Nevertheless, some 36 million pounds of toxic metals and 130 million pounds of toxic organics are released into lakes, rivers, and streams each year by municipal and industrial facilities. Because chlorinated hydrocarbons (see Chapter 13, Section A) and heavy metals persist in sediments and accumulate in tissues, fishing is banned and warnings are in effect against the consumption of fish in many regions of the United States where these pollutants occur.

Since the expiration of the CWA in 1982, reauthorization efforts have focused on correcting problems in the original legislation, particularly those programs dealing with waste discharge and pollution control. For example, while the original law was concerned with the reduction of pollution from point source discharges, it has been estimated that as much as one-half of water pollution comes from nonpoint sources such as pesticide-laden agricultural runoff and sewer overflow runoff from city streets and highways.

Several years in the making, the reauthorized package was passed by Congress in 1986, only to be vetoed by President Reagan in early 1987. The bill became law, however, when Congress promptly overrode the Presidential veto. The new legislation takes several major actions. It addresses the control of nonpoint sources of pollution, requires the EPA to publish revised and new water quality criteria, stresses new programs to combat water pollution from toxics, restricts the availability of waivers from national standards that had previously been easy to obtain by dischargers, and increases much needed funding for the construction of wastewater treatment facilities. Federal funding for sewage construction grants, however, ends in 1990.

Nevertheless, there are still major flaws in the water legislation. Amendments in 1977 to the CWA required the EPA to publish Ambient Water Quality Criteria for priority pollutants (those substances that Congress deemed most toxic), leaving it to the states to develop the standards. The EPA has published criteria for 126 priority pollutants; 109 criteria deal with the protection of human health and 34 criteria focus on the protection of aquatic life. But although these criteria have been published, few states have actually established standards for toxic pollutants or have incorporated standards into the regulation of toxic discharge. Without standards to be enforced, the law lacks substance.

Safe Drinking Water Act (SDWA)

The Safe Drinking Water Act was established in 1974 to ensure that public drinking water systems, which include surface water and groundwater, meet minimum standards for the protection of public health. The EPA is required to set standards for contaminants in drinking water. Furthermore, the law authorizes EPA to establish rules for the disposal of hazardous substances by injection into underground wells and to prohibit the development of new injection wells where underground drinking water systems are threatened.

By law, the EPA is currently required to regulate 83 potentially hazardous substances found in drinking water. Standards have been set for only 23 of these contaminants. Because the federal government has been slow to set standards, many states have developed their own, which vary from state to state and differ from federal standards. As a result, people living in different states are not uniformly protected. Despite state initiatives, standards or guidelines (either state or federal) have been established for less than half of the potentially toxic substances detected in groundwater. Reauthorized in 1986, the new SDWA requires the EPA to monitor public drinking water supplies for unregulated contaminants and to set deadlines for the issuance of standards. Until the standards are set, the law cannot be enforced.

Contamination of groundwater, which is

the primary source of drinking water for about 50% of the U.S. population, is a growing problem (see Chapter 6, Section B). The extent of contamination is uncertain, but recent reports indicate that the frequency may be considerably higher than previously thought in certain areas, such as farming regions. A survey in Iowa, for example, found that an alarming 70 to 80% of the wells surveyed were contaminated with pesticides.

The problem of groundwater contamination is addressed in a piecemeal fashion, with specific concerns amended to various existing legislation, such as CWA and RCRA. Attached to the reauthorized Superfund law, CERCLA, for example, is an amendment to RCRA that specifically requires that owners or operators of leaking underground petroleum storage tanks take necessary corrective action to protect human health and the environment, that is, to prevent groundwater contamination. As yet, however, there is no comprehensive statute that explicitly sets out a national policy on protecting groundwater and establishes the necessary uniformly applicable regulations.

D. Public Health and Safety

While protection of public health and safety is an inherent goal of all the major legislation under discussion, four statutes have been established to identify and regulate toxic substances and limit human exposure to these toxics in the workplace, in food, and in certain other consumer goods. These are the Toxic Substances Control Act (TSCA); the Occupational Safety and Health Act (OSHA); the Federal Food, Drug, and Cosmetic Act (FFDCA); and the Federal Insecticide, Fungicide, and Rodenticide Act (FIFRA).

Toxic Substances Control Act (TSCA)

Intended to protect public and environmental health, the Toxic Substances Control Act (TSCA) of 1976 was established to ensure the safety of new and existing chemicals. Because federal authority to deal with the overall life cycle of chemicals is fragmented, TSCA was enacted to fill the gaps left by the other laws.

Central to the law is the requirement that manufacturers submit certain information, called premanufacture notices (PMNs), on new products to the EPA for safety evaluation. Required information includes the chemistry of the substance, the proposed uses, the amounts to be produced or processed, the by-products, the number of workers to be exposed, the duration of exposure, and the method of disposal. Pertinent data on health or environmental effects are supplied at the manufacturer's discretion unless otherwise directed by the EPA. To assess whether the chemical, during its lifetime, will present an unreasonable risk of injury to people or the environment, the EPA can demand relevant toxicity data from the manufacturer. The law authorizes the agency to prohibit or limit the manufacture, production, distribution, use, importation, processing, and disposal of substances found to pose an "unreasonable risk to human health or the environment," chiefly on the basis of what the manufacturer chooses to disclose.

Unfortunately, the system of disclosure is haphazard. A study prepared by the Office of Technology Assessment found that only 10% of the premanufacture notices submitted to the EPA over a two-year period reported any information from tests used to estimate environmental effects. Furthermore, although about 50% of the premanufacture notices contained some data on *acute toxicity*, only 17% provided any information on the risks of cancers, birth defects, or mutations.

The EPA has been slow to test and regulate the vast numbers of chemicals in commercial production or use. According to a 1984 National Academy of Sciences report, there are very few data on the health effects of most chemicals in high-volume commercial use. Since 1976, only five chemicals or groups of chemicals have been regulated:

fully halogenated fluorocarbons, **dioxin, asbestos, polychlorinated biphenyls (PCBs),** and **vinyl chloride**, and these only after extensive debate. Moreover, despite evidence that vinyl chloride causes cancer in people, as well as in rats, mice, and hamsters, the EPA has proposed to relax the rules on the emissions of vinyl chloride.

In other instances where the effects are known and regulations to deal with the substances have been established, results are slow. In 1978, the manufacture, processing, and distribution of PCBs in commerce were banned, but some 500 million pounds of PCBs are still being stored or used. In 1979, highly specific rules for the disposal of PCBs became effective. But it was recently discovered that PCB-contaminated wastes were being dumped illegally into unlined pits in 12 states. Part of the problem is that the EPA is primarily a regulatory and administrative agency, not an enforcement agency. And TSCA places a large burden on the EPA in terms of technical expertise and managerial and legal resources.

Although TSCA expired in 1983 and needs extensive reworking, there has been no great effort to renew the law. Some of the central issues in reauthorization involve tightening up the data collection procedure, strengthening and expanding the testing program, and holding the manufacturer liable for damages.

Occupational Safety and Health Act (OSHA)

The primary purpose of the Occupational Safety and Health Act, enacted in 1970, is to protect workers from workplace hazards. Exposure to high levels of dangerous chemicals is generally more likely in the workplace than in the backyard, thus, the importance of its legislative goal is clear: to ensure that "no employee will suffer material impairment of health or functional capacity" from a lifetime of occupational exposure.

To achieve that goal, the act established the Occupational Safety and Health Administra-

tion (OSHA) to set health and safety standards, to enforce those standards through federal and state inspectors, and to educate the public. As a first step, the agency is authorized by law to set preliminary or consensus standards based on data and standards used by other agencies. It is expected to set permanent standards based on *criteria* documents and recommendations from the National Institute of Occupational Safety and Health (NIOSH). In addition, OSHA has the authority to issue emergency temporary standards in situations where a toxic or physically harmful substance poses grave danger.

The process of setting standards is a slow one. Despite nearly 20 years of effort, the agency has managed to set permanent standards (mostly derived from emergency standards) for less than two dozen substances of the hundreds recommended by NIOSH and the thousands of toxic substances that may warrant regulation. Instead, OSHA has a list of about 400 toxic substances with simple threshold limits, which have been adopted from lists provided mostly by private industrial hygiene organizations. Only recently were these promulgated as standards. The act has not been amended or modified since its passage. Its provisions are relatively clear, a characteristic that facilitates implementation. Delays in standard setting are due primarily to OSHA mismanagement and interagency squabbles.

Recognizing the need for improved, coordinated monitoring testing of toxic chemicals, OSHA proposed a Federal Cancer Policy in 1977. Its purpose is threefold: (1) to integrate scientific input and policy decisions on carcinogens, (2) to facilitate OSHA's standard-setting process, and (3) to coordinate the policies of OSHA, the EPA, the Food and Drug Administration (FDA), and the Consumer Product Safety Commission (CPSC) with the intent of reducing exposure to known man-made carcinogens to zero. Some analysts feel that the Federal Cancer Policy could have more far-reaching impacts on toxic chemicals than the Toxic

Substances Control Act. The proposed policy, put on hold in 1980 by the Reagan administration, may be resurrected by the Bush administration.

Federal Food, Drug, and Cosmetic Act (FFDCA)

Enacted in 1938, the Federal Food, Drug, and Cosmetic Act is the most extensive law of its kind in the world. Very broad in scope, the law is intended to ensure the purity, wholesomeness, safety, and cleanliness of food; the safety and effectiveness of drugs and medical devices; and the safety of cosmetics. At first glance, the law seems to cover everything from **aflatoxins**, diet pills, packaging materials, and toothpaste, to perfume, labeling requirements, animal growth hormones, heart pacemakers, and blood banks. But, the protective blanket is somewhat patchy in its coverage.

Food One of the principal regulations of the act relating to food safety specifically prohibits added or naturally occurring poisonous substances. To that end, food additives must meet certain safety criteria established by the FDA to be permitted in or on foods. A food additive is any substance that may become a component of food or otherwise affect the characteristics of the food. Substances that are intentionally added, such as preservatives, and those that inadvertently find their way into food from various sources, such as packaging materials and certain cookwares, are covered by the law.

Many additives, however, are specifically excluded from the testing and safety requirements of the food additives amendment. Not regulated as food additives are a large number of substances "generally recognized as safe" (GRAS) by qualified experts, but not necessarily on the basis of rigorous testing. Most of the additives on the GRAS list have been in use for a long time. Other additives are exempt on the basis of previous approval under the FFDCA, the Poultry Products Inspection Act, or the Meat Inspection Act. But previous approval is no assurance of safety on the basis of adequate testing. Pesticide residues in or on raw agricultural products, new animal drugs, and color additives—all technically fitting the definition of food additives—are regulated under other provisions of the law.

Moreover, while the law stipulates that articles coming into contact with food (in either home or commercial food establishments) may not impart flavor, color, odor, or toxicity to the food, ordinary housewares such as dishes, mugs, and storage containers are not included. Manufacturers are thus not required to submit safety data to the Food and Drug Administration. Consequently, contaminated dinnerware and cookware containing excessive levels of leachable **lead** and **cadmium**, for instance, have been marketed. Such items, however, are not exempt from the general safety provisions of the FFDCA; regulatory action can be and has been taken against items found to by unsafe—but only after lead-contaminated mugs, pitchers, or baking dishes have been sold and used.

Recently, one provision of the FFDCA, the Delaney Clause, has come under attack as being unreasonably restrictive. The Delaney Clause prohibits the EPA from setting a *tolerance* (maximum amount of a chemical residue legally permitted in a food) for any cancer-causing food additive, including pesticides, in processed foods. Thus, raw and processed foods are regulated differently. For example, for raw foods the EPA may (1) exempt a pesticide chemical from the requirement of a residue tolerance or (2) consider benefits as well as risks when setting tolerances, thus permitting a certain level of risk. In contrast, under the Delaney clause a zero risk standard has been employed for processed foods.

The problem is complex. Residues of some carcinogenic pesticides that are permitted on raw fruits and vegetables become more concentrated when these foods are processed. Such residues are illegal on or in foods to be processed. But as pointed out by a National Academy of Sciences (NAS) study, such a blanket prohibition does not distinguish between high-risk carcinogens and those that pose little risk. Moreover, many older pesticides have not been adequately tested and therefore cannot be evaluated with regard to carcinogenic risk. In effect, they are presumed innocent until proven guilty and continue to be used, some in large volume. In contrast, newer pesticides, which have been subjected to rigorous testing, are often not permitted on foods because some (even very small) carcinogenic risk has been found. Ironically, the risks associated with some of the newer pesticides may be substantially smaller than those for older, less well-tested chemicals.

Following publication of the NAS report in 1987, the EPA and Congress began grappling with a recommendation to adopt a uniform "negligible risk" standard to apply to both raw and processed food. (Determination of negligible risk depends on rigorous testing of older pesticides, a principal focus of the renewed FIFRA; see the next section.) Opponents argue that no level of cancer-causing pesticide is tolerable and, even more broadly, that all pesticide residues should be prohibited. The EPA recently changed the policy, arguing that the Delaney Clause only prohibits setting tolerances for cancer-causing substances that pose a significant risk. Residue levels in raw and processed foods will be treated similarly by the EPA. The FFDCA, however, has not been altered to reflect the EPA's policy change.

Cosmetics

The FFDCA requires that color additives in cosmetics (as well as in drugs and food) must be tested for safety and approved for use. Otherwise, the law does not specifically require that manufacturers test the safety of cosmetic products; it does, however, strongly urge safety determinations. Cosmetics not adequately tested must carry a warning label. There is no registration requirement for cosmetic ingredients; registra-

tion is voluntary and does not denote safety approval by the FDA. Several cosmetic ingredients are restricted or prohibited under the FFDCA. These include bithionol, **mercury** compounds, **vinyl chloride**, halogenated salicylanilides, zirconium (in aerosol cosmetics), **chloroform**, hexachlorophene, **formaldehyde**, and **chlorofluorocarbons (CFCs)**.

Drugs

New drugs are defined in the FFDCA as "articles intended for use in the diagnosis, cure, mitigation, treatment, or prevention of disease in man or other animals," and nonfood items are defined as "articles that are intended to affect the structure or any function of the body of man or other animals" (including weight reduction items). Both drugs and nonfood items as so defined must be reviewed and approved for safety and effectiveness by the FDA before being marketed. Certain foods or cosmetics for which therapeutic claims are made may be subject to the drug provisions.

Drugs are approved by the FDA on the basis of test results pertaining to safety and effectiveness that are submitted with a New Drug Application. Both the application and accompanying supporting data are usually submitted by the manufacturer. The process of approving new drugs and getting them on the market has been criticized as unnecessarily ponderous, as in the case of the AIDS drug AZT, which seems to retard the development of HIV symptoms. In contrast, the FDA has been blamed for approving inadequately or improperly tested drugs as in the case of L-tryptophan, a drug marketed for insomnia, depression, and weight control. The drug has subsequently been linked to a sometimes fatal blood disorder called eosinophilia-myalgia syndrome (EMS). As a result, the FDA has issued a recall of L-tryptophan.

The law specifies labeling requirements that include identification of active, habit-forming, or certain toxic ingredients; precautionary statements; usual or recommended dosage; and route of administration. Official drugs, that is, those listed in the United States Pharmacopoeia, the Homeopathic Pharmacopeia of the United States, or the National Formulary, must meet certain standards of strength, quality, purity, packaging, and labeling.

Federal Insecticide, Fungicide, and Rodenticide Act (FIFRA)

The nation's primary statute governing the sale and use of pesticides is the Federal Insecticide, Fungicide, and Rodenticide Act (FIFRA), passed in 1947. It was originally intended to protect farmers from ineffective and dangerous pesticides. Important amendments to FIFRA in 1972 shifted the emphasis from safeguarding the pesticide user to public health and environmental protection. FIFRA is intended to ensure that the use of a pesticide will not cause adverse environmental effects, defined as "any unreasonable risk to man or the environment, taking into account the economic, social and environmental costs and benefits of the use of any pesticide."

Specific requirements of the act include the registration of all pesticides based on health and safety test results; the classification of pesticides for general or restricted use; and the suspension (an immediate ban on production and distribution) or cancellation (a complete ban or a restriction in use) of those pesticides found to cause unreasonable adverse effects on the environment or people. A further provision concerning indemnification states that the EPA must compensate manufacturers for remaining stocks and pay for the cost of disposal, including storage and transport, of canceled or suspended pesticides. In addition, FIFRA directs the EPA to evaluate the approximately 600 active pesticide ingredients currently in use that were registered before November 1, 1984. These older ingredients, which account for most of the pesticides on the market, have not been adequately tested for their potential to cause cancer, genetic mutations, birth defects, sterility, infertility, nerve damage, or other chronic effects. If they meet the more stringent health and safety requirements, they can be reregistered by the EPA.

Several problems with existing regulations have been identified. One is the extreme slowness of the process of canceling dangerous pesticides. Under current rules, when new evidence arises to indicate that an in-use pesticide may be more harmful than previously thought, the EPA undertakes a *Special Review*, which involves examining existing data and calling for additional tests in keeping with the more stringent test requirements for newer pesticides. The EPA considers the risks and benefits and decides whether to cancel the older pesticide. The manufacturer can voluntarily withdraw the product or request a cancellation hearing. The entire process can take a dozen or more years—with the pesticide being sold and used all the while. Sometimes particularly troublesome pesticides are suspended while the cancellation process goes on.

Another problem has been the glacially slow reregistration process. To date, only 2% of the 600 or so older pesticides have been fully reevaluated. The Government Accounting Office (GAO) has charged that at its present pace, the EPA would not complete the task until well into the twenty-first century. Meanwhile, many questionable older pesticides continue to be used.

The FIFRA expired in 1984. After four years of struggle, in response to the widely recognized need to accelerate the retesting of older pesticide ingredients, in 1988 the 100th Congress passed a revised version of FIFRA calling for the completion of the process within nine years. The law sets up a system of fees to pay for reregistration. Furthermore, the new legislation addresses the method of compensating manufacturers and end users for canceled or suspended pesticides, which had been one of the major stumbling blocks in the reauthorization process and a significant problem for the EPA. Under the existing statute, the costs of compensation and disposal of canceled or suspended stocks have come out of EPA operating funds, which would otherwise have been used for regulating or reregistering pesticides. There have been charges that the EPA has dragged its feet in issuing warranted cancellation or suspension notices because of the high costs.

In the last few years the EPA has issued emergency cancellations for the following four pesticides: **ethylene dibromide (EDB)**, dinoseb, **2,4,5-T**, and silvex. To date, the federal government has paid more than $29 million in indemnification costs for ethylene dibromide and 2,4,5-T/silvex. Total costs, including disposal, for all four pesticides may run as high as $200 million. The revised law will permit compensation of farmers and other end users out of a U.S. Treasury Judgment Fund, rather than from the EPA budget. Moreover, manufacturers cannot be indemnified without specific Congressional appropriation.

Another major change in the law transfers the responsibility for transporting, storing, and disposing of suspended and canceled pesticides from the EPA to the manufacturers. The high costs associated with cancellation and suspension are partially attributable to the uncertainty concerning storage and disposal technologies. While the best disposal technology is debated or improved technology awaited, the chemicals must be stored, which is both costly and difficult. Dinoseb and EDB are both highly corrosive and must be kept in special containers.

In the recent effort to reauthorize FIFRA, several important but controversial issues were omitted from the final bill. Among the issues still to be addressed by Congress are groundwater protection from pesticide contamination, pesticide residues on foods, *inert ingredients*, the sale of U.S.-banned pesticides to other countries, and a farmer's liability for damages incurred by using a pesticide according to directions. Because authorization for the 1988 amendments expires in September, 1991, and because so many important issues were neglected, efforts to reauthorize and strengthen FIFRA continue.

E. Waste Management

The three laws discussed here specifically address various aspects of waste management. They range from the "cradle-to-grave" management of hazardous materials mandated by the Resource Conservation and Recovery Act (RCRA), to the cleanup of contaminated hazardous waste sites by the Comprehensive Environmental Response, Compensation, and Liability Act (CERCLA), to the regulation of the disposal of wastes in the oceans dictated by sections of the Marine Protection, Research, and Sanctuaries Act (MPRSA). Several other laws, notably the Toxic Substances Control Act (TSCA), and the Clean Water Act (CWA), have important provisions that address aspects of waste disposal, but overall their mandates are substantially broader (and thus were discussed in previous sections).

Resource Conservation and Recovery Act (RCRA)

The Resource Conservation and Recovery Act was enacted in 1976 and reauthorized in 1980 in the wake of the public outcry following disclosures of the toxic waste problem at Love Canal in Niagara Falls, New York. It regulates the management of hazardous wastes at each stage of their life cycle, from extraction to processing to final disposal, in short, from cradle to grave. The law requires the EPA to identify hazardous wastes, to establish standards for hazardous waste facilities, to track hazardous materials using a manifest system, and to regulate disposal facilities by issuing permits. The RCRA also defines and lists hazardous wastes. The Hazardous and Solid Waste Amendment (HSWA) of 1984 was an attempt to discourage most land disposal of certain hazardous wastes. One provision of the amendment specifically prohibits land disposal of **dioxin**-containing wastes and those containing high levels of **arsenic**, metals, and halogenated chemicals such as **PCBs**. Alternative waste treatment methods and technologies (such as incineration) have not yet been proven in terms of safety or effectiveness (see Chapter 16, Section C).

Recent newspaper stories about wandering garbage barges and contaminated groundwater make it clear that we are running out of suitable places to dump our waste and that we must develop a sensible, safe policy to address the problem. The RCRA expired in 1984 and is now up for reauthorization. Current versions of the bill stress the importance of waste reduction and encourage recycling. As the name of the act suggests, both notions were included in the original legislation, but the emphasis has been on handling existing hazardous wastes.

Congress is considering several major revisions to the existing law, including a tracking system for transportation, storage, treatment, and disposal of nonhazardous wastes similar to the system that applies to hazardous wastes. Another important provision of renewal efforts is a prohibition on disposal of household hazards, tires, yard wastes, and large household items in landfills. Current bills also include proposals to set minimum technical standards for municipal incinerator ash, industrial solid wastes, and large volume mining wastes. Moreover, standards for monitoring systems and for the construction of adequate containment in landfills and surface impounds have been suggested. Also, Congress must deal with the charges by various critics that the 1980 reauthorization was weakened by the insistence of the oil and gas industry that hazardous wastes produced by oil and gas drilling be exempted from regulation. Although a complete reauthorization package is not likely until 1992 or 1993, early Congressional action to regulate interstate shipments of garbage is expected.

Comprehensive Environmental Response, Compensation, and Liability Act (CERCLA)

The Comprehensive Environmental Response, Compensation, and Liability Act, more commonly known as the Superfund of 1980, authorized the federal government to respond to emergency spills of hazardous substances and leaks from toxic or hazardous waste treatment, storage, and disposal sites in response to the devastating discovery of vast quantities of toxic wastes at Love Canal in Niagara Falls, New York. It created a $1.6 billion fund for the cleanup of hazardous waste sites, such as Love Canal. The fund was generated from taxes on crude oil and 42 chemicals derived from petroleum plus an additional injection of funds from the government.

In a 1985 report called the Superfund Strategy, the Office of Technology Assessment (OTA), which provides scientific advice to the U.S. Congress, assessed the nation's Superfund program. It found several major problems. First, the EPA has vastly underestimated the magnitude of the toxic waste problem. The OTA estimates that as many as 10,000 waste sites would require priority cleanup. Since the widespread problem of leaking hazardous waste sites was first recognized a decade ago, the EPA has so far identified and scheduled for cleanup only about 1300 priority sites. Second, cleanup efforts have been meager. Of the 538 sites originally on the National Priority List, only 30% have received remedial attention and only 36 have been completely cleaned up. Moreover, OTA charges that contaminated material has been moved from problem sites and deposited in hazardous waste landfills that may become tomorrow's Superfund sites. Also, on-site containment may prove ineffective. A third problem is that efforts have focused chiefly on temporary cleanup measures, with little or no emphasis on permanent cleanup (such as groundwater cleanup) or long-term research and development of innovative technologies. Of the $1 billion spent to date, only $25 million have been spent on technological development.

Other recent reports charge that there has been serious mismanagement of the Superfund hazardous waste cleanup program. It is claimed that some contractors have charged exorbitant fees, that the EPA has not been aggressive enough in recovering Superfund money from polluters, and that the EPA has been lax in overseeing cleanup projects.

When the Superfund expired in September 1985, the cleanup at more than 200 sites was delayed for lack of funds. But concern about the problems of hazardous waste sites was sufficient to facilitate fairly quick reauthorization in 1986. The new legislation, called the Superfund Amendments and Reauthorization Act (SARA), represents a compromise between putting the full financial burden of cleanup on oil and chemical companies and a broad-based combination of business and public funding. SARA provides $9 billion for the period from 1987 to 1991. It emphasizes the importance of undertaking permanent cleanup or remedial actions, specifically those that reduce the volume, toxicity, or mobility of hazardous substances, pollutants, and contaminants. One provision of SARA amends the 1984 amendment to RCRA. As a result, states are required to inventory underground storage tanks containing petroleum and other regulated substances. Owners and operators of underground petroleum storage tanks are required to undertake corrective action to prevent leakage from these tanks.

In 1988, OTA released its assessment of how the Superfund program was being implemented under SARA. After studying 10 Superfund cleanup sites, OTA concluded that, contrary to SARA requirements, the Superfund program was not consistently selecting effective technologies to reduce the volume, toxicity, and mobility of contaminants. Moreover, OTA charged that impermanent solutions, namely, land disposal and containment of untreated wastes, were chosen with high frequency.

Marine Protection, Research, and Sanctuaries Act (MPRSA)

Sections of the Marine Protection, Research, and Sanctuaries Act, enacted in 1972, are col-lectively referred to as the Ocean Dumping Act. The law focuses exclusively on protecting the oceans by stipulating that alternative land-based disposal methods must be considered preferentially. It prohibits the transportation for dumping and/or the dumping of wastes into territorial seas or contiguous zones, unless specifically permitted by the EPA. Permits for dumping of municipal, industrial, and certain radioactive wastes into territorial waters are issued by the EPA only as long as the materials will not "unreasonably degrade" public health or the marine environment. Ocean dumping of high-level radioactive wastes is banned, and until January 1985, there was a two-year moratorium on ocean dumping of low-level radioactive wastes. At present, in the absence of a moratorium, Congress must approve requests for permits to dump low-level radioactive wastes. The U.S. Army Corps of Engineers is responsible for issuing permits for dumping of dredged materials, which may be dumped into the oceans in accordance with EPA's environmental criteria. Prevention of unlawful dumping is the responsibility of the EPA, the Corps of Engineers, and the U.S. Coast Guard.

Since the law was implemented, the EPA has successfully cut the volume of industrial wastes dumped in the ocean from 5 million tons to just over 2.5 million tons between 1973 and 1980. But the oceans are not yet safe. Since the expiration of the MPRSA in 1982, reauthorization efforts have been on the Congressional agenda. A few issues are particularly contentious. As land disposal problems and costs increase, there is growing pressure to dispose of wastes in the ocean. Stricter enforcement of air quality standards has led to a push to incinerate toxic substances at sea. Also at issue is the location of ocean dump sites: no one wants them too close to home. Hence, regional concerns are a major impediment to comprehensive and quick legislation.

In the closing days of the session, the 100th Congress passed a bill that would ban dumping of sewage sludge and municipal waste by

December 31, 1991. The Congress also approved reauthorization of other aspects of the MPRSA.

F. Additional Laws Recently Passed or Under Consideration

In addition to the major existing laws, several pieces of new or proposed legislation are worth noting. These deal with specific toxic substances or issues that have been inadequately covered by existing laws and are deemed of significant concern as health or environmental hazards. Passage of the proposed laws in some form is likely, although when Congress will reach final agreement is uncertain.

Radon

In late 1988, **radon** became a household word. The media gave major coverage to a 1988 EPA survey that suggested as many as eight million homes in the United States could contain excessive levels of radon activity. Spurred by the widespread concern regarding the extent of exposure to radon, the 100th Congress passed legislation, which amended TSCA, to create a national radon program. Important provisions included the following: determination of the extent of radon contamination in schools and federal buildings, development of improved methods of eliminating the gas, funding and technical assistance to state governments for radon control, certification of radon detection devices, and establishment of a radon information clearinghouse.

PCBs

The PCB Regulatory Improvement Act is intended to tighten up the regulation of **polychlorinated biphenyls (PCBs)** and to facilitate tracking of PCB waste from generator to final disposal. EPA regulations set an October 1988 deadline for retiring PCB capacitors and an October 1990 deadline for retiring many transformers. The bill is intended to provide safeguards during the period of peak disposal through 1993. If passed, it would require people responsible for disposal and storage to have insurance against accidents and cleanup costs. Normally PCBs are regulated under provisions of TSCA, but recent information about improper disposal indicates a need for more comprehensive rules. Thus, under the proposed legislation, PCBs would be subject to the more stringent RCRA regulations. A shift to RCRA authority is opposed by utility, waste treatment, and chemical industry groups, as well as by the EPA, which says it is unnecessary. At the time of adjournment, the 100th Congress was deadlocked over the issue of which federal law should regulate PCBs. In 1989, the EPA issued new regulations embodying many of the more stringent RCRA-based requirements of the proposed legislation.

Organotin

Another law, proposed in 1987, is the Organotin Antifouling Paint Control Act, which is intended to restrict the use and sale of tin-based chemicals, such as tributyltin (TBT). Used to prevent algae, barnacles, and other encrusting marine organisms from attaching to boat and ship hulls, the antifouling marine paints appear to be lethal to a variety of fish and shellfish species even at very low concentrations. Before adjourning in October 1988, the 100th Congress approved the bill to severely limit the organotin chemicals on some types of commercial and recreational vessels.

Lead

Congress is in general agreement that the standard for **lead** in drinking water needs to be tightened, but agreement as to how stringent the standard should be, how to achieve that standard, or who pays the costs of cleaning up the water supplies have been contentious issues. Efforts to reach agreement have been spurred on by the recent findings that nearly a million water coolers currently in use in schools and elsewhere have lead-lined tanks or lead parts that come in contact with the water. Shortly before adjournment, the 100th Congress passed a bill that would recall lead-lined tanks, prohibit lead in new water coolers, provide $90 million over the next three years to help schools find and reduce lead in drinking water, and fund state and local programs for screening the levels of lead in blood of children and infants.

Groundwater

There is strong Congressional support for comprehensive legislation to protect groundwater. Initial legislation efforts have focused on groundwater research. Proposed in 1987 and introduced in 1989, the Groundwater Research bill is intended to coordinate and improve research on problems of groundwater. If passed, it will establish a national groundwater quality assessment plan under the U.S. Geological Survey, initiate an EPA-directed program for groundwater protection, and direct the EPA to develop environmental profiles for groundwater contaminants. A major point of contention holding up passage is the EPA's refusal to permit the U.S. Geological Survey to be in charge of collecting the data that the EPA needs for regulatory purposes.

Oil Spills

For more than a dozen years there have been attempts to pass a comprehensive law covering liability and compensation for oil spills. Approval of major oil spill legislation was given added impetus following the 11-million-gallon spill from the Exxon tanker *Valdez*. The Oil Pollution Act became law in 1990 and requires that the spillers, rather than the public, pay the costs of cleanup. Oil companies are required to have sufficient insurance coverage to meet cleanup costs. Additional funds would be generated from a federal tax on oil. Moreover, spillers are liable for damages to property and natural resources, as well as for loss of earnings or other revenues as a result of damages. Additional funding would be made available by a federal tax on the oil industry. The new legislation requires double hulls on all new oil tankers and barges operating in U.S. waters, requires the president to ensure effective and immediate removal of an oil spill, and establishes a national planning and response system.

Summary

Strong legislation concerning toxic substances is vital for the protection of public health and the environment; it is fundamental to the nation's well-being. In the last two decades, there has been a continuing effort to develop a comprehensive policy and enforceable, meaningful laws regarding toxics. Significant progress has been made toward the goal of protecting the public and the nation's resources, but most assessments of the effectiveness of existing legislation note that many laws need reworking—to be strengthened, tightened, or made more inclusive. To that end, Congress moves slowly, often stalled by disagreements between industry and environmental interests. As mentioned, many major pieces of legislation have been allowed to expire and remain in limbo for years because of deep divisions among various interest groups, with industry too often lobbying most vigorously. The same forces that slow renewal of existing legislation also impede swift action on proposed new laws that are intended to address otherwise neglected or overlooked specific issues. Unfortunately, those issues and many of the laws that have been delayed in the reauthorization process are the ones most in need of speedy remedial attention.

G. The Right to Know about Toxics

As concern about the environmental and health effects of toxic substances has grown, the public has begun to demand more and better information about chemical risks present in the workplace, the community, the food supply, and consumer products. Everyone has a right to know about toxic hazards. Once they do, they can then accept risks or demand changes in toxics use. This information approach to toxics management reflects two important principles. Warnings about toxic exposures respect an individual's right to choose which risks to take and allow informed consent. Preventing potential problems by disclosing information and encouraging avoidance of risk controls toxics much more effectively than attempting to repair damage once it occurs.

A national right-to-know movement has evolved from local efforts by labor unions to inform workers about toxic risks and thereby prevent industrial disasters, as well as reduce reliance on toxic substances. The growth of this movement has been fueled by public education campaigns on toxic hazards and by the widespread perception that traditional regulatory controls on toxics have failed to protect people adequately. Information provided directly to people not only helps them avoid toxic hazards, but encourages them to support more effective regulatory controls at the local and federal level. This ground swell of "toxics populism" has transformed toxics management in the United States. How did the right-to-know movement originate? This section reviews it origins and discusses existing federal and innovative state laws that will provide Americans with extensive new information about chemical hazards in the coming years.

Workplace Right to Know

Labor unions concerned about the risks faced by workers in many industries were the first to assert their right to know about toxic hazards. Most workers have little information about chemicals used in production processes, and exposures to toxics in the workplace are often far greater than those received from food, water, consumer products, or outdoor air. From the union perspective, corporations have several incentives for not improving workplace health conditions or sharing information on hazards: the high costs of control, demands for higher wages to face workplace risks, and potential liability for illnesses that can be traced to occupational exposures. Management in many industries using **asbestos** and **vinyl chloride**, for example, had deliberately withheld information about significant health hazards from workers. One result is that an estimated 200,000 workers in the United States will die of asbestos-related diseases by the end of the century.

Early federal efforts to require industry to label chemicals and explain their hazards to those who handle them stimulated considerable opposition from the business community. These efforts ended in 1980 when the newly elected Reagan administration withdrew a chemical labeling rule that had been proposed by the Occupational Safety and Health Administration (OSHA). Disappointed by years of federal inaction, labor forces shifted their focus to progressive states and succeeded in passing state-level chemical hazard disclosure laws. California, for example, passed its right-to-know law in the wake of scandals about workers exposed without warning to the pesticide dibromochloropropane, which causes male sterility and cancer.

The attitude of the Reagan administration toward a federal rule shifted as it realized that providing information to workers could stimulate the marketplace to regulate toxics and reduce the need for direct federal regulation. It was thought that informed workers would demand higher wages, providing industry with an incentive to clean up workplaces. Businesses, concerned about the proliferation of different requirements in state laws, decided to support a uniform federal approach to chemical labeling that would preempt more stringent local laws. In 1983, OSHA issued a Hazard Communication Standard that required businesses to assess the hazards of chemicals they use and to distribute this information to educate employees about hazards in their workplace. The standard fell short of guaranteeing workers the right to refuse hazardous work. It was also initially limited to 14 million manufacturing workers, but a court order extended its coverage to an additional 60 million workers in 1987.

The success of this information approach to toxics regulation is difficult to assess. Workers now participate in training programs on toxics in the workplace and have access to *Material Safety Data Sheets (MSDS)* that describe the hazards of thousands of substances. But the accuracy of the information transferred as well as the ability of workers to understand and act on it is often questioned. Unless a union organization with health experts and bargaining power exists to transform the information into successful wage and safety demands, it is difficult for individual workers to change their workplace. Since less than 20% of the American labor force is unionized, it appears clear that the information approach alone cannot replace the traditional regulatory system of exposure standards and enforced controls.

Community Right to Know

From its inception, the worker right-to-know movement found allies among community members concerned about the presence of potentially dangerous industries in their neighborhoods. The first community right-to-know law was passed in 1981 in Santa Monica, California, following the discovery of **tetrachloroethylene** in municipal drinking water wells. Campaigns for disclosure emerged across the country, and many city ordinances and state laws have been enacted. Community right-to-know programs require inventories of hazardous substances used, stored, or generated as waste by local businesses, as well as establishing processes for emergency response planning and public education.

The industrial disaster at a Union Carbide pesticide plant in Bhopal, India, in December 1984 transformed the local movement of a community's right to know into a national constituency for a federal toxic disaster prevention and disclosure law. Over 2000 people had been killed by a cloud of methyl isocyanate gas—could such a tragedy occur as the result of toxics mismanagement in the United States? After it became clear that most communities had neither the information to assess the risks of such accidents nor plans to cope with them, Congress passed the Emergency Planning and Community Right-to-Know Act (EPCRA) of 1986.

EPCRA, also known as Title III of the Superfund Amendment and Reauthorization Act (SARA), establishes a basic right-to-know program for communities across the country and allows for more stringent local programs. Up to four million businesses are required to provide hazardous chemical inventory data to a hierarchy of local, regional, and state public committees. These inventories include information on hazardous chemical usage and storage needed to prepare emergency response plans for Bhopal-type accidents, as well as information on routine discharges of toxics that are permitted into air and water. Basic information about these discharges can be found in a computerized database called the Toxics Release Inventory (TRI), which is available through the National Library of Medicine.

The extension of the right-to-know movement from the workplace to the community is intended to create an informed citizenry, who can then participate more actively in toxics management debates. By arming communities with information, right-to-know programs can stimulate more effective control of toxic hazards (1) at the local level (by demanding improved safety planning from industry), (2) at the national level (by building a constituency for improving regulatory programs), and (3) in the marketplace (by increasing the demand for safer products).

The promise of community right to know is limited by several factors. Disclosures required by EPCRA began to be publicized in early 1989. Tremendous amounts of information are being generated, but much of it may be useless for accurately assessing health risks or may be difficult to understand without considerable expertise. Inventory data, for example, are not based on actual monitoring and are reported as an amount of annual emissions rather than as air or water concentrations to which people are exposed. As in the workplace, the success of the information approach to toxics regulation depends on the existence of organized groups with technical skills that can make use of the new information.

Right-to-know laws are catalyzing businesses to review their use of toxics and improve corporate management of health risks. Consumers of chemical products are seeking safer substances, sending a marketplace signal to producers. Simply disclosing information about toxic substances, however, has not provided sufficient incentive to generate the widespread innovations in production processes and shifts in consumer demand necessary to reduce overall reliance on toxic substances.

New State Innovations: The California Example

The federal programs providing for the right to know about chemical hazards have several important flaws. Neither the workplace nor community right-to-know laws place priorities on risks. An overwhelming amount of data is generated, but there is no systematic effort to communicate which hazards deserve to be corrected first. Entire categories of exposure that are of great concern to the public are not covered by these disclosure laws. For example, there is no right-to-know regulation about the presence of toxic chemicals in the food supply and consumer products.

Existing information programs have very few regulatory "teeth"—there is virtually no enforcement of the disclosure provisions of the Hazard Communication Standard or the EPCRA. Even more significant, once a warning has been provided about a chemical hazard, there is no requirement that action be

taken to reduce risks. If the producers and industrial users of hazardous chemicals do not feel marketplace or political pressures (from workers demanding higher pay, consumers demanding safer products, or both demanding the enforcement of environmental regulations), they do not need to change their toxics management practices.

Efforts to incorporate these concerns into an improved right-to-know system have occurred primarily at the state level, largely because the Reagan administration was hostile to attempts to extend federal regulatory programs. In the last five years, California has passed several laws that strengthen the information approach to toxics regulation and have served as a model for toxics reform in many states.

Two new California laws ensure that information disclosure results in concrete actions to control toxic hazards. EPCRA's approach to the threat of accidents like the one at Bhopal is disaster preparedness: communities plan for an adequate emergency response. California's Acutely Hazardous Materials Risk Management Act (1987) goes further and requires businesses to develop prevention programs that minimize accident risk. Rather than simply taking an inventory of stocks of hazardous chemicals, the California law requires businesses to publicize a "pessimistic" assessment of the off-site consequences of a major accident. This creates a public constituency that monitors a facility's risk reduction efforts.

EPCRA's approach to the risk from routine toxic emissions is simple disclosure: any plant's annual emissions of toxics to air and water become public knowledge. California's Air Toxics "Hot Spots" Information and Assessment Act (1987) requires high priority facilities to conduct risk assessments for their emissions and notify all exposed individuals that face significant health risks. By distributing understandable information (about cancer risks, for example, rather than pounds emitted per year) and focusing on the most serious environmental polluters, the California law directs the public's attention to the most pressing problems.

Concerned about the public health impact of the growing use of toxic chemicals and convinced that existing federal and state laws provided inadequate protection, California voters overwhelmingly adopted Proposition 65, the Safe Drinking Water and Toxic Enforcement Act, in 1986. The initiative statute expands the right to know about toxics to all potential routes of exposure.

Anyone who in the course of doing business exposes any individual to a chemical known to the state to cause cancer or reproductive toxicity must first provide clear and reasonable warning of the exposure. In California, it is no longer sufficient for a business to report its annual emissions to a local committee. Proposition 65 requires direct warnings to affected individuals prior to significant exposures occurring through the ambient environment, the workplace, food, or consumer products.

Proposition 65 adopts a preventive strategy for toxics management. The use of chemicals known to the state to cause cancer or reproductive toxicity will no longer be considered by government agencies "innocent until proven guilty" of harming public health. Proposition 65 shifts to businesses the burden of proving that exposures to known carcinogens or reproductive toxics do not pose health risks. Unless businesses can demonstrate that their use of chemicals poses no significant risk, discharges to sources of drinking water are prohibited and warnings must be provided prior to any other type of exposure.

Proposition 65 integrates the information and regulatory control approaches to toxics management, providing warnings about all significant risks and requiring restrictions on toxic discharges. Whether the law will by successful remains unclear, since its effectiveness will depend on how it is implemented. California's Health and Welfare Agency has exempted all exposures to carcinogens occurring through foods, drugs, and cosmetics from Proposition 65's warning requirement and is developing numerical limits on discharges that are less stringent than existing federal law.

Beyond its immediate political difficulties, the value of Proposition 65 as a model for toxics reform deserves further examination. Based on the information strategy, the law relies on market forces to induce changes in society's dependence on toxics. If products containing known carcinogens or reproductive toxics must be sold with a warning, this provides industry with a compelling incentive to reduce or eliminate their use of toxic chemicals. But if warnings are provided on all products containing more than trace amounts of toxic chemicals, without any information about the relative magnitude of the hazard posed by the exposure, the information strategy could backfire. Overwhelmed by warnings, consumers might conclude that "everything causes cancer" and refuse to pay attention to even important public health warnings. As with most federal and state efforts to establish a right to know about toxics, Proposition 65 has not succeeded in presenting information on which risks are really worth doing something about.

Proposition 65 shares an additional limitation of right-to-know legislation. A regulatory program that relies only on improving information in the marketplace may not prevent toxics problems. Proposition 65 requires warnings about exposures occurring through air, food, or consumer products, but it does not require an end to these exposures. To achieve its principal goal of protecting water supplies from toxic contaminants, Proposition 65 uses a traditional regulatory approach and simply bans their discharge.

Laws requiring the provision of information cannot solve all our toxics problems. They are unlikely to eliminate the need for many existing regulatory programs. The mix of information and control strategies adopted in Proposition 65 may serve as a model for future efforts to reform environmental regulation. An informed public can influence toxics management through the marketplace, as well as provide a supportive constituency for direct regulatory controls.

Further Reading

ARBUCKLE, J. G., and others. 1987. *Environmental Law Handbook*. 9th edition. Rockville, MD: Government Institutes, Inc.

COLBURN, T. E., DAVIDSON, A., GREEN, S. N., HODGE, R. A., JACKSON, C. I., and LIROFF, R. A. 1990. *The Great Lakes Great Legacy?* Washington, D.C.: The Conservation Foundation.

Environmental Protection Agency, Office of Toxic Substances. 1989. *The Toxics Release Inventory*. Washington, D.C.: USGPO.

U.S. Congress, Office of Technology Assessment. 1988. *Are We Cleaning Up? Ten Superfund Case Studies*. Special Report, OTA-ITE–362. Washington, D.C.: USGPO.

Copies of individual laws are available from the U.S. Government Printing Office, Washington, D.C.

PART TWO

A GUIDE TO COMMONLY ENCOUNTERED TOXICS

Acetic Acid

Other Names

Vinegar acid; ethanoic acid; ethyl acetate; *sec*-butyl acetate; 2-butanol acetate; *tert*-butyl acetate; *tert*-butyl ester; glacial acetic acid; methane carboxylic acid

Introduction

Acetic acid is a natural chemical found in apples, cheese, cocoa, grapes, milk, oranges, parsley, peaches, pineapples, raspberries, strawberries, and bay leaves. Vinegar is about 5% acetic acid. As a *GRAS*[1] substance, it is commonly used as a flavoring agent, during the pickling process, and to control the acidity in processed food. It is most often found in baked goods, cheeses and other processed dairy products, gelatins and puddings, chewing gum, liquor, condiments and relishes, and commercial gravies and sauces.

Although a natural substance, the acetic acid used in industry is manufactured from petroleum. Pure acetic acid is used in lacquer solvents, textile sizings, and paper coatings. It is also used to make various vinyl resins (the liquid used to make vinyl plastics) and dimethyl terephthalate (the main ingredient in polyester). Acetic acid is also a gasoline additive. It is also used in cosmetics such as freckle-bleaching lotions, hand lotions, and hair dyes.

Physical and Chemical Properties

Acetic acid is a colorless liquid or solid with a pungent, vinegar-like odor. It has a sharp, acid taste. Acetic acid is corrosive. When heated, it becomes a fire hazard.

Exposure and Distribution

About one million tons of acetic acid are manufactured in the United States annually, ranking it 35th among the chemicals produced here. It is widely distributed via pro-

[1] Italicized terms can be found in the Glossary.

cessed food, certain cosmetics, and gasoline vapors. Textile and paper workers, workers involved with plastics manufacture, and those who work with solvents are likely to be exposed to acetic acid at the workplace.

Health Effects

The toxicological properties of acetic acid at ordinary exposures are not well known, but at very high concentrations in the air, it is known to cause irritation to the eyes and throat and to depress the central nervous system. It is a severe irritant of the mucous membranes, skin, and eyes. Splashes on the skin can cause *dermatitis* and skin ulcers. Concentrated acetic acid splashed into the eyes can penetrate the cornea to cause swelling of the iris. Small amounts of highly concentrated acetic acid can severely burn the throat if swallowed.

Long-term exposure by humans to very high concentrations of acetic acid has caused blackened skin, bronchitis, chronic sore throat, and tooth damage.

Protection and Prevention

Harmful concentrations of acetic acid are rarely encountered in the home. It is, however, a widely used chemical in industry. If acetic acid is used in your workplace, request a *Material Safety Data Sheet (MSDS)* for specific information about how the chemical is used and how to avoid exposure.

Environmental Effects

Releases of acetic acid into urban air contribute to smog formation through the creation of **ozone**, which is a pollutant at the earth's surface.

Regulatory Status

Acetic acid is regulated by OSHA and the FDA. It is a GRAS substance.

Technical Information

Chemical formula: $C_2H_4O_2$
Molecular weight: 60

Amount released into environment: 74,000 tons/year

OSHA limit in workplace air: 10 ppm

Lethal concentration for humans in air: about 1000 ppm

Further Reading

PROCTOR, NICK H., HUGHES, JAMES P., and FISCHMAN, MICHAEL L. 1988. *Chemical Hazards of the Workplace*. 2d edition. Philadelphia: J. B. Lippincott Company.

Acetone

Other Names

Dimethyl ketone; 2-propanone; pyroacetic ether; ketone propane

Introduction

The solvent acetone is familiar to most people as fingernail polish remover. In the home workshop it is commonly used as a *solvent*; it is also used in glue and airplane dopes. It is widely used industrially as a solvent, in the production of lubricating oils, and as a raw ingredient used during the production of other chemicals such as **chloroform**, acrylic plastic, and methyl isobutyl ketone (a solvent used in plastics, pesticides, adhesives, and drugs). Nearly half of all acetone manufactured is used to make acrylic plastic.

Physical and Chemical Properties

Acetone is a clear liquid with a sweet, pungent odor. Some describe the odor as fragrant and mintlike. Acetone smells much like the related chemical **methyl ethyl ketone**. Acetone evaporates and catches fire easily.

Exposure and Distribution

Acetone is produced naturally by the body as a product of *metabolism*. It is also one of the top 50 chemicals manufactured in the United States. It ranked 43 in 1984, when about one million tons of it were manufactured. It is widely distributed in American homes, mostly as fingernail polish remover.

People are most likely to come into contact with acetone through the use of products containing acetone as a solvent, including certain paints, fingernail polish and finishes, fingernail polish removers, lacquer removers, and airplane dope.

Health Effects

Chronic low exposure to acetone is not considered to pose a health risk. The chemical has been widely used for many years, and few adverse health effects are associated with its long-term use, although frequent use can cause fingernails to dry and split.

High concentrations of acetone, however, can irritate the eyes and mucous membranes. Eye, nose, and throat irritations have been reported at air concentrations near the odor threshold, but this is unusual. More often, these symptoms are felt at much higher concentrations. Headache and light-headedness are reported by some people at air concentrations likely to cause throat irritation. Inhalation of very high concentrations can depress the central nervous system, causing dizziness, weakness, and loss of consciousness. Symptoms similar to drunkenness are also reported when high concentrations are inhaled. Such high concentrations in the air are not likely to be encountered by the average person. The presence of large amounts of acetone in the body can increase the liver *toxicity* of **carbon tetrachloride**.

The widespread use of fingernail polish and remover in the home makes acetone a common source of childhood poisoning. Ingestion of acetone causes central nervous system depression, high blood sugar levels, and high levels of acetone in the blood. These symptoms are similar to those observed in children with uncontrolled diabetes; thus, acetone poisoning is sometimes misdiagnosed as diabetes.

Acetone applied to the skin can cause drying or even slight reversible skin damage. Skin application of acetone can also increase the permeability of undamaged skin, potentially enhancing absorption of other, perhaps more dangerous chemicals. It can also cause peeling, splitting, or brittleness of exposed fingernails. Some people may be *allergic* to acetone when it is applied to the skin. The most common symptom of acetone allergy is *dermatitis*.

Protection and Prevention

Use acetone-containing products in a well-ventilated place. At workplaces where acetone is commonly used, such as a manicuring salon, be sure the work space has plenty of ventilation or is equipped with an exhaust fan. Request a *Material Safety Data Sheet (MSDS)* to get more information about how to avoid workplace exposure to acetone.

People who use acetone at home should try to avoid prolonged inhalation of vapors. Home workshops should be well ventilated when acetone is used. Keep acetone and acetone-containing products out of reach of children. If acetone is swallowed, seek medical attention immediately. Life-threatening symptoms of poisoning often appear hours after acetone is swallowed.

Regulatory Status

Occupational exposure to acetone is regulated by OSHA. The FDA also regulates the amount of residual acetone allowed as a result of making spice extracts. The EPA does not impose any emission or discharge limitations; however, significant acetone releases are subject to annual community right-to-know reporting.

Technical Information

Chemical formula: C_3H_6O
Molecular weight: 58
OSHA limit in workplace air: 750 ppm
FDA limit in spice extracts: 30 ppm residue
Acetone vapors can be smelled by most people when concentration in the air reaches 500 ppm. A concentration of 20,000 ppm in the air is dangerous.

Further Reading

Environmental Protection Agency. 1988. *Updated Health Effect Assessment for Acetone*. EPA–600/8–89–085. Cincinnati, OH.
National Institute for Occupational Safety and Health, U.S. Department of Health, Education, and Welfare. 1978. *Criteria for a Recommended Standard: Occupational Exposure to Ketones*. Washington, D.C.: Government Printing Office.

Acrolein

Other Names

Acrylaldehyde; propenal; allyl aldehyde; ethylene aldehyde

Trade Names

Aqualin; Aqualin-Biocide; Aqualin-Slimicide

Introduction

Acrolein is a strong, foul-smelling liquid used to make drugs, perfumes, food supplements, and resins. One use derives from its repugnant odor: small amounts are added to perfume methyl chloride gas. This gas, used as the working fluid in industrial refrigerators, cannot be smelled at dangerous concentrations. Acrolein is also used in military poison gas mixtures.

Physical and Chemical Properties

Acrolein is a colorless liquid at room temperature, but it is *volatile* so that people are most often exposed to it via inhalation. It has an acrid, choking odor.

Exposure and Distribution

Although used mostly at industrial sites, small amounts of acrolein can be found in the home. Acrolein is given off during cooking and is a component of tobacco smoke. Ordinary people can also be exposed to the chemical following accidental spills and leaks or by living near sites contaminated with hazardous waste. Most acrolein is made in Louisiana, then shipped around the country by rail and truck. Acrolein is among the most frequently encountered chemicals at EPA designated *Superfund* sites.

Health Effects

Acrolein is intensely irritating to the eyes and upper respiratory tract. Exposure to high concentrations in air can cause constriction of bronchial tubes and *pulmonary edema*. Although acrolein is capable of causing death at fairly low air concentrations, its horrible smell and irritating properties tend to protect people from fatal overexposure. One-half teaspoon of liquid acrolein can be fatal to an adult. Mice inhaling nonlethal concentrations of acrolein show suppressed antibacterial defense mechanisms in the lungs.

Acrolein can cause skin irritations and/or burns upon repeated or prolonged skin contact. If splashed in the eye, corneal damage, swelling of the eyelid, and a sticky discharge from the eye are likely.

The potential of acrolein to cause cancer has not been determined, but it is likely that it does. One of its *metabolites* causes cancer, and it is a positive *mutagen* to bacteria. Studies using animals to determine whether it causes cancer in mammals are sparse, and the results are mixed. These studies are difficult to carry out for acrolein because of the extreme acute *toxicity* of the substance. Injections of acrolein in pregnant mice have caused fetal malformations and death. But acrolein has not been linked directly with cancer or birth defects in humans.

Protection and Prevention

Exposure to dangerous amounts of acrolein are unlikely except by those who work directly with the substance. Workers who suspect that acrolein is used at their workplace should request a *Material Safety Data Sheet (MSDS)*. Accidental spills and Superfund sites are possible but uncommon sources of exposure for the average person.

Environmental Effects

Spills can kill exposed fish, land animals, and plants. Acrolein trends to break down quickly, and it does not bioaccumulate.

Regulatory Status

Acrolein is regulated by OSHA and the EPA. Spills and other accidental releases of acrolein must be reported to the EPA. Acrolein releases are subject to annual community right-to-know reporting, and the chemical is listed as a *hazardous air pollutant* in the 1990 Clean Air Act.

Technical Information

Chemical formula: C_3H_4O
Molecular weight: 56
Immediately dangerous to life and health (IDLH) in air: 5 ppm
OSHA limit in workplace air: 0.1 ppm

Further Reading

PROCTOR, NICK H., HUGHES, JAMES P., and FISCHMAN, MICHAEL L. 1988. *Chemical Hazards of the Workplace.* 2d edition. Philadelphia: J. B. Lippincott Company.

Aflatoxins

Introduction

Cancer risks to people exposed to industrial chemicals are often compared to cancer risks posed by eating peanut butter. This is because peanuts are susceptible to contamination by a particular mold that produces a cancer-causing by-product known as aflatoxin. But peanuts are not the only food that can become contaminated with aflatoxin. Many other grains and nuts are also susceptible to this mold, including corn, wheat, rice, cottonseeds, barley, soybeans, Brazil nuts, and pistachios.

Exposure and Distribution

The molds that produce aflatoxin are most likely to grow in warm, humid climates such as in the southeastern United States. But the warm, moist conditions favoring aflatoxin-producing mold can also be created in the field when rain falls on crops, such as corn and wheat, that are left in the field to dry. Aflatoxin-producing mold can also grow on plants damaged by insects or drought. Little is known about why or under what conditions the aflatoxin by-product is produced by the mold. Making matters worse, it is sometimes difficult to see the mold that causes the contamination. Thus, all susceptible crops are subject to routine testing for aflatoxin in the United States. But it is impossible to detect all of it.

For many years it was thought that aflatoxin was produced only when nuts, oilseeds, and grain were improperly stored. In fact, the duration of storage is an important factor as well. The longer agricultural products are stored in bins, the greater the chance that environmental conditions favorable to aflatoxin production will be created. The stored nuts or seeds may be inadvertently dampened, or the storage bin may not allow them to dry quickly enough to arrest the growth of mold, thus allowing pockets of mold growth to develop. In addition, bin hygiene on farms is often lax, allowing fresh grain to pick up mold spores from previously contaminated batches, thus perpetuating the problem.

Only recently was it recognized that food can become contaminated with aflatoxin-producing mold in the field. The mold grows on susceptible crops as the plants mature. Any stress to the growing plants, such as insect damage, drought, poor nutrition, or unseasonable temperatures, allows the mold to proliferate. It is well documented that aflatoxin is more common in poor quality cereals and nuts. While most of these low-grade products do not enter the human food market in the United States, they do enter the animal feed market, thereby contaminating animal products such as meat and milk with low levels of aflatoxin. People in developing nations are more likely to consume aflatoxin-contaminated food than are Americans. Not only are the storage facilities of poorer quality, but developing nations often ship their best quality grains and nuts abroad, leaving the indigenous population with a damaged product.

Animal feed contaminated with aflatoxin can be a problem. Cottonseed meal, a product often contaminated with high levels of aflatoxin, is banned for use as animal feed to protect both the animals and consumers from aflatoxin. (Cottonseed oil rarely contains any aflatoxin because the toxin sticks to the hulls of the seed.) Milk commonly becomes contaminated with aflatoxin. Powdered nonfat milk can contain eight times more aflatoxin than the original liquid product because the aflatoxin sticks to the milk proteins. Measurable levels of aflatoxin can be detected in some baby foods that incorporate dry milk to boost the protein content of the product. Fortunately, pasteurization, sterilization, and spray dry processing techniques can substantially reduce aflatoxin contamination of dried milk. Meat products are less of a problem than milk because little aflatoxin is carried over into animal flesh. In general,

an animal with detectable aflatoxin in the meat would be obviously sick and unsuitable for market. Pig liver and kidney tissues are exceptions to this rule. Chicken meat can also become contaminated with detectable levels of aflatoxin when the bird shows only mild ill effects (mouth sores and damaged kidneys and liver).

Health Effects

Aflatoxin has been called the most potent natural carcinogen known. It is a demonstrated dangerous carcinogen for several species of animals, including mice, fish, rats, marmosets, ducks, tree shrews, and monkeys. Cancers are found in these animals mainly in the liver, colon, and kidneys following ingestion of aflatoxin-contaminated food. Studies using rats indicate that males are more susceptible to cancer as a result of aflatoxin exposure. Nutrient imbalances also seem to predispose animals to cancer following aflatoxin ingestion.

Aflatoxin seems to cause liver cancer in people as well. Studies in East Africa found convincing correlations between aflatoxin ingestion and liver cancer. *Epidemiological* evidence indicates that men are more sensitive than women to aflatoxin exposure. Many scientists believe that a poor diet and previous liver disease can make people more susceptible to liver cancer resulting from aflatoxin exposure. Since malnutrition and hepatitis are common ailments among the East African people studied, it is likely that these people are more sensitive to liver cancer as a result of eating food contaminated with aflatoxin than the average American is. Nevertheless, the data were convincing enough to the FDA and EPA that these agencies have developed strict regulations to control levels in food and animal feed sold in the United States.

Aflatoxin can also cause acute poisoning. Severe liver disease has been seen in people who consume highly contaminated food. Children around the world exhibit symptoms similar to Ryes syndrome (fever, vomiting, coma, and convulsions) following ingestion of aflatoxin-contaminated food.

Protection and Prevention

Do not eat moldy food, particularly food susceptible to aflatoxin-producing molds, such as corn, peanuts, Brazil nuts, pistachio nuts, wheat, and rice. Peanut butter often contains aflatoxin, but the level of aflatoxin allowed in commercially prepared brands is strictly regulated. Be extra cautious about unroasted peanuts, particularly those sold unshelled or in bulk that are then roasted and ground into peanut butter on the premises. Peanuts and other nuts should be roasted before shipping and storage. Roasting helps to dry nuts, inhibiting the formation of mold.

People who handle bulk plant commodities such as grain, ground nut meal, oil seeds, and animal feeds, are at special risk for aflatoxin poisoning. Air concentrations of aflatoxin in such settings can reach levels high enough to cause measurable health problems. People who work in such environments should make sure that the workroom is well ventilated at all times.

Regulatory Status

The FDA strictly regulates the amount of aflatoxin allowed in food and animal feeds sold in the United States.

Further Reading

DENNING, D. W. 1987. Aflatoxin and Human Disease. *Adverse Drug Reaction and Acute Poisoning Review* 6(4):175–209.

Alachlor

Trade Name

Lasso

Introduction

Each year about 85 million pounds of alachlor are sprayed onto U.S. croplands, making it the single most widely used pesticide in the country. Alachlor is a selective *herbicide* used to control annual grasses and certain broad-leaved weeds. Although it is registered for use on 25 crops, about 98% of the total is accounted for by corn and soybeans. The remaining 1 or 2 million pounds are used on a variety of other crops including cotton, peanuts, beans, sunflowers, peas, and sugarcane. Since its registration in 1969, alachlor has been used liberally and is thus widely distributed and may pose risks to the public as a result of contaminated water and uptake by food plants.

Physical and Chemical Properties

Alachlor is a cream-colored or white solid that dissolves readily in acetone, benzene, and ethanol, but dissolves only slightly in water. It resists breakdown by *ultraviolet radiation*, but reacts with water under strongly acidic or alkaline conditions.

Exposure and Distribution

The primary pathway of human exposure to alachlor is thought to be direct contact, as occurs during mixing and applying. The 650,000 private farmers who apply roughly 70% of the 85 million pounds used in the United States are directly or potentially exposed to alachlor. Another 89,000 commercial applicators are exposed on the job to the pesticide. At present, the level of exposure to alachlor as a result of ingestion of contaminated foods is unknown. Only 10% of the residues of alachlor are detectable because the routine methods employed by the FDA only detect certain breakdown products. Because the detection methods are inadequate, actual residue levels are uncertain. The food *tolerances* established by the EPA are based on estimates of the residue levels. Consequently, existing tolerances may seriously underestimate exposure.

Moreover, some concern exists about the level of human exposure from consumption of drinking water contaminated with alachlor. Monitoring of both surface and groundwater systems has revealed substantial levels of contamination in some areas. For example, alachlor has been detected in groundwater in nine states—mostly corn-growing regions—in high concentrations. Evidence suggests that leaching from treated fields is particularly likely in very porous soils or those with reduced populations of microorganisms. In healthy soils, alachlor is broken down by microbial activity within 42 to 70 days, depending on conditions.

In plants, alachlor is taken up chiefly by germinating shoots rather than by the roots. Most of the herbicide is transferred within the plant to the growing parts (leaves, stems, and roots) rather than to the reproductive parts (flowers, fruits, and seeds). In animals, it appears to be rapidly metabolized and excreted in the urine and feces.

Alachlor is generally applied once during a growing season, chiefly by ground spraying. Until recently, aerial spraying was routine, but the producer voluntarily changed its recommendations to reduce applicator exposure. The herbicide is commonly used in conjunction with other herbicides, such as atrazine, **glyphosate**, **dicambe**, linuron, and dinoseb—many of which themselves pose toxic problems.

Health Effects

The EPA classifies alachlor as a probable human carcinogen (group B_2; see Chapter 3, Section B) on the basis of tests showing lung tumors in mice and stomach, nasal, and thyroid tumors in rats. There are no available data on human cancers related to alachlor exposure. Tests to determine whether alachlor causes mutations have generally proven negative, although one recent test was suggestive. Additional tests have been requested by the EPA. To date, there is no evidence that alachlor causes birth defects, although other reproductive effects have been observed. Furthermore, a two-year chronic exposure study in rats produced toxic effects in the liver and an irreversible, degenerative syndrome or lesion of the eye. There is some evidence that alachlor possibly causes allergic skin reactions.

Protection and Prevention

Containers of alachlor, like other pesticide containers, are extensively labeled to warn consumers of potential hazards and proper use. The labels carry the warning that the substance may be hazardous to health, which means that it causes tumors in laboratory animals. Consumers are warned not to contaminate bodies of water by improper disposal of the herbicide or cleaning of equipment. Protective clothing and proper handling are advised to reduce applicator exposure.

The structurally related herbicide metolachlor has been proposed as a suitable substitute for alachlor. Limited data from animal tests, however, suggest that it is also an animal carcinogen, albeit a less potent one. On the basis of limited test results, the EPA is considering classifying metolachlor as a possible human carcinogen (group C).

Regulatory Status

Because of its tumor-producing effects in test animals, alachlor is currently undergoing a *Special Review* to determine whether it can be reregistered. In the meantime, some restrictions on its use are in effect. It is prohibited in certain areas, such as Kern County, California, and regions east of the Mississippi River. Nor can it be used in areas with sandy or loamy soil. Aerial spraying is prohibited, and alachlor is prohibited on potatoes.

Technical Information

Chemical name: 2-chloro–2,6′-diethyl-*N*-(methoxymethyl)acetanilide
Chemical formula: $C_{14}H_{20}NO_2Cl$
WHO no observable effects level (rats and dogs): <200 mg/kg
Government standards for food tolerances:

lima beans	0.1	ppm
corn, fresh	0.05	ppm
eggs	0.02	ppm
peanuts	0.05	ppm
soybeans	0.2	ppm

Further Reading

Environmental Protection Agency. 1984. *Alachlor*. Special Review Position Document 1. Washington, D.C.
———. 1988. *Pesticide Fact Handbook*. Washington, D.C.

Aldicarb

Trade Name

Temik

Introduction

Aldicarb is one of the most toxic pesticides in use today. Registered for use in 1970, it is a *carbamate* insecticide, effective against not only a variety of insects but also mites and roundworms (see Chapter 14). It functions as a *systemic* poison, meaning that it is taken up by a plant's roots or leaves and circulated throughout the plant, making it available to sucking and chewing pests. Unlike many of its relatives, aldicarb is an acutely poisonous pesticide and is therefore not registered for home or garden use. It is, however, registered for use by certified applicators on a number of food crops, including sweet potatoes, peanuts, potatoes, oranges, sugar beets, pecans (in the Southeast only), some seed crops, soybeans, and sugarcane (in Louisiana only), and on cotton and ornamental plants. Residues have been detected in potatoes.

Several poisoning incidents involving the illegal use of aldicarb have been reported. In 1985, several hundred people were poisoned by eating watermelons containing residues of the insecticide. A similar rash of poisonings has been associated with contaminated cucumbers. Aldicarb is not registered for use on either watermelons or cucumbers.

Physical and Chemical Properties

The pesticide is relatively soluble in water, compared to other carbamates, and also dissolves fairly easily in organic solvents. Like many of its chemical relatives, it resists breakdown except in strongly alkaline solutions.

Exposure and Distribution

In California alone, some 200,000 pounds of aldicarb were used in 1984, more than 80% of which was applied to cotton. Because of its water solubility and systemic action, it is applied below the soil surface in granular form for uptake by the plant roots. Aldicarb leaches from the soil and has been found as a groundwater contaminant in New York, Florida, Wisconsin, Connecticut, Maine, Virginia, Maryland, and New Jersey. More than 1000 wells were found to be contaminated on Long Island at levels exceeding federal standards. In the most heavily contaminated well in Florida, the concentration was 30 times the legal limit. The problem is particularly acute in sandy, acidic soils under moist, warm conditions, all of which interact to reduce degradation and increase movement into groundwater.

In the laboratory, the insecticide has a *half-life* of one to two weeks. But under field conditions, the breakdown time varies with acidity, soil moisture, and temperature. Residues may persist up to ten weeks in the field. In plants and soils, some of the *metabolites* (metabolic products) of the insecticide are as toxic as the parent compound. In general, both aldicarb and its metabolites move through the soil, are readily absorbed by target and nearby plant roots, and move extensively throughout the plants.

Health Effects

Like many other carbamates, aldicarb reversibly inhibits the enzyme *cholinesterase*, as do its metabolic products (see Chapter 14). Aldicarb is distinguished by being one of the most acutely toxic pesticides in use, as indicated by the very small doses that are lethal. While it is rapidly and completely absorbed by the intestinal tract, most of it is excreted within 24 to 48 hours after exposure, primarily in the urine. Tests using rabbits and rats indicated that it is also readily absorbed through the skin, a factor that raises concern for fieldworkers who might be exposed to high levels of residues after crops are treated. Signs of poisoning in humans include dizziness, muscle weakness, stomach cramping, diarrhea, excessive sweating, nausea, vomiting, blurred vision, and convulsions.

In feeding experiments using mice and rats, aldicarb did not cause cancers, and it was found to be noncarcinogenic in skin tests in mice. *Mutagenicity* studies have been inconclusive, although some recent work suggests that aldicarb may potentially cause mutations. Other long-term health effects have not been demonstrated in laboratory tests, but some evidence suggests that it affects the immune system. *Epidemiological* studies tentatively point to a possible link between reproductive effects (in particular, an increase in spontaneous abortions) and contaminated well water. It is likely that aldicarb, like certain other carbamates, can be transformed to a carcinogenic nitroso derivative under the acidic conditions of the stomach.

Protection and Prevention

As in other cases of carbamate poisoning, atropine (administered by a physician) is helpful. Because of the toxicity of aldicarb and its ready movement from soils to plants, including neighboring food crops for which its use is not permitted, precautions, restrictions, and directions issued by the EPA must be followed carefully to avoid contamination of nontarget crops. Applicators and people involved in manufacturing the pesticide are warned to wear protective clothing, respirators, and goggles. The manufacturer has specifically prohibited the use of aldicarb in areas where drinking water has been contaminated. Since it is a systemic insecticide, residues of aldicarb probably cannot be eliminated by washing produce, although heat processing and cooking may reduce the levels.

Environmental Effects

Like certain other carbamates, including carbaryl, aldicarb is highly toxic to honeybees. Furthermore, it is very toxic to other wildlife, including some species of freshwater fish, invertebrates, and birds. At least one endangered bird species is threatened with extinction by environmental contamination with aldicarb. Consequently, the use of the pesticide is prohibited near the bird's habitat.

Regulatory Status

Aldicarb is restricted in use because of its environmental effects and mammalian toxicity. In 1984, the EPA began a *Special Review* of the insecticide on the basis of its toxicity and the presence of residues in food. As a result, the EPA has recommended banning the use of aldicarb on potatoes and imported bananas after concluding that it represents an unreasonable risk to children. Uses on ten other crops are allowed to continue. Recently, a scientific panel urged the California Food and Agriculture Department to ban the pesticide in the state. The recommendation was rejected, although tighter restrictions on the use of aldicarb were proposed. The pesticide has been banned in Wisconsin, Rhode Island, and New York, and at least temporarily in Florida. The manufacturer requested the withdrawal of aldicarb from use in potato farming on Long Island, New York.

Technical Information

Chemical name: 2-methyl–2-(methylthio)-proprionaldehyde-O-(methylcarbamoy)-oxime
Chemical formula: $C_7H_{14}N_2O_2S$
WHO no observable effects level (in rats): 0.125 mg/kg
Comparative ranking of acute toxicity of some of the most toxic pesticides in order of decreasing severity, based on comparison of the LD_{50} for rats: aldicarb > parathion > azinophos-methyl > dieldrin
Government standards for food tolerances:

bananas: 0.03 ppm
milk: 0.002 ppm
beef: 0.01 ppm
Drinking water (EPA recommended): 10 ppb
Acceptable Daily Intake: 0.003 mg/kg/day

Further Reading

HAYES, W. J., JR. 1982. *Pesticides Studied in Man.* Baltimore, MD: Williams and Wilkins.
MOTT, L., and SNYDER, K. 1987. *Pesticide Alert.* San Francisco: Sierra Club Books.

Aldrin and Dieldrin

Other Names

Aldrex; Aldrine

Trade Name

Octalene

Introduction

Used extensively since the late 1940s, the two commercial *organochlorine* insecticides, aldrin and dieldrin, are usually discussed together because of their close chemical relationship. Dieldrin is actually a conversion product of aldrin, formed by the addition of oxygen. The conversion to dieldrin occurs so readily in living organisms and in the environment that little aldrin remains following application. Hence, dieldrin is considered the primary toxic substance. It is one of the most *persistent* of all pesticides, remaining for years in soils, accumulating in the fatty tissues of living organisms, and consequently, concentrating in the food chain (see Chapter 14). Because of this persistence in soils, aldrin and dieldrin, like their close relatives, **chlordane** and **heptachlor**, effectively control soil insects, particularly termites. While no longer used in either form on food crops in the United States, residues of dieldrin from contaminated agricultural soils continue to be detected on or in foods, including carrots, corn, cucumbers, and sweet potatoes.

Physical and Chemical Properties

Aldrin is a light to dark brown crystalline solid with a mild chemical odor. It does not dissolve readily in water, but may react with a number of substances, including some strong acids, phenols, and certain metals. Although aldrin itself is nonflammable, fires in which aldrin (or any other chlorinated hydrocarbon) burns can release hazardous fumes of hydrochloric acid. Dieldrin that contains impurities is a buff to light tan, flaky material and is insoluble in water. The pure product is a white, crystalline solid that dissolves very slightly in water and quite well in certain solvents.

Exposure and Distribution

Highly effective and widely used, aldrin and dieldrin were approved for use on more than 40 agricultural crops and for soil treatment around various fruits, nuts, and vegetables until the early 1970s when restrictions were imposed on the use of persistent, chlorinated pesticides. During the period of intense agricultural use, aldrin and dieldrin were commonly detected air pollutants. Moreover, both marine and freshwater systems were widely contaminated; dieldrin has been found in all major U.S. river basins more often than any other pesticide. It has been estimated that dieldrin is considerably more persistent in water than other organochlorine pesticides, including **DDT** and **lindane**. According to the National Human Adipose Survey, dieldrin residues, which have been detected in the fatty tissues of nearly all people sampled, have dropped dramatically since the use of these insecticides has been limited.

Aldrin and dieldrin can enter the body through the skin, eyes, lungs, and *gastrointestinal tract*. In the United States, the potential for inhalation exposure is greatest for pesticide applicators and for people living in buildings where the pesticides have been used for termite control. Elsewhere in the world, workers engaged in the manufacture of the pesticides, agricultural and pest control workers who mix or apply the chemicals, and fieldworkers who enter fields following spraying run the risk of exposure via contact with the skin or through inhalation. Dieldrin still persists in agricultural soils in the United States and in other countries where its use is now banned or restricted, and it continues to be used on food crops in some areas of the world. Thus, consumers can still be exposed to residues on foods.

Health Effects

Rodent feeding tests and human poisoning cases indicate that aldrin and dieldrin are very acutely toxic when ingested and only slightly less toxic when absorbed through the skin. Severe poisonings, even fatalities, of humans have been reported. Like other organochlorine substances, these insecticides are toxic to the mammalian and insect nervous systems, producing a range of symptoms in humans including excessive irritability, headache, nausea, tremors, convulsions, coma, and even death following acute exposure. The onset of symptoms is rapid, usually within 15 minutes. In nonfatal cases of poisoning, recovery is generally complete, that is, there are no lingering effects. Long-term (chronic) exposure to low levels of the insecticides can cause skin irritation, weight loss, muscular twitching, and convulsions.

Animal test data indicate that aldrin and dieldrin cause liver cancer in several strains of mice and are therefore classsified by the EPA as probable human carcinogens (group B_2; see Chapter 3, Section B). Other studies reveal that aldrin produces liver and kidney damage in dogs and rats. At doses high enough to produce toxic effects, various reproductive effects have been observed, including decreased fertility, increased fetal deaths, and retarded growth. Other studies suggest that both insecticides cause changes in the immune system.

The EPA recently reviewed the results of tests for mutagenicity for both dieldrin and aldrin. Most of the tests of aldrin were negative, but the results in mammalian cells were inconclusive. Available data for dieldrin are insufficient to draw firm conclusions, but they do suggest that the insecticide does not cause mutations or damage DNA.

Protection and Prevention

The recommended immediate treatment in cases of dieldrin poisoning is much the same as for other chlorinated pesticides. If the substance has been ingested, vomiting should be induced, using Ipecac syrup if it is available. The victim should not be given milk or oily fluids. Contaminated skin or eyes should be flushed with water, and a physician should be contacted. Activated charcoal is sometimes given to absorb dieldrin from the digestive tract and promote excretion. Anticonvulsive drugs may be prescribed. Agricultural, pest control, and pesticide factory workers should wear protective clothing and breathing apparatus as described by the EPA to minimize exposure.

Consumers should be aware that, like other organochlorines, aldrin and dieldrin have an affinity for the outer layers or peels of fruits and vegetables, particularly root crops such as potatoes, beets, and carrots. Washing, peeling, and steaming can effectively remove a substantial amount of the residues. There is evidence, however, that some aldrin and dieldrin may be absorbed by plant roots and moved internally to other parts of the plants. Cooking and canning remove additional residues. Although organochlorines tend to concentrate in fats, evidence suggests that the process of refining vegetable oils removes most of the residues. This is not the case for certain dairy and other animal products since processing does not remove the pesticide residues. Reduction of the level of fat in cheese, milk, and meat can reduce organochlorine residues.

Environmental Effects

As with other toxic substances, a great deal of variation exists among species in their susceptibility to the acute toxicity and nonlethal chronic effects of aldrin and dieldrin. But, like other organochlorine insecticides that tend to concentrate in the food chain, these are particularly toxic to fish and birds that feed on them. Experimental tests suggest that both aldrin and dieldrin are toxic to various aquatic organisms at concentrations typically found in the environment.

Regulatory Status

In 1974, the EPA restricted the uses of aldrin and dieldrin because of dieldrin's persistence in tissues and soils. Since then, these pesticides have been registered only for treatment of nonfood seeds and for the control of termites. Although most countries now limit their use chiefly to termite control, agricultural uses are permitted in certain regions. For example, these insecticides were used against recent outbreaks of locusts in Africa and the Middle East.

Technical Information

Chemical names:
Aldrin: 1,2,3,4,10,10-hexachloro–1,4,4a,5,8,8a-hexahydro-endo–1,4-exo–5,8-dimethanonaphthalene
Dieldrin: 1,2,3,4,10,10-hexachloro–6,7-epoxy–1,4,4a,5,6,7,8,8a-octohydro-endo–1,4-exo–5,8-dimethanonaphthalene
Chemical formulas:
Aldrin: $C_{12}H_8Cl_6$
Dieldrin: $C_{12}H_8Cl_6O$
Residue levels in human fat:

1970: 0.16 ppm
1983: 0.06 ppm

Comparative ranking of acute oral toxicity of organochlorine pesticides in order of decreasing toxicity, based on comparison of the LD_{50} for rats by mouth: aldrin > dieldrin > lindane > heptachlor > DDT > chlordane
Government standards:
OSHA limit in workplace air: 0.25 mg/m^3
NIOSH limit: 0.15 mg/m^3

Further Reading

Environmental Protection Agency. 1987. *Carcinogenic Assessment of Aldrin and Dieldrin.* Washington, D.C.

Aluminum

Introduction

Until recently, aluminum was thought to be a fairly safe substance. It was known that aluminum dust could produce lung disease in workers and that patients undergoing *kidney dialysis* could suffer *dementia* from aluminum if ordinary tap water was used in the dialysis machine. But apart from these problems, it was not thought that aluminum posed a danger to the public at large. Two developments in recent years, however, have caused a re-evaluation of aluminum's safety. First was the discovery of high concentrations of aluminum in the brains of people suffering from *Alzheimer's* disease and certain other nervous system diseases. Second was the finding that acid rain washes aluminum out of soil and into freshwater, killing fish and perhaps raising the concentration in drinking water to levels that, in combination with aluminum from other sources, could become a health hazard.

Physical and Chemical Properties

Aluminum is the third most abundant element in the earth's crust (after oxygen and silicon) and by far the most abundant metal. It is not found in pure form, but is refined from the ores bauxite and cryolite. When purified, aluminum is a silvery white metal whose strength, light weight, and corrosion resistance make it suitable for a wide variety of applications. Aluminum does not dissolve readily in water that is *neutral* in acidity, but as water gets either increasingly *acidic* or *alkaline*, it dissolves more readily and therefore becomes more mobile in the environment. Aluminum combines with *organic matter* to form clumps or flocs and is sometimes used in water treatment as a flocculent to remove organic materials that might cause odor or taste problems. No physiological function for aluminum is known, and it is not required in the diet. Except in individuals with certain diseases, it is both poorly absorbed from the *gastrointestinal tract* and rapidly excreted by the kidneys.

Exposure and Distribution

Exposure to aluminum comes mainly from food and drink, not from air. A typical daily intake can range from several milligrams to about 100 milligrams, with 20 milligrams accepted as average. Aluminum is commonly found in the leavening agents used in cake mixes, frozen doughs, pancake mixes, self-rising flours, and home baking powders. It is also part of the anticaking agent used in table salt, nondairy creamers, and other dry powdered products. Processed cheese products (particularly the individually wrapped and sliced varieties) often contain aluminum in the emulsifiers used to make them smooth. Such cheeses can often double a daily intake with one slice. Some foods, such as tea, naturally contain high aluminum levels, and acidic foods, such as fruit juices and coffee, can dissolve aluminum from the cans they are stored in. Many individuals consume large quantities of such foods and food additives.

More important for many people than the intake from foods, however, is the ingestion of aluminum from several nonprescription drugs. Buffered aspirin and many *antacids* contain aluminum. These over-the-counter medications are often taken in large quantities and over long periods of time by people who use them. The aluminum content of some antacids ranges from 35 to over 200 milligrams per dose. At the maximum recommended dosage of 24 tablets or teaspoonfuls per day, a person could ingest between 840 and 5000 milligrams of aluminum per day; that is, between 42 and 250 times the average daily intake from all other sources combined. Fortunately for persons wishing to reduce aluminum consumption, at least 25 brands of aluminum-free antacids are currently on the market. Many aspirin formulas use aluminum-containing buffers to reduce the stomach irritation sometimes associated with aspirin use. Buffered aspirins have been especially marketed for arthritic patients who may consume 3 to 9 grams of aspirin daily to relieve arthritic pain and swelling. At this level of intake, the dose of aluminum from medication may range from 125 to 725 milligrams per day (that is, from 6 to over 35 times the average intake). Aspirins buffered with calcium carbonate and time-release formulas that do not contain aluminum are available.

Other sources of aluminum exposure are drinking water, some antidiarrhea agents and hemorrhoid medications, vaginal douches, antiperspirants, and lipsticks. Foods that are acidic, salty, or very alkaline can corrode the surface of aluminum pots, permitting some aluminum to enter the food. The scientific consensus appears to be that these sources of exposure are minor in comparison to the ones described earlier.

The concern over drinking water is that aluminum may be brought to relatively high levels because of the dissolving action of acid rain on soils, rocks, and the sediments at the bottoms of lakes and streams. The released aluminum washes into surface water and percolates into groundwater and may enter water supplies. In regions of the country most affected by acid rain (the Northeast, in particular), the aluminum content of surface water has increased as much as ten times since the turn of the century. While no health effects have yet been reported, problems may develop in the future if acidic water conditions become more widespread and severe.

The environmental distribution of aluminum is widespread because of its great abundance in the earth's crust. Table 16 presents a range of typical environmental levels. Concentrations tend to be high downwind of such industrial sources as coal-fired power plants, metal smelters, cement manufacturing plants, and waste incinerators, as well as in urban areas. Use of aluminum in the United States amounts to over 5 million tons per year. The major categories are packaging (29%), building materials (22%), transportation (21%), electrical (10%), consumer durables (7%), and other uses (11%).

Health Effects

Workers exposed to aluminum dust on the job, both in the aluminum fabricating industries and in the production of fireworks, explosives, and alumina abrasives, may develop a lung disease called *pulmonary fibrosis*. This is a thickening and scarring of the lung tissue around the inhaled particles and can lead to a breathlessness similar to *emphysema*.

Kidney disease can have various complications from aluminum poisoning. The kidneys are essential in removing whatever aluminum has been absorbed through the digestive tract. Their reduced functioning in disease and even during normal aging allows aluminum to build up in the body. The most severe complications have occurred in patients undergoing kidney dialysis (the filtering of blood in an external machine to remove waste and toxic products that are normally removed by the kidneys). When ordinary, untreated tapwater was originally used in dialysis machines, aluminum from the water could enter the patient's blood directly. As aluminum built up, a progressive brain disease developed called dialysis *dementia*. The disease is characterized first by disruptions of speech, followed by memory disorders, changes in personality, impaired reasoning ability, and disorientation; eventually convulsions and death would follow. With the discovery in the 1970s that aluminum was the cause of the disease, water used for dialysis was filtered to remove the aluminum, thereby largely preventing the disease. Other problems from the buildup of aluminum in kidney-impaired patients include easily fractured bones; disruptions of calcium, magnesium, phosphorus, and fluoride metabolism; and various forms of *anemia*.

Aluminum is now suspected, although not proven, to be a factor in the development of *Alzheimer's disease*. Alzheimer's disease is a progressive deterioration of the brain that occurs in elderly people. Lapses in memory and learning ability take place first, followed by progressive loss of muscular control; death is

TABLE 16 Environmental Concentrations of Aluminum

Medium	Concentration
Air	
Rural	50–500 ng/m^3
Urban	100–5000 ng/m^3
Water	
North American rivers	50 µg/L (12–2250 ppb range)
Acidic lakes and streams	100–800 µg/L
Drinking waters	>14 µg/L
Food	
Most unprocessed foods	<10 µg/g (10 ppm)
Tea (an accumulator plant)	up to 20,000 µg/g

the final result. The disease is insidious, and no cures or treatments are known. In patients who have died of Alzheimer's, the aluminum content of their brain cells has reached abnormally high concentrations. Moreover, the aluminum is not found everywhere in the brain, but just in those cells that have undergone the characteristic pattern of degeneration found in Alzheimer's victims. Another line of evidence comes from certain native populations on the Island of Guam in the Pacific. They too have high aluminum concentrations in the brain and suffer a rare neurological disorder similar to Alzheimer's. The soil from which these natives grow their food is rich in aluminum. Further evidence comes from laboratory studies. Experimental animals injected with aluminum also develop the same characteristic symptoms as Alzheimer's patients.

Aluminum may act by interfering with the normal *metabolism* of nerve cells, rendering them electrically silent and unable to conduct nerve signals. The fact that aluminum accumulates gradually over a lifetime, causing slow metabolic changes, corresponds with the fact that Alzheimer's disease develops in elderly people. Alternatively, aluminum may disrupt the delicate structures (neurotubules) within brain cells.

Nevertheless, aluminum has not been proven to be a cause of Alzheimer's; its accumulation could simply be another effect of the disease rather than its cause. The latest re-

search indicates that a *mutation* on a *gene* responsible for producing a particular brain protein (amyloid) causes it to build up, slowly leading to nerve cell death. Whether aluminum affects this process is not known at present. One bit of intriguing information, however, is that aluminum is normally carried through the bloodstream bound to a large carrier protein, which prevents aluminum's passage through the protective *blood-brain barrier*. In some Alzheimer's patients, this carrier protein is missing, perhaps allowing the much smaller aluminum ion easier penetration into the brain. Deciding which, if any, of these possible causes is correct awaits scientific research that is currently under way. In the meantime, since aluminum has no known physiological function, reducing its intake is prudent.

Protection and Prevention

Although it has not been proven to cause disease in healthy individuals, reducing the ingestion of aluminum is prudent for several reasons. First, the neurological disorders with which aluminum is associated occur in old age and thus may represent cumulative exposure over a lifetime. Reducing exposure may delay or prevent the onset of those disorders. Second, the treatment of kidney disease sometimes requires the use of aluminum-containing drugs. Reducing aluminum intake from other sources provides the physician maximum flexibility in choosing medications with less concern for possible aluminum-related complications. And third, aluminum itself may cause further damage to already weakened kidneys in the elderly.

To reduce aluminum consumption, select foods and food ingredients that are free of aluminum. For example, baking powders are available that do not contain aluminum. Compare ingredient labels among various brands of food whenever possible. People who frequently use antacids or buffered aspirin should ask their doctor or pharmacist to recommend aluminum-free formulas. Foods that are acidic (for example, tomatoes), salty, or alkaline (for example, oatmeal) should not be cooked in unlined aluminum pots and pans. (Aluminum containers lined with stainless steel or nonstick coatings can be safely used.) Check with the local water utility to see if aluminum is used in water treatment. If it is, find out whether it is being properly removed prior to distribution. Bottled nonmineral drinking water can be substituted if the aluminum content of the local water supply is high.

Environmental Effects

In regions of the world affected by acid rain, particularly Scandinavia, eastern Canada, and the northeastern United States, aluminum concentrations of surface water have increased above natural levels. This has happened because acidic rainfall and snowmelt dissolve aluminum out of soil and surface rocks and wash it into lakes and streams. The acidified water of the lakes and streams also dissolves aluminum from the bottom sediments. The high aluminum concentrations (up to ten times normal), together with the high acidity, have caused massive fish dieoffs. Aluminum acts on fish by clogging the gills (preventing breathing) and disrupting mineral metabolism. All of the lakes in many regions are devoid of fish life, and the variety of microorganism species has changed as well. Once gone, it is practically impossible to reestablish fish populations because of the changed water chemistry and absence of food sources.

Regulatory Status

Aluminum levels in the general air or drinking water are not regulated. Recommended limits on occupational air exposures to various aluminum compounds have been suggested by the American Conference of Governmental Industrial Hygienists. The EPA has established ambient water quality criteria for the protection of aquatic life (listed in the next section). Aluminum is on the *community right-to-know* list.

Technical Information

Chemical symbol: Al
Atomic number: 13
Atomic weight: 27
Ambient water quality criteria for protection of aquatic life:
  4-day average concentration: $<87\mu g/L$ (87 ppb)
  1-hour average concentration: $<750\mu g/L$ (750 ppb)
OSHA limits in workplace:
  aluminum metal dusts: 10 mg/m^3
  pyro powders: 5 mg/m^3
  welding fumes: 5 mg/m^3
  soluble salts: 2 mg/m^3
  soluble alkyls: 2 mg/m^3

Further Reading

Environmental Protection Agency. 1987. *Health Effects Assessment for Aluminum.* EPA/600/8–88–016. Springfield, VA: National Technical Information Service, U.S. Department of Commerce.

PERL, DANIEL P. 1985. Relationship of Aluminum to Alzheimer's Disease. *Environmental Health Perspectives* 63:149–153.

WILLS, MICHAEL R., and SAVORY, JOHN. 1985. Water Content of Aluminum, Dialysis Dementia, and Osteomalacia. *Environmental Health Perspectives* 63:141–147.

Ammonia

Other Names

Ammonia water; ammonium hydroxide

Introduction

Most people think of ammonia as a common household cleanser with a sharp, penetrating odor. While this is the source of several toxic hazards around the home, household ammonia solutions (5 to 10% ammonia dissolved in water) are an insignificant fraction of the total ammonia in use. By volume, ammonia is the fourth largest industrial chemical produced, over 80% of which goes to agricultural fertilizers. Industrial ammonia production, however, is dwarfed by the natural production of ammonia, which is part of nature's way of breaking down *organic matter* and recycling its components. Only in certain locations, such as animal feedlots or near chemical factories and chemical spills, do human activities create concentrations that greatly exceed *natural background levels*.

Physical and Chemical Properties

Ammonia is a colorless gas, less dense than air, with a penetrating odor. At high concentrations, ammonia in air can be explosive. Ammonia liquifies under pressure and is usually stored and transported as a liquid. The pure liquid is called anhydrous ammonia, meaning "without water." It readily dissolves in water to form a strongly *alkaline* solution, capable of causing *caustic* burns. Mixing household ammonia solution with bleach to concoct a more effective cleaning solution produces *chloramines*, gases that are more dangerous than either straight ammonia or bleach fumes alone. Other mixtures made at home can also release ammonia gas.

Exposure and Distribution

Household exposures to ammonia are dangerous in three situations: (1) when cleaning without adequate ventilation; (2) accidental eye and skin contact and accidental swallowing; and (3) mixing ammonia with *lye*, **sodium hydroxide**, or bleach (*sodium hypochlorite*) to form cleaning solutions. Inadequate ventilation permits ammonia fumes, ordinarily innocuous, to build up to levels that can cause symptoms to develop. Ovens, cabinets, and shower stalls are places of restricted air flow that often require placing your head inside to clean effectively, which can lead to toxic exposures.

As previously mentioned, the most serious household exposures occur when ammonia cleaning solutions are mixed with other products. Stirring lye or sodium hydroxide into ammonia cleanser releases toxic quantities of ammonia gas. Chloramine gases are produced when bleach, which contains chlorine, is mixed with ammonia. Chloramines are dangerous because they are not well absorbed by the protective *mucous membranes* of the upper respiratory tract and are inhaled deep into the lungs. There they turn back into ammonia and hypochlorous acid, which can then react with the unprotected cells of the small air exchange sacs (alveoli). The consequences are described under the section on Health Effects.

Accidents occurring during transport and storage of ammonia also pose a hazard. Leaking valves and misconnected hoses are responsible for numerous exposures each year, particularly in the agricultural industry, where concentrated ammonia solutions are pumped from tanker trucks to farm vehicles for spreading on fields. First- and second-degree burns are common, and loss of eyesight occasionally results. Mass evacuations and exposures to the public are rare events but do occur. While no comprehensive national figures are available on effects of chemical accidents, limited data indicate that ammonia spills are second only to **chlorine** in numbers of injuries, deaths, and evacuations caused. Fortunately, only a few dozen injuries and several deaths appear to be caused each year, mostly to persons involved with the spills (workers and drivers).

Production of ammonia is about 15 million tons per year. Fertilizers account for 80% of use (as ammonia and ammonium compounds), followed by production of plastics, fibers, and resins (10%), explosives (5%), animal feed (1.5%), pulp and paper (0.6%), and rubber (0.5%). Ammonia and its compounds are also used as cleaning fluids and as scale-removing agents and in food as leavening agents, stabilizers, and flavoring. These compounds include ammonium bicarbonate, ammonium carbonate, ammonium hydroxide, ammonium phosphate, and ammonium sulfate.

Ammonia is not an *ambient* pollutant; that is, ordinary concentrations in the environment are not harmful. The concentrations in the air vary with underlying land use. In general, urban levels are higher than rural ones, except in areas of intensive animal husbandry and/or use of organic manures. Drinking water concentrations are low because of the conversion of ammonia to chloramines during chlorination treatment. The chloramines produced are not thought to present a hazard because they are swallowed rather than inhaled. Groundwater ammonia levels are low, except for shallow groundwater reserves near areas of intensive use or accumulation, such as fertilized crop lands and feedlots. The amount of ammonia from ammonium salts added to food is vastly outweighed by the intestinal production of ammonia during the digestion of proteins in foods. Table 17 shows typical ammonia concentrations in various media.

Health Effects

Ammonia is an irritant that affects the skin, eyes, and respiratory passages. Ingestion can cause corrosive effects to the mouth, esophagus, and stomach. The symptoms of ammonia exposure are a burning sensation (in the eyes, nose, and throat), pain in the lungs, headache, nausea, tearing, coughing, and an increased breathing rate. The concentrations that produce these symptoms are shown in Table 18.

Inhaling concentrated ammonia fumes or chloramines irritates the deep lung tissues. *Pulmonary edema* (fluid in the lungs) and *pneumonia* can result; permanent structural change may occur in severe cases. In the few reported instances of home exposures serious enough to require hospitalization, the patients recovered within several days to weeks. Gaseous ammonia quickly dissolves on moist body surfaces, causing alkaline burns. Contact with liquid anhydrous ammonia results in second-degree burns with formation of blisters. Weaker ammonia solutions can produce *inflammation* and mild burns.

Eye contact with concentrated ammonia gas or anhydrous liquid ammonia is very serious. Damage occurs within 5 to 10 seconds. Without immediate flushing followed by prompt medical treatment, permanent damage and often complete blindness will result. Eye exposure to less concentrated ammonia fumes causes mild burns that usually heal well, but which also require immediate medical treatment. The ammonium compounds in foods are generally considered to be safe. There is no indication that ammonia produces chronic, low-level effects such as cancer, birth defects, or mutations.

Protection and Prevention

Adequate ventilation when using household ammonia cleansers is important. Mixing of several cleaning products should not be attempted; in particular, ammonia should never be mixed with lye, sodium hydroxide, or bleach. When applying ammonia followed by a chlorine-containing product on a surface (for example, when cleaning mildew from ceramic tile), a thorough rinse of the first solution should be made before applying the second product to prevent the formation of dangerous chloramine gases. Protective clothing (including rubber gloves, long sleeves, and glasses or goggles) should be worn when using ammonia.

Splashes to the skin and eyes should be

TABLE 17 Ammonia Concentrations in Various Media

Medium	Concentration
Air	
Urban, gas	5–25 $\mu g/m^3$
Nonurban, gas	2–6 $\mu g/m^3$
Urban, particulates	4–5 $\mu g/m^3$
Nonurban, particulates	1 $\mu g/m^3$
Water	
Most surface waters	<0.18 mg/L (0.18 ppm)
Near urban areas	0.5 mg/L (0.5 ppm)
Near intensive farms	12 mg/L (12 ppm)

TABLE 18 Concentrations of Ammonia That Produce Adverse Health Effects

Health Effect	Concentration in Air
Odor threshold (detection)	3.5 mg/m^3 (5 ppm)
Odor threshold (recognition)	35 mg/m^3 (50 ppm)
Throat irritation	280 mg/m^3 (400 ppm)
Cough	1200 mg/m^3 (1700 ppm)
Life threatening	1700 mg/m^3 (2400 ppm)
High mortality	>3500 mg/m^3 (>5000 ppm)
Taste threshold (in water)	35 mg/L (35 ppm)

treated by thorough rinsing with water (for 5 to 10 minutes). Saturated clothing should be removed to prevent continued skin contact. If breathing of fumes causes symptoms to develop, immediately go out into the fresh air. A doctor should be consulted if symptoms worsen and in all cases of eye contact.

Environmental Effects

Ammonia (NH_3) adds nitrogen (N) to the environment. In areas that cannot handle the added nitrogen, disruptions to the ecosystem will result. These include toxic effects on plants, fish, and animals and changes in the balance of species. In general, such effects are seen only in close proximity to specific concentrated sources of ammonia, such as animal feedlots and sewage and industrial outfalls. However, in areas of dense population, ammonia can have a regional effect on nearby bodies of water. Fertilizer runoff and possibly nitrates in rainfall are affecting coastal waters along much of the eastern seaboard, in effect, fertilizing estuaries, marshes, and shallow waters and stimulating growth of unwanted species, which may affect commercial fisheries. Although ammonia is a base, it actually acidifies soil by its rapid conversion to **nitrate** (NO_3), releasing hydrogen ions just like other acids.

Regulatory Status

The EPA has set environmental limits on ammonia in water for the protection of human health and aquatic life. The ambient water quality criterion for aquatic life is lower because ammonia is a greater threat to aquatic life than to human health. Various states have set limits at or below the EPA guidelines. The Food and Drug Administration (FDA) regulates the ammonium compounds in food. Specific compounds are *generally recognized as safe (GRAS)* and are allowed in baked goods at levels not to exceed so-called good manufacturing practices. Regulations governing the maximum allowable ammonia concentration in industrial air also have been adopted to protect workers. Ammonia is on the *community right-to-know* list.

Technical Information

Chemical formula: NH_3
Molecular weight: 17
U.S. ambient water quality criterion for human health protection: 35 mg/L
Recommended water quality criterion for protection of aquatic life: 0.02 mg/L
OSHA limit in workplace air: 17.5 mg/m^3 (25 ppm)

Further Reading

Environmental Protection Agency. 1987. *Health Effects Assessment for Ammonia.* EPA 600/8–88–017. Springfield, VA: National Technical Information Service, U.S. Department of Commerce.
National Research Council. 1979. *Ammonia.* Committee on Medical and Biological Effects of Environmental Pollutants. Subcommittee on Ammonia. National Academy of Sciences. Baltimore: University Park Press.
World Health Organization. 1986. *Ammonia.* Environmental Health Criteria No. 54. Geneva.

Arsenic

Introduction

Arsenic, the familiar poison of legend and literature, is a naturally occurring chemical element. It is used mainly in pesticides and wood preservatives, and it is responsible for lung cancer, skin cancer, and other diseases in people exposed to it. Arsenic is increasing in the environment mainly from air pollution and by seepage from hazardous waste dumps.

For centuries, arsenic compounds have been used as medicines and tonics for control of such diseases as syphilis and amebic dysentery. With the introduction of penicillin and other antibiotics in this century and the growing awareness of arsenic's hazard, such uses have been largely discontinued. Some usage still occurs, however, particularly in veterinary medicine, where organic arsenic formulations are used as feed additives to enhance growth in poultry and swine. Discontinuance of the additives several days before slaughter allows the residues to be excreted, and the practice is believed to be safe.

Physical and Chemical Properties

Arsenic is a metallic-like substance recovered from copper smelter dust and processed to a white powder. The toxicity of arsenic depends on its form, with *inorganic* arsenic being much more toxic than *organic* arsenic. Most human exposure occurs from food and is predominantly in the less hazardous organic form. Exposure to the more harmful inorganic form is discussed in the next section. Arsenic and **selenium** are antagonistic toxins: exposure to one reduces the adverse effects of the other.

Exposure and Distribution

Most human exposures (by weight) are to arsenic in food (70%), a result of natural occurrence, pesticide residues, and antibiotics given to commercial livestock. Meat, fish, and poultry contain the highest concentrations, and seafood is particularly enriched. But most of the arsenic in food is in a complex organic form that is believed to be toxicologically *inert*. Drinking water (29%) and air (1%) provide relatively smaller exposures, but in the more harmful inorganic form. Cigarette smokers receive an added dose of inorganic arsenic, directly to the lung, because arsenic is present in tobacco leaves and is released into the smoke when tobacco is burned. Children have greater exposure from drinking water because they drink more in proportion to their body weights than do adults. Other groups with high exposures are workers in the smelter and arsenic chemical manufacturing industries, farm workers, and carpenters working with preserved woods. Table 19 gives estimated arsenic exposures for a wide variety of groups in the population.

Most inorganic arsenic dispersed in the environment is a result of human activities: metal ore smelting, coal burning, and the production and use of pesticides. In the immediate vicinity of smelters and arsenic pesticide factories, air and soil levels are elevated. Children in these areas are particularly prone to arsenic exposure because of the extra time spent playing outdoors and on contaminated soils. The highest arsenic levels are found around cotton gins, where cotton wastes contaminated with pesticide residues are released to the local environment. The EPA estimates that as of 1978, 40,000 people lived in areas with arsenic concentrations in the air at least 100 times greater than the national average, that 500,000 people lived in areas with air concentrations at least 10 times greater, and that 3 million people lived in areas with levels greater than the national average.

Coal burning produces the largest quantity of arsenic waste of any industry because of the large amount of coal burned and the fact that arsenic is a trace contaminant of coal. Some of the arsenic is released through the smokestack along with the other stack gases, but the majority is landfilled with the collected *fly ash* and *bottom ash*. Arsenic emitted from the stack is believed to be responsible for the widespread and increasing contamination of much of the United States, which is now showing up as increasing concentrations in the nation's rivers. The collected ash, as well as arsenic-containing slag from copper smelting, are buried in hazardous waste landfills. Studies now show that arsenic is gradually migrating away from such pits and appearing in nearby groundwater.

Some areas of the western United States experience high levels of arsenic in groundwater because of naturally high concentrations in the underlying rocks. Fortunately, relatively few people receive drinking water from these sources. Arsenic levels are also high in agricultural areas where arsenic pesticides are used, the drift from spraying operations and erosion of contaminated soils reaching the local surface waters. Typical concentrations of arsenic in various environments are provided in Table 20.

Arsenic is mixed with other ingredients for use as wood preservatives (68%), pesticides and drying agents for cotton (23%), glass decolorizers (4%), and other uses (5%). A small amount of high-purity arsenic metal is used in semiconductors. Since the 1985 closure of the ASARCO smelter in Tacoma, Washington, no arsenic has been produced in the United States. The entire consumption of 20,000 tons per year is imported.

Health Effects

Lung cancer from inhaling arsenic and skin cancer from swallowing it are the two most dangerous effects of arsenic exposure for the general population. Poisoning as a result of accidental contamination of food products and other disorders from chronic, low-level exposures are also significant. Lung cancer from breathing arsenic is an occupational disease for workers in the smelting industry and the arsenic pesticide manufacturing industry. Elevated rates of lung cancer have also been observed for people living in the vicinity of

TABLE 19 Selected Arsenic Exposure Scenarios for Specific Human Subpopulations[a]

	Exposure Scenarios (μg/day)									
Exposure Medium	General Population	Smokers in General Population	Child	High Fish Consumption	High Wine Consumption	Woodworker	High Activity Woodworker	Contaminated Well Water Consumption	Worst Case	Maximum Fish Consumption
Water	5	5	2.5	5	5	5	5	1000	1000	5
Food and fish	21	21	11	21 + 1000	21	21	21	21	21 + 1000	21 + 10,000
Wine and liquor	0.01	0.01	—	—	500	—	—	—	500	—
Air	0.06	0.06	0.06	0.06	0.06	0.06	0.06	0.06	6	0.06
Cigarettes	—	90	—	—	—	—	—	—	90	—
Soil	—	—	20	—	—	—	—	—	20	—
Exposure to wood	—	—	—	—	—	260	500	—	500	—
Totals	26	116	34	1026	526	286	526	1021	3137	10,026
Per kg/day	0.4	2	8	15	7	4	7	15	44	143

[a]Data do not distinguish between organic and inorganic forms of arsenic.

Source: Environmental Protection Agency. 1982. *An Exposure and Risk Assessment for Arsenic.* EPA-440/4-85-005. Springfield, VA: National Technical Information Service, U.S. Department of Commerce.

TABLE 20 Arsenic Concentrations in Various Media

Medium	Concentration	Medium	Concentration
Air		Soil	
Remote	0.0004 µg/m^3	Natural background	<10 mg/kg
Urban	0.003 µg/m^3	Near airborne sources	up to 380 mg/kg
Near smelters	0.03 µg/m^3	Food	
Water		Meats, eggs, and milk	0.01–0.03 mg/kg
Surface	91% <10 µg/L	Vegetables and fruits	0.01–0.03 mg/kg
Well	1.9–21.5 µg/L	Cereals, nuts, and sugars	0.01–0.04 mg/kg
Near landfills	0.04–5.8 mg/L	Fish and shellfish	0.07–1.47 mg/kg

such factories. Calculations based on these high-level exposures and projected to the population at large indicate that as many as 50,000 lung cancer cases may develop in the entire current U.S. population as a result of arsenic in the air and in tobacco smoke.

Nonfatal skin cancers have been observed in certain groups consuming well water containing high arsenic levels. Projections based on these exposures would seem to indicate that hundreds of thousands of people could develop skin cancer as a result of the current levels of arsenic in drinking water. These projections are suspect, however, because a prevalence this great should already be evident in the general population, and it is not. While United States skin cancer rates are high and rising, they are almost certainly due to exposure to **ultraviolet radiation** in sunlight, not to arsenic ingestion. Nevertheless, the fact that arsenic levels are increasing both in surface water and in groundwater near hazardous waste sites gives ample cause for concern about a future outbreak of arsenic-related skin disorders.

The International Agency for Research on Cancer places inorganic arsenic in its highest classification of cancer-causing substances (Group I), indicating that sufficient evidence exists to judge arsenic as a producer of human cancers. The Cancer Assessment Group of the Environmental Protection Agency puts arsenic in the top one-fourth of 54 chemicals ranked for their potency in producing cancer and places it in Group A, its highest category of cancer-causing chemicals (see Chapter 3, Section B).

Other disorders resulting from chronic arsenic exposure are, in decreasing order of importance, noncancerous skin *lesions*, peripheral nerve effects, and cardiovascular changes. Skin disorders include increased *pigmentation*, wart-like lesions on the palms and soles, and transverse white lines across the nails. Nervous system effects begin with tingling and numbness of the soles and palms and progress to a widespread and painful *neuritis* of the upper and lower limbs. Peripheral vascular changes occasionally leading to gangrene have also been reported. Most of these nonfatal conditions subside after exposure has ceased.

Acute arsenic poisoning is characterized by severe *gastrointestinal* damage resulting in vomiting and diarrhea and general vascular collapse leading to shock, coma, and even death. Several hundred deaths from accidental contamination of food have occurred in Japan, but no cases have been reported in the United States.

Protection and Prevention

Unfortunately, there is little one can do directly to avoid the hazards of arsenic exposure, except to stop cigarette smoking and avoid second-hand smoke. Most cases of acute poisoning are the result of accidental contamination of food or water, situations over which one has little or no control.

Chronic, low-level exposures are greatest around smelters and arsenic factories. To the extent one can move away from these areas, exposures can be reduced. Since children are at highest risk in the general population, careful monitoring of their play areas, particularly in the vicinity of these sources, would be prudent. Handwashing before eating is helpful.

Proper disposal of empty pesticide and wood preservative containers should be practiced. Containers should be triply rinsed with water, and the rinse water applied in the same manner as the full-strength solution. The empty container can then be disposed of in the trash. Unused pesticides or preservatives should be given to a friend to use, taken to a proper disposal center, or returned to the manufacturer or dealer if possible. Under no circumstances should they be flushed down the drain or placed in the trash.

Since there is evidence that arsenic is gradually accumulating in the environment, sources of arsenic emissions must be carefully controlled. This is an area of governmental regulatory policy. The public can express their concern to elected representatives and to regulatory agencies that effective policies be enacted and that regulators do their job.

Environmental Effects

Arsenic is toxic to plants in high concentrations. Orchards with a long history of arsenic pesticide use slowly lose their fertility as arsenic builds up in the soil. Eventually the trees may become totally unproductive. Damage to barley and alfalfa has been noted as well.

Regulatory Status

Inorganic arsenic is listed as a hazardous air pollutant by the EPA. This means that special precautions must be taken to prevent its release from industrial sources. The EPA also limits the concentration of arsenic in drinking water. OSHA regulates worker exposure to organic arsenic compounds in air. Arsenic is on the EPA *community right-to-know* list.

Technical Information

Chemical symbol: As
Atomic number: 33
Atomic weight: 75
Maximum permitted level in drinking water: 50μg/L(50 ppb)
OSHA limit in workplace air: 0.5 mg/m^3

Further Reading

Environmental Protection Agency. 1984. *Health Assessment Document for Inorganic Arsenic.* EPA–600/8–83–021F. Springfield, VA: National Technical Information Service, U.S. Department of Commerce.

————. 1982. *An Exposure and Risk Assessment for Arsenic.* EPA–440/4–85–005. Springfield, VA: National Technical Information Service, U.S. Department of Commerce.

National Academy of Sciences. 1977. *Arsenic.* National Research Council. Committee on Medical and Biological Effects of Environmental Pollutants. Washington, D.C.: National Academy Press.

Asbestos

Introduction

Asbestos is a broad term applied to a group of naturally occurring fibrous mineral compounds. These compounds have been used extensively in the building trades and have resulted in tens of thousands of cases of lung cancer and fibrous lung disease in asbestos workers. As many as 15 million schoolchildren and 3 million school workers have the potential to be exposed because of the installation of asbestos-containing materials in public buildings between 1945 and 1978. The EPA has already banned the use of asbestos in many products and will phase out all other uses over the next ten years.

Physical and Chemical Properties

Asbestos fibers are small and odorless, often invisible except through a microscope, and indestructible in most uses. They can be transported on clothes and other materials, and they have aerodynamic features that allow them to be suspended and resuspended easily in the air and to travel long distances. Once released, asbestos fibers are difficult to detect and contain, and they readily enter the surrounding air. People are thus exposed not only at the time and place of release, but long after the release and far from its source. There is constant renewal of risk because asbestos fibers reenter the atmosphere repeatedly over time.

Two forms of asbestos fibers are common: chrysotile and amphiboles. Chrysotile fibers are curly, tend to clump together, and are more easily rejected by the body. Amphiboles are smooth, needle-like fibers with pointed ends that are readily taken into the lungs. Most of the asbestos used in schools and other buildings is chrysotile and may therefore pose less of a hazard than the amphiboles that shipbuilders and other workers were exposed to in the past. At the present time, however, no scientific consensus has been reached on this point, and all asbestos that is flaking or crumbling should be viewed with concern.

Exposure and Distribution

People inhale asbestos when they breathe air in which fibers are suspended. This is the main route of exposure. Approximately half of inhaled fibers are cleared from the lungs and swallowed, exposing the throat and digestive system. Asbestos can also be swallowed in drinking water, which it enters either from naturally occurring rock sources (such as serpentine) or by deterioration of asbestos–cement pipe used in conduits. The hazard from drinking water asbestos has only recently been investigated and is not well understood.

Asbestos fibers are released at all stages of the mining, use, and disposal of asbestos products. The EPA estimates that approximately 700 tons per year are released into the air during mining and milling operations, 100 tons per year during product manufacture, and about 18 tons per year from landfills. Installation and maintenance of asbestos products (for example, sanding and buffing) also release fibers, as does demolition of buildings containing asbestos materials. Asbestos fireproofing materials were sprayed in schools and other buildings during the years from 1945 to 1978; asbestos-containing plaster and decorative ceiling tiles were also installed then. In many cases, these materials are now beginning to flake and crumble, releasing fibers to the air in the buildings. Asbestos levels are elevated near freeways, presumably due to release from asbestos brake linings.

The National Academy of Sciences (NAS) estimates the typical concentration of asbestos in urban air to be approximately 0.0004 fibers per milliliter, which works out to be over 10,000 fibers in the air of a typical room. The NAS also estimates that a person with a typical exposure in an urban area faces a lifetime risk of between 1 in 100,000 and 29 in 100,000 of developing cancer as a result of asbestos in air both indoors and outdoors. The difference in risk depends on sex (women face less risk than men) and on whether a person smokes. Given a U.S. urban population of 180 million people, this risk estimate translates into 1,800 to 52,200 expected cancers from asbestos. The specific risk estimates are listed in the Technical Information section.

Health Effects

Asbestos is known to cause lung and bowel cancer as well as noncancerous lung diseases. EPA considers asbestos a known human carcinogen (group A; see Chapter 3, Section B). The life-threatening conditions repeatedly identified are lung cancer, mesothelioma, and asbestosis. Lung cancer is responsible for the largest number of deaths from asbestos exposure. For cancer, there is no safe dose, that is, any exposure increases risk and the risk increases in proportion to both the level and duration of exposure. In addition, asbestos and tobacco smoke have a strong *synergistic* interaction in producing lung cancer: asbestos exposure appears to multiply by a factor of five rather than simply adding to the underlying lung cancer risk from smoking. Most people who develop lung cancer die from it within two years of diagnosis.

Mesotheliomas are a group of rare human cancers caused almost exclusively by exposure to asbestos. These cancers occur in the membranes (mesothelia) that line body cavities. Mesotheliomas can occur in the lung (pleural mesotheolioma) and in the abdomen (peritoneal mesothelioma). Most people who develop mesothelioma die within the first two years after diagnosis, often having been in constant pain.

Asbestosis involves the fibrosis (development of excess fibrous connective tissue) of the lung and its surrounding membrane. There is no effective treatment and it is often disabling or fatal. It is more uncommon than lung cancer or mesothelioma at exposures lower than the current OSHA workplace standard, and it is not certain whether asbestosis occurs as a result of nonoccupational exposures.

Protection and Prevention

In the home, asbestos is found in vinyl floor tiles and vinyl sheet flooring; patching compounds and textured paints; certain ceiling compounds installed between 1945 and 1978; stove and furnace insulation; some furnace, oven, and stove door gaskets; pipe, wall, and ceiling insulation; certain appliances; and some roofing shingles, siding shingles, and siding sheets. The identification of asbestos should be left to a professional; plumbers, building contractors, or heating contractors can often make a visual determination. Laboratories are also able to analyze samples for asbestos. The most important thing to know is that unless the material is deteriorating or unless remodeling is contemplated that could release asbestos fibers, asbestos in place is best left alone. If work must be done, use a contractor trained in safe asbestos-handling procedures.

The Consumer Product Safety Commission has established a hotline for information about asbestos removal procedures, asbestos testing laboratories, and where to get respirators for individuals wishing to do the work themselves. (See the National Hotline section at the back of this book for this and other asbestos hotline numbers.)

Regulatory Status

The EPA regulates asbestos in the environment and in manufactured goods. It recently banned the use of asbestos in asbestos–cement pipe and fittings, in roofing and flooring felts, in vinyl asbestos floor tile, and in fireproof clothing. These items, as well as previously banned consumer patching compounds and artificial emberizing compounds that release asbestos fibers, can no longer be sold. Asbestos use in all other products is to be phased out over a seven-year period. Asbestos is listed as a *hazardous air pollutant* in the 1990 Clean Air Act, requiring the EPA to set

TABLE 21 Cancer Risk for Various Groups at Two Asbestos Exposure Levels

Group	Expected Cancers per 100,000 People	
	Median Exposure (0.0004 fiber/cm^3)	High Exposure (0.002 fiber/cm^3)
Lung cancer		
Male smokers	29.2	146
Female smokers	10.5	52.4
Male nonsmokers	2.7	13.2
Female nonsmokers	1.4	6.8
Mesothelioma, all groups	15.6	78

Source: Risk from Exposure to Asbestos. 1986. *Science* 234:923.

emission standards. It is also on EPA *community right-to-know* list.

The EPA is setting standards for removal of asbestos in public schools. The regulation for controlling releases from asbestos mines, mills, and manufacturing facilities makes use of the "best practicable control technology currently available" combined with "no visible emissions." OSHA regulates workplace exposures.

Technical Information

OSHA limits in workplace air:
 Current: 2 fibers/cm^3
 Proposed: 0.5 or 0.2 fiber/cm^3

EPA proposed drinking water standard:
 7.1 million fibers/L exceeding 10μm in length

Table 21 shows the cancer risk for various segments of the population.

Further Reading

Environmental Protection Agency. 1986. Asbestos: Proposed Mining and Import Restrictions and Proposed Manufacturing, Importation, and Processing Prohibitions. *Federal Register* 51(19):3738–3759.

National Research Council. 1984. *Nonoccupational Health Risks of Asbestiform Fibers.* Washington, D.C.: National Academy Press.

U.S. Consumer Product Safety Commission. 1982. *Asbestos in the Home.* Washington, D.C.: Government Printing Office.

Aspartame

Other Names

N-L-Aspartyl-L-phenylalanine–1-methyl ester; 1-methyl-N-L-aspartyl-L-phenylalanine

Trade Names

Equal; NutraSweet

Introduction

The sweetener aspartame was discovered by accident in 1965. Eventually the compound was proved to be better tasting than many of the alternatives on the market, and it was thought that it would have an excellent chance of surviving rigorous toxicity testing. In fact, it has been the subject of more than 100 scientific studies, making it one of the most studied food additives on the market. But is it safe? Critics believe that many of the studies used by the FDA to approve the use of aspartame are tainted by excessive food industry support. For example, in one study, an animal tranquilizer known to protect laboratory animals from one of the predicted toxic effects of aspartame was used during toxicity testing.

Physical and Chemical Properties

Aspartame is an odorless white powder that is soluble in water and alcohol. It does not dissolve well in fats and oils. When heated or kept moist, it tends to break down, eventually losing its sweet taste (although soft drink manufacturers have learned to slow the process down).

Exposure and Distribution

Adults can be exposed to aspartame by consuming diet soft drinks, various low-calorie desserts, and any foods sprinkled with the sweetener. It has all but replaced saccharin, mainly because consumers seem to prefer the taste of aspartame. Children are also large consumers of this chemical, undoubtedly influenced by their parents' choices. The National Center for Health Statistics estimates that almost 40% of children up to the age of nine regularly drink soft drinks containing artificial sweeteners.

Health Effects

Reviews of aspartame toxicity ordered by the FDA show no adverse health effects among the laboratory animals tested. One of its breakdown products, diketopiperazine, has also been subjected to toxicological testing, with no adverse health effects identified.

Nevertheless, complaints about aspartame account for 80% of the telephone calls received on the FDA food additives hotline. (**Sulfites** account for another 15%.) The most common complaint about aspartame is that it causes severe headaches among sensitive individuals. But the FDA has been unable to prove that this is indeed the case. The FDA did find that some people break out in hives following aspartame ingestion. In addition, aspartame can cause severe problems for people with phenylketonuria (PKU) disease.

Despite the lack of evidence regarding toxic effects of aspartame, some scientists are concerned because aspartame contains an amino acid called aspartate that in large doses is known to stimulate the brain excessively. (**MSG** contains the amino acid glutamate that has a similar effect on the brain.) This overstimulation can damage the brain, perhaps leading to neurological diseases. Studies also indicate that children, especially infants, might be particularly vulnerable to brain damage caused by aspartate-induced overstimulation of neurons in the brain. Some scientists suggest that pregnant women should avoid ingesting aspartame because infant laboratory animals seem particularly vulnerable to brain damage caused by excessive stimulation to the brain brought about by aspartate.

Protection and Prevention

Almost all adult exposure to aspartame is voluntary. It can be avoided by reading the labels on all low-calorie or reduced calorie products before purchasing them. Parents who wish to err on the side of caution (as we advocate often in this book) should not allow their children to use aspartame. Because of a child's small body weight, aspartame doses per pound of body weight can easily be two to three times higher than that of an adult drinking the same amount of artificially sweetened soft drink.

Regulatory Status

As a condition of FDA approval of aspartame, the manufacturer is required to monitor the consumption of aspartame in food products. Products using aspartame must carry a label to warn people with PKU disease that the product contains phenylalanine.

Technical Information

Chemical formula: $C_{14}H_{16}N_2O_5$
Molecular weight: 292

Further Reading

JANSSEN, P. J. 1988. Aspartame: Review of Recent Experimental and Observational Data. *Toxicology* 50(1):1–26.

Asphalt

Other Names

Bitumen; tar

Introduction

Asphalt, a residue of the petroleum refining process, is frequently encountered in the environment because it is widely used for road paving. It is also used for roofing; for lining canals and other water-containing structures; as a protective coating for water mains and the undersides of automobiles; and in batteries, industrial adhesives, and electrical insulation. Most of the world uses the term "bitumen" to refer to what we in the United States call "asphalt." The term "tar" is often used to describe both asphalt and coal tar, but it is important to distinguish petroleum tars, such as asphalt, from coal tars and coal tar products such as **creosote**. Generally the health hazard of petroleum tars is far less than that of coal tar products.

Physical and Chemical Properties

Asphalt is a black or dark brown substance with an unmistakable aromatic odor that is particularly noticeable when the asphalt is heated. Depending on temperature and its specific chemical composition, asphalt can be gooey or solid. Some solid forms are brittle and others are rubbery. Their actual chemical composition is quite complex, consisting of a variety of both heavy and light *hydrocarbon* compounds.

Exposure and Distribution

Annual worldwide production of asphalt is currently a little more than 100 million tons, with the large majority of this used for road surfacing. Because heated asphalt emits far more potentially toxic ingredients (light *aromatic hydrocarbons*) than do cooled-off road surfaces or roofs, the largest public exposures are to road workers and roofers. The general public is exposed primarily when passing by road construction sites where hot asphalt is being poured and leveled or when entering a building undergoing asphalt roofing work. Workers in industries using or producing asphalt are potentially subject to accidental skin contact with splashed hot asphalt, which presents a burn hazard that far exceeds the toxic hazard.

Health Effects

Laboratory studies with test animals show that persistent contact of asphalt on skin can cause cancer and that long-term exposure to asphalt fumes can cause respiratory problems. But at levels the public is likely to encounter, and even at levels to which road workers are exposed, the *epidemiological* evidence suggests that asphalt fumes do not pose a significant health hazard.

Protection and Prevention

While the health hazard is slight, those concerned about asphalt can try to avoid spending time near road construction sites and in buildings with newly prepared asphalt roofing substances.

Regulatory Status

Exposure of the general public to asphalt is unregulated.

Further Reading

World Health Organization. 1982. *Environmental Health Criteria Report No. 20: Selected Petroleum Products*. Geneva.

Azinophos-Methyl

Trade Name

Guthion

Introduction

Introduced in 1953, azinophos-methyl is a long-lasting *organophosphate* insecticide, acaricide (mite killer), and molluscide (slug and snail killer) that is used extensively in agriculture. Approximately 70% of this pesticide is used on vegetables, ornamentals, cotton and orchard crops, such as peaches, apples, and almonds. Azinophos-methyl is used on a total of about 80 food crops. Its persistence, or resistance to breakdown, is related to its complex structure. When it does break down, it forms many diverse products that are difficult to detect as residues on or in food products. Consequently, azinophos-methyl is used less commonly than other organophosphates on food crops. Nevertheless, despite detection problems, it has been detected on apples and pears.

Azinophos-methyl is a major component of *Integrated Pest Management* programs (see Chapter 14, Section F) in a number of fruit-growing states because it is only slightly toxic to important predators of the pests of fruits. Since it is, however, highly toxic to many other nontarget species, azinophos-methyl is being replaced by the less toxic synthetic pyrethroids.

Physical and Chemical Properties

In its pure form the insecticide is a white, crystalline solid, but the technical grade of the material that is generally available forms a brown waxy solid. It can be broken down by acids and cold alkaline solutions.

Exposure and Distribution

About 2.5 million pounds of azinophos-methyl are applied as sprays or dusts to the foliage of noncitrus tree crops and cotton and are thus regionally limited. The Northwest region (Oregon, Washington, and Idaho) produces the largest fraction of orchard crops in the United States, while the Southwest (Texas, New Mexico, Arizona, and Colorado) constitutes the primary cotton growing region. Fieldworkers and residents of these areas are potentially exposed to the pesticide in the air, soil, and water. Because azinophos-methyl residues persist for quite a while, it is also likely that consumers in other parts of the country are exposed to the insecticide on fruits and vegetables treated with it.

Health Effects

Azinophos-methyl is *acutely* toxic for humans when ingested, but not quite as toxic as **parathion**. Readily absorbed through the skin, as are many other organophosphates, it is considerably less toxic than parathion, but much more toxic than **malathion**. Like other organophosphates and certain carbamate pesticides, azinophos-methyl inhibits the normal function of *cholinesterase*, an enzyme involved in the transmission of nerve signals (see Chapter 14, Section B). Typically, cholinesterase inhibition produces symptoms that resemble those of heat stroke, heat exhaustion, pneumonia or other serious respiratory infection, gastroenteritis, or low blood sugar; however, it can generally be distinguished on the basis of laboratory tests. Signs and symptoms of poisoning can include any of the following: headache, nausea, abdominal cramps, diarrhea, muscular weakness, low blood pressure, paralysis, inability to coordinate muscular activity, and cardiac irregularities. Because of its toxicity, azinophos-methyl has been associated with numerous poisoning incidents. Severe poisoning can lead to convulsions, cessation of breathing, and death.

Because data from animal tests and human *epidemiological* studies are inadequate or lacking, this insecticide cannot be assessed in terms of its cancer-causing ability, although some studies suggest that it may cause cancer in rats. Not enough evidence exists to determine whether it causes mutations, birth defects, or reproductive problems.

Protection and Prevention

By law, containers of the pesticide must carry a warning label indicating its toxicity to people and wildlife and listing precautions for proper use and handling, such as wearing protective clothing and disposing of it properly. Since the residues remain on the surface of the fruits, they can be washed off. Both cooking and heating will reduce residue levels.

Treatment of poisoning is similar to that for other organophosphates. First-aid responses should include giving artificial respiration if breathing stops, maintaining an open airway, and if the victim is conscious, inducing vomiting. If the chemical is in the eyes or on the skin, flushing with water is recommended. Generally, medical treatment will include the administration of atropine. Some physicians will also administer an oxime, such as pralidoxime.

Environmental Effects

Azinophos-methyl is acutely toxic to fish and wildlife, although species susceptibility is highly variable. Container labels are required by law to carry information on endangered species by area, county, and state.

Regulatory Status

This pesticide is available for use by certified applicators and is not available for household use. Moreover, there are restrictions on reentry periods for fieldworkers and crop rotations. For example, since azinophos-methyl is not registered for use on root vegetables, there is a 6-month restriction on planting root crops in areas treated with this insecticide. For all other crops for which its use is not registered, there is a 30-day restricted period.

Technical Information

Chemical name: O,O-dimethylphosphodith-
ioate-S-ester with 3-(mercaptomethyl)–
1,2,3-benzotriazine–4(3H)-one

Chemical formula: $C_{10}H_{12}N_3O_3PS_2$

OSHA limit in workplace: 0.2 mg/m^3

Further Reading

National Academy of Sciences. 1987. *Regulating Pesticides in Food: The Delaney Paradox.* Washington, D.C.: National Academy Press.

Barium

Introduction

Barium metal is a natural component of the earth's crust; it is widespread but found at low concentrations. Barium sulfate is used as an X-ray contrast medium for the digestive tract. It is not absorbed and is considered safe in this application. Other more toxic barium compounds are used in rat poisons, fireworks, paints, and plastics. The accidental swallowing of these products, usually by children, and the mistaken use of toxic barium chemicals instead of barium sulfate in radiology, although rare, have been reported.

Physical and Chemical Properties

Barium is a silvery-white, shiny metal. It burns in air, producing a red flame, and reacts violently with water. Because barium is so reactive, it is usually found combined with other elements to form compounds. In nature it occurs primarily as barium sulfate. Barium chloride is the most toxic barium compound; paradoxically, it was used in medicine for its stimulating action on heart muscle and nerve activity. Within the body, barium behaves like calcium and accumulates in bone.

Exposure and Distribution

Exposure to barium comes mainly from food and to a lesser extent from water. The average daily intake for an adult is about 0.75 mg, of which 90% comes from food. Water concentrations of barium are generally low, ranging from 0.001 to 0.172 milligram per liter, but about 150,000 people in the United States who receive water from public systems are supplied with water containing more than 1.0 milligram per liter (1 ppm). Various communities served by private wells in Illinois, Kentucky, Pennsylvania, and New Mexico are reported to have drinking water concentrations of more than ten times the federal barium limit for public supplies. For these people, a majority of their barium exposure comes from drinking water. Less than 20% of swallowed barium is absorbed. The average person inhales about 1 microgram of barium per day, a much lower exposure than from drinking water.

Health Effects

Absorbed barium causes strong and prolonged contractions of all muscles, including the digestive tract and heart. The result is violent bowel movements, vomiting, severe abdominal pain, excessive salivation, muscle twitching, elevation in blood pressure, and changes in heart activity. Muscular weakness follows and eventually paralysis of the limbs and respiratory muscles, which can lead to death from *respiratory arrest*. A fatal dose of barium chloride is 1 gram; toxic effects can be seen after swallowing 0.2 to 0.5 grams. Other barium compounds (carbonate, hydroxide, nitrate, acetate, and sulfide) are not as toxic as barium chloride, requiring up to 15 grams to be ingested for life-threatening consequences.

Chronic exposure to barium occurs from drinking water in certain areas. Several studies of communities from such areas show a slightly elevated death rate from heart disease; other studies show no effect. But even in those communities with elevated heart disease death rates, no clear link to barium has been established. Animal studies show rises in blood pressure (*hypertension*) with long-term barium exposure. No information has been reported on the relationship of barium to *mutations*, cancer, or birth defects.

Barium appears to act by altering the membranes in muscle and nerve cells, preventing the flow of potassium both in and out. This leads to excessive excitability in these tissues. All signs of acute barium toxicity, except hypertension, are relieved by intravenous potassium injection.

Protection and Prevention

Barium-containing products are not commonplace. Ordinary precautions to prevent children from touching potentially hazardous products, such as rat poisons, should be taken (for example, store them in childproofed or locked cupboards or on high shelves). For the few communities in which barium concentrations in drinking water are high, switching to bottled water may reduce exposure.

Regulatory Status

The EPA limits the concentration of barium in drinking water at 1.0 milligram per liter (1 ppm). Surveys of public water supplies consistently show barium concentrations at much lower levels than the federal limit, both at the water utility and at consumer taps. A recent review by the National Academy of Sciences (NAS) suggests the barium in drinking water is not as harmful as originally believed because it is less well absorbed from the *gastrointestinal tract* than previously thought and that a level of 4.7 milligrams per liter would be a safe federal standard. Barium is on the EPA *community right-to-know* list. Occupational exposures to barium are regulated by OSHA by limiting the concentration of *soluble* barium compounds in factory air.

Technical Information

Chemical symbol: Ba
Atomic number: 56
Atomic weight: 137
Federal drinking water standard: 1.0 mg/L (1ppm)
OSHA limit in workplace air: 0.2 mg/m^3

Further Reading

Environmental Protection Agency. 1985. *Drinking Water Criteria Document for Barium (Final Draft)*. PB86–118031. Springfield, VA: National Technical Information Service, U.S. Department of Commerce.

National Academy of Sciences. 1982. *Drinking Water and Health, Volume 4*. Washington, D.C.: Safe Drinking Water Committee, National Research Council

———. 1977. *Drinking Water and Health, Volume 1*. Washington, D.C.: Safe Drinking Water Committee, National Research Council.

Benomyl

Trade Name

Benlate

Introduction

Introduced in 1967, the *fungicide* benomyl is notable for its effectiveness against a broad spectrum of fungal pests and its *systemic* action, meaning that it is absorbed through the leaves or roots and moves to other parts of the plant, generally the growing parts. Because the fungicide is taken up by the plant, it protects plants and controls disease more effectively and over a longer period of time than chemicals that remain on the surface of the plant. Not only is benomyl one of the first successful systemics, but it is also useful against a greater variety of fungi than many newer ones. It is registered for use on more than 100 fruit, vegetable, and field crops, such as rice, as well as on lawns and turf.

Benomyl is related to the carbamate pesticides, which include **aldicarb** and **carbaryl**, but it does not produce the toxic effects on the nervous system that are typical of most other carbamates. That is, it does not inhibit the enzyme *cholinesterase*, which is essential in the proper transmission of nerve signals (see Chapter 14, Section B).

Physical and Chemical Properties

Benomyl is a white crystalline powder with a faint acrid odor. At room temperature it is nonvolatile. It is fairly insoluble in water, but dissolves readily in **chloroform**.

Exposure and Distribution

About three million pounds of benomyl are used in the United States annually, roughly one-third of which is applied to tomatoes, rice, apples, grapes, and citrus. Benomyl is sprayed onto foliage, applied to soils, used for dipping fruits and roots, and used in a combination product with another carbamate to treat seeds. One advantage of using benomyl

or one of the other benzimidazoles (see Technical Information section) is that these newer systemic fungicides can be applied less frequently and at lower rates than such nonsystemics as **captan** and the **ethylenebisdithiocarbamates**, or EBDCs. Thus, in theory, hazards to wildlife and the environment are reduced.

Health Effects

The EPA has classified benomyl as a probable human carcinogen (group B_2; see Chapter 3, Section B) on the basis of test results. Both benomyl and carbendazim (a *metabolite* of benomyl) have been linked to an increased incidence of cancer of the lymph glands in female mice, and benomyl and another of its metabolic products are associated with liver cancer in both male and female mice. Moreover, benomyl appears to cause mutations in some test systems, birth defects in rats, and reproductive effects in rats, including an increase in fetal death and reduced sperm counts.

Laboratory studies and use experience indicate that benomyl and other benzimidazoles are of moderate to low acute toxicity when ingested. They do not accumulate in tissues and are almost entirely eliminated within 24 hours. Although the benzimidazoles themselves do not inhibit cholinesterase, one breakdown product of benomyl does so irreversibly and is comparable in potency to the breakdown products of the *organophosphate* pesticides. Certain people appear to be particularly sensitive to benomyl and develop *dermatitis* following exposure.

Protection and Prevention

For several species of pests, particularly rice blast and stem rot, there are no registered alternatives to benomyl. Nor do agricultural practices, water management, or crop rotations control these diseases. In the production of fruits and vegetables, however, other fungicides can be used effectively. But several of these, such as **captan** and the **EBDCs**, are undergoing scrutiny by the EPA for health effects, while certain newer, promising systemics such as **fosetyl Al** are registered only for limited use.

Benomyl is one of many pesticides that cannot be detected by the routine testing methods used by the FDA when it samples produce for residues. Moreover, because it is a systemic pesticide, it cannot be washed off the surface of the produce. Undue occupational exposure can be reduced by the use of protective clothing, which must be worn by people handling and working with the fungicide.

Environmental Effects

A major drawback to using benomyl is that it is especially toxic to a variety of organisms, including earthworms, honeybees, and certain species of fish. Toxicity to fish varies greatly with species; catfish are especially sensitive. As a result, continued use of benomyl for certain purposes, such as in flooded rice paddies, hinges on field studies to determine whether residues can escape into aquatic systems.

A large number of fungal species have developed *resistance* to benomyl (see Chapter 14, Section D). To counter problems of pest resistance, the manufacturer recommends using less fungicide in treatments and timing fungicide application more carefully. Some growers use benomyl in combination with captan or one of the EBDCs or only at selected times, such as postharvest, in an attempt to slow the development of resistance.

Regulatory Status

Benomyl is undergoing a *Special Review* by the EPA on the basis of evidence of adverse effects on nontarget species and hazards to wildlife, in addition to data showing *mutagenic, teratogenic,* reproductive, and more recently, carcinogenic effects. As of 1989, numerous *tolerances* have been established for both raw and processed agricultural products, although the EPA is reviewing its tolerance policy.

Technical Information

Benomyl is closely related to three other agricultural fungicides—carbendazim, thiabendazole, and thiophanate-methyl—together called the benzimidazoles. Carbendazim is not only a commercial fungicide, but is also the principal metabolite of both benomyl and thiophanate-methyl. Thus, it is thought to be the component that actually kills fungi. Thiabendazole is used to treat people and animals for various parasites, such as pinworms, hookworms, and roundworms.

Chemical name: methyl–1-(butylcarbamoyl) 2-benzimidazole carbamate

Chemical formula: $C_{14}H_{18}N_4O_3$

NAS estimated risk from lifetime dietary exposure: 7.2×10^{-6}

OSHA limit in workplace air (considered safe for people who are not sensitive): 1.4 mg/kg/day

Further Reading

HAYES, W. J., JR. 1982. *Pesticides Studied in Man*. Baltimore, MD: Williams and Wilkins.

National Academy of Sciences. 1987. *Regulating Pesticides in Food: The Delaney Paradox*. Washington, D.C.: National Academy Press.

Benzene

Other Names

Benzol; carbon oil; coal tar naphtha; cyclohexatriene; phenyl hydride; pyrobenzole

Trade Name

Benzin

Introduction

While pumping gasoline, struggling through an organic chemistry class, or cleaning paint brushes, most of us have encountered the compound benzene. First delineated in 1865, the benzene ring structure is the basic chemical building block for both naturally occurring and synthetic organic compounds (including many of the substances in this book). In living organisms, the benzene ring is a common component of crucial substances, such as vitamins, sugars, and enzymes, which are involved in normal biochemical processes. Man-made benzene, derived from petroleum and coal, is produced in enormous volume—about 4.6 million tons in the United States annually—as a feedstock in the synthesis of a diverse array of commercial products. Benzene is found in paints, oils, resins, paintbrush cleaners, adhesives, aspirin, deodorants, oven cleaners, **asphalt**, explosives, pesticides, plastics, detergents, dyes, synthetic rubber, and many other products. In addition, it is a natural constituent of and an additive to gasoline and jet fuel (gasoline is 1.8 to 5.0% benzene by volume). Benzene is an effective replacement for lead in gasoline, boosting the octane levels in unleaded fuel. As lead is phased out, more benzene is being used. Premium unleaded gasoline contains as much as 3% benzene.

Physical and Chemical Properties

At room temperature, pure benzene is a clear, *volatile*, colorless liquid. An easily detectable and recognizable (but not unpleasant) odor characterizes benzene and the myriad of compounds containing the benzene ring. Consequently, chemists call this class of compounds the *aromatics*. Pure benzene readily separates from water and, at room temperature, floats on the water surface. It evaporates quickly, but not as quickly as rubbing alcohol. Classified as a highly flammable liquid by the Department of Transportation, benzene can be ignited over a wide range of temperatures. In addition, dangerous chemical reactions result when benzene is mixed with oxidizing agents such as chlorine, liquid oxygen, and sodium peroxide.

Exposure and Distribution

Because it occurs in so many products, benzene is widely distributed in air and water. It is released into surface water in municipal and industrial wastewater discharges. It has been found as a contaminant of groundwater as a result of leaching from hazardous waste sites and leaking from underground gasoline storage tanks. It is a constituent of emissions from motor vehicles and from major chemical manufacturing and refining industries, all of which were thought to be the principal sources of exposure to benzene until very recently. The California Air Resources Board cited motor vehicles as the source of 80% of *ambient* benzene in the state. A Washington-based public interest group released a report in 1990 charging that the greatest cancer risk from benzene is associated with inhaling the fumes while filling the gas tank. The EPA estimates the chance of developing cancer from a lifetime of self-service refueling is about 8 in 100,000.

However, studies in which people carried personal air quality monitors throughout the course of a normal day revealed that the major source of exposure to benzene is cigarette smoking. Although cigarettes emit a relatively small amount of benzene compared to industrial emissions, smokers directly breathe the 30 metric tons of benzene released annually by cigarettes. Nonsmokers, too, are exposed to higher levels of benzene from cigarettes and other indoor sources than from industrial sources.

OSHA estimates that 240,000 industrial workers—principally those working in the petroleum and coal industries—are routinely exposed to benzene in the workplace. NIOSH estimates that as many as two million workers in the United States may be potentially exposed to significant levels of benzene. Under current OSHA standards, there is reason to believe that workers exposed to benzene run some, perhaps substantial, risk of contracting and/or dying of leukemia. Previous standards, changed in 1987 despite industry objections, permitted a leukemia-induced death rate of 95 per 1000 workers based on an assumed lifetime occupational exposure.

Health Effects

Exposure via inhalation, skin, or eye contact can cause upper respiratory tract irritation, *dermatitis,* or eye irritation, respectively. If benzene is aspirated into the lungs, it can cause *pulmonary edema* and hemorrhage. Because benzene is poorly absorbed through the skin, it is unlikely to cause systemic effects if it comes into contact with the skin. *Acute exposure* following ingestion or excessive inhalation depresses the central nervous system resulting in headache, dizziness, nausea, convulsions, coma, and possibly death.

The International Agency for Research on Cancer classifies benzene as a carcinogen. Aplastic *anemia,* changes in the production of red and white blood cells in the bone marrow, and other effects on the blood are associated with chronic exposure to benzene. Bone marrow changes can occur several years after exposure has ceased. *Epidemiological* studies link chromosomal aberrations and leukemia to benzene exposure.

Protection and Prevention

OSHA requires a well-ventilated work area, protective clothing, and goggles for workers exposed to high levels of pure benzene. As with most chemicals, people should avoid direct contact. If benzene is spilled or splashed onto the skin, wash promptly with soap and water. If the chemical gets into the eyes, flush immediately with water. Excessive inhalation should be treated by getting the person into fresh air immediately. If benzene is ingested, do not induce vomiting nor give either epinephrine or alcohol. Vomiting increases the risk of aspirating the chemical, which can cause pulmonary edema or hemorrhage. In all cases other than minor skin contact, a physician should be notified.

A variety of approaches to reduce the volume of benzene released to the environment can be adopted. These include reducing gasoline consumption by increasing the fuel efficiency of automobiles and by driving less, reducing spillage and leakage from gasoline pumps at service stations, and replacing underground storage tanks that leak. In fact, reauthorized Superfund legislation has mandated replacement of all underground tanks that are leaking petroleum (see Chapter 17).

Since benzene is an important component of oil-based paints and solvents, using substitutes for these products can reduce both emissions and exposure. For example, a little "elbow grease" is an effective, if more labor intensive, substitute for chemical paint removers. And not only do water-based products perform as well as their oil-based counterparts, but they are less toxic and easier to clean up. Much of the hazardous waste in this country's landfills comes from discarded household products, many of which contain benzene. Instead of throwing old paint, oil, or gasoline cans in the garbage or pouring their unused contents down the drain (an illegal practice in most areas), check with your local refuse collection agency about proper disposal. Waste oil can be reclaimed, and some wastes are accepted by industrial waste handlers. Some local agencies even conduct hazardous waste roundups as a public service. The EPA recommends commercial incineration as a suitable disposal method.

Environmental Effects

Although benzene-containing petroleum products are deliberately introduced to aquatic systems to control weeds, benzene is unlikely to be a significant contaminant of surface water since it readily evaporates into the atmosphere. Nor does it adsorb strongly to soil particles. Moreover, microorganisms in soil and aquatic sediments break down the benzene ring. However, benzene is a long-term contaminant of groundwater because it cannot readily evaporate underground, and since little microbial activity occurs in underground water, it is not degraded.

Regulatory Status

Benzene is listed as a *hazardous air pollutant* in the 1990 Clean Air Act, requiring the EPA to set emission standards. The EPA has also established standards for benzene levels in drinking water and criteria for ambient freshwater and saltwater. The "action" level for benzene in drinking water in California is considerably lower than the maximum permitted under federal regulations. OSHA has issued standards for workplace exposure. Land disposal of benzene products is prohibited under the Resource Conservation and Recovery Act (1984). Benzene is on the EPA's *Community Right-to-know* list.

Technical Information

Chemical name: benzene
Chemical formula: C_6H_6
OSHA limit in workplace air: 3.3 mg/m^3
OSHA short-term (5-minutes) limit:
   16.5 mg/m^3
Lowest observable effects level:
   ambient freshwater: <5300 µg/L
   ambient saltwater: <5100 µg/L
   EPA maximum contaminant level in drinking water: 5 µg/L
   EPA maximum contaminant level goal in drinking water: 0 µg/L

Further Reading

Agency for Toxic Substances and Disease Registry. 1987. *Toxicological Profile for Benzene.* Washington, D.C.: U.S. Public Health Service.

WITTCOFF, H. A., and REUBEN, B. G. 1980. *Industrial Organic Chemicals in Perspective. Part 1: Raw Materials and Manufacture.* New York: John Wiley.

———. 1980. *Industrial Organic Chemicals in Perspective. Part 2: Technology, Formulation, and Uses.* New York: John Wiley.

Benzo[*a*]pyrene (B[*a*]P)

Other Names

B[*a*]P; BAP; BP; benz[*a*]pyrene; benzo-*alpha*-pyrene; 3,4-benzopyrene

Introduction

When tobacco, foods, garbage, wood, coal, or petroleum products are burned, one of the most hazardous pollutants given off is benzo[*a*]pyrene, or B[*a*]P. B[*a*]P has no known commercial uses; it is an unwanted by-product of combustion, particularly when the combustion occurs at a temperature too low to burn the fuel completely. B[*a*]P is also found in coal tars and coal tar derivatives such as **creosote**. Relatively small amounts are found in **asphalt**. While no adequate tests have been performed on humans to determine the health risks of B[*a*]P, numerous tests on mice, rats, and other animals show that this substance is a toxic hazard. There are indications that the inhalation of B[*a*]P in tobacco smoke is a major reason why cigarette smoking causes cancer.

Physical and Chemical Properties

In pure form at room temperature, B[*a*]P is a yellow solid consisting of plate- or needle-shaped crystals. In quantities found in the environment, it has no detectable odor. When it is formed from the burning of tobacco, fuels, or other substances, it is usually released into the atmosphere attached to smoke particles. B[*a*]P is only slightly soluble in water; it binds to many forms of *organic matter*.

Exposure and Distribution

Forest fires are a natural source of B[*a*]P, but human activities are the major source of this substance. Moreover, naturally produced B[*a*]P is distributed widely throughout the environment, whereas B[*a*]P produced by people is more concentrated in the air that people breathe. For the general public, the greatest exposures to B[*a*]P are from cigarette smoking, breathing air contaminated by smokers, wood burning in woodstoves and fireplaces, and cooked foods. The most intense exposures to B[*a*]P, however, occur in the workplace, particularly around coke ovens, creosote factories, meat-smoking factories, and trash incinerators. Some restaurant kitchens may also be sites of workplace exposure.

In comparison with rural air, typical urban air has roughly 10 to 100 times the concentration of B[*a*]P. A smoke-filled room is likely to have roughly 50 times the concentration that urban air has. However, some of the highest levels of B[*a*]P have been found in Third World village huts where firewood or coal is inefficiently burned for heating and cooking; the levels here can be 1000 or more times those found in urban air. B[*a*]P released to the atmosphere during combustion is later deposited with rain and falling particles; hence, it can be found in drinking water, soil, and vegetable crops far from its sources. Available evidence suggests that B[*a*]P *bioconcentrates* in *food chains*. It can enter the body by inhalation, ingestion, or direct contact with the skin.

Health Effects

Available evidence from animal tests indicates that B[*a*]P impairs reproduction in mice by causing birth defects and reduced body weight of newborn animals. These tests show that direct contact with skin can cause skin lesions and that inhalation can cause bronchitis. Animal tests also show that cancer can be induced by inhalation, ingestion, or skin contact with B[*a*]P. These tests are conducted using doses of B[*a*]P that are thousands or more times greater than those likely to be received by humans. Because of the clearcut results from animal tests and the absence of any direct information from *epidemiological* studies concerning the ability of B[*a*]P to cause cancer in humans, the EPA has classified this substance as a probable human *carcinogen* (group B_2; see Chapter 3, Section B).

Protection and Prevention

The best way to reduce exposure to B[*a*]P is to avoid cigarette smoking and avoid breathing second-hand smoke. Reducing consumption of smoked foods also helps, as does avoiding unnecessary breathing of smoky air from wood fires. Replacement of a smoky wood stove or fireplace with an efficient wood stove, designed to reduce the leakage of smoke into the living quarters, will also lower exposure to B[*a*]P.

Regulatory Status

Regulations often refer not to B[*a*]P alone but to all the *polycyclic aromatic hydrocarbons (PAHs)* or all the *volatile* coal tar products, of which B[*a*]P is considered to be among the most toxic. The World Health Organization (WHO) has a recommended upper level for PAHs in drinking water. An OSHA regulation limits the average amount of all volatile coal tar products that a worker can be exposed to over an 8-hour period in the workplace. It has also defined an advisory level for B[*a*]P that is 1000 times more stringent than its regulated level for all airborne coal tar products. The EPA has formulated guidelines relating the risk of cancer to the level of B[*a*]P in drinking water.

Technical Information

Total U.S. emissions of B[*a*]P by source:

coal burning	600 tons/year
coke production	200
forest fires	150
wood burning for heating and cooking	70
vehicles	2
cigarettes	0.05

B[*a*]P emission rates per unit of activity:
gasoline powered automobiles
0.5–1.0 µg/km

diesel cars and light trucks
1–3 µg/km
heavy duty trucks
10–30 µg/km
small coal stoves
50 mg/kg of coal
wood stoves and fireplaces
0.1–10 mg/kg of wood
cigarette smoking
0.1 µg per cigarette
inhaled per cigarette
0.03 µg
food (typical diet)
50 ng/day

Typical U.S. environmental concentrations of B[*a*]P by location:
nonurban outdoor air
0.1–1.0 ng/m³
urban outdoor air
0.2–20 ng/m³
smoke-filled room
100 ng/m³
drinking water
0.3–2.0 ng/L
rural surface soils
100–1000 µg/kg

WHO limit for aromatic hydrocarbons in domestic water supply: 0.2 µg/L

OSHA limit in workplace air (coal tar volatiles): 0.2 mg/m³

OSHA advisory level in workplace air: (B[*a*]P): 0.2 µg/m³

EPA estimates for lifetime risk of cancer from B[*a*]P in drinking water:

1 in 10^7 at 0.28 ng/L
1 in 10^6 at 2.8 ng/L
1 in 10^5 at 28 ng/L

The NAS estimates that the long-term risk for nonsmokers of dying from lung cancer increases above the background risk by roughly 5% for every additional nanogram per cubic meter of B[*a*]P in the air routinely breathed. This is equivalent to saying that if 300,000 people are exposed to an extra nanogram per cubic meter of B[*a*]P over their lifetime, then on average one extra death from lung cancer will occur in that group because of this additional exposure.

Further Reading

Agency for Toxic Substances and Disease Registry. 1987. *Toxicological Profile for Benzo[a]pyrene.* Washington, D.C.: U.S. Public Health Service.

Beryllium

Introduction

Beryllium, an industrial metal, causes a chronic lung disease called berylliosis and is believed to cause lung cancer. Most reported cases of berylliosis occurred among workers in the fluorescent lamp industry, in which beryllium was once used in lamp phosphors. The removal of beryllium from phosphors in 1949 and the tightening of occupational health and safety standards at the same time largely eliminated the beryllium hazard in industry. Exposure of the general population occurs as a result of air pollution, but is not considered to be a significant hazard at this time.

Physical and Chemical Properties

Beryllium is the lightest of all solid and chemically stable elements. It is number 4 in the periodic table of the elements and has properties similar to aluminum. It is exceptionally resistant to corrosion and extremely hard. Used in metal alloys, it provides improved resistance to metal fatigue, vibration, and shock.

Exposure and Distribution

In typical residential environments, roughly 70% of beryllium exposure occurs from drinking water, 30% from food, and only fractions of a percent from air and dust. An adult in the United States typically takes in about half a millionth of a gram per day (400 to 450 nanograms per day); however, less than 1% of swallowed beryllium is absorbed from the *gastrointestinal tract*. Certain occupational settings and proximity to factories that use beryllium can increase exposures in a few cases. But the tightening of industrial safety and hygiene regulations (such as washing workers' garments at the factory) have made such exposures much less common. Beryllium has also been detected in tobacco smoke, perhaps doubling the exposure to smokers. The information on this subject is scanty, however.

Coal and fuel oil contain beryllium as a trace contaminant. Burning of these energy sources releases beryllium oxide into the air and accounts for 99% of U.S. emissions, which total approximately 200 tons per year. Released on small particles that remain airborne for an average of 10 days, beryllium oxide then falls to the ground, either in rain or snow or as dry particles. The oxide is very difficult to dissolve and does not move readily in soil or surface waters. It is therefore unlikely to *bioconcentrate* in *food chains*. Because beryllium is a contaminant of coal, it is also found in the ash left when coal is burned. Ash is disposed of in landfills, which could become a source of beryllium contamination of nearby groundwater. Very little data are available on this subject. Sewage sludge incineration is also emerging as an important source of beryllium emissions.

Typical beryllium levels are given in Table 22.

Beryllium is used primarily in metal alloys (mainly with copper), which account for 75% of total consumption. The alloys go into instruments, aircraft parts, springs, electrical connectors, and other industrial components. Beryllium incorporated into ceramics used for high heat conductivity accounts for 15% of its use. The ceramics are used in electrical insulators and rocket nozzles. Pure beryllium metal accounts for the last 10% of total consumption, used in missile and rocket parts, aircraft, heat shields, and nuclear weapons.

Beryllium ore is mined in the United States exclusively at Spor Mountain, Utah, and is processed in Delta, Utah. This source supplies 85% of the domestic consumption of 300 tons per year of beryllium metal.

Health Effects

Beryllium is primarily a threat to the lungs. In the 1940s, *acute poisoning* of workers was common, causing chemical pneumonitis, a chemically induced *inflammation* of the respiratory tract. After exposure ended, the condition often improved in several weeks without treatment, although some deaths occurred. Only 15 cases of acute poisoning are known to have occurred in the United States since 1950, and no cases have been reported since 1968.

Chronic exposure to beryllium causes chronic beryllium disease (berylliosis), an inflammatory *lesion* of the lungs, accompanied by the formation of nodules or granules around the deposited particles. Characteristic *immune system* responses also occur. The disease is almost entirely restricted to workers who have been exposed on the job; to their families, who may have been exposed to beryllium particles brought home on clothing; and to nearby residents of factories using beryllium. There can be a long *latency period* (up to 25 years after exposure) followed by the onset of symptoms, including shortness of breath, weight loss, weakness, chest pain, and constant hacking cough. Complications include *fibrosis* of the lungs, *emphysema*, and death.

Approximately 1000 cases of berylliosis have been reported in the United States, mainly among workers exposed before 1949. In the general population, 65 cases of berylliosis have been reported, 42 from air pollution in the vicinity of two beryllium-emitting plants and 23 from household exposure to dust brought home on work clothes. No new cases have been reported for workers exposed after 1972 or for the general population since the introduction of air quality and work hygiene standards in 1949. These figures may be underestimates, however, because of the misdiagnosis of certain lung conditions that are in reality berylliosis. It is possible that workers in some industries are currently exposed to levels of beryllium that are causing harm.

Beryllium most likely causes lung cancer in humans, although the evidence is not conclusive. An elevated occurrence of lung cancer is associated with beryllium-related occupations. But the association is weak, and

TABLE 22 Beryllium Concentrations in Various Environments

Medium	Concentration
Ambient air	<0.001–0.28 ng/m^3
Highest measured urban value (Dallas, 1979)	0.40 ng/m^3
Natural waters	0.01–1.0 µg/L (0.01–1 ppb)
Soils	0.6–6.0 µg/g

the studies contain flaws. The International Agency for Research on Cancer (IARC) considers the available information to provide "limited" evidence of carcinogenicity in humans; the Cancer Assessment Group (CAG) of the EPA considers the evidence to be "inadequate" for a conclusion of human cancer production. Animal studies are far more definitive, however, leading both the IARC and the CAG to conclude that the evidence is "sufficient" for cancer production in animals. On the overall strength of available evidence, the EPA classifies beryllium as a probable human carcinogen (group B$_2$), placing it in the lower third of 55 chemicals tested and ranked for potency in producing cancer. Studies on the ability of beryllium to produce *mutations* and reproductive effects have been inconclusive.

Protection and Prevention

The general public presently is not at high risk from beryllium; no new "neighborhood" cases of berylliosis have been reported since the 1940s. However, the gradual accumulation of beryllium in the environment from power plant emissions and hazardous waste landfills may change this assessment in the future. People with respiratory symptoms who may also have been exposed to beryllium on the job should seek medical attention and mention the possibility of beryllium exposure at the time a medical history is taken.

Regulatory Status

Beryllium levels are not regulated in water or in the general air, although the EPA designates beryllium as a hazardous air pollutant in the 1990 Clean Air Act. It is on the EPA *community right-to-know* list. Workplace exposures are regulated by OSHA.

Technical Information

Chemical symbol: Be
Atomic number: 4
Atomic weight: 9
OSHA limits in workplace air:
  8-hour time-weighted average: 2 µg/m^3
  acceptable ceiling concentration: 5 µg/m^3
  acceptable maximum peak above the acceptable ceiling concentration for an 8-hour shift: 25 µg/m^3 for 30 min. maximum

Further Reading

Agency for Toxic Substances and Disease Registry. 1988. *Toxicological Profile for Beryllium.* Washington, D.C.: U.S. Public Health Service.
Environmental Protection Agency. 1986. *Health Assessment Document for Beryllium.* EPA–600/8–84–026B. Springfield, VA: National Technical Information Service, U.S. Department of Commerce.

BHT and BHA

Other Names

Butylated hydroxytoluene (BHT); butylated hydroxyanisole (BHA)

Introduction

BHT and BHA are preservatives. Developed in 1947 to check *oxidation* in rubber products, these chemicals are now widely used in consumer and food products. BHT and BHA have recently been suggested as herpes self-treatment medications and as substitutes for vitamins A and E. These uses have not been demonstrated to be effective.

BHA and BHT are used in a wide variety of products. Although consumers are most aware of BHT as a food additive, less than 5% of it is actually used in the United States in food. Most of it is used as an *antioxidant* in rubber and plastic (85%) and in liquid petroleum products such as gasoline and motor oil (9%). BHT is also used in a wide variety of cosmetic products, insecticides, synthetic detergents, asphalt floor tiles, paints, and inks.

Physical and Chemical Properties

BHT and BHA are synthetic chemicals in the form of colorless, odorless, and tasteless gases. These chemicals work by slowing the rate at which fats and oils react with oxygen. This oxidation reaction is the process that causes fats and oils to become rancid or rubber and plastics to become brittle. BHA and BHT are soluble in animal fats, vegetable oils, many solvents, ketones, alcohols, and linseed oil. They are slightly soluble in water.

Exposure and Distribution

The highest concentrations of BHT and BHA in edible products are found in chewing gum and active dry yeast, but large amounts of these products are not eaten. Consumers are likely to eat the highest quantities of BHT and BHA in prepared snacks, frozen convenience foods, and prepared cereal products. Many of these foods have a high percentage of fat, which needs to be protected from oxidation. Meats are not allowed to be treated with BHT and BHA, with the exceptions of frozen pork sausage and freeze-dried products.

BHT and BHA are often added to a product's packaging material rather than to the food itself. The preservative then vaporizes inside the package during storage. Antioxidant concentrations are similar to those found by adding BHT or BHA directly to the food.

Health Effects

Long-term animal studies indicate no health problems associated with BHT and BHA at levels consumed in the normal diet. The National Cancer Institute Carcinogenesis Technical Report considers the chemical to be safe at such normal levels. However, rats fed low levels of BHT show reduced weight gain. Liver enlargement, increased adrenal gland weights, and increased cholesterol levels in the blood have also been reported in test animals fed moderate doses of BHT for their entire lives. There are also scattered reports of an increased incidence of lung tumors in BHT-treated mice. But at the same time, it has also been shown that BHA protects against the cancer-causing properties of several chemicals. Some people think that a drop in U.S. stomach cancer rates can be attributed to the use of BHT and BHA. However, most scientists attribute this drop to overall improvements in food preservation over the last 80 years. On the one hand, it may be that low doses of BHT and BHA do not cause cancer but rather hasten tumor development in animals that already have cancer. On the other hand, some researchers have found that large doses of BHT and BHA cause cancer, hemorrhage, liver enlargement, and lung damage. Liver enlargement seems to be temporary.

Self-treatment doses of 100 to 1000 times normal daily exposure are sometimes recommended by self-styled healers and nutritionists. After eating such high levels, people have reported short-term stomach cramps, vomiting, dizziness, and loss of consciousness, particularly when taken on an empty stomach. Studies using animals dosed at these high levels indicate that absorbed BHT and BHA are rapidly excreted in the urine and are unlikely to accumulate in the body. Other studies indicate that BHT and BHA do accumulate in fat tissue.

Considerable uncertainty on both sides of the BHT/BHA safety issue is evident in the scientific literature. This uncertainty should be weighed against strong evidence that rancid fats and oils (unprotected by BHT and BHA) are unhealthy. A one-time consumption of rancid food can cause diarrhea. Continued consumption leads to deficiencies of vitamins E and A, liver enlargement, and poor growth rates in children. Very rancid oil may be fatal and can cause severe respiratory problems and symptoms of muscular dystrophy.

Protection and Prevention

Since BHT and BHA are not allowed in fresh foods, exposure can be minimized by avoiding processed foods, particularly those high in fat or oil. Self-treatment for herpes and the substitution of BHT or BHA for vitamins A and E should be avoided in light of uncertainty about the long-term health effects of high doses and the lack of evidence that such applications work.

Regulatory Status

BHT and BHA are regulated by the FDA at levels such that the average person, following a normal diet, is unlikely to eat more than 0.5 milligram of BHT and/or BHA per kilogram of body weight. This is considered a normal exposure.

Technical Information

FDA standards: Most foods are regulated according to the amount of fat or oil contained in the product. In general, 200 ppm BHT and/or BHA by weight of the fat or oil contained in the product are allowed. Some foods are exempt from this overall standard and have individual limits, as follows:

beverage and dessert mixes
  90 ppm (by weight)
breakfast cereal
  50 ppm (by weight)
dry potato products
  50 ppm (by weight)
rice
  33 ppm (by weight)
unsmoked dry sausage
  30 ppm (by weight)
chewing gum base
  1000 ppm (by weight)
active dry yeast
  1000 ppm (by weight)

Further Reading

ALLEN, J. C., and HAMILTON, R. J., eds. 1982. *Rancidity in Foods*. New York: Applied Science Publishers.

GOSSELIN, R. E., SMITH, R. P., and HODGE, H. C. 1984. *Clinical Toxicology of Commercial Products*, 5th edition. Baltimore: Williams and Wilkins.

Bis(chloromethyl)ether

Other Names

BCME; dichloromethyl ether; *sym*-dichloromethyl ether; chloro(chloromethoxy)methane; oxybis(chloromethane); dimethyl–1,1-dichloro ether; chloromethyl ether

Introduction

Bis(chloromethyl)ether or BCME was once used extensively during the manufacture of plastics and other chemicals. But it is rarely used today because it is a potent cancer-causing agent. Nevertheless, it is still found in toxic waste dumps, and it is produced in small amounts whenever **formaldehyde** and **hydrochloric acid** combine. BCME is one of a family of chemicals known as chloroalkyl ethers. Other chemicals in this family include bis(2-chloroethyl)ether (BCEE) and chloromethyl methyl ether (CMME). These chemicals have similar chemical and toxicological properties to BCME, although they are not as potent. They are used primarily during the production of plastics and resins and in research laboratories. BCEE is commonly used during textile processing and paint manufacture. It has been detected in the drinking water of several highly industrialized areas, probably as a result of spills and improper waste disposal practices. BCME is often found as a contaminant of these related compounds, particularly of CMME.

Physical and Chemical Properties

Bis(chloromethyl)ether is a colorless liquid with a suffocating odor. It evaporates easily and breaks down rapidly when it comes into contact with water. It easily catches fire when exposed to heat or flame, emitting toxic **chlorine** fumes.

Exposure and Distribution

Although BCME is normally considered an occupational hazard only, it is found in hazardous waste dump sites. But the most likely means of exposure is inhalation of BCME vapors in the workplace whenever CMME is used, or in situations where formaldehyde and hydrochloric acid mix. Industries that use hydrochloric acid and formaldehyde together include textile production, particle board and paper production, and biological and chemical research laboratories. Very low levels of BCME have been detected in drinking water in areas of high industrial activity. This is most likely the result of spills and improper waste disposal.

Health Effects

Bis(chloromethyl)ether is a known human carcinogen, responsible for cancers of the mucous membranes, skin, and lungs. Lung cancers have been reported in rats that have inhaled very small amounts of BCME. BCME has also been linked to human lung cancer. CMME is also known to cause cancer in humans.

Low concentrations of BCME are irritating to the eyes and skin, and it is readily absorbed into the mucous membranes. *Acute exposures* can cause edema, pulmonary congestion, eye damage, reduced lung function, cough, difficulty in breathing, and the coughing up of blood. Chronic low-level exposures can cause a nagging cough and decreased lung capacity. It can also be absorbed through the skin to cause lung cancer. Target organs are the lungs, eyes, and skin.

Protection and Prevention

People should assume that BCME is present whenever they are working with CMME and whenever, in the course of manufacturing, formaldehyde and hydrochloric acid mix. Measures should be taken to avoid inhaling fumes from such industrial processes.

Environmental Effects

The chemical breaks down rapidly in the environment. Since very small amounts of BCME are created at any one time, the chemical is unlikely to pose a threat to the environment upon accidental release. However, it tends to *bioaccumulate* in fish, indicating that it can be passed along the *food chain*.

Regulatory Status

Bis(chloromethyl)ether is one of 13 carcinogens regulated by OSHA without permissible exposure limits. Worker exposure to BCME and CMME is controlled through the use of engineering, work practices, and protective clothing. If BCME is used or formaldehyde-hydrochloric acid reactions are common at work, request a *Material Safety Data Sheet (MSDS)* to get more information about exposure routes and suggested protective measures. BCME is listed as a *hazardous air pollutant* in the 1990 Clean Air Act. It is also on the EPA *community right-to-know* list.

Technical Information

Chemical formula: $O(CH_2Cl)_2$
Molecular weight: 115
ACGIH average limit in workplace air:
  0.001 ppm

Further Reading

Agency for Toxic Substances and Disease Registry. 1988. *Toxicological Profile for Bis-chloromethyl Ether*. Washington, D.C.: U.S. Public Health Service.

Cadmium

Introduction

Cadmium is a rare element mined in association with **zinc**. Discovered in 1817, it was rarely used until about 50 years ago. But today, cadmium is widely used in a myriad of products and industrial processes. It is used to galvanize metal parts, as a pigment in paints and plastics, in rechargeable **nickel–cadmium batteries**, and as a catalyst and preservative in the plastics industry. Many special-purpose alloys and solders are formulated with cadmium. Ceramic glazes, oil paints, and other art supplies often contain cadmium-based pigments.

Significant amounts of cadmium can be released into the atmosphere during volcanic eruptions, but the most important sources of atmospheric cadmium contamination are the burning of fossil fuels (especially coal), municipal and medical waste, and sewage sludge. Cadmium and zinc mining, metal processing, electroplating, plastics and dye manufacturing, the manufacture and disposal of nickel-cadmium batteries, municipal waste-water treatment, and application of phosphate fertilizers are all sources of cadmium in soil, water, and sediments. From these sources cadmium is taken up by plants and animals and enters the food supply.

Physical and Chemical Properties

Cadmium is a soft, silvery metal that keeps its metallic luster when exposed to the environment. It is not a mechanically strong metal, but it is highly resistant to corrosion. Although chemically similar to zinc, it is not known to be an essential human nutrient.

Cadmium tends to stick to fly ash, dust, soil particles, and sediments. It is particularly attracted to fly ash and clay soils. Thus, cadmium that is released into the air as a result of combustion tends to stick to emitted ashes. These can stay in the atmosphere for a week or more. In this way, cadmium originating from combustion sources can be distributed over a wide area before settling to the ground. Once on the ground, cadmium tends to attach to clay particles near the soil surface. The metal then moves unchanged through the environment, attached to dust particles, taken up by plants, or washed into storm drains and surrounding waters. Cadmium washed into rivers, lakes, and estuaries is strongly attracted to sediments or organic material from which it enters the aquatic *food chain*.

Exposure and Distribution

Small concentrations of cadmium are found in rocks and soil all over the world, so that almost everyone is exposed to low levels of cadmium in their air, water, and food. People who live in urban or industrial environments are routinely exposed to cadmium levels well over a thousand times higher than those of their rural ancestors. Cadmium is a trace contaminant in fertilizers and is slowly but steadily building up in agricultural soils. This may become the most important source of cadmium in the future. Currently, food contributes 80 to 90% of the cadmium dose received by most people.

Flounder, mussels, scallops, oysters, and crab usually contain the highest concentrations of cadmium among marine species. Many plants readily take up cadmium from the soil. Thus, fruits, vegetables, grains, and tobacco grown in cadmium-laden soil will often contain significant concentrations of the metal. Food and drink contamination may also arise as a result of using water from pipes soldered with cadmium-containing materials or from dissolution of cadmium from pottery painted with cadmium-containing pigments. Antique cadmium-plated cookware and serving dishes can release enough cadmium to cause acute symptoms of poisoning.

Smoking is another significant source of exposure. The blood of heavy smokers shows on average twice the amount of cadmium normally found in nonsmokers. Unlike **lead**, however, cadmium concentrations in breast milk are extremely low, even when the mother has been exposed to significant levels of the metal.

In addition to exposure associated with eating and smoking, cadmium in urban and industrial air can be a significant source of exposure. Air concentrations of cadmium tend to be the highest around smelters, near incinerators, and along highways. Cadmium-containing bottom and fly ash from incinerators and power plants may become a source of exposure from improper disposal in landfills.

Health Effects

Inhaled cadmium is associated with lung cancer in people. The EPA classifies it as a probable human carcinogen (group B_1, see Chapter 3, Table 5). Although cadmium-induced lung cancer has been formally linked only to the heavy concentrations normally associated with occupational exposure to cadmium fumes, there is growing concern that cadmium can cause lung cancer at concentrations of those found in the air around smelters and some incinerators. Chronic exposure to low levels of cadmium may also result in progressive lung diseases such as *emphysema* and *chronic bronchitis*.

Chronic exposure to cadmium is also associated with a wide range of other diseases, including heart disease, anemia, skeletal weakening, depressed immune system response, and kidney and liver disease. Cadmium-caused kidney disease is the most thoroughly studied of these. Most of these chronic diseases arise from the fact that until 50 to 60 years of age, cadmium is continuously accumulated in the human body, particularly in the kidney, after which time soft tissue concentrations begin to decline. In most cases, kidney function is not affected until cadmium concentration reaches a critical level. Then, signs of kidney dysfunction become apparent. At this time the excretion of cadmium increases dramatically, but unfortunately, the kidney damage is irreversible. It is this accumulation of cadmium in the kidneys that is of special concern because particular groups of people in the United States (because of dietary and smoking habits, occupation, or location) are exposed to relatively high levels of cadmium daily.

High levels of cadmium in the body are also associated with brittle bones. In Japan, where the population ingests very high levels of cadmium relative to the United States, the cadmium-caused combination of brittle bones and kidney damage is called Itai-itai (Ouch-ouch) disease. Fortunately, this painful disease is rare, even in Japan.

Ingestion of highly contaminated food and drink leads to vomiting, diarrhea, and in severe cases, shock. High concentrations of cadmium in the air can cause chest pain, coughing, and lung problems as well as chills, muscle aches, nausea, vomiting, and diarrhea 4 to 10 hours following exposure. Such concentrations can also be highly irritating to the lungs, causing immediate coughing and pain. But high concentrations of cadmium that have not caused lung irritation can be fatal, sometimes hours or even days following exposure.

Protection and Prevention

Cadmium is widely dispersed in the environment and in different products. This implies that the best way to minimize exposure to cadmium is to push for its reduced use. Nevertheless, one can take certain steps to minimize exposure. Limit your intake of foods known to have elevated levels of cadmium, including liver and kidney products, flounder, mussels, scallops, oysters, and vegetables grown using sewage sludge fertilizers (particularly lettuce, cabbage, spinach, carrots, potatoes, rice, and wheat). Do not cook or store food in antique kitchenware, unless you have had the pieces tested for safety. Avoid tobacco smoke. Follow the suggestions outlined in Chapter 8, Section B, about the proper handling of cadmium-containing art

materials. Do not allow children to use art supplies containing cadmium.

Research is in progress to determine whether cadmium-induced kidney and bone damage is less likely when adequate amounts of protein, calcium, zinc, and vitamin D are included in the diet. The results of these studies are still unclear.

While exposure to cadmium cannot be absolutely avoided, people who are concerned about cadmium in the environment can try to limit purchase of disposable plastics and reduce the amount of garbage they generate, particularly if their community relies on a municipal waste incinerator. Do not put nickel–cadmium batteries in the garbage: save them for disposal when household toxic wastes are collected so that the nickel and cadmium can be recycled. Support efforts to limit the use of municipal and hospital waste incinerators. Alternatives to burning medical waste are available, and the volume of medical waste generated can be reduced by using fewer disposable products. Push for emission controls on existing incinerators; cadmium emissions are easily controlled. If you operate a business that uses cadmium, investigate alternative processes and treatments that minimize or eliminate the element. Industrial workers who suspect that they are exposed to cadmium at the workplace should request a *Material Safety Data Sheet (MSDS)*.

Environmental Effects

Cadmium is strongly accumulated by organisms at all levels. It is not metabolized and passes unchanged along the *food chain*. Cadmium has the potential to concentrate in the food chain, but studies conducted so far show limited *bioconcentration*. In addition, few species show any adverse health effects as a result of contact with cadmium, except in areas of extremely high concentration.

Regulatory Status

Cadmium has not yet been subjected to strict regulation. The EPA listed the metal as a

TABLE 23 Typical Concentrations of Cadmium

Source	Rural Areas	Urban/Industrial Areas
Agricultural soils	1 µg/g	
Rural air	0.003–0.62 ng/m^3	5 ng/m^3
Sediments	1.0 µg/g	0.6–4.1 µg/g
Coastal waters	0.01 µg/L	0.15 µg/L
Freshwater	0.1–1.2 µg/L	1–36 µg/L
Fruits and vegetables	0.01–0.15 mg/kg	0.3–0.5 mg/kg

hazardous air pollutant, in the 1990 Clean Air Act. The EPA recently set forth drinking water standards for cadmium which went into effect December 1990. However, no standards exist or are planned for waters in rivers, lakes, and estuaries. Most routine industrial releases of cadmium must be reported to the EPA under community right-to-know guidelines. Spills of over 10 pounds must also be reported to the EPA. The FDA regulates the cadmium content of agricultural fertilizers.

Technical Information

Chemical symbol: Cd
Atomic number: 48
Atomic weight: 112.4
Table 23 shows typical concentrations of cadmium from a variety of sources.
Daily dose information:
　United Nations tolerable daily dose:
　　60–70 µg
　American typical daily intake: 20 µg
　Japanese typical daily intake: 40–50 µg
EPA drinking water standard: 5 µg/L

Further Reading

Agency for Toxic Substances and Disease Registry. 1988. *Toxicological Profile for Cadmium.* Washington, D.C.: U.S. Public Health Service.

Caffeine

Introduction

Caffeine can be considered the most popular drug in the United States. Almost everyone is voluntarily exposed to it during their lifetime. Caffeine is included in this book because it is so widely encountered. It provides an interesting counterpoint when evaluating the chemicals we are involuntarily exposed to daily.

Physical and Chemical Properties

In its pure form, caffeine is a white, odorless, bitter powder that resembles cornstarch in appearance. It is moderately soluble in water at body temperature and readily soluble in boiling water.

Exposure and Distribution

Caffeine is found naturally in coffee, tea, chocolate, kola nuts, mate leaves, and several other plant seeds, barks, and leaves. It is thought to provide plants with some protection from insects, fungi, and bacteria.

Coffee beans and tea leaves account for most of the caffeine consumed, but not all is consumed in coffee mugs and tea cups. Caffeine extracted during the decaffeination of coffee is saved for use in other products such as soft drinks and drugs. The following list shows the distribution of caffeine use in the United States (as of 1982).

Coffee	60%
Tea	16%
Soft drinks	16%
Drugs	6%
Chocolate	2%

Nearly all of the caffeine found in soft drinks is added during manufacture. Soft drinks usually contain about one-fourth of the caffeine normally found in an equivalent amount of coffee and about half that normally found in an equivalent amount of tea.

Health Effects

Caffeine stimulates the central nervous system, heart, and respiratory system. Exactly how it does this is unknown. Apart from sleep disruption, the clearest effect on laboratory animals of regular doses of caffeine (equivalent to one or two 6-ounce cups of coffee) is an increase in general body movement. Few studies on humans have focused on body movement alone, but examinations of caffeine's effects on work output and athletic performance have revealed that two or three 6-ounce cups of coffee can prolong the amount of time an individual can perform physically exhausting work. The quality of such work is not improved. Also, no improvement in intellectual ability is associated with the use of caffeine. In fact, caffeine seems to worsen performance that involves short-term memory.

Sleep disturbances are experienced by most people who drink a cup of strong coffee within an hour of bedtime. The most noticeable effects are an increase in the amount of time it takes to fall asleep and a reduction in total sleep time. But what effects are there on the heavy coffee drinker who only drinks in the morning and afternoon? Some evidence suggests that heavy caffeine users are more easily aroused by sudden noises, exhibit increases in body movements during sleep, and complain of poorer quality sleep than people who abstain. Whether the quality of sleep is actually poorer is still subject to debate among researchers.

Caffeine reaches almost every part of the body and therefore has the potential to affect most body functions. In fact, it can produce acute effects on the cardiovascular system, the digestive system, energy expenditure, and frequency of urination. Heavy caffeine use may also adversely affect behavior. Caffeine significantly increases blood pressure in people who have been without the drug for several days. But complete tolerance to this effect develops quickly. Caffeine does have a tendency to induce arrhythmias or palpitations in the hearts of susceptible individuals. But it has also been shown to increase the rate and improve the depth of breathing in other users. Heavy caffeine use is also associated with high cholesterol levels, but the reason for this is unknown.

Coffee drinking increases the secretion of acid into the stomach, but caffeine may not be the culprit. Other components of the brew, such as tannic acid, may be responsible for stomach upset. However, caffeine is known to slow the emptying of the stomach's contents into the small intestines and the passage of material through the small intestine, while emptying of the large intestine is speeded up. These effects may contribute to stomach upset and to ulcers of the stomach and small intestine. Coffee and tea can inhibit absorption of some nutrients, particularly iron. In addition, caffeine's ability to increase urination by as much as 30% for up to 3 hours after ingestion can cause such nutrients as calcium, magnesium, and sodium to be flushed from the body.

Caffeinism is the name given to symptoms associated with very heavy daily caffeine use. These symptoms include frequent urination, jitters, agitation, irritability, muscle twitching, lightheadedness, rapid breathing, rapid heartbeat, palpitations, upset stomach, loose stools, and heartburn. Seldom do all these symptoms occur together. Some of these symptoms also result from stress. Some believe that when stress and heavy caffeine use are a daily part of a person's life, the effects may be additive. Caffeine and emotional stress can cause higher than normal levels of adrenaline in the body, and the combination of caffeine and competitive stress is reported to cause delirium. Caffeine also interferes with relaxation training. People who use caffeine are able to learn the relaxation techniques just as quickly as nonusers, but they find it more difficult to maintain a state of relaxation under stress.

The evidence connecting caffeine and cancer is not convincing. Recent studies, however, suggest a link between heavy caffeine beverage use and bladder cancer in men. A much publicized 1979 report suggesting that benign breast tumors in women disappeared when caffeine was removed from the diet has not been supported by later studies. Nevertheless, stories in the press continue to report the disappearance of benign breast tumors after caffeine has been removed from the diet. It is too early to dismiss the effect completely. It may be that caffeine is not the cause of these benign tumors or of cancer itself. Study of other components in coffee and tea that may be responsible for cancers is under way.

No direct evidence exists that caffeine use during pregnancy gives rise to birth difficulties or birth defects. Evidence from animal studies, however, suggests that caffeine may have the capability to cause birth defects in some species of mammals. No *epidemiological* data are available. Nevertheless, many health professionals suggest that caffeine intake should be limited during pregnancy, especially during the first trimester.

Protection and Prevention

Adults are usually aware of their caffeine intake. Exceptions include the ingestion of caffeine in drugs and in some soft drinks. The best defense against unintentional caffeine use is to read the labels on nonprescription drugs and soft drinks. Caffeine is found in many commonly used pain relievers and appetite suppressants, stimulants, diuretics, cold remedies, and cola soft drinks. Some prescription drugs also contain caffeine. Ask your pharmacist about the caffeine content of pain relievers in particular.

Children are mostly unaware of their caffeine use. Parents should pay close attention to the soft drinks that their children consume. Children and teenagers consume half of all soft drinks sold. The amount of caffeine in their bloodstream after drinking a soda containing caffeine may be higher than an adult might expect because of the child's small body. Caffeine-free soft drinks are becoming easier to find, and their use for children is encouraged.

Environmental Effects

It is thought that the natural caffeine found in plants inhibits the effects of molds, bacteria, and fungi. For the most part, plants have developed a resistance to their own poison. However, as caffeine-bearing plants age, the soil around them becomes increasingly rich in caffeine, eventually becoming sterile. For this reason, coffee plantations tend to degenerate after 10 to 25 years.

Regulatory Status

The FDA regulates caffeine use in processed foods and drinks and in commercial drugs. There are no specific limitations beyond "good manufacturing practice."

Technical Information

Chemical names: 3,7-Dihydro–1,3,7-trimethyl–1H–purine-2,6-dione; 1,3,7-trimethylxanthine
Chemical formula: $C_8H_{10}N_4O_2$
Molecular weight: 194

Further Reading

GILBERT, RICHARD J. 1986. Caffeine, the Most Popular Stimulant. *The Encyclopedia of Psychoactive Drugs.* New York: Chelsea House Publishers.

Captan, Captafol, and Folpet

Trade Names

Merpan; Difolotan; Phaltan

Introduction

Introduced in 1949, 1961, and 1962, respectively, the *fungicides* captan, captafol, and folpet are discussed together here because of their structural, functional, and toxicological similarities. Structurally, the three are closely related to the now banned drug thalidomide, which was found to cause birth defects. Consequently, their ability to cause birth defects has been very well studied. Until recently, they had been considered among the safest pesticides and were widely recommended to householders for use in lawns and gardens. Together the three are the most widely used fungicides in the United States, with some 18 million pounds applied annually. They function to protect the surface of foliage and fruit and are nontoxic to the plant.

About 10 million pounds of captan are applied to 83 different food crops ranging from fruit and vegetable crops to seed crops. It has probably been recommended for more diseases of deciduous fruit trees, such as apples, almonds, and peaches, than any other fungicide. Residues of the pesticide have been detected on five common foods: apples, cherries, grapes, strawberries, and watermelons. About 30% of the strawberries and 18% of the grapes tested contained residues, albeit generally at levels below the *tolerances* (the allowable maximum residue level). Captan is also applied to manufactured items such as blankets, rugs, mattresses, flooring materials, oil-based paints, and leather goods. And it is the most heavily used fungicide around the home.

About 6 million pounds of captafol are used in agriculture to control diseases of apples, cherries, tomatoes, potatoes, and rice and in the timber industry to reduce fungal infestations in logs and wood products. It has

34 food crop uses. Folpet, although used in much smaller quantities than either captan or captafol, has a wide range of applications. Some 1.5 million pounds are used annually in agriculture on apples, avocados, cucumbers, blueberries, lettuce, squash, and ornamentals and in the manufacture of interior and exterior paints and coatings.

Physical and Chemical Properties

Captan, a white crystalline material, dissolves only slightly in water and not at all in petroleum oils. It resists breakdown except under *alkaline* conditions. Similarly, captafol, also a white crystalline solid, is essentially insoluble in water. It will, however, dissolve slightly in most organic solvents. Like captan, it breaks down under strongly alkaline conditions.

Exposure and Distribution

In agriculture, captan is applied as a spray or mist in solution or as a dry dust. Although it does not appear to be toxic to plants and works chiefly on the plant's surface, it can be absorbed by both the roots and leaves and transported to other parts of the plant. Little is known about the *metabolism* of the fungicide by plants or whether it is likely to *bioaccumulate*. Nor is much known about the environmental fate of captan, except that in dry form it resists breakdown. Residues of the fungicide tend to remain as superficial deposits on crop surfaces for a fairly long time, which means that consumers may be exposed to the pesticide on treated fruits and vegetables.

The environmental fate (or distribution) of captafol is uncertain. As a consequence, it is difficult to estimate possible human exposure levels. It is known that captafol is stable under ordinary environmental conditions and decomposes only very slowly under *acidic* conditions. It apparently does not leach from the soil. Uptake and metabolism by plants are probably similar to that of captan. Less information about the behavior of folpet in the environment or in organisms is available.

Health Effects

The EPA has classified all three fungicides as probable human carcinogens (group B_2) on the basis of animal test data (see Chapter 3, Section B). Captan and folpet are linked to specific rare intestinal tumors in mice. In rats, captan produces kidney tumors; captafol causes cancer in rats and mice. Several breakdown products of captafol have been isolated from animal tissues. The major single metabolic product of both captan and captafol is tetrahydrothalimide, a suspected carcinogen.

Experimental studies indicate that captan does not cause birth defects in mammals or birds, but that captafol may cause other adverse reproductive effects in birds and rats. In certain tests using mammalian cells and microorganisms, captan caused mutations, but it is thought that in the intact organism the fungicide would be detoxified. Few conclusions have been drawn about the long-term effects of folpet since there are large gaps in the available data.

In general, these fungicides have a low *acute toxicity* when ingested. While both captan and captafol are skin irritants, the degree of effect is significantly different. Captan has been used successfully to treat several kinds of fungal *dermatitis*. In contrast, a high incidence of skin irritation among farmers using captafol on citrus trees has been reported. The effect can be quite severe, ranging from rashes and itching to edema and elevated blood pressure. Captafol causes liver abnormalities, edema, and high blood pressure in rats and irreversible eye damage on contact. Of possible relevance to human health is the observation that protein-deficient rats were far more susceptible to the effects of captan than to any other pesticide tested. Evidently the lack of adequate protein enhances the *mutagenic* activity of the fungicide.

Protection and Prevention

Although captan has been readily available for household use, captafol is available only to certified applicators. Users are cautioned to avoid contaminating bodies of water with these fungicides and, for captafol, to rotate crops in accordance with EPA restrictions. As for all pesticides, the EPA requires that container labels carry precautionary information concerning the application, handling, and disposal of these chemicals.

Environmental Effects

Captafol is highly toxic to both cold and warm water fish species and is slightly less toxic to freshwater aquatic invertebrates. Captan is moderately toxic to a variety of aquatic organisms. Evidence suggests that captafol is likely to impair reproduction in birds, although the data are incomplete. At present, there is no evidence of impaired reproduction associated with captan, but other effects cannot be ruled out. Captan appears to be particularly toxic to sheep and cattle. The effects of folpet are uncertain.

Regulatory Status

Currently, captan, captafol, and folpet are under *Special Review* by the EPA because of their carcinogenicity in mammals and toxicity to aquatic species. The EPA has banned the use of captan on 42 fruit and vegetable crops and has continued registration for use on 24 other crops, including lettuce, cherries, apples, and tomatoes. Captan is listed as a *hazardous air pollutant* in the 1990 Clean Air Act and it is on the EPA *community right-to-know* list.

Technical Information

Chemical names:
captafol: 3*a*,4,7,7*a*-tetrahydro–2–1,1,2,2-tetrachloroethylthio-(1*H*)-isoindole–1,3(2*H*)-dione; tetrachloromethylmercaptocyclohexane dicarboximide

captan: 3*a*,4,7,7*a*-tetrahydro–2-trichloromethylthio-(1*H*)-isoindole–1,3-(2*H*)-dione; *N*-(trichloromethylthio)4-cyclohexen–1,2-dicarboximide
folpet: *N*-(trichloromethylthio)-phthalimide
Chemical formulas:
captan: $C_9H_8Cl_3NO_2S$
captafol: $C_{10}H_9Cl_4NO_2S$
folpet: $C_9H_4Cl_3NO_2S$
Comparison of dose-related toxicity in rats based on the LD_{50} lethal dose:
captan: >12,600 mg/kg
captafol: 2500–6200 mg/kg
Government standards for food tolerances:
captan: 0.25–100 ppm
captafol: 0.02–50 ppm
OSHA limits in workplace air:
captan threshold limit value: 5 mg/m^3
captan occupational intake: 0.7 mg/kg/day
captafol threshold limit value: 0.1 mg/m^3
captafol occupational intake: 0.014 mg/kg/day

Further Reading

HAYES, W. J., JR. 1982. *Pesticides Studied in Man.* Baltimore, MD: Williams and Wilkins.
National Academy of Sciences. 1987. *Regulating Pesticides in Food.* Washington, D.C.: NAS Press.

Carbaryl

Trade Names

Sevin; Hexavin; Dicarbam

Introduction

Introduced in 1956, carbaryl is one of the oldest and most widely used *carbamate* pesticides in the world. It is a *broad spectrum* insecticide, controlling 100 to 150 species, but it is virtually ineffective against houseflies, certain aphids, and spider mites. Carbaryl primarily kills insects on *contact*, but it can be absorbed by the plant and can kill plant-eating insects.

Carbaryl has a number of proven uses. First, because it is not particularly toxic to mammals when ingested or absorbed through the skin, it is registered for home use and is therefore a major active ingredient in many common household and garden pesticide products, including pet flea powders. Also, as an agricultural insecticide, it is used to protect various citrus, nut, fruit, vegetable, and forage crops. Because of its short *half-life*, carbaryl is registered for use on crops right up until harvest. Nevertheless, residues have been detected on harvested bananas, corn, grapefruit, oranges, peaches, and watermelons. In a campaign that gained a considerable amount of publicity, carbaryl has been used extensively in efforts to wipe out the gypsy moth, a pest that has been found throughout the United States. In the eastern United States, the gypsy moth has severely damaged both deciduous and evergreen forests, resulting in the death of millions of trees.

Physical and Chemical Properties

In its pure form, carbaryl is an odorless, white crystalline solid. It is slightly soluble in water, and under normal storage conditions, carbaryl is unlikely to decompose in the presence of heat, light, or water.

Exposure and Distribution

An estimated 100,000 workers who are involved in either the manufacture or application of carbaryl risk possible health effects from on-the-job exposure to high concentrations or large quantities of the insecticide. Normally the general population is exposed to carbaryl in much smaller quantities and in less concentrated form in products available for home use. But because carbaryl is commonly applied to crops and forests by aerial spraying, the insecticide can end up in drinking water, backyard vegetable gardens, and pastures. Although some carbaryl is consumed as a residue on foods or as a contaminant of groundwater, the principal routes of entry are inhalation and absorption through the skin.

In the environment, carbaryl is rapidly decomposed by sunlight under aqueous conditions. Because it is only slightly soluble in water, it is not very mobile in soils; nevertheless, it has been detected in groundwater.

Health Effects

Carbaryl, like many other carbamate pesticides and the *organophosphate* pesticides, affects the nervous system in a complex way by inhibiting the normal function of *cholinesterase*, an enzyme crucial to the normal transmission of signals in the nervous system (see Chapter 14, Section B). Exposure to airborne concentrations permitted by the government causes a substantial (about 25%) reduction in enzyme activity. Actual symptoms, however, are generally not seen until the enzyme is inhibited by 30% or more. The range of symptoms exhibited by people who have been exposed to excessive carbaryl includes tearing of the eyes, nasal discharge, sweating, abdominal cramps, nausea, tremors, difficulty in breathing, and convulsions.

Mammals convert carbaryl fairly readily to less toxic compounds, which are excreted in the urine. Because the pesticide does not accumulate in the tissues, the effect of carbaryl is generally reversible, which means that once the exposure is stopped, the effects stop.

At present, there is no strong evidence of long-term adverse effects of prolonged exposure to carbaryl, although laboratory studies show that the insecticide may cause birth defects in dogs and cancer in various test organisms. Several reproductive effects, including a decrease in the number of both offspring and sperm produced, have been reported for rats given very high doses, several thousand times greater than the amounts recommended for human consumption. Carbaryl itself does not appear to cause mutations, but like other carbamates, it can interact with **nitrates** under acidic conditions (similar to those found in the human stomach) to form **nitroso**-carbaryl, which can cause both cancers and mutations.

Protection and Prevention

The specific antidote (to be given by a physician) for carbaryl poisoning is atropine. It is recommended that vomiting should be induced and large quantities of water be given if carbaryl is ingested. If the chemical contacts skin or eyes, the area should be flushed with water immediately. Agricultural workers, fumigators, nursery workers, and people engaged in the manufacture of the insecticide are advised to wear protective clothing, including long-sleeved shirts, long pants, and gloves, and to use respirators. Precautions for home use of available carbaryl-based products are given on the container and should be followed carefully. Like other pesticides, carbaryl should be disposed of as a hazardous waste; it should not be rinsed down the drain or put out for routine trash collection.

For certain pest species, such as the gypsy moth, alternatives to carbaryl exist and have been used successfully. For example, outbreaks of the gypsy moth have been suppressed by the biological insecticide *Bacillus thuringiensis*, which selectively kills only moth and butterfly caterpillars. It does not adversely affect other nontarget species. Another biological control agent is a virus (with the trade name Gypchek) that only affects the gypsy moth; it does not affect other insects. No adverse effects on fish, birds, mammals, or people have been reported from use of this virus.

Environmental Effects

Although carbaryl appears to be relatively less toxic than many other pesticides currently on the market, there is an important drawback to its extensive use. Like several other carbamates, it is extremely toxic to honeybees—the principal pollinators of many agricultural crops (see Chapter 14, Section D). Thus, careless or ill-conceived (particularly aerial) spraying programs have the potential for reducing agricultural production. The problem has been recognized, and formulations of carbaryl that are less toxic to honeybees are being developed.

Regulatory Status

The EPA has set tolerance (permissible) limits for residues on foods and animal fodder, while the OSHA has established a standard for occupational exposure. Although no federal regulations have been put into law regarding safe levels in drinking water, the National Academy of Sciences and the National Research Council have calculated a safe level. The Food and Agriculture Organization and the World Health Organization of the United Nations have established an acceptable level for human consumption. Carbaryl is listed as a *hazardous air pollutant* in the 1990 Clean Air Act, requiring the EPA to set emission standards. It is also on the EPA *community right-to-know* list.

Technical Information

Chemical name: 1-naphthyl methyl carbamate
Chemical formula: $C_{12}H_{11}NO_2$
Comparative ranking of acute toxicity of car-

bamate pesticides in order of decreasing severity, based on comparison of the oral LD_{50} (lethal dose) for rats: aldicarb > propoxur > carbaryl > ethylenebisdithio carbamates > benomyl

Government standards:

EPA food tolerances: 0–12 ppm

Residues on animal fodder: 100 ppm

OSHA limit in workplace air: 5 mg/m^3

Acceptable daily intake: 0.01 mg/kg of body weight

Further Reading

HAYES, W. J., JR. 1982. *Pesticides Studied in Man.* Baltimore, MD: Williams and Wilkins.

Carbon Black

Other Names

Furnace black; colloidal black; thermal black; channel black; acetylene black; activated carbon; actibon; carboraffin; gas black norite; opocarbyl; ultracarbon

Introduction

Carbon black is the black stuff you get on your hands when you read the newspaper. But only 1% of the amount manufactured is used as a pigment in inks and paints. Most of it (65%) is added to the rubber used in making tires, allowing them to last up to 10 times longer. Another 29% is used to make other types of rubber and plastic. Carbon black is also used as a deodorizer and in filters to remove impurities from food, water, and other chemicals.

Physical and Chemical Properties

Carbon black is a black powder that is nearly pure carbon.

Exposure and Distribution

Nearly 1.5 million tons of carbon black are manufactured in the United States annually, making it one of the top 35 chemicals produced. People come into contact with carbon black every day as the part of the black grime associated with reading the newspaper and driving the car. It is the most common pigment used in paints and inks. Carbon black exposure is also likely in the workplace. It is used in the manufacture of batteries, cement, ceramics, plastics, rubber, paper, and ink. Some water purifying systems use activated carbon, or carbon black, to remove impurities from water. It works because many impurities readily stick to carbon.

Health Effects

No health hazards are associated with inhaling or ingesting small amounts of carbon black. Inhaling air contaminated with visible amounts of it can cause coughing and mucus build-up, but these symptoms rapidly disappear once heavy exposure stops. Long-term exposure to high concentrations of carbon black can cause permanent lung damage and temporary skin irritation. Although carbon black by itself has not been shown to cause cancer, the cancer-causing properties of **benzene** extracts taken from carbon black are well documented.

In addition, simultaneous exposure to *polycyclic aromatic hydrocarbons (PAHs)*, such as **benzo[*a*]pyrene**, and carbon black can lead to health problems. PAH is strongly attracted to carbon black particles. If the contaminated carbon black particles are released into the environment, they can travel away from the source of PAH contamination, where they can be inhaled by unsuspecting people. The carbon black serves as a vehicle for the PAH allowing it to travel farther from its source than it normally could. Once released from the carbon black inside the lungs, the PAH can cause health problems. In addition, the carbon black used to make tires can be contaminated with impurities, which can lead to health problems if inhaled every day. There is no evidence that carbon black from other sources poses a significant health hazard. For example, because of better ink formulations and press technology, the grime from newspapers no longer contains heavy metals. Even if carbon black particles do have cancer-causing chemicals stuck to them, they are usually tightly bound and are not easily broken free, even in the presence of hot and cold water, stomach acid, or blood plasma.

Protection and Prevention

When possible, avoid places where carbon black and PAHs are emitted simultaneously, such as areas with heavy automobile traffic.

Regulatory Status

The FDA has banned carbon black from food and drugs because of the PAH it contains.

OSHA has set limits on the amount of carbon black allowed in workplace air.

Technical Information

OSHA limit in workplace air: 3.5 mg/m^3
 In the presence of PAH: 0.1 mg/m^3

Further Reading

National Institute for Occupational Safety and Health. 1978. *Criteria for a Recommended Standard: Occupational Exposure to Carbon Black.* Number 78–204. Washington, D.C.: U.S. Government Printing Office.

SHREVE, R. N., and BRINK, J. A., JR. 1977. *Chemical Process Industries.* 4th edition. New York: McGraw-Hill.

Carbon Monoxide

Introduction

Carbon monoxide is a poisonous gas emitted from car tailpipes and other sources of fire. It can attain lethal levels in enclosed garages and is sometimes used in suicides. Cigarette smoke and dense traffic create the most significant exposures for the general public. Carbon monoxide is responsible for a larger number of severe chemical poisonings than any other single agent, mostly from improper use of indoor appliances, such as using cooking stoves for heating purposes.

Physical and Chemical Properties

Carbon monoxide is a nonirritating, colorless, tasteless, and essentially odorless gas. It forms by the incomplete combustion of organic matter (gasoline, wood, and tobacco) and is given off in the exhaust from tailpipes, furnaces, chimneys, and wood stoves.

Carbon monoxide causes harm by depriving the body of oxygen. When breathed, it preferentially binds to blood *hemoglobin*, displacing oxygen at the binding site. It also hinders the release of oxygen at the tissues. *Carboxyhemogobin (COHb)* is the name of the complex formed by carbon monoxide and hemoglobin. The percentage of COHb in the blood is the best indicator of exposure.

Exposure and Distribution

Cigarette smoking causes the largest human exposure to carbon monoxide. The COHb content in an average nonsmoker is about 0.5%, while in a smoker it is ten times higher, about 5% (but levels up to 12% have been reported). Even in the most polluted environments, the COHb of nonsmokers rarely exceeds 2%. Exposures tend to be higher in winter than in summer because of the extra fuel burned for space heating and because of more time spent indoors, where carbon monoxide is a component of indoor air pollution (see Chapter 5, Section C).

Carbon monoxide is present wherever significant burning occurs. For example, forest fires produce enormous quantities, but fires tend to be irregular and the gases dissipate with the prevailing winds. The highest concentrations to which people are routinely exposed (other than smoking) occur in densely populated urban areas with high traffic congestion. The air in and around congested city streets and urban freeways contains high levels of carbon monoxide, particularly at rush hours when traffic comes to a halt. Smoking cigarettes in a enclosed car during rush hour traffic can bring the concentration of carbon monoxide in car air to well over twice the national standard for protection of human health. Enclosed, unventilated parking garages, buildings along city streets, and heavily traveled tunnels contain the highest levels, as shown in Table 24.

On a national scale, transportation accounts for 67% of outdoor emissions, followed by combustion of fuels for heating and electrical power production (12%), industrial processes (8%), and other sources (13%). Over the ten years from 1979 through 1988, emissions of carbon monoxide have declined by 25%, and outdoor air quality (as measured by a system of government monitoring stations) has improved by 28%. Nevertheless, over 30 million people live in counties in which the air quality violates the national standard for protection of human health. The cities with the most severe carbon monoxide problems are Los Angeles, Denver, Washington, D.C., New York, Las Vegas, Spokane, Washington, and the Steubenville-Weirton, Ohio-West Virginia area, but many other congested urban areas are nearly as bad.

Health Effects

The symptoms of carbon monoxide poisoning, such as might be experienced by drivers stuck in rush hour traffic, include headache, dizziness, drowsiness, and nausea. More severe exposures cause vomiting,

TABLE 24 Carbon Monoxide Levels in Various Locations

Location	Carbon Monoxide Concentration (ppm)
City freeway, halted traffic	> 44
Closed car, with cigarette smoking	>87
Enclosed, unventilated garage	>100
Heavily traveled tunnels	>200 (1-hour maximum)
General nonsmoking exposure	<20–50
Certain occupations	>100

collapse, coma, and even death, depending on the degree of oxygen deprivation. Suicidal or accidental death from running a car in an enclosed garage or from using an unvented, poorly tuned combustion appliance indoors results from depression of the central nervous system to the point where breathing is stopped (*respiratory arrest*).

The body systems most affected are the ones most dependent on a steady supply of oxygen: the brain, the heart, and in pregnant women, the developing fetus. People who are inherently vulnerable to carbon monoxide poisoning are those with reduced heart and lung (*cardiopulmonary*) functioning, such as the elderly, who typically suffer from some degree of narrowing of the arteries (*atherosclerosis*). Other vulnerable groups include fetuses and young infants, who are in critical stages of brain and nervous system development; individuals with chronic *bronchitis* or *emphysema*, who have difficulty compensating for reduced blood oxygen by breathing harder and more frequently; and others with various blood disorders such as *anemia*. Over 40 million people are in these vulnerable groups.

Recent biomedical research has established that low levels of carbon monoxide exposure, typical of poorer quality urban air, lead to more frequent and prolonged angina attacks in people with heart disease, cause reductions in the capacity for work and athletic performance, and may trigger heart attacks by reducing the oxygen supply to the heart. The EPA has judged the evidence for this last possibility as inconclusive at this time, while acknowledging the plausibility of a connection.

Effects on the central nervous system of moderate exposures to carbon monoxide include losses in attentiveness, visual perception, manual dexterity, learning ability, and performance of complex neurological tasks such as driving. Particularly troublesome is the suggestive but not conclusive evidence that drivers in fatal auto accidents often have elevated carboxyhemoglobin (COHb) levels. One problem with the existing neurological research is that only relatively high levels of COHb (over 5%) have been studied. Whether or not the slight elevations in nonsmokers caused by typical pollution conditions create problems has not been investigated. A second problem is that only healthy young adults have been studied. What the consequences might be in more sensitive groups, such as those with preexisting nervous system diseases (for example, senility) or reduced oxygen-carrying capacity (for example, anemics), are unknown.

Damage to development in fetuses and young children has also been postulated. Newborns of mothers who smoke, thereby subjecting their unborn babies to reduced blood oxygen, tend to have reduced birth weights, slowed development after birth, and a higher frequency of sudden infant death syndrome (SIDS). However, the numerous toxic substances present in tobacco smoke make it difficult to pinpoint carbon monoxide as the cause of these problems.

Protection and Prevention

Smoking causes the greatest human exposure. Eliminating smoking is the most important reduction in hazard, as it is for reduction of numerous other toxic effects. When combustion takes place, adequate ventilation is mandatory. This is true for warming cars up in garages, using wood stoves and gas ranges, and venting exhaust gases from home furnaces, water heaters, wood stoves, and fireplaces. Joggers, bikers, and other exercisers should avoid places and times of traffic congestion for their daily workouts.

First-aid for highly exposed people involves removing them immediately from the source of exposure, providing fresh air, and administering artificial respiration if necessary. If no permanent injury was caused by the oxygen deprivation, the effects of carbon monoxide poisoning are totally reversible.

Environmental Effects

Humans appear to be both the most exposed and the most sensitive species to typical levels of carbon monoxide air pollution.

Regulatory Status

Carbon monoxide is one of the six air pollutants for which the EPA is required to periodically review and revise the standards for protection of human health and welfare. The latest cycle of review ended in September 1985. The EPA left the existing primary health standard intact (see Technical Information section), but it erased the secondary standard for protection of welfare effects (including effects on crops, vegetation, and statuary). The reason given was that no *welfare* (nonhealth) effects were expected at the levels of carbon monoxide currently found outdoors. New human health studies at lower exposure levels were being conducted at the time of the standards review, and the results of that work are expected to influence the next periodic evaluation. Exposures in the workplace are regulated by OSHA.

Technical Information

Chemical formula: CO
National Ambient Air Quality Standards:
  8-hour average: 9 ppm (10 mg/m^3)
1-hour average: 35 ppm (40 mg/m^3)
OSHA limit in workplace air: 55 mg/m^3
  (50 ppm)

Further Reading

Environmental Protection Agency. 1985. Review of the National Ambient Air Quality Standards for Carbon Monoxide: Final Rule. *Federal Register* 50(178):37,484–37,501.
———. 1984. *Revised Evaluation of Health Effects Associated with Carbon Monoxide Exposure: An Addendum to the 1979 EPA Air Quality Criteria Document for Carbon Monoxide.* EPA–600/8–83–033F, Final Report. Washington, D.C.
National Research Council. 1977. *Carbon Monoxide.* Washington, D.C.: Committee on Medical and Biological Effects of Environmental Pollutants, National Academy of Sciences.

Carbon Tetrachloride

Other Names

Methane tetrachloride; carbona; tetrachloromethane; perchloroethane

Trade Names

Freon 10; Halon 104; Mecatorina

Introduction

Most carbon tetrachloride is used to manufacture fluorocarbon propellants. It is also a valuable general purpose cleaner, used as a solvent for oils, fats, lacquers, varnishes, rubber, waxes, and resins. Carbon tetrachloride is also used during manufacture of paints and plastics. It was once used in home cleaning fluids and in fire extinguishers for home use, but these uses have been discontinued.

Physical and Chemical Properties

Carbon tetrachloride is a clear, colorless liquid with a sweet, ether-like smell.

Exposure and Distribution

This chemical is widely distributed in industry. About 500,000 tons of carbon tetrachloride are manufactured each year. Once a common household solvent, it was removed from the consumer market following information about its toxicity. Concerns about its toxicity and environmental effects have also encouraged industry to avoid using carbon tetrachloride whenever possible.

Major sources of release of carbon tetrachloride to the environment have traditionally been carbon tetrachloride production, the use of pesticide *fumigants* on grain, chlorinated paraffin wax production, and fluorocarbon production. Since the EPA has canceled the use of grain fumigants containing carbon tetrachloride, emissions are expected to decrease significantly. In addition, better control technologies are expected to reduce emissions still further.

Nevertheless, the EPA estimates that 10% of the country's groundwater may be contaminated with carbon tetrachloride at levels near or above the water quality standard. This is because carbon tetrachloride, spilled onto soil, easily leaches into groundwater, where it remains for years. In addition, carbon tetrachloride remains widely distributed in the air, primarily because it takes nearly 50 years to break down once it is released into the atmosphere. Carbon tetrachloride is also known to migrate into drinking water from polyvinyl chloride (PVC) water supply pipes. The National Research Council estimates that the average person takes in small amounts of carbon tetrachloride daily from air (62%), water (23%), and food (15%).

Health Effects

Carbon tetrachloride can cause adverse health effects when it is inhaled, ingested, or absorbed through the skin. The liver, kidneys, and lungs are most sensitive to overexposure. This information is based on numerous studies using animals. Exposure to high doses of carbon tetrachloride in the air can be fatal. Dizziness, vertigo, loss of coordination, mental confusion, abdominal pain, vomiting, and diarrhea are common symptoms of overexposure. Heart arrhythmias, convulsions, and coma may also occur. Even if an exposure causing these symptoms is not fatal, it can lead to liver and kidney damage within a few days. Harmful changes in the blood can also occur. Unfortunately, the sweet odor of carbon tetrachloride does not provide satisfactory warning of overexposure.

Liquid carbon tetrachloride splashed in the eye causes painful but minimal damage. Prolonged or repeated skin contact with the chemical may result in blistering or skin irritation. Single oral doses of carbon tetrachloride can be fatal at low doses. Even if no ill effects are reported immediately after swallowing the substance, kidney and liver changes still can occur.

Repeated inhalation of nonlethal levels of

carbon tetrachloride causes nausea, vomiting, dizziness, drowsiness, and fatigue. These chronic exposures can also cause abnormalities of the eyes, such as reduced visual field. Chronic ingestion of abnormally high concentrations of carbon tetrachloride in contaminated water can affect the liver, kidneys, and nervous system. Prolonged exposure to carbon tetrachloride can cause an abnormal accumulation of fat in the liver. This condition, known as fatty liver, causes distortion of the liver, but rarely affects liver function. Fatty liver disappears completely several weeks after carbon tetrachloride exposure ceases.

Carbon tetrachloride probably also causes cancer. Animal studies demonstrate that it produces liver cancer in mice and rats. But studies examining cancer rates among humans exposed to carbon tetrachloride are inconclusive. Most short-term tests for mutagenicity have been negative. Nevertheless, the EPA considers carbon tetrachloride to be a probable human carcinogen (a B_2 substance according to the classification in Chapter 3, Section B). Although no evidence is available to prove that carbon tetrachloride causes birth defects, preliminary studies indicate that pregnant women who are regularly exposed to carbon tetrachloride vapors may risk damage to the fetus.

Protection and Prevention

Although carbon tetrachloride has been removed from the consumer market, many previous users still have bottles of the solvent in their homes. These should not be used. Dispose of the unused portions during hazardous waste roundups, when available in your community. Carbon tetrachloride can be removed from contaminated drinking water by using activated carbon filters or by boiling. But keep in mind that carbon tetrachloride boiled out of your drinking water simply goes into your household's air. The carbon tetrachloride found in outside air is nearly impossible to avoid. Carbon tetrachloride is widely used in the workplace; request a *Material Safety Data Sheet (MSDS)* if you suspect that carbon tetrachloride is being used.

Environmental Effects

Unlike other chlorinated compounds, carbon tetrachloride does not appear to *bioaccumulate* in animals or in food chains. However, chemical reactions involving carbon tetrachloride are known to deplete stratospheric ozone (see Chapter 11).

Regulatory Status

Carbon tetrachloride is regulated by OSHA, the EPA, the FDA, and the Consumer Product Safety Commission. It is listed as a *hazardous air pollutant* in the 1990 Clean Air Act, requiring the EPA to set emission standards. Moreover, since carbon tetrachloride is known to deplete stratospheric ozone, the 1990 Clean Air Act also stipulates that production and use of the chemical be phased out by the year 2000. Carbon tetrachloride is on the *community right-to-know* list.

Technical Information

Chemical symbol: CCl_4
Molecular weight: 154
Amount released into the environment: 28,000 tons/year
Odor threshold: 0.5 mg/L in water
EPA drinking water standard: 5 ppb
OSHA limit in workplace air: 10 ppm

Further Reading

Agency for Toxic Substances and Disease Registry. 1988. *Toxicological Profile for Carbon Tetrachloride*. Washington, D.C.: U.S. Public Health Service.

Environmental Protection Agency. 1984. *Health Assessment Document for Carbon Tetrachloride*. Springfield, VA: National Technical Information Service, U.S. Department of Commerce.

Carrageenan

Other Names

Irish Moss; Fulcelleran

Introduction

The food additive carrageenan is derived from a class of seaweeds known as Rhodophycae, or the red seaweeds. While carrageenan does not appear to be toxic, it is included here because it is widely used and sometimes its use is questioned by consumer advocates. The use of these seaweeds in food and medicine has been known in Ireland, the South Pacific Islands, and Japan for centuries. Its use in the United States began in 1835. Not until after World War II, when it replaced Japanese Isinglass (agar), did it become common in processed foods. Today, it is used as a thickener, stabilizer, and emulsifier in many processed foods, including chocolate drinks, pressure-dispensed whipped cream, syrup, confections, evaporated milk, cheese products, ice cream, sherbet, popsicles, salad dressing, and artificially sweetened jellies and jams.

Physical and Chemical Properties

Carrageenan is a sulfated polysaccharide containing 20 to 40% sulfur (measured in dry weight). It has a seaweed-like odor, gluey texture, and salty taste. It is soluble in hot water.

Exposure and Distribution

Carrageenan is used in many processed foods as a thickener. Processed foods are the most common route of exposure for most people.

Health Effects

No obvious adverse health effects are seen among populations using red seaweed as a food source. However, animals fed purified carrageenan have developed several problems. Carrageenan can produce intestinal ul-cers in several species of laboratory animals. When added to the feed of pregnant animals, it tends to decrease the number of live births and result in immature or abnormal skeletal structures. Carrageenan also tends to increase the permeability of blood vessels and inhibit the formation of chemicals that trigger the body's immune system. It is poorly absorbed from the stomach and intestines, but it can nevertheless become concentrated in the liver, kidney, and spleen.

A final health-related issue concerns nutrition. Excessive consumption of carrageenan can cause nutritional deficiencies because it is used as a thickener in many "junk" foods in place of more nutritional eggs and cream. However, these foods, whose properties carrageenan is trying to imitate, are high in calories and cholesterol.

Protection and Prevention

Exposure can be minimized by avoiding processed foods that contain the chemical. Read the labels on processed foods before purchasing.

Regulatory Status

Carrageenan remains on the FDA *generally recognized as safe (GRAS)* list. While the FDA Select Committee on GRAS Substances has stated that no evidence is available to demonstrate a hazard to public health at current use levels, uncertainties still exist. Therefore, additional studies are being carried out.

Further Reading

International Agency for Research on Cancer. 1982. Carrageenan. *IARC Monograms*, vol. 31. Lyon, France.

Cesium-137

Other Names

^{137}Cs; radioactive cesium

Introduction

Cesium-137 is a *radioactive isotope* of the element cesium that is produced in nuclear power plants and from the explosion of nuclear weapons. A related isotope, cesium-134, usually accompanies it and will be discussed here as well. The element cesium has no known value as a trace nutrient. Radioactive cesium has figured prominently in three important news stories about radiation hazard.

First, in the 1960s, the isotope was found to be highly concentrated in the Eskimo population—as much as 100 times higher than in people living at lower latitudes. Investigation revealed that a sizable fraction of the cesium-137 released from nuclear weapons tests in the atmosphere during the 1950s and early 1960s was deposited on the Arctic tundra. Prevailing high-altitude northerly winds had transported the material there. The isotope was subsequently incorporated into lichens growing on the tundra. When caribou ate the lichens, the process of *bioconcentration* began, leading to higher levels of the isotope in the caribou than in the lichens. Eskimos, eating caribou meat, bioconcentrated it further (see Chapter 10, Section A).

Second, radioactive cesium was one of the substances of major concern in the aftermath of the 1986 nuclear power plant accident at Chernobyl in the Soviet Union. The third event occurred in 1987 in a village in Brazil. A discarded container of cesium-137 that had been used as a source of radiation for medical treatment was found and opened by townspeople. At least a dozen people died and many others came down with serious radiation illness after playing with the material out of fascination with its seemingly magic glow.

Currently, radioactive cesium is receiving increased attention because it is likely to be used in a new technology for preserving foods; the benefits and risks of this use of radiation are discussed in Chapter 15, Section H.

Physical and Chemical Properties

Cesium is a blue, volatile solid. It is relatively soluble in water and binds very strongly to soil particles. Its chemical properties resemble those of the other alkaline elements such as sodium and potassium; thus it can be found uniformly throughout the body, not concentrating in any one particular organ or type of tissue. Cesium-137 has a half-life of 30 years and decays by emitting a *beta particle*. Its *decay product* is barium-137, which is also radioactive. Cesium-134 has a half-life of 2.3 years and also decays by emitting a beta particle.

Exposure and Distribution

Radioactive cesium would be virtually absent from the environment were it not for nuclear weapons testing, nuclear power production, and the use of nuclear isotopes in medicine. Weapons testing has resulted in the release to the environment of thousands of times more radioactive cesium than that from the nuclear power industry. The major pathway of human exposure to radioactive cesium released from weapons testing and nuclear reactor accidents is a deposition from the atmosphere to the soil, uptake by grains, and subsequent concentration in grazing animals. Because cesium binds strongly to soils, plant uptake is by direct absorption into the leaves rather than by root uptake. Consumption of milk, meat, and grains accounts for most of the human exposure, while fruits, vegetables, and fish are relatively less important sources. Marine fish are usually about 100 times lower in cesium-137 than are freshwater fish because potassium, which is more abundant in seawater, blocks uptake of cesium by marine organisms. In the body, radioactive cesium is rapidly taken up in the bloodstream and is distributed to virtually all tissues. An adult human excretes ingested cesium-137 within a few months, while the corresponding time for infants is a few weeks.

Nuclear reactors operating normally release to the environment about one part in a million of the cesium-137 formed in the reactor core. This results in about the same amount of radioactivity in the environment as is produced by radioactive **strontium-90**. During normal operations, most of the radioactive cesium that is released from reactors exits with liquid wastes rather than as a gas vented to the atmosphere. Thus, the major pathway for human ingestion of this relatively small source of environmental radioactivity is by eating freshwater fish.

Health Effects

The most likely cause of death from acute exposure to high levels of cesium-137 is destruction of bone marrow. The symptoms of lower exposures are similar to those from other whole body sources of radiation (discussed in Chapter 15, Section G).

Protection and Prevention

First and foremost, remember the Brazilian episode and keep away from glowing powders or any substance in a container labeled with the international symbol for radiation hazard.

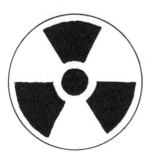

In the event of a serious exposure to radioactive cesium, patients are often advised to ingest prussian blue, which binds to cesium and helps to prevent absorption into the bloodstream from the *gastrointestinal tract*.

Regulatory Status

In the United States, the general restrictions on radiation exposure apply to radioactive cesium; they are given in Table 13 (in Chapter 15).

Technical Information[2]

Chemical symbol: ^{137}Cs
Atomic number: 55
Atomic weight: 137

The decay of cesium-137 produces a *beta particle* with a maximum energy of 1.18 million electronvolts (MeV) and a *gamma ray* with maximum energy of 0.66 MeV. The decay produces barium-137 as a daughter *isotope*, which is also a beta emitter and poses an additional hazard.

Nuclear weapons testing resulted in the release of nearly 10^{18} *becquerels* of radioactive cesium. (See Chapter 15, Section E for a clarification of the units used here.) By 1980, less than 1% of this remained in the atmosphere, about half of what was released was deposited on the ground and still remains there, while the remainder has decayed. From all the nuclear weapons tests, a total dose of about 5×10^5 person-sieverts has been delivered, or 0.1 millisievert per person. (For a discussion of the health implications of this, see Chapter 15, Section G.)

From normal operation of the world's nuclear reactors during the 1980s, radioactive cesium has been released to the environment at the rate of about 4×10^{13} becquerels/year. The dose to humans from environmental exposure to cesium-137 is roughly 2×10^{-12} person-sieverts/becquerel released. Thus, the 4×10^{13} becquerels released annually from routine nuclear power operations result in a global dose of about 100 person-sieverts per year. Divided by the global population of 5×10^9 people, this amounts to a negligible dose per person per year.

[2]For a discussion of the meaning of the units of radiation used below, see Chapter 15, Section E.

The accident at the Soviet Union's nuclear power facility at Chernobyl in 1986 resulted in the release of about 4×10^{16} becquerels of radiation from cesium-137 and cesium-134. Estimates of the total number of fatal cancers expected to result worldwide from this release of radiation vary from a few thousands to hundreds of thousands depending on the assumptions made about the geographic distribution, the environmental fate, and the potency of the radioactive material.

Further Reading

ROSS, M. 1975. The Transportation of Radioactive Wastes: The Possibility of Release of Cesium. In *The Nuclear Fuel Cycle*. The Union of Concerned Scientists. Cambridge, MA: MIT Press.
World Health Organization. 1983. *Environmental Health Criteria Report No. 25: Selected Radionuclides*. Geneva.

CFCs

Other Name
Chlorofluorocarbons

Trade Names
Freon; Halon

Introduction
Chlorofluorocarbons, or CFCs, were developed in 1930 at General Motors to replace the toxic and corrosive cooling agents that were widely used in refrigerators at the time. Thomas Midgley, a GM employee, came up with a "wonder chemical" that was almost nontoxic, nonflammable, stable, cheap, and had the correct volatility to replace all other refrigerants. The market for CFCs grew quickly, even beyond refrigeration. Today, CFCs are used as solvents and aerosol propellants, for foam production, for sterilization, and for fire-fighting. In 1986, over 300,000 tons of CFCs were produced in the United States.

But the so-called wonder chemical has a dark side. CFCs are slowly causing the depletion of stratospheric ozone, thus thinning the layer of atmosphere that protects the earth from the sun's harmful **ultraviolet radiation** (see Chapter 11). In addition, CFCs are responsible for about one-fifth of the gases that cause global warming. In light of these problems, several industrialized nations are calling for restricted use of CFCs; du Pont, who makes CFCs, has agreed to stop all production by the year 2000.

Halons are a closely associated class of chemicals that are used for special situation fire-fighting. They have three to ten times the ozone-depleting potential of CFCs. Halon production is estimated to be on the order of 20,000 tons annually, and demand for these chemicals is growing.

Physical and Chemical Properties
Chlorofluorocarbons are odorless, colorless gases that are extremely stable. Therefore,

they are able to make their way to the stratosphere before being broken down by the intense ultraviolet radiation found 20 to 30 miles above the earth's surface. As CFCs break down, chemical reactions occur that transform ozone molecules, consisting of three oxygen atoms (O_3), into ordinary two-atom oxygen molecules (O_2). In this way, the ozone layer in the stratosphere is destroyed.

Exposure and Distribution

Chlorofluorocarbons are widely distributed. The United States uses about one-third of the one million tons produced worldwide each year. All but the most specialized industrial refrigerators use CFCs as the working fluid, but this accounts for less than 6% of CFC use in the United States. Foam production, vehicle air conditioning, and solvent applications account for most CFC use. The Investor Responsibility Research Center recently estimated that the average home refrigerator contains 0.5 pounds of CFCs in the cooling system and an additional 2.5 pounds in the foam wall insulation used to keep it cold inside. Many foams, particularly those used for insulation, are made using CFCs. Much of the CFCs used during manufacturing remains trapped in the bubbles of the foam, which accounts for the good insulation properties of the foam. Foam manufacture accounts for over 20% of the CFCs used in the United States.

More than 20% of the CFCs purchased are used for solvents, mostly in the electronics industry. Even though banned in the United States, CFCs should not be overlooked as an aerosol propellant. Worldwide, aerosols account for more than one-fourth of all CFCs used.

All vehicular air conditioners use CFCs. In fact, over one-fourth of all CFCs used in the United States go into automobile and truck air conditioning. This high proportion used in vehicles can be explained by four factors. First, automobile air conditioners

leak. Second, when vehicle air conditioners are serviced, the CFCs contained in the cooling unit are often released into the atmosphere, then replaced with fresh. Third, vehicles are poorly insulated, so that the average car typically has as much cooling capacity as an entire house. Finally, a vehicle has a shorter useful lifespan than does the average refrigerator or home air conditioner. Leftover CFCs are often just thrown away with the car.

People are likely to inhale measurable quantities of CFCs at work, especially in places where CFCs or CFC-containing products are manufactured, serviced, or used. Beauty shops (many cosmetic products still contain CFC propellants), fire extinguisher servicing companies, auto body shops, air conditioner and refrigerator servicing companies, electronics manufacturing firms, foam blowing shops, and firms where insulating foams are used to manufacture products are typical sites where CFCs may be found.

Health Effects

CFCs are not very toxic. But this blanket statement is misleading because CFCs are a class of over a dozen individual chemicals. In general, all CFCs cause central nervous system depression following overexposure. Heart palpitations have been reported among human volunteers exposed to high concentrations of CFCs in air. Breathing high concentrations of CFCs over prolonged periods has reportedly caused death due to heart failure among fire fighters and those who deliberately inhale CFCs. The doses at which these symptoms appear vary among the individual CFCs. Recent studies indicate that some CFCs may cause mutations. But so far, no studies have found CFCs to cause cancer.

Protection and Prevention

While under most circumstances CFC fumes are not harmful to a person's health, there are other compelling reasons to avoid CFC use (as discussed in Environmental Effects).

Consumers can reduce their use of CFCs by avoiding insulated products made from foams manufactured using CFCs. These can be found in home insulation products, packaging material, marine flotation devices, and single service foam containers (such as egg cartons, fast food containers, food trays, insulated drinking cups, and ice chests). Rigid foam is available that makes use of little if any CFCs. These can be recognized by their beaded texture. DOW Chemical completely phased out CFCs from its Styrofoam products at the end of 1989. These foam products without CFCs or paper products can be substituted for CFC-containing foams. Many soft foams are also manufactured using CFCs. These are predominantly used in furniture, bedding, carpet underlays, and automobile seats and dashboards. These types of foam are more difficult to avoid. However, furniture, bedding, and carpet pads are available that make use of fiber fills or laytex foams.

Consumers should also consider foregoing automobile air conditioning. Air conditioners that are not used regularly leak CFCs more readily than those used often. Before buying a car with air conditioning, think about how often it will actually be needed.

Slightly reformulated CFCs, called HCFCs, should be widely available soon. These destroy only a fraction of the ozone that CFCs do. If given the choice, buy products that use these compounds (when other substitutes are not available).

Environmental Effects

The problems with CFCs are primarily environmental. CFCs destroy the stratospheric ozone layer that protects people from harmful ultraviolet rays from the sun (see Chapter 11). Already, holes and breaks in the ozone layer are apparent to scientists. Without the ozone layer's protective shield, skin cancer and eye damage are more likely among people, and the marine food chain could be profoundly disrupted. In addition, CFCs are responsible for about one-fifth of the greenhouse gases emitted into the atmosphere every year (see Chapter 11, Section A).

Regulatory Status

When it became evident that CFCs were responsible for stratospheric ozone destruction, the United States government, reacting to pressure from consumers, banned CFCs from most aerosol products. This happened in 1978. The United Nations spearheaded an international attempt to restrict the production and use of CFCs, culminating with an International agreement known as the Montreal Protocol. The Clean Air Act of 1990 is consistent with provisions of the Montreal Protocol, and in some ways goes beyond it. The Clean Air Act calls for a phase out of production and use of ozone depleting chemicals. CFCs will be phased out by the year 2000; exceptions are authorized for medical devices and certain exports to developing nations. Additionally, the act requires that the EPA issue regulations by 1992 that set requirements for recycling and disposal. A ban on venting during appliance repair will also begin in 1992.

Recently, the State of Vermont banned the registration of automobiles that make use of CFCs in their air conditioning systems, starting with 1993 models.

Despite these cuts, ozone destruction by CFCs is not likely to cease in the near future. First of all, the agreement does not call for a ban of CFCs, only a cut. In addition, CFC emissions will continue from sources already in the marketplace, such as old refrigerators, foam materials, and vehicles. Finally, developing countries, who use few CFCs now, are allowed under the Montreal Protocol to increase their per capita consumption of CFCs. It is possible that declining emissions from the industrialized world may be offset by growth in CFC emissions from the developing world.

Technical Information

Chemical formulas for common CFCs and Halons:

CFC-11: trichlorofluoromethane, CCl_3F

CFC-12: dichlorofluoromethane, CCl_2F_2

CFC-113: 1,1,2-trichloro–1,2,2-trifluoroethane, CCl_3CF_3

Halon 1202: difluorodibromomethane, CF_2Br_2

Halon 1301: trifluoromonobromomethane, CF_3Br

HCFC-22: chlorodifluoromethane, $CHClF_2$

U.S. production of CFCs and Halons: 330,000 tons/year

Further Reading

BRODEUR, PAUL. 1986. Annals of Chemistry: The Ozone Layer. *The New Yorker Magazine.* June 9.

COGAN, DOUGLAS, C. 1988. *Stones in a Glass House: CFCs and Ozone Depletion.* Washington, D.C.: Investor Responsibility Research Center.

Chlordane

Trade Names

Velsicol–1068; Octachlor; Chlorkil; Ortho-chlor

Introduction

Chlordane is an effective *contact* insecticide used in the United States in agriculture (until 1978) and to control soil pests, particularly termites. It belongs to a group of closely related *organochlorines,* which includes **aldrin, dieldrin,** endosulfan, and **heptachlor.** Commercial- or technical-grade chlordane is actually a mixture of several forms of chlordane and heptachlor; the insecticidal activity is due to the joint toxicity of the components. Like many other organochlorines, chlordane is highly *persistent* in soils, which makes it both very useful in termite control and a potential threat to public health and the environment. Although no longer used in agriculture, chlordane residues are still detectable in previously treated soils and in some food crops grown in those soils.

Physical and Chemical Properties

Commercial-grade chlordane is a viscous, light yellow to amber colored liquid, which is insoluble in water. It will dissolve in most organic solvents, such as **benzene** and **acetone.**

Exposure and Distribution

Chlordane does not leach from soils but rather clings to soil particles. Since it does not break down readily, residues are found years after application. In comparison with other organochlorine insecticides, chlordane is less persistent in soils than **DDT,** dieldrin, and **lindane,** but slightly more persistent than heptachlor and aldrin. Chlordane accumulates in aquatic sediments, where it has been found in high concentrations. The levels in the water itself, however, are relatively low.

This insecticide is readily absorbed by the mammalian skin, lungs, and digestive tract. It is rapidly metabolized, but eliminated only slowly. Although it does not tend to accumulate in high levels in tissues, chlordane breakdown products and heptachlor epoxide have been found in human milk and fetuses. In its monitoring program, the National Human Adipose Survey shows that levels of oxychlordane and heptachlor epoxide in human tissues remained essentially unchanged from 1970 through 1983. In contrast, levels of banned or highly restricted organochlorines, such as DDT and dieldrin, have declined substantially.

In plants, chlordane concentrates in oil seed crops, and like aldrin and dieldrin, it has an affinity for the outer parts or peels of root crops. A recent survey of pesticide residues on foods revealed that chlordane was one of the five most frequently detected residues on potatoes. Since some residues evidently remain on foods, consumers may ingest some chlordane. In the United States, however, exposure to chlordane primarily results from applications to control termites. Studies have shown that both pest control workers and those living in treated buildings and homes may be exposed to significant levels.

Health Effects

Chlordane is moderately toxic when absorbed by the skin, lungs, or digestive tract. Some cases of human poisoning have been reported. Since chlordane is toxic to the nervous system, as are other organochlorines, symptoms of poisoning are similar. They include headache, dizziness, abdominal disturbances, nausea, vomiting, mental confusion, muscle twitching, tremors, convulsions, and ultimately death in extreme cases. The EPA classifies chlordane as a probable human carcinogen (group B_2; see Chapter 3, Section B) on the basis of tests showing that it causes liver cancer in mice and rats. Data assessing its ability to cause *mutations* are inadequate; in some tests mutations occurred, while the results of other tests were negative. Rabbits given high doses of chlordane showed no evidence of adverse reproductive effects, including birth defects.

Protection and Prevention

To prevent poisoning following ingestion, the victim should be induced to vomit, using Ipecac syrup or large quantities of water. No milk or oily fluids should be given. To prevent problems following contact with the skin or eyes, the area should by flushed thoroughly with water and contaminated clothing removed. In cases of poisoning, a physician should be contacted. Various *barbiturates* (for example, sodium amytal) may be prescribed. Residues on foods can be reduced by peeling, washing with a little detergent, or cooking. Canning also seems to reduce residues.

Environmental Effects

Generally, chlordane does not appear to be toxic to terrestrial plants at normal application rates, but like DDT and other organochlorines, it is toxic to marine and freshwater algae, even at low concentrations. It reduces populations of aquatic invertebrates and is particularly toxic to marine mollusks, such as clams, but seems to be less toxic to fish than related compounds (with the exception of heptachlor). The toxicity of chlordane to aquatic organisms is temperature dependent, so it may be more of a problem in the tropics than in temperate regions.

Chlordane depletes soil fertility by inhibiting the growth and function of soil microorganisms and is highly toxic to earthworms. Certain bird species seem to be less susceptible to chlordane than to some other organochlorines, especially aldrin and dieldrin. Evidently, this insecticide is only slightly toxic to vertebrates, but it shows some variability in tissue accumulation. Various studies, however, have found no detectable residue levels in birds and very low levels in fish.

Regulatory Status

In 1978, the EPA canceled all agricultural uses of chlordane. Since 1983 it has been registered for use only for soil application to control termites. In 1987, the EPA canceled the use of chlordane for application in home interiors when it found that indoor air concentrations of the pesticide were quite high. Chlordane is listed as a *hazardous air pollutant* in the 1990 Clean Air Act, requiring the EPA to set emission standards. It is also on the EPA *community right-to-know* list.

Technical Information

Chemical name: 1,2,4,5,6,7,8,8 '-octachloro–2,3,3*a*,4,7,7*a*-hexahydro–4,7-methano-(1*H*)-indene

Chemical formula: $C_{10}H_6Cl_8$

Residue levels in human fat (oxychlordane):
  1972   0.10 ppm
  1983   0.09 ppm

EPA lethal dose (LD_{50}) for rats:
  oral: 280 mg/kg
  skin: 600 mg/kg

OSHA limit in workplace air: 0.5 mg/m^3

WHO recommended temporary acceptable daily intake: 0.001 mg/kg

Further Reading

World Health Organization. 1984. *Environmental Health Criteria No. 34*. Geneva.

Chlorine, Hydrogen Chloride, Hydrochloric Acid, and Hypochlorite

Introduction

Chlorine is a toxic gas that most people hear about when an occasional freight train derails or a tanker truck overturns, spilling its load. Actually, chlorine and chlorine-containing compounds are everywhere, appearing in such common household products as bleach, cleansers, and table salt (sodium chloride); in plastics (polyvinyl chloride), aerosol propellants (**chlorofluorocarbons**), and pesticides; and throughout the body in all nerve and muscle tissues. During World War I, chlorine was briefly used for chemical warfare, but it was not well suited to this purpose and was replaced by other chemicals. Current toxic exposures tend to come from accidental spills and from the improper use of household products. Because the hazardous properties of chlorine, hydrogen chloride, hydrochloric acid, and hypochlorite are related, they are treated as a group here.

Physical and Chemical Properties

Chlorine is a natural chemical element (atomic number 17), which at room temperature is a greenish-yellow gas with a pungent smell. Heavier than air, chlorine is easily liquified under pressure and is usually stored and transported that way. It is very reactive, combining readily with most elements to form compounds. This property accounts for the fact that it rarely occurs in nature in its pure form. Pure chlorine is made by separating it out of chlorine compounds. Volcanic eruptions are the only natural source of chlorine gas, and the quantities emitted are small.

Chlorine will dissolve in water to form hypochlorous acid, hypochlorite ion, and hydrochloric acid. Bleach is sodium hypochlorite. Hydrogen chloride is a colorless gas, also with a pungent smell. It is recovered as a byproduct of the industrial use of chlorine gas.

It dissolves readily in water to form hydrochloric acid, a strong *acid*.

Exposure and Distribution

Accidental spills and leaks during transport and storage are the greatest exposure hazards. It is not uncommon for neighborhoods bordering such spills or even whole towns to require evacuation. Chlorine and hydrochloric acid rank first and third, respectively, in causing injuries and deaths from large accidents that involve industrial chemicals. Fortunately, the actual number of serious consequences is usually small. In the years 1983 and 1984, for example, transportation accidents involving chlorine caused a total of 3 deaths and 46 injuries; no deaths were reported from hydrochloric acid.

Household bleach contains chlorine in the form of a weak sodium hypochlorite solution. Hypochlorite itself can be dangerous (see Health Effects), but the more serious problems arise when bleach is mixed with other products in an attempt to improve its cleaning power. When mixed with acid, bleach produces chlorine gas. Some toilet bowl cleaners and rust removers contain enough acid to release large quantities of chlorine gas upon mixing. Vinegar apparently is not acidic enough to release chlorine, although conflicting reports have been published. As a matter of caution, vinegar should not be mixed with bleach. **Ammonia** reacts with bleach to release *chloramines*, toxic gases that penetrate and injure the deep tissues of the lung. (See the entry on ammonia for more details on chloramines.)

Chlorine and hypochlorite are also used extensively as drinking water and swimming pool disinfectants and in sewage treatment. When properly used, no health hazard exists from the chlorine in these applications. However, chlorine will react with *organic matter* in drinking water to produce cancer-causing *trihalomethanes*. (This subject is discussed in detail in the entry on **chloroform** and in Chapter 6, Section A.)

The misapplication of chlorine and hypochlorite in swimming pools has resulted in cases of excessive acidity, of children inhaling the vapors from solid hypochlorite pool tablets, and of urine and ammonia levels high enough to react and release chloramines. Proper pool maintenance avoids these conditions. No cases have been reported of pool chlorine vapors causing serious health problems.

Of all industrial use of chlorine and hydrochloric acid, 80% is in the production of chlorinated *hydrocarbon* compounds (solvents and cleaning agents), pesticides, and plastics (polyvinyl chloride or PVC). The pulp and paper industry is the second largest user (16%), where chlorine is used to bleach or whiten pulp for paper stock. Water treatment is the remaining major use (4%). Hydrochloric acid is released in major quantities by coal combustion and the burning of paper and plastics in municipal waste. There is no evidence, however, that these sources produce human health effects or that the hydrochloric acid released makes a major contribution to acid rain. Industrial production of chlorine totals 10 million tons per year, and hydrochloric acid, 2.5 million tons per year.

Health Effects

Chlorine is a strong irritant to the *mucous membranes* of the eyes, nose, throat, airways, and lungs. Symptoms include tearing, coughing, choking, headache, and dizziness. Severe exposure can produce *pulmonary edema* and death, usually delayed for several hours after exposure. Immediate death can be caused by reflex closure of the airways (bronchospasm) and suffocation, if the concentration is high enough. A single chorine gas exposure can produce signs of obstructive airway disease (narrowing of the airways by contraction of the surrounding muscles), indicated by breathing difficulties and wheezing noises. This condition usually resolves itself with medical treatment, although there is some disagreement whether lasting damage is done.

There is a slight increase in the risk of bladder cancer and possibly of colon and rectal cancers in long-time users of chlorinated water supplies. The increase in risk is most apparent in nonsmokers because cigarette smoking increases the chances of these same cancers so that the effect of chlorination, while surely present, is hard to detect.

Hydrogen chloride gas rapidly turns to hydrochloric acid on contact with moisture on the skin, in perspiration, and in mucous membranes. Most of the ensuing damage is caused by the acidity, which can often be tasted as a sharp stinging sensation even before it can be smelled. Similar to chlorine, irritation is mainly to the eyes, nose, throat, and airways, but also to the mouth and skin. At levels below the threshold for smell or taste, hydrochloric acid can cause sneezing, laryngitis, chest pain, hoarseness, and a feeling of suffocation. Skin burns, *inflammation*, and *ulceration* of the *nasal septum* can also occur. Erosion of tooth enamel has been reported in workers and also in competitive swimmers in pools where improper chlorine treatment raised acidity levels.

Hypochlorite in bleach is a corrosive substance, capable of damaging skin, eyes, and other membranes. According to statistics from poison control centers, an unexpectedly high number of children accidently swallow laundry bleach each year. Relatively few fatalities are reported, probably because of the immediate vomiting that is usually produced. Damage to the esophagus and stomach can occur. Administering acids such as vinegar to neutralize the hypochlorite only worsens the damage because the heat and gases produced can release chlorine gas into the respiratory tract.

The World Health Organization concludes that apart from accidents, there is no health risk to the general population from exposure to chlorine, hydrogen chloride, or hydrochloric acid. Cancer, mutations, and birth defects have not been associated with any of them.

Protection and Prevention

Locations downwind of chlorine spills receive the highest concentrations. Evacuations from major spills should be to upwind and lateral locations. Individuals who are exposed should be removed immediately from the site and should receive medical attention.

Home exposures can be minimized by not mixing chlorine-containing products with other substances, such as ammonia or vinegar. Another approach is to substitute cleansers using oxygen bleach for products containing chlorine. Adequate ventilation should be maintained while cleaning. Should respiratory symptoms develop (such as breathing difficulties and prolonged coughing) or throat or eye burning begin, a doctor should be contacted.

Environmental Effects

Chlorine is an effective *biocide*, capable of killing plants, bacteria, algae, and fungi. For this reason it is widely used in the disinfection of drinking water. Hydrogen chloride and hydrochloric acid are toxic to plants, causing leaf burns and internal damage. Effects are significant only in the vicinity of spills and localized sources of pollution (for example, chemical factories).

Regulatory Status

Occupational exposures to chlorine and hydrogen chloride are regulated by federal standards. There are no drinking water or ambient air quality regulations. Chlorine and hydrogen chlorine are listed as *hazardous air pollutants* in the 1990 Clean Air Act, requiring the EPA to set emission standards. It is also on the EPA *community right-to-know* list.

Technical Information

Chemical symbols or formulas:
   chlorine: Cl
   hydrogen chloride: HCl
   hydrochloric acid: HCl aq

hypochlorite: HOCl
sodium hypochlorite (bleach): NaOCl
OSHA limits in workplace air:
chlorine: 3 mg/m^3 (1 ppm)
hydrogen chloride: 7 mg/m^3 (5 ppm)

Further Reading

GOSSELIN, ROBERT E., SMITH, ROGER P., and HODGE, HAROLD C., editors. 1984. Hypochlorite. In *Clinical Toxicology of Commercial Products*, 5th edition. Baltimore, MD: Williams and Wilkins.

National Research Council. 1976. *Chlorine and Hydrogen Chloride*. Washington, D.C.: National Academy of Sciences.

World Health Organization. 1982. *Environmental Health Criteria No. 21: Chlorine and Hydrogen Chloride*. Geneva.

Chloroform

Other Names

Trichloromethane; methenyl chloride; methane trichloride; methyl trichloride; formyl trichloride

Trade Names

Freon 20; R 20; Refrigerant 20

Introduction

Just about anyone who drinks chlorinated water, swims in a pool filled with chlorine-treated water, or uses products made from chlorinated water is exposed to low levels of chloroform. This is because the **chlorine** used to disinfect drinking water reacts with naturally occurring organic material, such as rotting leaves, in the water to form chloroform. Chloroform can also be found in the air in urban and industrial areas, the result of paper and pulp manufacturing, automobile exhaust, tobacco smoke, plastics burning, and evaporation from polluted rivers and lakes. Although chloroform is no longer used as a general anesthetic, it still has industrial applications as a *solvent* and an extracting agent and as an intermediate in the manufacture of fluorocarbons, dyes, and drugs. It is also used as the working fluid in industrial refrigerators. Some consumer products may still contain chloroform. The most likely candidates include cough syrups, toothpaste, liniments, glue, and pesticides.

Physical and Chemical Properties

Chloroform smells and tastes sweet. This solvent does not catch fire easily and is not explosive. The liquid evaporates easily.

Exposure and Distribution

Annual chloroform production in the United States is about 150,000 tons. It is produced in West Virginia, Texas, Kansas, Kentucky,

New Jersey, and California. It is shipped mostly by rail and barge in bottles, fiberboard boxes, metal drums, and tank cars. But manufactured chloroform is not the primary source of human exposure because over 2000 tons of chloroform are unintentionally created during the chlorination of drinking water.

Nearly 70% of people in the United States are served by chlorinated municipal drinking water. Most of the chloroform found in water is due to chlorination. Other sources of chloroform in water are municipal wastewater, which is often treated with chlorine before release, and the pulp and paper industry, which uses chlorine to bleach paper pulp. Chloroform can even be detected in rainwater in areas where the air is heavily contaminated with the chemical.

Chloroform-contaminated air can be found in rural, urban, and industrial areas, as well as inside the home. Pulp and paper bleaching are responsible for the largest proportion of chloroform released into the air, but a wide variety of activities also emit chloroform. These include the manufacture of chemicals and drugs, **TCE** (trichloroethylene) degradation, evaporation from chlorinated cooling water, grain fumigation, automobile exhaust, tobacco smoke, and evaporation from swimming pools and fountains. Very little chloroform is spilled directly onto the land. Possibly the most significant source of airborne chloroform to the average person is the shower. Chloroform readily evaporates from chlorinated hot water, and concentrations can become quite high in the air of an enclosed shower stall. Indoor air can also become contaminated with chloroform as a result of using cleaning and laundry products containing chlorine bleach. Although typical concentrations inside the home are similar to those found in urban outdoor air, people taking a shower can be exposed to concentrations 10 to 100 times this while showering.

Interestingly, soft drinks sometimes contain levels of chloroform above those normally found in water. These are thought to result from the use of water taken from industrial taps during their manufacture. Other foods also contain small amounts of chloroform, including seafood, dairy products, meat, fats and oils, vegetables and fruit, bread, and mother's milk. Although it appears that dietary intake of chloroform in some cases may be substantial, not enough information is available to assess average intake rates.

Health Effects

Chloroform is a narcotic at very high doses. Symptoms of dangerous overexposure include dilation of the pupils, a warm feeling, and paralysis, possibly followed by death. Dizziness, mental dullness, abdominal pain, nausea, vomiting, headache, slowed respiration, decreased blood pressure, fatigue, unconsciousness, and eye and skin irritation have also been attributed to very high doses of chloroform.

Chronic exposure to high, but not immediately life-threatening, concentrations can lead to fatigue, anorexia, anemia, weakness, blurred vision, memory loss, tremors, enlarged liver, jaundice, and kidney damage. The liver and kidney are most vulnerable to permanent damage due to chronic chloroform exposure.

Numerous *epidemiological* studies have found a relationship between drinking chlorinated water and cancer of the bladder and large intestine. But chloroform has never been isolated as the sole or primary cause of these cancers. High doses of chloroform are reported to cause kidney and liver cancer in laboratory animals exposed for their entire lifetimes. But some scientists believe that these cancers follow organ damage that occurs in animals only after very large doses of chloroform. Other scientists believe that chloroform promotes the growth of existing cancers rather than actually causing the cancers. *Ames test* results have been negative. In spite of these disagreements, the EPA considers chloroform a probable human carcinogen (group B_2; see Chapter 3, Section B). Chloroform is toxic to the fetus, but it apparently does not cause birth defects in the animal species that have been tested.

Overweight people retain more chloroform than do thin people because chloroform can be stored in body fat. When an overweight person inhales chloroform, it is quickly removed from the bloodstream to be stored in body fat. The bloodstream never becomes saturated with chloroform. When exposure stops, chloroform stored in body fat is slowly released, thereby continuing the original exposure. In thin people, the bloodstream quickly becomes saturated with chloroform because there is less fat to absorb the chemical. Even if more is inhaled, it has nowhere to go and the excess is simply exhaled.

Laboratory animals given alcoholic beverages show significantly increased levels of chloroform and changes in their livers. Similar changes are observed in test animals given ethanol and chloroform together.

Protection and Prevention

Avoiding chloroform is nearly impossible given its wide distribution in air and water. Nevertheless, exposure can be minimized by ensuring that rooms where hot water is used, particularly the shower stall, are well ventilated. The air inside swimming pool or hot tub enclosures can also contain high levels of chloroform. An activated carbon filter installed on the cold water pipe going into the hot water heater can significantly decrease chloroform concentrations both in the hot water and inside the house. Since carbon filters located at the tap can be installed only on the cold water pipe, they are not as effective at combating the problem of chloroform contaminating indoor air.

Alternatives to using chlorine to disinfect water do exist, but they are expensive and form other toxic by-products. Until the consequences of using alternative disinfection techniques are better understood, chlorine will remain in use.

Environmental Effects

Although chloroform evaporates rapidly when spilled on land, it can leach into groundwater where it will remain for several months or even years. Evaporation from still water is quite slow, but it will evaporate quickly from flowing water or if it is stirred or sprayed. Chloroform remains in the atmosphere for several months before it is *photochemically* degraded. For this reason, emissions into the air are likely to spread over large areas.

Regulatory Status

The EPA regulates the amount of chloroform found in water. Chloroform is included in regulations governing trihalomethanes, a group of chemically related compounds that includes chloroform. WHO suggests a drinking water guideline for chloroform alone that is about one-third the trihalomethane level allowed in the United States. Therefore, regulations concerning chloroform in water are expected to undergo revision. The FDA banned chloroform from cosmetics and drugs in 1976. The chemical was banned from food in 1983, but small amounts of chloroform are allowed to leak into food from packaging material. So far, there are no regulations concerning chloroform concentrations in ambient air. However, it is listed as a *hazardous air pollutant* in the 1990 Clean Air Act, requiring the EPA to set emission standards. It is also on the EPA *community right-to-know* list.

Technical Information

Chemical formula: $CHCl_3$
Molecular weight: 119
Ambient air concentrations in highly urban areas: 0.0005 ppm
Average daily intake from air (estimated): 0.0071 mg

Average daily intake from water: 0.064–0.136 mg

Occupational exposures from inhaled air: 7–170 ppm

Acute health effects air levels:

headache, dizziness, sleepiness: 50–150 ppm

irritation to mucous membranes, nausea, irregular heartbeat: 150 ppm

liver and kidney damage: 15,000 ppm

death: >15,000 ppm

Chronic health effects air levels:

fatigue, headache, memory loss (inhaled regularly): 100 ppm

cirrhosis (inhaled over extended periods): 100 ppm

OSHA limit in workplace air: 10 ppm

EPA limit in drinking water: 10 mg/L

Odor threshold for chloroform: 200–300 ppm

Further Reading

Agency for Toxic Substances and Disease Registry. 1988. *Toxicological Profile for Chloroform.* Washington, D.C.: U.S. Public Health Service.

Chromium

Introduction

Chromium is a metal widely used in chrome-plated steel and stainless steel. It has the unique property of being required for human health in one form, while being among the strongest known causes of lung cancer in another form. It is usually ranked second after **benzene** as a major toxic air pollutant. Small chrome-plating shops near residential neighborhoods and power plant cooling towers are the two major sources of hazardous exposures.

Physical and Chemical Properties

Chromium is found in nature in three stable forms: chromium metal, chromium(III), and chromium(VI). Chromium metal is element number 24 in the periodic table of the elements. It occurs widely in the ore chromite, from which it is refined. Chromium metal is extremely resistant to chemical attack (corrosion and oxidation), which accounts for its use in stainless steel and chrome plating. Chromium(III) and chromium(VI) are forms of chromium that combine with other elements to form compounds. (The Roman numeral refers to a property called valence which determines the types of compounds or chemical reactions a substance can participate in.)

Chromium(III) (or trivalent chromium) is the form most widely encountered in the environment. It is the more stable of the two and is required for human health, participating, along with insulin, in maintaining proper blood sugar levels. Chromium(VI) (or hexavalent chromium) is the more important commercial form because of its chemical properties, but it can produce both immediate adverse health effects and lung cancer. Chromium(VI) is rapidly transformed by *organic matter* into chromium(III) so that significant quantities of chromium(VI) are almost always the result of human releases.

Exposure and Distribution

Most people are exposed only to chromium(III) (the necessary kind) in food and to a lesser extent in water. Air makes a relatively small contribution, except in the vicinity of certain factories. The typical daily adult intake of chromium ranges from 0.03 to 0.1 milligrams, over 90% of which comes from food. Formula-fed infants, however, receive over 99% of their chromium intake from the water used to reconstitute the formula. This example illustrates the point that levels of substances in drinking water considered safe for adults can possibly be hazardous to formula-fed infants, whose entire nutritional intake is based on drinking water. Parents of formula-fed babies should ascertain the quality of their local water supply, and if questionable, they should switch to another source of water for making up formula or should use ready-to-drink varieties. No adverse effects have been reported for ordinary exposures to chromium(III). The National Academy of Sciences considers an adequate yet safe intake of chromium to be 0.05 to 0.20 milligrams per day.

Chromium(VI), the dangerous form, is used in metal finishing (chrome plating), chromium chemicals production, chromium pigments for paints and textiles, leather tanning, and some wood preservatives (chromated copper arsenate). It is also used in electrical power plant cooling towers to prevent corrosion in the cooling loops. Drift from cooling towers can be an important source of chromium(VI) in the vicinity of electrical power plants. Chromium(VI) is also released when municipal refuse is incinerated and when sewage sludge and waste from electroplating and chromite refinery operations are disposed. Solid waste containing chromium(VI) can become a hazard when disposed of in landfills because this form of chromium is very mobile in groundwater, whereas chromium(III) is not. Concentrations of chromium(VI) can be high in factories in any of the previously mentioned industries and in the vicinities of such factories. Typical environmental levels of chromium are shown in Table 25, but unfortunately, a breakdown between hazardous and nonhazardous forms is not available.

Steel production, combustion of coal and oil, and chromium chemicals production release the most total chromium into the air. Electroplating operations, leather tanneries, and textile manufacturing are the largest sources of water releases. Chromium chemical plants and chromite ore refineries are the largest sources of chromium-containing solid wastes. Total consumption of chromium in the United States is approximately 500,000 tons per year, of which 60% goes to metallurgical uses, 21% to chemicals production, and 18% for use in lining furnaces (refractory uses).

Health Effects

Chromium metal appears to be biologically inert and no harmful effects have been reported. Chromium(III) is required for health, and all ordinary exposures are considered to be safe. Chromium(VI) compounds are responsible for the majority of all adverse effects of chromium.

Chromium(VI) can produce liver and kidney damage, internal hemmorhage, *dermatitis*, respiratory damage, and lung cancer, although dramatic cases of chromium poisoning are rarely seen today because of improvements in industrial safety and hygiene. Only six cases of *acute poisoning* have been reported since 1935, but most were fatal regardless of treatment. Longer-term exposures to the respiratory tract and skin can produce perforated and ulcerated *nasal septa*, *inflammation* of the nasal passages, frequent nose bleeds, and skin *ulcers*. These effects are usually seen after industrial exposures. A more common response is an allergic skin reaction (allergic contact dermatitis) after exposure to chromium in such diverse products as leather, cement, brewery yeast, wood preservatives, priming paint, glue, and paint

TABLE 25 Environmental Levels of Chromium

Medium	Concentration	Comments
Air		
Remote	0.005–1.1 ng/m^3	Chromium(III) and chromium metal
Urban	5.2–160 ng/m^3	Highest level in Baltimore, MD
Near cooling towers	50 ng/m^3	
Water		
Remote surface water	<5 µg/L	
Surface drinking water	<5–17 µg/L	
Tapwater	0.4–8 µg/L	
Contaminated groundwater	220 µg/L	
Water near cooling towers	2500–2750 µg/L	
Food		
Most foods	0.02–0.51 µg/g	Often higher in acidic foods
Wine	0.45 mg/L	
Beer	0.3 mg/L	
Spirits	0.135 mg/L	

pigments. Such reactions can often be successfully treated with hydrocortisone creams or ascorbic acid (vitamin C) solutions.

Lung cancer is now known to be a potential consequence of breathing chromium-(VI) compounds. The EPA places chromium-(VI) among the top one-fourth of substances ranked for carcinogenic potency and classifies it in group A, which means sufficient evidence of causing human cancer (see Chapter 3, Section B). Workers in the chromium chemicals industry in the United States, Great Britain, West Germany, and Japan show a clear association between chromium exposure and lung cancer. Laboratory experiments further confirm that chromium(VI) compounds (or their reactive intermediates within cells) can damage genetic material. Other studies on laboratory animals show that this form of chromium can cause fetal malformations and reproductive problems.

Protection and Prevention

Avoiding long-term proximity to factories that produce or use chromium chemicals, to power plant cooling towers, and to municipal refuse incinerators will reduce exposure to chromium(VI). Stainless steel and refractory steel production facilities, chrome-electro-plating operations, and other major industrial facilities are also sources of chromium and should be avoided to the extent possible. Most chrome-plating shops are small operations that are widely dispersed in urban areas and are sometimes in close proximity to residential neighborhoods. Children should not be allowed to play near these businesses or on playgrounds nearby because the soils may be contaminated.

Unusual skin rashes that appear after contact with products containing chromium can usually be treated with topical medications, and further contact with the suspected product should be avoided. Adequate clothing (long sleeves, pants, and gloves) may be sufficient to eliminate skin exposure. Acute exposures that might occur in a laboratory, in an industrial facility, or by accidental swallowing of chromated wood preservative must be immediately treated by trained medical personnel.

Environmental Effects

Chromium does not *bioconcentrate* in *food chains*. Naturally occurring chromium has been associated with soil infertility only in a few places because of high concentrations. Chromium in the form of chromate chemicals is particularly toxic to plants, however, and chromium salts should be avoided in all plant growing media. Chromium(VI) is toxic to aquatic life, and water quality standards have been established for the protection of aquatic species. Because chromium(VI) is rapidly transformed to nonhazardous chromium(III) in the environment, a hazard exists only in the vicinity of direct discharges to water bodies.

Regulatory Status

Federal water quality standards are established by the EPA for the protection of human health and for the protection of aquatic life. Chromium is listed as a *hazardous air pollutant* in the 1990 Clean Air Act, requiring the EPA to set emission standards. It is also on the EPA *community right-to-know* list. Occupational exposure standards set by OSHA are also in force for regulating worker exposure to various chromium compounds in factory air.

Technical Information

Chemical symbol: Cr
Atomic number: 24
Atomic weight: 52
Adequate and safe dietary intake level:
   50–200 μg/day
Primary drinking water standard (health protection): 50 μg/L (50 ppb)
Ambient water quality criteria (protection of aquatic life):
    freshwater: 11 μg/L (11 ppb)
    saltwater: 50 μg/L (50 ppb)
OSHA limits in workplace air:
   chromium(VI): 50 $\mu g/m^3$
   chromium(III): 0.5 mg/m^3

Further Reading

Environmental Protection Agency. 1985. *Health Assessment Document for Chromium, Final Report.* EPA 600/8–83–014F. Washington, D.C.
National Research Council. 1974. *Chromium.* Washington, D.C.: Committee on Biologic Effects of Atmospheric Pollutants, National Academy of Sciences.

Creosote

Other Names

Creosotum; creosote oil; brick oil; coal tar creosote

Introduction

As a wood preservative, creosote prevents or slows decay and increases the life expectancy of the wood by a factor of five or more. Its primary use as a wood preservative is on railroad ties and utility poles, but it is used extensively on construction lumber, fence posts, plywood, and foundation materials. When used as a wood preservative, creosote is actually a mixture of chemicals produced by the distillation of wood or coal tar. The composition varies depending on the source and may contain phenol, cresols (methyl phenol), creosols, and other **benzene**-based aromatic chemicals.

Creosote has a number of diverse secondary uses. It is a waterproofing agent, an animal dip, a constituent of fuel oil, a lubricant, and an intermediate in chemical manufacturing. It is used as an antiseptic, a disinfectant, an antipyretic, an astringent, and a germicide.

Physical and Chemical Properties

Creosote is a flammable, heavy, oily liquid with a characteristic sharp, smoky smell. It has a caustic, burning taste. Pure creosote is colorless, while the industrial grade is brownish.

Exposure and Distribution

Wood preservatives are used in large quantities; creosote and two other wood preservatives, inorganic **arsenic** compounds and pentachlorophenol, account for about one-third of all agriculturally and industrially used pesticides (fungicides) in the United States.

A large number of construction workers and a smaller number of do-it-yourself householders throughout the country may be exposed to creosote when working with treated wood since the primary route of exposure is through skin contact. Workers who treat the wood by applying the creosote are exposed routinely to much higher levels.

Health Effects

Ranked by the EPA as a probable human carcinogen (group B_1; see Chapter 3, Section B), creosote causes both cancer and mutations in laboratory tests. Both direct contact with the liquid and exposure to the vapors can cause progressive burning, itching, discoloration, ulceration of the skin, and ultimately, gangrene. It produces eye injuries, can increase the skin's sensitivity to the sun, and may cause skin cancer. *Acute systemic effects* include headache, vomiting, vertigo, hypothermia, convulsions, respiratory difficulties, and death. One chemical constituent of creosote, cresol, is very corrosive to all tissues.

Protection and Prevention

The Consumer Awareness Program requires information to be provided to consumers about proper handling of treated wood products. It recommends against using creosote-treated wood in proximity to food, animal feed, and public drinking water. People are advised not to burn creosote-treated wood. Applicators must wear protective clothing, special face masks or goggles, respirators, and gloves. If creosote is used on wood that will come into contact with bare skin, such as in outdoor furniture or play gyms, two coats of urethane or shellac sealer must be applied. A sealer should also be applied to treated wood used in areas where inhalation exposure may occur, such as in barns and stables.

The only effective alternatives to creosote as a wood preservative are pentachlorophenol and inorganic arsenic compounds, both of which pose health or environmental problems. One alternative to creosote-treated wood is to substitute concrete or even plastic posts. Also, those types of wood that are considerably more resistant to rot can be used in place of less resistant wood.

Regulatory Status

No federal criteria have been set for creosote levels in water, and there are no air standards. NIOSH, however, recommends a workplace exposure level that has yet to be adopted by OSHA. In 1978, the EPA initiated a *Special Review* of creosote based on its carcinogenicity. As a result, rather than banning the chemical, the EPA proposed a set of regulations intended to reduce exposure. Creosote is listed as a *hazardous air pollutant* in the 1990 Clean Air Act, requiring the EPA to set emission standards. It is also on the EPA *community right-to-know* list. Creosote is a restricted-use pesticide, meaning that it may be applied only by certified applicators.

Technical Information

Chemical names of creosote components: cresol, phenol
NIOSH recommended limit: 0.1 mg/m^3

Further Reading

Environmental Protection Agency. 1988. *Pesticide Fact Handbook*. Washington, D.C.

2,4-D

Trade Names

Agrotect; Rider; Lawn-keep; Super D Weed-one; Weed-B-Gone; Weedone

Introduction

The herbicide 2,4-D is a close chemical relative of two other phenoxy acids, **2,4,5-T** and 2,4,5-TP (Silvex), both of which have gained considerable notoriety as a result of being contaminated with highly toxic **dioxin** or TCDD. Although pure 2,4-D does not contain TCDD, it can be contaminated with dioxin during the manufacturing process and has been intentionally combined with 2,4,5-T in some of its formulations.

Introduced in 1944, 2,4-D was the first hormone-like weed killer. The *herbicidal* action of 2,4-D is relatively selective; it is toxic to a wide variety of broad-leaved plants, but generally does not affect grasses, such as cereal crops, ornamental lawns, and pasture forage. Physiologically, 2,4-D behaves like natural plant hormones, called auxins, that regulate plant growth. Its toxicity is due to its ability to interfere with normal plant growth processes. In addition to its use as a weed killer, it is used in low doses to control a variety of developmental processes in broad-leaved plants, such as ripening of fruit and root development.

Since its introduction, 2,4-D has become the most extensively used herbicide in the world. In 1985, agriculture and forestry applications in the United States accounted for nearly 40 million pounds of 2,4-D, which is a substantial decrease from the 1975 levels of about 60 million pounds.

Physical and Chemical Properties

The herbicide is a corrosive white powder that is slightly soluble in water, aqueous alkali, and alcohols, but insoluble in petroleum oils. For convenience in application, it is often converted to an oil-soluble form.

Exposure and Distribution

Because 2,4-D is used so extensively both in agriculture on important crops, such as corn, wheat, sorghum, oats, barley, and sugarcane, and in forestry management to control terrestrial and aquatic weed species, there is a considerable potential for widespread distribution and subsequent exposure to the herbicide. As with many other pesticides, the method of application and the physical and chemical properties of 2,4-D determine its distribution. Available in several different forms, it can be applied by aerial spraying, ground spraying, or direct injection into individual plants. The water-soluble salt formulations are readily taken up by the roots of plants, although the oil-soluble forms are more readily absorbed by plants and, as a result, are more effective against target species.

In all plants, 2,4-D is readily metabolized, but the end-products differ among species. In tolerant species, such as corn, the herbicide is converted to an inactive, nontoxic form, whereas in susceptible species the *metabolite* is the active form. Studies on animals indicate that 2,4-D generally undergoes little *metabolism*, is excreted rapidly, and thus does not tend to *bioaccumulate*.

There are, however, other important implications for nontarget species associated with the use of each of the formulations. Certain 2,4-D forms are very volatile and can inadvertently come into contact with nearby nontarget plant species. More significantly, aquatic systems are particularly vulnerable to inappropriate or careless use of these formulations, which are moderately or highly toxic to phytoplankton, aquatic invertebrates, and fish. In contrast, the salt form, although more soluble in water, is only slightly toxic to aquatic organisms other than plants and is of low toxicity to birds.

In most soils and water, 2,4-D is relatively nonpersistent since it readily undergoes biological and nonbiological degradation. Of course, physical and chemical properties of the soil or water (such as *pH*, organic content, temperature, and moisture content) influence the process of degradation and thus the duration of exposure time. For example, under alkaline conditions (pH > 7.0), the most important and rapid mechanism for the loss of 2,4-D appears to be hydrolysis (a reaction with water), while under more acidic conditions (pH < 7.0) the slower process of vaporization may be more significant. An important implication of this is that a decrease in the pH of the water (as is occurring in many lakes and streams in the United States as a result of acid rain) causes an increase in the breakdown time of the herbicide, thus prolonging the exposure time. Microbial activity, which is the primary means of breakdown, is maximized in soil by conditions of warm temperatures, high moisture content, and high organic content. Although the herbicide does not *adsorb* strongly to soils, meaning that it is fairly mobile, it does not appear to pose a serious migration problem into streams and lakes.

Studies indicate that the levels of 2,4-D to which agricultural and forestry workers and nontarget species, such as rabbits, deer, and fish, are normally exposed during or following application are considerably lower than those producing toxic effects.

Health Effects

Although this herbicide has been studied extensively, a review by the International Agency for Cancer Research (IARC) concluded that there were insufficient data to assess the cancer-causing ability of 2,4-D. Both testing and reporting were deemed inadequate. It does not cause *mutations* in most microbial test systems, but there is some evidence of mutagenicity in cultured mammalian cells and insects. There have been repeated reports of reproductive problems associated with exposure to 2,4-D, but studies on sheep, rats, and hamsters have failed to show clearly that it causes birth defects. Possibly the observed birth defects attributed to 2,4-D may have been caused by impurities in the for-

mulations. There is, however, evidence that 2,4-D is toxic to developing embryos.

When ingested in large doses, 2,4-D is of moderate *acute toxicity* to mammals, causing *gastrointestinal* irritation, spasms of the heart muscle, and central nervous system depression. It is a skin and an eye irritant, and prolonged inhalation causes coughing, dizziness, and temporary loss of coordination. Tests of subacute toxicity indicate that prolonged exposure to relatively low levels of 2,4-D can produce a variety of responses ranging from a reversible loss of coordination to stomach ulcers and even death.

Protection and Prevention

Agricultural workers and people who manufacture the herbicide are undoubtedly exposed to higher levels than the general public. All precautions prescribed by the EPA and the manufacturer should be observed when using and handling the chemical. Protective clothing should be worn. At present, it is uncertain to what extent the public is exposed, but it is likely that some residues remain on harvested foods. Therefore, it is prudent to wash all fresh produce. Despite laboratory evidence of adverse reproductive effects in mammals that argues for cautious application and reduced use of 2,4-D, there have been numerous citizen complaints concerning careless spraying practices by the U.S. Forest Service.

Environmental Effects

Studies of the environmental effects of 2,4-D indicate that careless or inappropriate use may pose serious problems for nontarget species. As previously mentioned, it is quite toxic to aquatic invertebrates and fish, although the toxicity varies among species. The herbicide is used routinely to kill water hyacinths in ponds and lakes and to clear weeds along drainage and irrigation ditches—both of which normally contain a diverse community of aquatic organisms that may be adversely affected by high concentrations of 2,4-D.

The U.S. Forest Service is a primary consumer of 2,4-D, using it extensively in its habitat improvement programs and forestry and rangeland management programs. Because 2,4-D has been used so extensively, many target plant species have developed *resistance* to it. Moreover, there is evidence that 2,4-D enhances the toxic effects of certain unrelated *insecticides.* It has been found to increase the toxicity of **DDT** to fruit flies and of **parathion** to mosquito larvae. Perhaps more important, the addition of even a small amount of **carbaryl**, which is itself not particularly toxic to fish, greatly increases the toxic effects of 2,4-D on rainbow trout, sockeye salmon, and green sunfish—all nontarget species.

Regulatory Status

Concerns about the possible carcinogenicity of 2,4-D prompted the EPA to initiate a *Special Review*. The review process was halted in 1988. 2,4-D is listed as a *hazardous air pollutant* in the 1990 Clean Air Act, requiring the EPA to set emission standards. It is also on the *community right-to-know* list.

Technical Information

Chemical name: (2,4-dichlorophenoxy)acetic acid
Chemical formula: $C_8H_6O_3Cl_2$
OSHA limit in workplace air: 10 mg/m^3
EPA water quality criterion for human health: 100 µg/L
WHO acceptable daily intake: 0.3 mg/kg

Further Reading

U.S. Forest Service. 1984. *Pesticide Background Statements. Vol. I. Herbicides.* Agricultural Handbook No. 633. Washington, D.C.: U.S. Department of Agriculture.

Daminozide

Trade Names

Alar; Kylar; B-Nine; Aminozide

Introduction

Daminozide, or Alar, has been the focus of a great deal of public attention since the mid-1980s following disclosures that (1) it is suspected of causing cancer; (2) its principal breakdown product, UDMH (unsymmetrical 1,1-dimethylhydrazine), is known to cause tumors in test animals; and (3) both commonly remain as residues on fruits (chiefly apples) and other produce. Moreover, assurances by growers and the FDA that residue levels are very low have been questioned since neither Alar nor UDMH can be detected by the FDA's routine testing procedures for pesticide residues, although suitable detection methods are available. Since the initial outcry, some supermarket chains claim to sell no apples treated with Alar. Similarly, many manufacturers of apple juice and apple sauce no longer use Alar-treated fruit.

A 1987 study by the Natural Resources Defense Council (NRDC) claimed that 38% of the U.S. apple crop is treated with Alar, particularly such varieties as Red and Golden Delicious, MacIntosh, Jonathan, and Stayman. In fact, apples are the primary recipient of the vast bulk of daminozide used in the United States, accounting for about 75% of the volume. Residues have been detected not only on fresh produce, but also on various processed foods, including apple juice, peanut butter, cherry pie filling, and concord grape juice. Alarmingly, the chemical tends to concentrate in processed food, resulting in higher residue levels in apple sauce, apple juice, and dried apples than in fresh apples. Moreover, UDMH is produced during processing and concentrates similarly.

Alar made headlines again in early 1989 with the release of a new report by the NRDC which pointed out that young children are at greater risk from residues of Alar (and other agricultural chemicals) than the general public because of dietary and metabolic differences between children and adults. In response, schools across the nation removed apples from their lunch menus and the demand for *organically grown* produce soared. Growers, insisting that apples are safe and that only 5% of the nations apple crop is treated with daminozide, launched a campaign to counter the effects of the NRDC report. Heeding public pressure, the manufacturer voluntarily withdrew Alar from the market.

Although commonly referred to as a pesticide, daminozide is actually a plant growth regulator, controlling both vegetative and reproductive growth. Introduced in 1967, it is used on orchard crops, primarily apples, but also peaches, pears, prunes, cherries, and nectarines. It is also used extensively on peanuts. Alar has limited use on cantaloupes, brussels sprouts, tomatoes, and grapes in some regions. By controlling reproductive growth, the chemical slows fruit ripening, prevents fruit from dropping prematurely, and allows the fruit to develop a deeper, more uniform color.

Physical and Chemical Properties

Daminozide is a white, crystalline solid. It is soluble in water and methanol, but insoluble in **xylene** and certain other *solvents*. In the environment, it leaches from the soil and resists being broken down by sunlight. It degrades readily under aqueous conditions to UDMH, which means that solutions are unstable and should not be stored for more than 24 hours.

Exposure and Distribution

About 825,000 pounds of daminozide are used annually in the United States, with apples and peanuts accounting for 600,000 and 125,000 pounds of the total usage, respectively. As mentioned, consumption of raw and processed foods, particularly apples, can account for significant exposure to daminozide and UDMH.

Daminozide is rapidly absorbed by the leaves, stems, and roots of plants and is transported to other parts of the plant; it accumulates in roots and fruits. It does not, however, accumulate in rotational (that is, nontreated, successive) crops because it does not persist in soil. It is broken down by microbial action as well as by water. Consequently, the potential for groundwater contamination is minimal. In dairy cows, most of the ingested residues of daminozide are rapidly excreted in the urine and feces.

Health Effects

Several studies indicate that both Alar and UDMH cause cancer, although the data are incomplete. A 1987 study by the National Academy of Sciences estimated the risk of either benign or malignant tumor formation associated with exposure to daminozide to be considerably greater than the one in one million risk that is considered acceptable by the EPA. There is insufficient information to determine whether Alar or UDMH causes mutations, reproductive effects, birth defects, or other adverse effects, although evidence to date suggests that it is neither a *mutagen* nor a *teratogen*. Alar, however, is of low acute toxicity both orally and dermally.

Protection and Prevention

Because daminozide breaks down so readily to UDMH when in solution, special handling is required. Solutions must be used within 24 hours after being mixed to prevent production of the contaminant. Although Alar is no longer being sold in the United States, there are no restrictions on sales and use of remaining stocks. Thus, consumers should not assume that growers are no longer using the chemical. Since the recent uproar, however, more and more growers claim that they no longer use Alar. People who are concerned about exposure to Alar can buy apples and other produce grown by state-certified organic growers. Many supermarket chains, responding to the public's concerns, advertise that their produce is tested for residues or that they buy only from farmers who do not use daminozide.

Environmental Effects

Daminozide is not acutely toxic to fish or to terrestrial wildlife nor does it accumulate in fish. The ecological effects of the breakdown product UDMH cannot be assessed because data are unavailable.

Regulatory Status

Daminozide is classified as a general use pesticide; there are no restrictions on its use. A cautionary statement on container labels, however, warns users to use solutions within 24 hours of mixing.

Since 1985 when the EPA proposed to cancel all uses of daminozide on food (a position it retracted soon after), the safety of the growth regulator has been under scrutiny. The EPA has moved slowly to deal with Alar, deciding to disallow any new registration of products containing daminozide but not banning existing stocks. In 1989, the usually very lengthy *Special Review* process began to determine what further regulatory action is warranted. The EPA intends to cancel the registration of Alar, but that will take one or two years to conclude. In the meantime, the manufacturer, Uniroyal, has voluntarily withdrawn Alar from the U.S. market, although it will continue to sell the product overseas.

Technical Information

Chemical names: butanedioic acid mono (2,-2-dimethylhydrazine); succinic acid 2,2-dimethyhydrazine
Government standards for food tolerances: permitted on apples: 20ppm

on dried tomatoes: changed from 40 ppm to 0.5 ppm

Further Reading

Environmental Protection Agency. 1988. *EPA Pesticide Fact Sheet 26: Daminozide*. Washington, D.C.
———. 1985. *Daminozide Special Review Position Document 2/3/4*. Washington, D.C.
MOTT, L., and SNYDER, K. 1987. *Pesticide Alert*. San Francisco: Sierra Club Books.
SEWELL, B., and WHYATT, R. 1989. *Intolerable Risk: Pesticides in Our Children's Food*. New York: Natural Resources Defense Council.

DDT

Other Name

Dichlorodiphenyltrichloroethane

Trade Names

Anofex; Dinocide; Neocidol

Introduction

First synthesized in 1873, the insecticidal properties of DDT were not discovered until 1939. DDT quickly gained wide popularity, appearing to be a miracle pesticide: highly effective against a broad range of insect pests, inexpensive to manufacture, and evidently safe for people and other mammals. Although credited with saving millions of human lives by controlling the insects that spread malaria, yellow fever, typhus, and other often fatal diseases, DDT eventually became the focus of a long-term controversy and the symbol of a miracle gone awry.

Because of their *persistence* in the environment, DDT and certain other *organochlorine* pesticides and related compounds (such as **PCBs**) pose a serious and unacceptable threat to nontarget species, including people. They tend to *bioconcentrate* (particularly in aquatic organisms); they accumulate in fatty tissues; and they are transferred through the *food chain*. The well-publicized link between high levels of DDT in birds and subsequent reproductive problems (such as thin-shelled eggs) made DDT a household word.

Although no longer registered for use in the United States, DDT is used in agriculture and disease-control programs in other parts of the world. DDT residues continue to be detected in human tissues, in soils, in groundwater, in marine and freshwater sediments, and on fresh fruits and vegetables. In a recent U.S. survey, DDT was the most frequently found residue on carrots and potatoes. In fact, 22% of the carrots tested contained DDT residues. It was also detected on onions, sweet potatoes, and spinach.

Physical and Chemical Properties

Pure DDT is a white, tasteless, almost odorless, crystalline solid. It is highly insoluble in water, but readily dissolves in fat, **benzene**, and **chloroform**. The less pure form, or technical grade, of DDT is white, waxy solid with a characteristic sickly-sweet smell.

Exposure and Distribution

During its heyday, DDT was used in enormous quantities worldwide and distributed nearly everywhere. Residues have been found in human and animal tissue samples, including human breast milk, from even the most remote areas of the world. The two major residues or breakdown products of DDT are DDE, which is stored in tissues more tenaciously than DDT and is the most commonly found DDT product in human tissue, and DDD (itself also a minor insecticide often referred to as TDE or tetrachlordiphenyethane). In the United States, the National Human Adipose Survey has monitored tissue levels of DDT, its breakdown products, and six other organochlorine pesticides since 1970. Both here and elsewhere, there has been a dramatic decline in the levels of DDT detected in tissues following the steady drop in DDT use.

DDT can be absorbed by the lungs and the *gastrointestinal* system. It is not readily taken up by the skin, however, which may account for its fairly good safety record despite often careless handling. As with most pesticides, DDT manufacturers, applicators, and field-workers run the greatest risk of exposure.

Despite a U.S. ban on its use in 1972, DDT continues to be detected on agricultural products and other food items. In a survey of fresh produce done 12 years after its banning, DDT was the most common contaminant. In another more comprehensive survey, DDT residues were among the most frequently detected on five different food crops. Residues continue to be found in some food fish, crabs, and wild ducks. Recently, increasing levels of DDT (DDE) residues have been detected in migratory birds, bats, insects, and fish in certain areas of the country, chiefly New Mexico and Texas. The source is uncertain; migratory species possibly pick up DDT in Mexico and other southern wintering sites. There has been some speculation that U.S. farmers are illegally obtaining DDT from Mexico. The most likely reason for the presence of DDT in foods is its persistence in soils and sediments. In California, for example, DDT residues have been found in all sampled soils having a prior history of DDT usage.

Additional explanations of detectable DDT have been suggested. Residues may be linked to the widespread use of dicofol and chlorobenzilate, two newer structurally related *acaricides* both of which are contaminated with DDT as a result of the manufacturing process. (Registration of dicofol, which contains 7% or more of DDT, was recently suspended.) Also, some imported food most likely contains residues of DDT since it is still used for agricultural purposes elsewhere.

Health Effects

Like other organochlorines, DDT is primarily toxic to the nervous systems of mammals and insects. In mammals, signs of poisoning include numbness of the face, headache, fatigue, delayed vomiting, abnormal susceptibility to fear, unrest, confusion, excessive irritability, sensitivity to stimuli, tremors, and convulsions. Death can result from heart or respiratory failure. The onset of symptoms generally occurs several hours following DDT consumption, but may be more rapid, occurring within 30 minutes of a large dose. Recovery is complete in animals that survive. Death occurs in 24 to 72 hours. The range and progress of symptoms exhibited by human test volunteers and victims of accidental and suicidal ingestion are similar to those displayed by test animals.

The EPA classifies DDT as a probable human carcinogen (group B_2; see Chapter 3, Section B). There is some evidence that it causes mutations in mammalian cells, and it seems to cause adverse liver effects, independent of and in addition to liver cancer. Various reproductive effects, including decreased fertility, changes in sex organs, and altered metabolism of female hormones (which may be associated with eggshell thinning in birds) have been found in different species.

Protection and Prevention

In cases of poisoning, the victim should be induced to vomit using Ipecac syrup or water; do not offer milk or oily liquids. Contaminated skin or eyes should be flushed with water, and contaminated clothing should be removed. A physician should be contacted, who may prescribe an anticonvulsive drug. Like residues of other organochlorine insecticides, most DDT residues probably remain on the outer surface of fresh fruit and vegetables and can be removed by washing with a little detergent, rinsing, peeling, and cooking. There are effective substitutes for DDT in the control of malaria-carrying mosquitoes. The organophosphate **malathion** and the carbamate propoxur are safer alternatives, but both are prohibitively more expensive than DDT.

Environmental Effects

Because DDT persists for years in soils and sediments, its long-term effect on such soil organisms as fungi, bacteria, slugs, and earthworms has been well studied. Apparently, soil organisms are not adversely affected over the long term, but declines in numbers may occur in some species shortly after application. Slugs and earthworms, however, bioconcentrate DDT, show adverse affects, and indirectly threaten the animals that feed on them.

Aquatic organisms bioconcentrate DDT from the surrounding water considerably more efficiently than do soil organisms. Fish, for example, have been found with levels of

DDT (actually DDE) in their tissues many hundreds of thousands of times greater than found in the water. Scientists have carefully studied the apparent link between high levels of DDT in fish and aquatic organisms, the precipitous decline in the number of certain fish-eating bird species, and the subsequent recovery of those bird populations following the reduction in DDT use. During the period of intensive DDT use, fish contained high levels of DDT and related pesticides. Certain species of birds that fed on the contaminated fish, including eagles, ospreys, brown pelicans, and peregrine falcons, suffered enormous reproductive losses. The birds produced eggs with very thin shells that were easily crushed in the nest. Evidently the organochlorines interfered with the formation of normal eggshells.

There are several other less well known effects. DDT is directly toxic to fish species. Newly hatched fish seem to be considerably more sensitive to DDT and other organochlorines than either eggs or adults—at concentrations that typically occur after land application. Moreover, U.S.–Canadian studies of fish and bird populations in the Great Lakes region suggest that DDT (and certain other chlorinated hydrocarbons) may be associated with observed problems of development in the young of the species. The extensive use of DDT in agriculture and for the control of disease-carrying insects has led to the development of insect *resistance* to a number of pesticides and to a resulting reduction in pesticide effectiveness (see Chapter 14). Most of these impacts of DDT on nontarget species are indirect. In contrast, honeybees are highly susceptible to DDT on direct contact.

Regulatory Status

After years of debate, DDT was banned in the United States in 1972. It continued to be produced here until 1976. DDE is listed as a *hazardous air pollutant* in the 1990 Clean Air Act, requiring the EPA to set emission standards.

Technical Information

Chemical name: 1,1-trichloro–2,2-bis(p-chlorophenyl)ethane

Chemical formula: $C_{14}H_9Cl_5$

Residue levels in human fat
   (1970): 7.95 ppm
   (1983): 1.67 ppm

Comparative ranking of toxicity of organochlorine insecticides, in order of decreasing toxicity, based on the lethal dose (LD_{50}) of rats given DDT by mouth: aldrin > dieldrin > lindane > heptachlor > DDT > chlordane

OSHA limit in workplace air: 1 mg/m^3

Further Reading

Colborn, T. E., Davidson, A., Green, S. N., Hodge, R. A., Jackson, C. I., and Liroff, R. A. 1990. *Great Lakes: Great Legacy?* Washington, D.C.: Conservation Foundation.

Mott, L., and Snyder, K. 1987. *Pesticide Alert.* Natural Resources Defense Council. San Francisco: Sierra Club Books.

National Academy of Sciences. 1987. *Regulating Pesticides in Food.* Washington, D.C.: National Academy Press.

Diazinon

Trade Name

Spectracide

Introduction

Generally considered safe, diazinon has been used extensively for the control of insects in and around the home, on lawns and gardens, on pets, and in stables since its introduction in the early 1950s. It is also used to control pests of fruits, nuts, tobacco, vegetables, Christmas trees, and rice in the soil and on foliage. It is also effective against DDT-resistant flies.

Diazinon is an *organophosphate* which shares some similarities with **azinophos-methyl** and chlorpyrifos. Considered relatively safe, diazinon preparations can be contaminated with another commercially available organophosphate insecticide called sulfotepp, which is considerably more toxic than pure diazinon. Sulfotepp can be formed during the synthesis of diazinon, but generally constitutes less than 1% of the preparation.

Physical and Chemical Properties

Pure diazinon is a colorless liquid with a faint odor. It dissolves slightly in water. While diazinon is stable under alkaline conditions, it breaks down slowly in water and acid solutions. It is sensitive to heat, degrading quickly at boiling temperature.

Exposure and Distribution

Diazinon is the third most widely used organophosphate insecticide in the United States. It is applied as either a spray or a dust. Residues of the pesticide have been found on various fresh foods, including bananas, carrots, cauliflower, cherries, and onions.

Health Effects

There is considerable variation in species susceptibility to the toxic effects of diazinon. It is moderately toxic to rats and slightly less so to mice by both oral and dermal routes of exposure. In comparison with other organophosphates, diazinon is less toxic than **parathion** and more toxic than **malathion**. Diazinon does not appear to cause cancer, although the data are limited. Some test results suggest that it may cause *mutations*. When injected into chicken eggs, it produces birth defects in the chicks, but none in the young of rabbits receiving oral doses of the pesticide. In some tests using mice, there was evidence of adverse behavioral effects in the offspring.

Like other organophosphates and some *carbamate* pesticides, diazinon interferes with the activity of the enzyme *cholinesterase*, which is involved in the normal transmission of nerve signals. During normal *metabolism*, most organophosphates are detoxified. Diazinon, however, produces toxic metabolic products, also capable of inhibiting cholinesterase. Signs of poisoning, which include headache, intestinal cramps, excessive secretions, and spasms of the bronchial tubes, are easily confused with those of heat stroke, heat exhaustion, low blood sugar, gastroenteritis, and pneumonia or other severe respiratory infections. Laboratory tests to determine the cholinesterase level are often needed to diagnose diazinon poisoning. Mild cases of poisoning can resemble asthma. Unlike malathion and most other organophosphates, diazinon does not interact with other organophosphates to enhance their toxicity.

Protection and Prevention

The EPA cautions users to follow directions on the pesticide container label, to avoid breathing the spray or mist, and to avoid contact with the skin or eyes. Diazinon should not be applied near water sources that are being used by people or livestock and should be kept out of all water bodies. Chemical treatment of diazinon-containing wastes with acids is recommended in contrast to the procedure used for most other organophosphates, which are broken down with alkali. Although this insecticide typically remains on the surface of plants, it is unknown whether residues of the pesticide can be removed by washing with water.

Environmental Effects

Serious environmental problems are associated with the use of diazinon. It is very toxic to birds, particularly ducks and geese, and to various species of fish, aquatic insects, and other invertebrates. In scattered incidents throughout the country, mostly on golf courses, more than 20 species of birds have been killed inadvertently. Consequently, it has been banned for use on golf courses and sod farms.

Regulatory Status

In 1986, the EPA began a *Special Review* of all products containing diazinon because of its toxicity to nontarget avian species. This was a first step in considering cancellation of all uses, not just on golf courses and sod farms.

Technical Information

Chemical name: O,O-diethyl–2-(isopropyl–6-methyl–4-pyrimidinyl) phosphorothioate
Chemical formula: $C_{12}H_{21}N_2O_3PS$
WHO no observable effects level per body weight in rats: 0.1 mg/kg
WHO no observable effects level per body weight in dogs, humans, and monkeys: 0.02–0.05 mg/kg

Further Reading

Environmental Protection Agency. 1986. *EPA Pesticide Fact Sheet 96: Diazinon*. Washington, D.C.
HAYES, W. J., JR. 1982. *Pesticides Studied in Man*. Baltimore, MD: Williams and Wilkins.
World Health Organization. 1984. *Environmental Health Criteria No. 63: Organophosphate Pesticides*. Geneva.

Dicamba

Trade Names

Banex; Banvel; Brush Buster

Introduction

Like the phenoxy acid herbicides **2,4-D** and **2,4,5-T**, dicamba regulates plant growth, alters leaf and root development, and interferes with normal flowering mechanisms. One advantage of dicamba use is that it is effective against those species that are resistant to 2,4-D. Until recently, it had been considered a suitable alternative to the high-risk phenoxy acids 2,4,5-T and silvex, which were restricted in the late 1970s and, more recently, canceled entirely as a result of contamination with **dioxin**. Dicamba can also become contaminated with dioxin during the manufacturing process, but only with a less toxic form. Recent findings indicate that dicamba is contaminated with dimethyl**nitrosamine** (DMNA), which causes tumors in animal test systems.

Dicamba is generally nontoxic to a wide variety of nontarget species and is used extensively in agriculture and forestry, but it is particularly toxic to conifers and some legumes, such as beans and peas. Introduced about 1965, it has been applied annually to control broad-leafed weed and brush species and some annual grassy weeds. It is particularly useful in controlling weeds of cereal crops and sugarcane and in established grasslands. Dicamba can move to various parts of the plant following absorption through the roots or leaves.

Physical and Chemical Properties

The pure material is a white, crystalline solid, while the technical grade is a pale, buff-colored, crystalline solid. Dicamba in its various forms is soluble in water, stable under acidic conditions, and resistive to breakdown when exposed to water and air under normal conditions.

Exposure and Distribution

In the United States, some three million pounds of dicamba are applied annually, usually in combination with other herbicides such as 2,4-D. Application is by ground or aerial spraying, by injection into tree stumps, or by distribution of granules at the base of the plants. In agriculture, dicamba is used to control weeds in the production of grains, corn, sorghum, sugarcane, asparagus, and forage crops. The U.S. Forest Service accounts for a substantial percentage of total U.S. consumption of dicamba, using it to control both deciduous trees and shrubs (those that lose their leaves, such as maples) and conifers, as well as to kill weeds.

Dicamba is taken up by both the roots and leaves of plants, but the ease and rate of absorption, movement, and *metabolism* in the plant vary greatly from one species to another. In animals, dicamba does not *bioaccumulate* to any appreciable extent, nor is it rapidly metabolized. Most of it is excreted unchanged.

Under a fairly broad range of conditions, dicamba is very stable. It is resistant to breakdown by acids, alkalis, light, oxidation, and water, and thus it is moderately *persistent* in soils (3 to 12 months). This means that it can be used to control pest species for a full season, in theory requiring less frequent applications. The primary mechanism of degradation of dicamba in both soil and water appears to be by microbial activity, which is strongly influenced by *pH*, moisture, and temperature. For example, in acidified lakes without functioning microbial populations, no dicamba degradation occurs.

The herbicide does not readily adsorb to soil particles; it is quite soluble in water and therefore tends to be fairly mobile in soils. The rate of leaching depends in a complex way on pH. Despite its great ability to move through soils, dicamba residues have been found in water samples only infrequently and in very low concentrations. The contaminant, DMNA, volatilizes very quickly, within a matter of a few hours, and readily breaks down in the presence of light. Therefore, little is likely to remain on plant surfaces or in soils.

Health Effects

The long-term health effects of dicamba are uncertain at present. Initial tests had revealed no cancer-causing activity, but these tests have been declared invalid and the EPA has requested new tests. Moreover, as previously mentioned, dicamba has been found to be contaminated with DMNA, a known potent carcinogen. As a result, the EPA is considering restrictions on the use of dicamba.

Other tests for long-term effects indicate that dicamba is not *mutagenic*. Studies on rats show no birth defects or other reproductive impairment, but both have been observed in rabbits at relatively low doses. Dicamba is classified as slightly toxic in *acute toxicity* tests when administered by mouth and as a mild skin irritant in skin exposure tests. Inhalation tests indicate that it is a slight health hazard (category III) that warrants caution in handling.

Protection and Prevention

There are several alternative herbicides that can be used. For example, effective in the production of sugar are **glyphosate**, **paraquat**, and **2,4-D**, each of which has its own set of benefits and disadvantages. If dicamba is ingested, a physician should be notified and vomiting induced with water or Ipecac syrup. As with any pesticide, caution in handling and using dicamba is recommended to reduce chances of exposure.

Environmental Effects

Laboratory studies show that dicamba has a low toxicity to invertebrates and microorganisms, with a few exceptions. Some soil organisms have reduced growth rates when exposed to dicamba, and some aquatic invertebrates appear to be relatively more sensitive than others. In general, the herbicide is only slightly toxic to most marine and freshwater relatives of crabs and lobsters. Similarly, it seems to be slightly toxic to those fish and amphibian species that have been tested, although it should be noted that the number of species tested is quite small. As mentioned, however, it is extremely toxic at low concentrations to certain kinds of plants, such as the pea family and conifers, many of which are grown as crops.

Regulatory Status

Use is restricted to prevent water contamination. Dicamba may not be used in such a way that irrigation or domestic water supplies are contaminated. The EPA is presently reviewing available data on possible health effects.

Technical Information

Chemical name: 3,6-dichloro-*o*-anisic acid or 2-methyl–3,6-dichlorobenzoic acid
Chemical formula: $C_8H_6Cl_2O_3$
Government standards for food tolerances:
   sugarcane: 0.1 ppm
   asparagus: 3.0 ppm
Residue levels found on sugarcane:
   0.445 ppm
(Note the difference between the level of residue allowed to remain on sugarcane and the amount that has actually been detected.)

Further Reading

Federal Register. 1984. Vol. 49, no. 235. Washington, D.C.: U.S. Government Printing Office.
HAYES, W. J., JR. 1982. *Pesticides Studied in Man*. Baltimore, MD: Williams and Wilkins.

Dichlorvos

Trade Names

No-Pest Strip; Vapona

Introduction

The insecticidal action of dichlorvos was discovered in 1955. It is actually a gaseous breakdown product of another *organophosphate* insecticide called trichlorfon. Because it vaporizes so readily, dichlorvos is impractical for use on field crops, but it is used on pesticide strips to control insects in closed spaces, such as grain storehouses, mushroom houses, tobacco warehouses, greenhouses, restaurants, and other food-handling establishments. It is also impregnated in dog and cat flea collars. It is used to spray aircraft to prevent accidental introduction of unwanted pest species. Like other organophosphates, dichlorvos inhibits key enzymes involved in the transmission of nerve signals. No changes in enzyme activity, however, have been reported in people exposed to the typical concentrations used to kill unwanted insects in airplanes, particularly those arriving from tropical countries. Moreover, this insecticide is sufficiently selective that it is used in the treatment of certain internal parasites (roundworms) in people and other animals.

Physical and Chemical Properties

The pure material forms a colorless to amber-colored liquid with a mild chemical odor. It is slightly soluble in water, but decomposes rapidly under aqueous or moist conditions. Both strong acids and bases break it down readily. The vapor diffuses rapidly throughout closed spaces.

Exposure and Distribution

Dichlorvos is a commonly used insecticide, available to the householder as a liquid spray or impregnated in no-pest strips and flea collars. Its extensive use and effectiveness over a period of several months has led to wide-spread human exposure, which has become a cause of concern.

Health Effects

Recent evidence from two-year animal tests strongly suggests that dichlorvos causes cancer, although previous results were negative. In humans, however, a particularly high cancer risk seems to be associated with exposure to No-Pest Strips in the home. The EPA estimates a 1 in 100 chance of getting cancer from a lifetime exposure to levels typically released by the strips. Dichlorvos does not seem to cause birth defects in tests with rabbits and rats. Some bacterial tests suggest that this insecticide may cause *mutations*, but tests using mice and fruitflies were negative. While there have been a few reports of sterility associated with exposure to dichlorvos, most evidence indicates that there are no reproductive effects except at dose levels lethal to the mother.

Dichlorvos is moderately toxic to mammals; it is less *acutely toxic* than **parathion**, but more toxic than **malathion**. Symptoms of poisoning from this and other organophosphates vary from headache, nausea, and abdominal cramps to muscular weakness, cardiac irregularities, and cessation of breathing. Numerous instances of accidental human poisoning resulting in death following ingestion or dermal contact have been reported. Generally, symptoms develop quickly, and in nonfatal cases of poisoning, recovery from symptoms is rapid. Dichlorvos is *metabolized* and excreted in humans very rapidly; it does not *bioaccumulate*. It also does not transfer to milk when fed to cows.

Protection and Prevention

Treatment for poisoning is similar to that for other organophosphates: maintaining an open airway, artificial respiration, and administering counteractive drugs, such as atropine and pralidoxime, which interacts positively with atropine.

Environmental Effects

Dichlorvos enhances the toxicity of malathion, but only to a slight extent. It appears to have a beneficial effect in pregnant pigs; the birth weights and weights at weaning of young are increased.

Regulatory Status

Dichlorvos is undergoing a *Special Review* because of the estimated human cancer risk—one of the highest risk levels for any substance—from exposure to dichlorvos vapors. Dichlorvos is listed as a *hazardous air pollutant* in the 1990 Clean Air Act, requiring the EPA to set emission standards. It is also on the EPA *community right-to-know* list.

Technical Information

Chemical name: O,O-dimethyl-O,2,2-dichlorovinyl phosphate or 2,2-dichlorovinyl phosphate
Chemical formula: $C_4H_7Cl_2O_4P$
WHO no observable effects level in humans: 0.033 mg/kg
OSHA limit in workplace air: 1 mg/m^3

Further Reading

HAYES, W. J., JR. 1982. *Pesticides Studied in Man*. Baltimore, MD: Williams and Wilkins.
World Health Organization. 1984. *Environmental Health Criteria No. 63: Organophosphate Pesticides*. Geneva.

Dioxane

Other Names

1,4-Dioxane; *p*-dioxane; *p*-dioxan; di(ethyl-ene oxide); diethylene dioxide; diethylene ether; diethylene oxide

Trade Name

Holcomb's Window Cleaner

Introduction

Dioxane is an important commercial *solvent.* It is also used as a stabilizer during the manufacture of industrial paints. In some biology laboratories it is used to remove water from tissue samples, which are then studied under the microscope. It should not be confused with the similarly named chemical contaminant **dioxin**.

Physical and Chemical Properties

Dioxane is a synthetic organic compound with no known natural sources. It has a faint, pleasant, alcohol-like odor that can be recognized at low concentrations, but people tend to get used to the smell. The vapors are not irritating until dangerous concentrations are in the air. Pure dioxane is a colorless, volatile liquid that is heavier than water. The vapors are quite flammable and easily react with other chemicals used in industrial settings. It can be explosive when mixed with air. Dioxane is not easily broken down by microorganisms, although it does degrade upon prolonged exposure to light.

Exposure and Distribution

Production of dioxane in the United States averages a little less than 3000 tons annually. It is manufactured in the eastern and southern regions of the United States and shipped primarily via rail and truck in bottles, cans, and metal drums. Contact with high concentrations of dioxane is most likely at job sites where it is used, although the public may be exposed to it as a result of accidents or spills during shipping. Some consumer products make use of dioxane, most notably Holcomb's Window Cleaner.

Although dioxane has not been included in federal and state surveys of drinking water, it has been reported to occur in both surface water and groundwater. Distribution and average concentrations of the chemical in water are unknown. No information on its occurrence in food or air appears to be available.

Health Effects

Dioxane is readily absorbed through the skin, lungs, and *gastrointestinal tract.* It is a moderately *acute toxin,* but symptoms of overexposure may be delayed for hours following exposures that had erroneously been considered negligible. It easily penetrates the skin, and large amounts spilled on the skin or clothing can be life threatening. Dioxane spilled on the skin can be irritating. It can also make the skin dry with no other signs of irritation, but if it is allowed to remain on the skin or clothing, smarting and reddening of the skin may result. Some people show an *allergic* response when their skin comes into contact with dioxane.

The vapor can be irritating to the eyes, nose, and throat. Inhaled vapors can cause a slight smarting of the eyes or respiratory system if the chemical is present at high concentrations. Symptoms disappear when exposure to the chemical stops. Overexposure may also cause eye irritation and can permanently injure the cornea. Dioxane can also be inhaled in sufficient amounts to cause *systemic* intoxication, narcosis, *pulmonary edema*, and even death. The kidney and liver can be damaged as a result of acute inhalation exposure to dioxane. Dioxane can also cause kidney and liver damage if swallowed.

Chronic exposure to dioxane is also hazardous. Prolonged skin exposure can cause a rash or burn. Repeated exposure to levels that do not cause overt symptoms can lead to slowed central nervous system function and to liver and kidney damage. These symptoms may be delayed because the chemical has a tendency to accumulate in body tissue. Dioxane has been shown to cause liver and nasal cancers in laboratory rats and mice when low doses are administered orally over a long time. *Epidemiological* data indicating that dioxane is a human carcinogen are not available. The EPA has classified dioxane as a probable human carcinogen (a B_2 substance according to the classification in Table 5 of Chapter 3). Some evidence suggests that dioxane may suppress immune system function.

When dioxane is present in chlorinated water, a highly toxic compound is formed. One researcher found that chlorination of dioxane increased its toxicity 1000 times. Therefore, never pour unwanted dioxane down the drain.

Protection and Prevention

Dioxane is most likely to be encountered at the workplace. If solvents are used at work, be sure to learn the names of those used. Wear protective clothing when required. Request a *Material Safety Data Sheet (MSDS)* if solvents are part of your workplace environment. Avoid buying window cleaners that contain dioxane. Should you inhale, swallow, have skin contact with, or spill dioxane, get medical attention immediately. Remember that damage due to overexposure may be delayed by several hours.

Environmental Effects

The environmental fate of dioxane can only be estimated on the basis of the chemical's physical properties. Few actual measurements exist. Dioxane can be expected to evaporate from soil and surface water and to move easily through soil. This property, combined with dioxane's slow microbial degradation, implies that spilled dioxane could pose a toxic threat to groundwater supplies if concentrations were high enough.

Regulatory Status

Dioxane is listed as a *hazardous air pollutant* in the 1990 Clean Air Act, requiring the EPA to set emission standards. OSHA has set standards regarding maximum average concentrations found in workplace air. Dioxane is subject to *community right-to-know* reporting.

Technical Information

Chemical formula: $C_4H_8O_2$
Molecular weight: 88
Lowest reported lethal dose for humans:
    (oral): 500 mg/kg
    (inhaled for one week): 470 ppm

Further Reading

Agency for Toxic Substances and Disease Registry. 1988. *Toxicological Profile for 1,4-Dioxane.* Washington, D. C.: U.S. Public Health Service.
SAX, N. I. 1988. *p*-Dioxane. *Dangerous Properties of Industrial Materials Report*, January/February. New York: Van Nostrand Reinhold.

Dioxin

Other Name

TCDD

Trade Names

Agent Orange; Silvex

Introduction

Dioxin is thought to be one of the most toxic chemicals ever made by humans. The basis for this is animal testing, which reveals that the size of the dose of dioxin that can cause disease in some animals is lower than that for any other man-made chemical. Very low doses are also suspected to cause human illness.

Dioxin is an unavoidable by-product in the manufacture of certain herbicides such as **2,4,5-T**. In industrial processes involving the use of **chlorine**, dioxin is often inadvertently formed; one important example of such a process is the bleaching of paper, including that used in milk cartons. Dioxin can also be formed when organic wastes that contain chlorine are burned; the general mix of plastics found in municipal waste is likely to contain such organics. There are no known beneficial uses of dioxin.

The use of the herbicide Agent Orange (which is contaminated with dioxin) to defoliate the jungle during the Vietnam War resulted in the first public awareness of the hazards of dioxin because of claims that some of the soldiers, Vietnamese people, and domestic animals exposed to it became ill. The explosion at the chemical plant in Seveso, Italy, in 1976, which exposed thousands of people to dioxin, and the discovery of dioxin in toxic wastes at Times Beach, Missouri, further sparked public concern about this substance. There is still considerable debate about the magnitude of the actual risk dioxin poses to people, and as yet there is no widely accepted evidence that serious harm actually resulted from the exposures just mentioned.

There are a large number of different types of dioxin, but TCDD is believed to be the most dangerous, and the word "dioxin" in the popular press usually refers to this one type. Furans are a related group of chemicals, and the information provided here about dioxin is broadly applicable to the furans as well.

Physical and Chemical Properties

Dioxin occurs in the environment in quantities too small to be detected by odor or appearance. Herbicides that contain it are difficult to recognize unless labeled containers show the trade names Agent Orange or Silvex or indicate that 2,4,5-T (the chemical abbreviation for the herbicidal agent that contains dioxin) is present.

Dioxin will persist for many years in soil or in animal tissue, but in sunlight it degrades within a day or so to what are believed to be harmless products. Dioxin cannot be flushed away easily from contaminated surfaces because it is not very soluble; it probably accumulates in the fatty tissue of animals (see Chapter 10, Section A).

Exposure and Distribution

Exposure of the general public and especially of workers in herbicide factories to dioxin can result from skin contact with herbicides containing it. This used to be the major exposure route of concern, but the concentration of dioxin in 2,4,5-T is about 1000 times less today than it was during the Vietnam War because of improvements in the manufacturing process. That fact, plus the identification of other mechanisms by which dioxin can be released into the environment, have recently shifted attention to other sources. One exposure pathway is breathing of, or skin contact with, the fumes and ash that result from burning municipal garbage, particularly if the garbage contains polyvinyl chloride or other organic substances containing chlorine. Eating contaminated fish, particularly those living downstream of paper pulp mills, is an additional source.

Recently, there has been considerable publicity directed at bleached paper and cardboard food containers, which often contain trace amounts of dioxin that can contaminate the food they contain. Milk cartons are of particular concern, and an evaluation of this risk has recently been released by the FDA. Their regulatory finding is summarized under the Regulatory Status section. Cardboard containers for juices and microwave dinners are also possible sources of dioxin in food. Disposable diapers, tampons, and toilet paper made from bleached paper are additional potential sources of exposure to dioxin. Dioxin is also found in waste water discharged from industrial plants that bleach paper or that use chlorine in other ways, such as in certain metallurgical processes, and in the manufacture of certain wood preservatives, such as pentachlorophenol.

Health Effects

Symptoms of human exposure include chloracne (a skin eruption resembling acne), headaches, dizziness, digestive disorders, and generalized aches and pains. Chloracne can result from exposure to as little as one-billionth of an ounce of dioxin. Some recent *epidemiological* studies indicate that exposure to larger amounts of dioxin can result in at least one type of cancer (soft tissue sarcoma) in people, but not all epidemiological studies support this claim. Quantitative and widely accepted dose–response information is also lacking. Animal studies reveal that exposure to dioxin can result in various types of cancer, liver and kidney ailments, fetal death, and birth deformities. But the minimum dose of dioxin needed to cause cancer in animals varies by as much as a factor of 5000 from one species to another, so drawing conclusions from these studies about the sensitivity of people is difficult. The FDA estimates that for every one million average milk drinkers in the United States, five will get cancer as a result of dioxin in milk containers, but a reduction in this risk is pending (see Regulatory Status section).

Protection and Prevention

No antidote for dioxin is known. As for all herbicides, those contaminated with dioxin should be disposed of properly. If possible, stay sufficiently far from areas where herbicides are used or organic wastes are being burned to avoid fumes and fallout. Since garbage incineration is being proposed in many urban areas, readers may want to discuss with local political leaders and scientists the risks and benefits of this method of waste processing (see also Chapter 16). Do not use herbicides such as Agent Orange or Silvex that contain 2,4,5-T. Avoid use of chlorine-bleached paper and cardboard products when possible. (Even if the dioxin threat from this source ultimately proves to be negligible, such action will reduce the toxic threat from chlorine-containing bleaching agents, as well.) Substitutes for the use of chlorine in the paper-bleaching process exist. Products made in this way are increasingly available and should be used. Do not eat fish caught from waters contaminated with the discharge from paper pulp mills.

Environmental Effects

Exposure to dioxin can cause cancers, birth defects, and fetal death in domestic and wild animals.

Regulatory Status

Currently all herbicidal products containing 2,4,5-T (and hence, dioxin) are banned by the federal government for most uses, but are still permitted on rangelands and rice fields. Dioxin is also regulated under the Clean Water Act. One type of dioxin, 2,3,7,8-tetrachloro-dibenzo-*p*-dioxin, is listed as a *hazardous air pollutant* in the 1990 Clean Air Act, requiring the EPA to set emission standards. In 1989, the FDA ordered that by 1992, manufacturers of milk cartons must alter the bleaching process to greatly reduce dioxin levels in cardboard containers.

Technical Information

Chemical name: 2,3,7,8-tetrachlorodibenzo-p-dioxin

The full name of the ingredient in Agent Orange that contains dioxin is 2,4,5-trichlorophenoxyacetic acid (abbreviated 2,4,5-T). The dioxin-containing ingredient in Silvex is 2–2(2,4,5-trichlorophenoxy)propionic acid (abbreviated 2,4,5-TP). Polychlorinated biphenyls (**PCBs**) may also contain TCDD.

The highest levels of dioxin found in discharge waters from paper pulp mills are about 0.5 part per trillion. Typical concentrations of dioxin in bleached paper products range from undetectable up to about 10 parts per trillion. Fish found downstream of paper pulp mills can contain nearly 200 parts per trillion of dioxin, with levels of 50 parts per trillion not uncommon. As of 1989, milk in cardboard containers in the United States contained dioxin at levels of several hundredths to nearly one part per trillion. It is estimated that the current daily intake of dioxin in the United States averages about 20×10^{-12} grams per kilogram of body weight.

Further Reading

American Medical Association. 1981. *The Health Effects of "Agent Orange" and Polychlorinated Dioxin Contaminants.* Chicago.
GALSTON, A. W. 1979. Herbicides: A Mixed Blessing. *Bioscience* 29(2):85–94.
TSCHIRLEY, F. 1986. Dioxin. *Scientific American* 254(2):29–35.

Di(2-ethylhexyl)phthalate

Other Names

DEHP; 1,2-benzenedicarboxylic acid; bis-(2-ethylhexyl) ester; phthalic acid; bis(2-ethylhexyl) ester; BEHP; bis(ethylhexyl) ester; bis(2-ethylhexyl)phthalate; di(2-ethylhexyl)-orthophthalate; di(ethylhexyl)phthalate; dioctyl phthalate; DOP; 2-ethylhexyl phthalate; octyl phthalate; phthalic acid; dioctyl ester

Trade Names

Bisoflex 81; Bisoflex DOP; Compound 889; DAF 68; Ergoplast FDO; Eviplast 80; Eviplast 81; Fleximel; Flexol DOP; Good-Rite GP 264; Hatcol DOP; Kodaflex DOP; Mollan O; Nuoplaz DOP; Octoil; Platinol AH; Platinol DOP; Pittsburg PX–138; Reomol DOP; Reomol D 79P; Sicol 150; Staflex DOP; Truflex DOP; Vestinol AH; Vinicizer 80; Witcizer 312.

Introduction

Di(2-ethylhexyl)phthalate or DEHP is a chemical added to plastic to make it soft and flexible. It is one of several chemicals that are used to keep plastic soft, but DEHP is the one to which people are most likely to be exposed. More than one-third of the weight of many soft plastics may be DEHP. It is widely used in consumer products such as imitation leather, rainwear, footwear, upholstery foams, flooring, tablecloths, shower curtains, food packaging materials, and children's toys. Unfortunately, plasticizers such as DEHP do not become a permanent part of the plastic product in which they are used. Almost 2000 tons of DEHP are lost from plastic products each year, eventually to be deposited into the air, water, and soil. A similar amount is released into the atmosphere every year during the manufacture of plastic and plastic products.

Physical and Chemical Properties

Di(2-ethylhexyl)phthalate is a clear, oily liquid with a slight odor that is commonly associated with the smell of plastic. It is not very soluble in water, but it is highly soluble in fat. Because of these properties, foods (or other materials) that have a high level of fat or oil tend to pull DEHP from their packaging into the wrapped product.

Exposure and Distribution

This chemical has been detected in air, water, and soil, as well as in food, blood, and plasma stored in plastic containers made with DEHP. The most significant route of exposure for the average person is through contaminated food. Food, particularly that which is high in fat, is easily contaminated with DEHP when stored in plastic containers. Water brought into the house in polyvinyl chloride pipes can also become contaminated with DEHP. Moreover, DEHP is a ubiquitous contaminant. Low concentrations are found almost everywhere in the air, water, soil, and food. Indoor air can also become contaminated with low levels of DEHP as a result of *outgassing* from plastic products.

People who must rely on dialysis treatments or who receive transfusions of large quantities of blood stored in plastic containers are exposed to much higher doses of DEHP than the average person. DEHP tends to migrate into blood or other body fluids collected or transported in plastic containers and tubes. Another highly exposed group of people are workers who formulate or process plastics. There are more than 600,000 people in the United States that receive larger than average doses of DEHP from dialysis, regular blood transfusions, and occupational exposure.

Health Effects

Very few acute health problems are caused by DEHP, even when high concentrations are inhaled. It is mildly irritating when spilled on the skin. However, long-term exposure to DEHP is associated with liver damage and testicular injury. Moreover, DEHP has been shown to cause liver tumors in rats and mice. Humans may be less susceptible to cancer caused by DEHP exposure because the chemical is *metabolized* differently in humans than it is in rodents. However, not enough data are available to evaluate possible cancer risks adequately in humans.

Protection and Prevention

In today's world, it is difficult to avoid soft plastics, but with a little effort and creative thinking, it is possible. Most DEHP exposure can be avoided by not storing food in plastic containers and poly bags. Be particularly careful not to use plastic containers for food storage that were not designed to be used with food, such as baby bathtubs, plastic garbage cans, and sweater storage boxes. Don't use plastic food wrap, especially in the microwave (heat accelerates DEHP outgassing). Don't buy large soft plastic items such as shower curtains and foam-filled furniture. There are good substitutes for most of these plastic products such as glass containers, waxed paper, cotton shower curtains, and polyester- and down-filled furniture. Exposure to some DEHP in food is probably unavoidable, however, because the use of DEHP-containing plastic tubing in food processing is widespread. Diets high in **zinc** may protect against testicular injury from chronic high DEHP exposure.

Throwing out soft plastics does not solve the problem, however, because DEHP leaches into groundwater and outgasses into the air from landfills. It is best to avoid bringing soft plastic home at all.

Environmental Effects

It tends to accumulate in sediments and adhere to particulate matter.

Regulatory Status

The FDA stipulates that materials containing high levels of DEHP cannot be used to store foods that are high in fat because of DEHP's tendency to migrate into fatty material. However, these containers are often used for imported food, food that is not high in fat, and food stored at home in reused plastic containers. DEHP is on the EPA *community right-to-know* list. It is also listed as a *hazardous air pollutant* in the 1990 Clean Air Act, requiring the EPA to set emission standards.

Technical Information

Chemical formula: $C_{24}H_{38}O_4$
Molecular weight: 390
Amount produced: 3–4 million tons/year
Amount released by industry into environment: 3200 tons/year
Typical exposure levels for consumers:
    from food: 0.3 mg/day
    from water: 0.002 mg/day
    from ambient air: 0.0004 mg/day
Typical exposure level for plastic workers:
    0.3 mg/day average (in addition to ambient sources)
OSHA limit in workplace air: 5 mg/m^3

Further Reading

Agency for Toxic Substances and Disease Registry. 1988. *Di(2-ethylhexyl)phthalate*. Washington, D.C.: U.S. Department of Health.

EBDCs: Mancozeb, Maneb, Metiram, and Zineb

Other Name

Ethylenebisdithiocarbamates

Trade Names

Dithane M–45; Dithane M–22 or Manzate; Polyram; Dithane Z–78

Introduction

The four pesticides mancozeb, maneb, metiram, and zineb are discussed as a group because of their close structural and functional similarities. Together they constitute a subclass of the *carbamate* pesticides called the ethylenebisdithiocarbamates (EBDCs). The four EBDCs share properties with several other dithiocarbamate pesticides and the drug Antabuse (disulfiram), which is used in the treatment of alcoholism. Introduced between the 1930s and the 1960s, the EBDCs are the mostly widely used group of fungicides in the world, accounting for about 57% of fungicide use worldwide. In the United States alone more than 30 million tons of EBDCs are used each year. They are *broad spectrum* fungicides (effective against a wide variety of fungi) that are not absorbed by the plant, but nevertheless control nearly all the leaf diseases of vegetables in the United States. The EBDCs are used on a variety of fruits, vegetables, and small grains, including raisins, cereal grains, brans, apples, potatoes, grapes, corn, wild rice, tomatoes, onions, citrus crops, and animal feeds. Maneb is used on some 56 crops, while mancozeb is used on 44 crops.

This group of fungicides has a number of additional desirable characteristics. They are inexpensive and generally nontoxic to plants, and there is no evidence that the target species have developed *resistance* to the pesticide. They are compatible with a number of other pesticides, which gives them a broader range of use. The EBDCs are effectively employed in some *Integrated Pest Management* programs. They are not without risks, however. The EBDCs are readily metabolized by living organisms and degraded in the environment to ethylene thiourea (ETU), a potent cancer-causing agent.

Physical and Chemical Properties

The EBDCs contain one or more atoms of either manganese or **zinc** attached to otherwise similar organic structures, but they differ considerably in their physical properties. Maneb and zineb, for example, are structurally identical except that maneb contains manganese whereas zineb is zinc based. Maneb, a yellow, crystalline solid, is moderately soluble in water and stable under normal storage conditions, but it decomposes readily when exposed to moisture or acids. In contrast, zineb is a light-colored powder that is only slightly soluble in water and unstable in light, heat, and moisture. The solubility of mancozeb, which consists of maneb joined to a zinc ion, is unknown. The common breakdown product and contaminant of all the EBDCs, ethylene thiourea, is soluble in water.

Exposure and Distribution

The EBDCs are applied chiefly as dusts and sprays to protect the surface parts of plants. In the United States, about 16 million pounds of mancozeb are applied annually, mostly as foliar sprays, and another 10 million pounds of maneb are used. Together they account for about 85% of total EBDC consumption. Mancozeb is used primarily on apples, potatoes, and tomatoes. Also, about 80% of the onion acreage in the United States is treated with mancozeb.

Although about one-third of all the fruit and vegetable crops in the United States are treated with EBDCs, they are among the large group of pesticides that cannot be detected on or in foods using routine FDA testing methods. Nor does the primary metabolic product, degradation product, and contaminant ETU show up in the routine tests. Therefore, it is uncertain to what extent people are exposed to the EBDCs and ETU, although it is thought likely that the primary route of exposure to the general population is through contaminated fruits and vegetables. In aqueous conditions, about half the ETU residue will break down in one to two days. It has the potential to *leach* from soils.

Health Effects

In animal studies, the EBDCs have an extremely low *acute toxicity*. Nevertheless, signs of poisoning have been observed following high doses, including tremors, gastrointestinal problems, decreased coordination, and decreased kidney function.

All are classified as probable human carcinogens (group B_2) by the EPA, chiefly because of the inevitable presence of ETU. An increase in lung and liver cancers in mice and in thyroid cancer in rats has been associated with the EBDCs. Moreover, this group of fungicides appears to cause birth defects as well. Studies show that the EBDCs are toxic to the thyroid gland; the smallest doses that produce any detectable effect will affect the thyroid. The contaminant and breakdown product, ETU, is an even potent more cause of cancers, birth defects, and thyroid disorders. Both maneb and zineb are linked to an increase in various reproductive effects, including sterility and stillbirths.

Interaction with alcohol greatly increases the toxicity of EBDCs, which could pose a problem for farm or factory workers exposed to relatively high levels of the fungicides. The EBDCs can cause inflammation of the skin and/or irritation of the mucous membranes. Some kinds of anemia have been found in workers exposed to zineb.

Protection and Prevention

Protective clothing is required for all applicators and others handling the pesticides.

Labels on pesticide containers carry a warning of acute aquatic toxicity. There are registered, effective alternative fungicides for nearly all EBDC uses, but they are more expensive, sometimes prohibitively so, particularly in humid, moist regions, and not without risks. Because the fungicides are not absorbed by the plant, it is likely that residues can be removed by washing and/or peeling fresh produce. There is no special antidote; in cases of poisoning the symptoms are treated. But because of the similarities between the EBDCs and Antabuse, alcohol should not be given in cases of poisoning.

Environmental Effects

This group of pesticides is acutely toxic to various aquatic organisms, particularly cold water fishes and certain invertebrates, and therefore poses a serious hazard to the environment. Toxicity varies with species; the EBDCs are of moderate acute toxicity to warm water fishes.

Regulatory Status

Residue *tolerances* (maximum amount permitted in or on food) have been established for about 150 food items, but none for milk, meat, and eggs even though the EBDCs are applied to animal feed and can be expected to show up in animal products. Nor have any tolerances been established for ETU, although it has been detected on agricultural products. Evidence linking EBDCs with tumors, birth defects, and acute toxicity to various aquatic organisms has triggered a *Special Review* to determine whether to continue existing registration and use standards.

Technical Information

Chemical names:
  mancozeb: manganese, 1,2-ethanediyl-
          bis(carbamo-dithioate) ×
          zinc
  maneb: manganese, 1,2-ethanediyl-
          bis(carbamo-dithioate)

metiram: mixture of zinc ethylene-
          bis(dithiocarbamates) and
          ethylenebisdithiocarbamic
          acid cyclic anhydrosulfides
zineb: zinc ethylenebisdithiocar-
          bamate

Chemical formulas:
  mancozeb: $C_4H_6MnN_4S_4[Zn]$
  maneb: $C_4H_6MnN_4S_4$
  zineb: $C_4H_6ZnN_2S_4$

Comparative toxicities based on the LD_{50} or LC_{50} of mancozeb to different species:
    LD_{50} for rats: >5000 ppm
    LC_{50} for trout: 0.46 ppm
    LC_{50} for bluegill: 1.54 ppm
    LC_{50} for daphnia: 0.58 ppm

Further Reading

Environmental Protection Agency. 1987. *EPA Guidance for Reregistration of Pesticide Products Containing Mancozeb as the Active Ingredient.* Washington, D.C.

HAYES, W. J., JR. 1982. *Pesticides Studied in Man.* Baltimore, MD: Williams and Wilkins.

MOTT, L., and SNYDER, K. 1987. *Pesticide Alert.* San Francisco: Sierra Club Books.

Ethylene Dibromide (EDB) and Ethylene Dichloride (EDC)

Trade Name

Dowfume (EDC)

Introduction

Ethylene dibromide (EDB) gained a great deal of notoriety a few years ago when residues of the probable cancer-causing *fumigant* were detected on foods. As a result of the uproar, the use of EDB as a pesticide was banned. A similar *organochlorine*, ethylene dichloride (EDC), is also an effective fumigant. Both have been used since the mid-1920s to kill insects, insect eggs, and certain microorganisms in grain elevators, warehouses, buildings, soils, and green houses, as well as in packaged products such as breakfast cereals, dried fruits, and grains. EDB, however, has been used much more extensively than EDC.

Ethylene dibromide and ethylene dichloride share not only a very similar chemical structure, but also similar properties, uses, and effects. The narcotic properties of EDC have long been recognized; in fact, it was used as an anesthetic as far back as 1848. These narcotic effects are actually the basis of the fumigant activity of both EDB and EDC. Since the 1920s, both EDB and EDC have been used as **lead** scavengers in gasoline containing tetraalkyl lead compounds. About 90% of the EDB used has been to prevent the buildup of lead in car engines. This use is declining as lead is being rapidly phased out of gasoline. Both EDB and EDC have been found as groundwater contaminants and appear to cause cancer.

While a major use of EDB has been as a fumigant, the primary use of EDC is as an industrial solvent and in the production of **vinyl chloride**, a known carcinogen.

Physical and Chemical Properties

EDB and EDC are heavy liquids with a **chloroform**-like odor. They become gases at temperatures greater than 40°F. The two compounds are similarly stable (meaning they do not easily decompose), noncorrosive, and only slightly soluble in water. EDC is highly flammable. Because fumigants can be lethal to people at very low doses, they are often intentionally spiked with a substance that has a strong tear gas effect to serve as an indicator or warning of exposure. The two compounds are commonly mixed with **carbon tetrachloride**.

Exposure and Distribution

According to 1982 estimates, about 3.5 million tons of ethylene dichloride were produced domestically that year. Of that, approximately 84% was used to produce vinyl chloride. EDC is an intermediate in the production of various chlorinated *solvents*. Other minor uses include grain fumigation, textile and polyvinyl chloride (PVC) cleaning, metal degreasing, and the manufacture of paints, varnish removers, and soaps.

EDC can enter the environment through atmospheric emissions, waste effluents to waterways, and land disposal of liquid and solid wastes. Its high volatility suggests that it evaporates quickly from soil and water and that much ends up in the atmosphere via this route. Roughly one-half of the atmospheric emissions are released directly at production sites, where outdoor air concentrations have been found to be high. Dispersed applications, such as the volatilization of paints and the fumigation of grains, account for about one-third of the atmospheric emissions.

While concentrations of EDC and EDB detected in groundwater and surface waters are generally low (ranging from less than 1.0 to 10 $\mu g/L$), there is evidence that they can *leach* from soils into groundwater. Because evaporation rates from underground water are low, EDC and EDB can accumulate in *aquifers* used for drinking water. Given current projections of increased production of EDC, continuing contamination of groundwater is likely. Moreover, it has been suggested that EDC is produced in domestic water supplies as a result of chlorination. But the low levels in drinking water and food appear to pose little risk for the general public.

The primary route of exposure to EDC is by inhalation of polluted air. Because of the relatively high *ambient* concentrations, people living in the vicinity of production and use facilities face a greater risk of exposure to significant levels of ethylene dichloride than the general population. In women exposed at the workplace, it has been found that EDC accumulates in breast milk and remains there for about 18 hours following exposure.

Health Effects

Tests show that EDC is readily absorbed from the *gastrointestinal tract*, and there are numerous reports of poisoning in humans as a result of accidental or suicidal ingestion. Tests and case studies of responses to skin exposure are inconclusive, although rash and skin irritation are commonly associated with skin contact.

EDB is highly *acutely toxic* both orally and dermally, much more so than EDC. The symptoms of poisoning by EDB and EDC resemble those caused by various related *halogenated hydrocarbons* and include any of several central nervous system and gastrointestinal problems such as dizziness, nausea, headache, vomiting, diarrhea, dilated pupils, weak pulse, cyanosis, and unconsciousness. Poisoning deaths result from circulatory and respiratory failure. Liver and kidney damage and usually reversible changes in the cornea of the eye have been linked to exposure to EDC and EDB. EDB is also irritating to mucous membranes.

In mammals, the normal *metabolism* of EDC produces *metabolites* (including chloroacetaldehyde, chloroacetic acid, and chloroethanol) that appear to be several times more toxic than the parent compound. The metabolic products bind more strongly to DNA than does EDC; such binding reactions are involved in the development of *mutations*, birth defects, and cancers. Although EDC metabolism in humans has not been

well studied, it is assumed to be similar to that in rats and mice.

On the basis of animal test results, the EPA has listed EDC as a group B_2 carcinogen (see Chapter 3, Section B). It causes cancer in dietary tests with both rats and mice and causes mutations in bacteria, plants, *Drosophila*, and mammalian cells, but it does not appear to cause reproductive or developmental effects at concentrations below those that would be toxic to the mother. There is insufficient *epidemiological* evidence to determine whether EDC causes birth defects or reproductive effects in humans.

Ethylene dibromide appears to be a more potent carcinogen than EDC, presumably because of its greater ability to bind to DNA and cellular proteins. The carcinogenicity of EDB is enhanced by certain dietary substances and drugs (such as disulfiram), which inhibit a particular enzyme system involved in the metabolism of EDB. Both mutations and reproductive effects are caused by EDB in test systems.

Protection and Prevention

Fumigants are able to penetrate not only the skin and the membranes that line the respiratory and gastrointestinal tracts, but also rubber and plastics used in protective clothing. Moreover, ordinary respirators are not very effective. Workers engaged in the manufacture or application of EDC or EDB should avoid coming into contact with these compounds, either through skin contact or inhalation, by following stringent precautions detailed by the EPA and the manufacturer. If the skin or eyes are contaminated, they should be washed or flushed with water immediately.

Environmental Effects

In the atmosphere, EDC is expected to react with other chemical compounds and thus break down fairly rapidly. Some of the breakdown products (such as chloroacetyl chloride) may persist long enough to react with **ultraviolet radiation**, producing **chlorine**, which contributes to the destruction of the Earth's protective ozone layer.

Because EDC is excreted relatively rapidly once absorbed and because its high volatility makes it generally unavailable for excessive uptake, it is unlikely to *bioaccumulate* to any significant extent. In contrast, recent evidence suggests that EDB is far more persistent (up to 20 years) in topsoil than predicted on the basis of its volatility and water solubility. In laboratory experiments, residues of EDB become tightly bound to or entrapped in soils.

Regulatory Status

Ethylene dibromide is no longer in use as a pesticide because of its carcinogenicity. In 1983, the EPA issued emergency suspension orders (an unusual move taken against only four pesticides to date) on all soil treatments with EDB, along with a phase-out of fruit and vegetable fumigation. The action came nearly a decade after studies revealed that EDB causes cancer and birth defects in test animals. Certain uses were permitted while the EPA considered cancellation. Finally in 1984, registration for all major uses of EDB was canceled and all existing stocks were recalled for disposal. Moreover, under the Clean Air Act, EDC is listed as a *hazardous air pollutant*. It is also on the *community right-to-know* list.

Technical Information

Chemical names:

  EDB: 1,2-dibromoethane
  EDC: 1,2-dichloroethane

Chemical formulas:
  EDB: $C_2H_4Br_2$
  EDC: $C_2H_4Cl_2$

Comparative toxicity (LD_{50}, oral):
  EDB: 117–146 mg/kg
  EDC: 670–850 mg/kg

OSHA limits in workplace air:

	EDB	EDC
average over 8 hours	20 ppm	50 ppm
maximum ceiling for 5 minutes in any 3-hour period	30 ppm	100 ppm
	50 ppm	200 ppm

Further Reading

Environmental Protection Agency. 1985. *Health Assessment Document for 1,2-Dichloroethane (Ethylene Dichloride)*. North Carolina: Research Triangle Park.

———. 1983. *Ethylene Dibromide Special Review Position Document 4*. Washington, D.C.

HAYES, W. J., JR. 1982. *Pesticides Studied in Man*. Baltimore, MD: Williams and Wilkins.

Ethylene Glycol

Other Names

1,2-Dihydroxyethane; 1,2-ethanediol; ethylene alcohol; ethylene dihydrate

Trade Names

Dowtherm SR 1; Fridex; Macrogol 400 BPC; Norkool; Ramp; Tescal; Ucar 17; Zerex

Introduction

Ethylene glycol is familiar to almost every car owner as automobile antifreeze, but it is also used in a wide range of other products such as polyester, cosmetics, paints, ink, glues, wood stains, tobacco products, and automobile brake fluid. It is also used for manufacturing countless other chemicals, and it is a popular industrial *solvent*, making ethylene glycol one of the top 20 chemicals in production volume. It is of historical interest as well because the 1935 Federal Food, Drug, and Cosmetic Act was passed after the deaths of many people who had taken a drug sweetened with ethylene glycol.

Physical and Chemical Properties

Ethylene glycol is a clear, colorless, syrupy liquid with a sweet taste. It is capable of absorbing about twice its weight in water. It evaporates slowly at room temperature, but once heated to temperatures typical of automobile engines, it readily evaporates.

Exposure and Distribution

Ethylene glycol is widely distributed in American homes, and it is found in high concentrations in most motor vehicle antifreeze and brake fluids. Cosmetics, particularly those with a creamy texture, often contain it. Ethylene glycol formulations are also likely to be encountered at industrial and manufacturing sites, auto wrecking yards, service stations, and other locations where automobiles are used and serviced. It is also found in low concentrations in urban air.

Health Effects

Ethylene glycol is a dangerous poison. While it does not evaporate fast enough at room temperature to pose a health risk, some chronically exposed people report headaches and throat irritation upon inhalation of vapors. Nevertheless, dangerous amounts of ethylene glycol can be quickly inhaled when the chemical is heated. In addition, ethylene glycol *aerosol* can become attached to airborne dust, allowing dangerous amounts of the chemical to be inhaled and enter the bloodstream. Although liquid ethylene glycol produces no significant irritation when spilled on the skin, it is extremely dangerous when swallowed. Lethal doses range from about one-half cup for adults to a few tablespoons for children and pets.

During the first 12 hours following overexposure, the exposed person appears drunk, although no alcohol odor is evident on the breath. If large amounts are inhaled or swallowed, convulsions and coma will also occur. Other signs of overexposure to ethylene glycol include irregularities of the eye, such as rapid eye movement, paralysis of the eye muscles, and blurred vision. Reflexive movement may also be slowed, or body muscles may twitch rapidly. After about 12 hours, high blood pressure, rapid heartbeat, and shallow rapid breathing are experienced. If the patient is still alive after 24 to 72 hours, irreversible kidney damage begins to occur. The severity of all these symptoms depends on the amount of ethylene glycol absorbed after exposure to the chemical. Anyone who has swallowed ethylene glycol or inhaled hot vapors must be seen by a doctor immediately. Ethylene glycol exposure does not appear to cause cancer or birth defects. It was found to be nonmutagenic in the *Ames test*.

Protection and Prevention

Most ethylene glycol poisoning incidents occur among children and pets since they are attracted to its sweet taste. Antifreeze and brake fluid leaks from motor vehicles are common sources of exposure, so all fluids that leak from a car should be cleaned up. Children should not be allowed to play in garages or storage areas where automobiles or auto supplies are kept. Children should also not be allowed to play in vacant lots where cars or trucks are stored because ethylene glycol spills, although invisible, will make the soil taste sweet. Automobile antifreeze and brake fluids are being developed that do not contain ethylene glycol, with the most promising substitute being the related, and seemingly less toxic, propylene glycol. Cosmetics that contain ethylene glycol will list the ingredient on their labels.

Environmental Effects

Wildlife is attracted to the sweet taste of ethylene glycol, so spills onto the soil or street should be cleaned up immediately. Its vapors contribute to the formation of urban **ozone** pollution.

Regulatory Status

The FDA does not allow ethylene glycol to be used in foods or drugs. Because of its toxicity, the FDA has warned cosmetics manufacturers not to use it in creams that may be spread over large areas of the body (such as sunscreens). OSHA regulations specify an air concentration ceiling level that may not be exceeded at any time. Ethylene glycol is on the EPA *community right-to-know* list. It is also listed as a *hazardous air pollutant* in the 1990 Clean Air Act, requiring the EPA to set emission standards.

Technical Information

Chemical formula: $C_2H_6O_2$
Molecular weight: 62
Amount evaporated from U.S. automobiles: 50,000 tons/year
Adult lethal dose (LD_{50}): 3–4 oz
Regulatory information:
   OSHA ceiling value in air: 50 ppm
   FDA: may only be used in some cosmetics and in packaging adhesives

EPA: routine emissions must be reported annually; spills into waterways must be reported

Further Reading

ARENA, JAY M., and DREW, RICHARD H., eds. 1986. *Poisoning: Toxicology, Symptoms, Treatments*. Springfield, IL: Charles C. Thomas, Publisher.

LINNANVUO-LAITINEN, M., and HUTTUMEN, K. 1986. Ethylene Glycol Intoxication. *Clinical Toxicology* 24:167–174.

Ethylene Oxide

Other Names

Dimethylene oxide; 1,2-epoxy ethane; oxirane; EtO

Introduction

Ethylene oxide is an important industrial chemical used as a *fumigant,* to sterilize medical and dental instruments, and during the manufacture of other chemicals. It is one of the top 25 chemicals produced in the United States, with nearly three million tons of it manufactured in 1986 alone. Ethylene oxide may also be emitted during combustion of organic materials and from natural biological processes.

Most ethylene oxide is used to manufacture **ethylene glycol** (which is used in automotive antifreeze and to make polyester) as well as various detergents, *solvents,* adhesive additives, and polyurethane foam. Although sterilization uses account for only a small fraction of the ethylene oxide used, it is the most likely source of exposure for the average person. Ethylene oxide is used to sterilize delicate medical instruments that would be otherwise destroyed by heat and hot water sterilization systems. It is also used to eliminate pests from books, furniture, textiles, and cosmetic and dairy packaging. It is sometimes used to sterilize beehives.

Physical and Chemical Properties

Ethylene oxide is a colorless, flammable gas at room temperature. It has an ether-like odor. Exposure leaves a peculiar taste in the mouth. It dissolves easily in water and various organic solvents.

Exposure and Distribution

People exposed to the highest concentrations of ethylene oxide are those that work in industries where ethylene oxide is used, stored, or transported. These industries include chemical manufacturing, companies that fumigate spices, health care facilities, some museums and libraries, pharmaceutical and medical device manufacturers, some furniture makers, specialty gas transportation companies, and chemical distribution companies. Transport and storage companies are included in this list because small amounts of the gas easily leak from storage facilities. Significant ethylene oxide residues have been found on instruments sterilized in ethylene oxide.

People who do not work directly with ethylene oxide can be exposed to it via outdoor air near hospitals that use ethylene oxide sterilizers or near factories and distribution companies that use or store the chemical. Ethylene oxide residues are also found in tobacco smoke and in some foods. The group of food additives known as polysorbates, and an ethylene oxide polymer used in beer, are suspected of *outgassing* ethylene oxide into food.

Health Effects

Inhaling high levels of ethylene oxide can cause central nervous system depression, respiratory tract and mucous membrane irritation, vomiting, loss of coordination, and convulsions. Recurrent exposure to moderately high doses causes similar symptoms. Skin and eye contact with liquid or gaseous ethylene oxide causes burning. Repeated contact with the gas may cause the formation of cataracts. Some people develop an *allergy* to ethylene oxide.

Ethylene oxide causes various forms of cancer in laboratory animals. Evidence from studies on both animals and humans suggests that ethylene oxide is capable of causing leukemia, stomach cancer, brain tumors, and possibly breast cancer. Ethylene oxide has also been shown to cause genetic damage in several tests, including those conducted with bacteria, rodents, and monkeys. It thus appears to be a *mutagen.* Limited data on humans support this conclusion. Ethylene oxide appears to pose a risk to the fetus as well. It caused birth defects in mice, rats, and rabbits at doses that did not cause ill effects in the mothers. Exposure may cause an increased risk of spontaneous abortions in humans.

Protection and Prevention

People who work in hospitals or other health care facilities that use ethylene oxide sterilizers should try to avoid areas where the sterilizers are routinely used. Operators of such equipment should be sure to follow all operating procedures carefully. Pregnant women should be particularly careful to avoid areas where ethylene oxide is used. All workers who think that they may be handling ethylene oxide should request a *Material Safety Data Sheet (MSDS)* to learn more about potential hazardous and protective measures available to them.

It is more difficult to avoid ethylene oxide in outdoor air. The area around a hospital is likely to contain more ethylene oxide in the air than other areas of a city. People who routinely work with ethylene oxide might want to avoid buying a house next to a hospital that uses ethylene oxide sterilizers.

Regulatory Status

Ethylene oxide concentrations at the workplace are regulated by OSHA. Ethylene oxide is on the EPA *community right-to-know* list. It is also listed as a *hazardous air pollutant* in the 1990 Clean Air Act, requiring the EPA to set emission standards.

Technical Information

Chemical symbol: C_2H_4O
Molecular weight: 44
Emissions from typical large city hospital: 2 tons/year
Typical exposures from outdoor air:
  urban air: 50 ppt (parts per trillion)
  near places that manufacture, store, or use large quantities of ethylene oxide: 160–17,000 ppt
  near rural hospitals: 9 ppt
Other exposures:
  from food: 10 μg/day
  from tobacco smoke: 140 μg/day (for the smoker)
OSHA limit in workplace air: 1 ppm

Further Reading

World Health Organization. 1985. *Environmental Health Criteria No. 55: Ethylene Oxide.* Geneva.

Extremely Low Frequency Electromagnetic Fields

Other Names

ELF fields; low frequency electromagnetic fields; high-voltage transmission lines (HVTLs); high tension wires

Introduction

Exposure to extremely low frequency electromagnetic fields or ELF fields is practically inescapable in today's society. Such fields exist wherever alternating current (ac) flows along transmission lines or into electric appliances. Electricity produced by batteries is not alternating (it is direct current, or dc) and does not produce ELF fields; therefore, it is not of concern to us here. Intense electric shocks, which can cause severe burns, muscular spasms, brain dysfunction, and death, are also not what concerns us here. Such shocks result from the direct passage of a strong electric current through the body. ELF fields also penetrate the body, but they instead induce tiny electric currents. Any health damage produced by ELF fields is far more subtle than that resulting from a serious electric shock.

Extremely low frequency fields have been proposed for use by the U.S. Navy for undersea communication with submarines. In medicine, they are occasionally used to stimulate growth of bone tissue to repair fractures. ELF fields are also used in cathode ray tubes, which create the images on computer terminal screens.

Physical and Chemical Properties

Extremely low frequency fields can be detected without special instruments only if they are intense enough to wiggle hairs on the body, create a humming noise, or produce **ozone** (which can be detected by its pungent odor). With the exception of the intense fields produced in the immediate vicinity of high-voltage transmission lines (HVTLs), the ELF fields encountered in the ordinary environment are not directly detectable by the senses. ELF fields are usually defined to be those at or below 60 cycles per second. Electricity in the United States is transmitted at 60 cycles per second (or 60 hertz, in technical jargon), which means that the electric and magnetic fields produced by the current flowing in the wires turn around 60 times every second. In much of the rest of the world, electricity is transmitted at 50 cycles per second. This frequency range is well below that of radio and television signals and microwaves, which are discussed in the entry on **Microwave and Radio Frequency Radiation**.

Exposure and Distribution

The major exposure to ELF fields by the general population results from living near electric transmission lines and using such appliances as personal computers and electric blankets. Electricity is transmitted cross-country along high-voltage transmission lines. Within a town or city, the voltage is reduced in a series of steps. By the time it enters your house, it is reduced to about 110 volts, but along some sections of city streets, the voltage is higher than that. The closer you live to HVTLs, the more intense the ELF field you receive from electric transmission. At the ground just beneath an HVTL, the electric field strength is typically about 10 to 100 times as great as that found in the immediate vicinity of common household appliances. The typical ELF electric field exposure from all household sources is small compared to that received by some workers in the electric power industry or in industries where huge electric motors are used.

In contrast to electric fields, magnetic fields produced a few inches away from household electric currents are stronger than those from HVTLs at the ground just below the transmission lines. But people tend to spend much more time near transmission lines (especially the ones along the street in front of typical homes) than they do near turned-on appliances, so the total exposure to magnetic fields from transmission lines generally exceeds that from appliances.

People spending much of their workday in front of computer terminal screens are likely to be receiving more exposure to ELF fields from this source than from all other sources combined. The earth's natural background ELF fields, which result mainly from magnetic pulsations within the Earth and from thunderstorms, are roughly one-millionth as strong on average than those occurring in the vicinity of household electric wires.

Health Effects

Many studies seeking to characterize the extent of biological damage from ELF fields have been carried out using cell cultures, laboratory animals, human volunteers, health data for workers in electric industries, and broad health surveys of the general population. Results to date are contradictory and, in some cases, beset with difficulties in interpretation due to improper experimental design and use of statistics. Test tube studies of cell response to ELF fields indicate that hormonal secretion, calcium exchange, and tissue growth could be affected by ELF fields comparable in strength to those found in many homes and workplaces. These studies suggest that it is the magnetic field, not the electric field, within an ELF field that is particularly hazardous. Laboratory studies using live animals (mice, rats, and monkeys) and human volunteers show highly differing responses depending on the type of animal and even the particular experiment. No solid and consistent pattern of evidence indicates a risk to humans at average ELF field levels found in the home or ordinary workplace.

Epidemiological surveys, in contrast, do suggest that the incidence of childhood cancers is greater among children living near power lines carrying high currents. But these studies leave unanswered the question of whether the cancer rate might be higher be-cause children living near power lines are more likely to be exposed to other potentially cancer-causing substances such as automobile exhaust. Moreover, information on differences in magnetic field strength from one home to another are difficult to obtain because the fields vary during the day. Other studies indicate that the incidence of birth defects and miscarriages afflicting pregnant women who spend a considerable part of the workday in front of a computer screen is significantly greater than average. Despite the uncertainties and contradictions, all the studies taken together suggest that there is reason to be concerned about ELF fields. Sufficient evidence has now accumulated to warrant caution about spending large amounts of time exposed to the ELF fields from high-voltage overhead wires, huge motors, electric blankets, or computer terminal screens.

Protection and Prevention

Some exposures to ELF fields can and should be easily avoided. While the health risk of not doing so may turn out to be negligible, a "better safe than sorry" philosophy motivates the following suggestions. Users of electric blankets should turn on the blanket, warm the bed, and then turn it off before getting into bed. Avoid jogging or hiking trails that go directly underneath HVTLs. Do not buy a home located near an HVTL right-of-way. Try to sit at least two feet away from a computer screen. Protective lap shields are available for pregnant women who sit at computer terminals all day.

Environmental Effects

Effects on wild animals, including interference with bird migration, have been suggested, but as yet no definitive evidence is available that demonstrates either a hazard or the absence of a hazard.

Regulatory Status

The combination of studies that have been done to date has led some nations and some

TABLE 26 Electric Fields Encountered in Typical Household Situations

Situation	Average Electric Field (volts per meter)
Average over typical households	1–10
One foot from toasters, irons, TVs, hair dryers	30–60
One foot from electric broilers	130
Covered by an electric blanket	Up to several thousand but variable over body
Directly below an HVTL	10,000

TABLE 27 Magnetic Fields Encountered in Typical Household Situations

Situation	Average Magnetic Field (milliteslas)[a]
A few inches from soldering guns and hair dryers	1–2
A few inches from other appliances	0.1–1
On ground below an HVTL	0.035

[a] A tesla is a unit of magnetic field; a millitesla is one-thousandth of a tesla; 10,000 tesla is equal to one gauss, another unit of magnetism.

states in the United States to adopt regulations governing exposure of electric industry workers to ELF fields. In the United States, regulations in some states place an upper limit of about 10,000 volts per meter on the magnitude of an ELF electric field that is permissible anywhere at ground level within the right-of-way for HVTLs. These right-of-ways are strips of land about 100 yards wide that are set aside beneath the HVTLs. Meeting these regulations is not a difficulty for power companies. In the Soviet Union, there are regulations for workers in the industries that require high ELF exposures. There is no limit on how long a worker can be exposed to an ELF field of 5000 volts per meter, but at 10,000 and 20,000 volts per meter, workers can be exposed no more than 180 minutes per day and 10 minutes per day, respectively. In addition, the Soviet Union restricts household ELF fields at less than 1000 volts per meter.

Technical Information

ELF fields generate electric currents in the human body. Electric fields result in what are called leakage currents, and from household appliances these currents are typically in the range of 1 to 1000 microamperes. (An ampere is a unit of electrical current.) Magnetic fields can induce electric currents in the body, and typical values in the home are between 1 and 1000 microamperes. Tables 26 and 27 show typical electric and magnetic fields encountered in a household.

Further Reading

BRODEUR, P. 1989. *Currents of Death: Power Lines, Computer Terminals, and the Attempt to Cover Up Their Threat to Your Health.* New York: Simon and Schuster.

Congressional Office of Technology Assessment. 1989. *Biological Effects of Power Frequency Electric and Magnetic Fields.* Washington, D.C.: U.S. Government Printing Office.

World Health Organization. 1984. *Environmental Health Criteria Report No. 35: Extremely Low Frequency (ELF) Fields.* Geneva.

Fluoride

Introduction

Few public health measures have sparked as much heated debate as the fluoridation of public water supplies. Since the practice began in 1945, there have been two vigorously argued points of view. On one side are dental and public health officials who argue that fluoride in drinking water is a proven method to reduce the incidence of dental caries (cavities) and that it is safe. On the other side are numerous environmental and consumer groups, as well as many scientists and concerned citizens, who state that public fluoridation forces everyone served by such community water systems to consume fluoride, whether willing or not; that the safety of long-term, low-level consumption of fluoride has not been established; and that other equally effective measures to reduce dental decay in children, the high risk group, are available. No simple answer to all of these issues is available, but the best evidence suggests that fluoridation, when practiced according to recommended guidelines, does not produce major health effects and can be beneficial. At the same time, overconsumption of fluoride by small children occurs frequently, can lead to mottling of the teeth, and should be avoided.

Chemical and Physical Properties

Fluoride is a compound of the element fluorine, a highly reactive, yellowish green gas. Hydrogen fluoride gas and hydrofluoric acid are both extremely dangerous substances, causing severe burns on contact, respiratory damage if inhaled, and eye irritation. These substances ordinarily are found only in industry, but are sometimes used in rust removers. Sodium fluoride is the compound used to treat water supplies. It can also be found in tablets, liquids, rinses, gels, toothpastes, and lozenges for the prevention of tooth decay. Toothpastes may also contain fluoride as stannous fluoride or the most widely used sodium monofluorophosphate.

Exposure and Distribution

Most fluoride exposure comes from drinking water (75 to 90% of daily intake), with the remainder coming from food. In areas where the water approaches the federal limit for fluoride and for infants and children (who consume more fluids in proportion to their body weights than do adults), the drinking water contribution can approach 100%. However, as water fluoridation is increasingly practiced, foods processed with fluoridated water make up a greater fraction of the food supply, thereby increasing the contribution made by foods to daily intake. Some scientists have suggested that this increase in exposure to fluoride means the level of fluoride in water can be reduced without compromising anticavity benefits.

Fluoride occurs naturally in drinking water at varying concentrations depending on the local geology. Virtually all public drinking water contains less than 2 ppm (2 mg/L) fluoride, whether intentionally fluoridated or not. In many cases, the water is less than 1 ppm fluoride, which is the level considered optimum for cavity prevention without undue side effects. Communities with less than this optimum amount have often decided to treat their water with fluoride to bring it up to this level. Nearly 60% of public water systems have fluoride at the optimum level, either naturally or by treatment.

Fluoride exposure also occurs in children by swallowing small amounts of toothpaste while brushing their teeth and by swallowing fluoridated mouthwash. Infants may receive high exposures from infant formulas with high fluoride levels. Each of these exposures daily can lead to excessive fluoride intake. Tea plants naturally accumulate fluoride from soil, and drinking large quantities of tea will raise a person's intake. In fact, the only documented U.S. cases of severe health effects from fluoride were in two people who drank large amounts of tea over several decades made from water with extremely high natural fluoride levels.

Health Effects

Before we examine the health problems of fluoride, let's look at the health benefits. Unquestionably, the intake of small, recommended amounts of fluoride provides partial protection against tooth decay (dental caries). There is also evidence that small doses of fluoride can help stimulate bone growth in patients with *osteoporosis*.

Recent surveys show that cavities in U.S. schoolchildren have declined 36% since 1980 and that half have never had tooth decay. These results are attributed to increased use of fluoride in water, toothpaste, and mouthwash. Optimal water fluoridation provides a range of protection against tooth decay of 50 to 60%. School water fluoridation programs, fluoride supplements, and use of fluoridated salt all provide a similar range of protection. Topical treatments, such as brushing with a fluoridated toothpaste, rinsing with a fluoridated mouthwash once per week, and dentist-applied formulations, reduce cavities by 25 to 35%. The best protection comes from a combination of swallowed (systemic) and topical treatments. The World Health Organization, however, advises that there is no justification for using more than one systemic measure at any one time, and that if an optimal systemic program is in place, only one topical application should be used.

But what about the potential damages to health from fluoride? Acute poisoning has been reported from the accidental swallowing of large quantities of fluoride compounds and following the improper operation of water fluoridation equipment. The symptoms are *gastrointestinal* illness, nausea, and vomiting. Death can result if the quantities ingested are large enough (5 to 10 grams is considered a lethal dose for an adult). Long-term exposure to high levels of fluoride in drinking water can lead to a serious condition called severe skeletal fluorosis, or crippling fluorosis. In this disease, fluoride causes irregular bone deposits to form, which can lead to severe pain in joints and eventual crippling. This condition might develop only after decades of drinking water with several times the legal limit of fluoride.

Mottling of the teeth (dental fluorosis) is the most widespread effect of fluoride. As tooth enamel forms in childhood, prior to the eruption of the teeth, exposure to excessive fluoride can cause staining or streaking of the enamel surface. In its mild form, dental fluorosis is characterized by white, opaque areas on the tooth surfaces; in severe form, it shows up as brown stains and severe pitting of the teeth. Mild and moderate dental fluorosis are not believed to alter the strength or longevity of the teeth and are considered to be mainly cosmetic effects. At this time, it has not been shown that even severe dental fluorosis leads to more rapid wear of tooth enamel in people, although this has been observed in cattle drinking highly fluoridated water.

The degree of dental fluorosis depends on the amount of fluoride exposure up to about age 8. At drinking water levels recommended for optimum benefit (1 ppm), mild and moderate mottling can be expected in a small proportion of children (less than 10%). At the current federal limit (4 ppm), moderate fluorosis might affect about 30% of exposed children. Less than 1% of the U.S. population is exposed to water with fluoride greater than 2 ppm.

There is no currently accepted, valid evidence that fluoride causes cancer, birth defects, or genetic damage to offspring. A 1990 review by the U.S. Public Health Service of 50 human *epidemiological* studies and animal studies concluded that there was no evidence that fluoride causes cancer in humans. This review was made after a study by the U.S. National Toxicology Program showed that four male rats fed high doses of fluoride over their lifetimes developed a rare form of bone cancer.

Protection and Prevention

Overexposure to fluoride during childhood, with the possibility of mottling of the teeth, can be avoided by limiting the additional intake of fluoride. If the public water supply is fluoridated, bottle-fed infants should not be given fluoride supplements. Only small, pea-sized amounts of toothpaste should be given to young children, who should be instructed not to swallow it and should be monitored during brushing. Fluoride mouthwash should not be given to children under the age of 6, who might swallow it. If the water supply is not fluoridated and the natural concentration is less than 1 ppm (ask the local water supplier), these precautions are not as important. Recent surveys have shown, however, that nonfluoridated communities are experiencing nearly the reduction in tooth decay that fluoridated communities are, indicating that fluoride in the food supply is reaching them. Therefore, monitoring of young children's intake of fluoride even in nontreated areas is warranted.

Utilities that supply public drinking water are required to notify their customers if the fluoride concentration exceeds 2 ppm. At such levels, the possibility of moderate to severe dental mottling increases, and consumers can switch to bottled water to lower their risk.

Environmental Effects

Atmospheric releases of fluorides from certain industries have resulted in serious adverse effects on local vegetation and animals.

Regulatory Status

The EPA regulates the fluoride concentration in public drinking water supplies. In 1985, the EPA raised the legal limit (Recommended Maximum Contaminant Level) of fluoride to 4 ppm from 2 ppm, using the rationale that any increased dental fluorosis is not an adverse health effect under the meaning of the Safe Drinking Water Act, but rather a cosmetic effect. A Secondary Drinking Water Standard to protect against the *welfare effect* of dental mottling is maintained at 2 ppm, requiring public utilities to notify their customers if water concentrations exceed this level.

Technical Information

Chemical symbol of fluorine: Fl
Atomic number of fluorine: 9
Atomic weight of fluorine: 19
Chemical formula of sodium fluoride: NaF
Primary drinking water standard for health protection: 4 mg/L (4 ppm)
Secondary drinking water standard for welfare protection: 2 mg/L (2 ppm)
Optimum concentration to prevent dental decay while avoiding dental mottling: 1 mg/L (1 ppm)
Lethal dose (LD_{50}) for an adult: 5–10 g

Further Reading

Environmental Protection Agency. 1985. National Primary Drinking Water Regulations: Fluoride. *Federal Register* 50(93):20,164–20,175.

LEVERETT, D. H. 1982. Fluorides and the Changing Prevalence of Dental Caries. *Science* 217:26–30.

MURRAY, J. J., ed. 1986. *Appropriate Use of Fluorides for Human Health*. Geneva: World Health Organization.

Food Colors

Other Names

Blue No. 1; FD and C Blue No. 1; Brilliant Blue

Blue No. 2; FD and C Blue No. 2; Indigotine; Indigo Carmine

Green No. 3; FD and C Green No. 3; Fast Green

Red No. 3; FD and C Red No. 3; Erythrosine

Red No. 40; FD and C Red No. 40; Allura Red AC

Yellow No. 5; FD and C Yellow No. 5; Tartrazine

Yellow No. 6; FD and C Yellow No. 6; Monoazo; Sunset Yellow

Introduction

To many people, the addition of color to food represents the absurdity of chemical additives. Yet manufacturers claim that people will not buy processed food that is not colored. Although there is a trend away from using synthetic food colors in processed food, the American food industry nevertheless puts over 3000 tons of food color into processed foods every year. Yet only about 10% of food consumed in the United States contains synthetic food colors. This entry discusses all the food colors together to avoid unnecessary repetition. Nevertheless, it should be remembered that each food color has individual toxicological properties.

Physical and Chemical Properties

Synthetic food colors are manufactured from molecules derived from petroleum or coal tar. Tiny amounts of coloring agents can tint huge vats of product. Most synthetic colors do not fade during processing and storage, giving them a decided advantage over natural coloring agents.

Exposure and Distribution

Synthetic food colors are found in a wide variety of products. They are most commonly used in soda, candy, dessert mixes, commercially prepared baked goods, sausages (including hot dogs), toothpaste, and other cosmetics. Red No. 40 and Yellow No. 5 and No. 6 account for over 90% of the food dyes used in the United States. Using data provided by the FDA, one consumer group calculated that some children consume as much as 3 pounds of food dye by their twelfth birthdays. It should be noted that a larger selection of dyes are available for use in drugs and cosmetics than are allowed in food.

Health Effects

There is no doubt that very high doses of most of the synthetic food dyes that the FDA has approved for use are capable of causing cancer. That fact has been proved in many laboratory tests using mice, rats, rabbits, and sometimes monkeys. So the question is not whether food dyes are capable of causing cancer, but at what doses. Table 28 shows the adverse health effects, including cancerous tumors, that are associated with very high doses of the seven legal food colors.

The FDA maintains that because so little of the cancer-causing dye is actually used to color food, the amount ingested by the average person is insignificant. That is, dyes are not a major hazard. Although the Delaney Clause of the Food, Drug, and Cosmetic Act bans the use of all carcinogenic agents in food, the dyes continue to be used. Primarily because of the food color issue, the FDA has reiterated that it will accept the use of food additives that pose a "negligible risk" to the consumer. This means that on the basis of a quantitative health risk assessment, the risk of getting cancer from eating food colors is less than one in a million. The negligible-risk approach requires that data describing the ability of a chemical to cause cancer are available and that it is possible to translate high-

TABLE 28 Health Effects of Very High Doses of the Legal Food Colors

Food Color	Health Effects
Red No. 3	Thyroid tumors, chromosomal damage
Red No. 40	Lymphatic tumors
Blue No. 1	Chromosomal damage
Blue No. 2	Brain tumors
Green No. 3	Bladder tumors
Yellow No. 5	Thyroid and lymphatic tumors, allergy
Yellow No. 6	Kidney tumors, chromosomal damage, allergy

dose animal data to low-dose human risk. Not all people agree that this is possible. For now, consumers must exercise their freedom of choice about the use of food colors, as well as other food additives such as **saccharin** and **aspartame**. Choice, in turn, implies that consumers must be educated about the possible hazards of the food they purchase.

Protection and Prevention

Food colors can be avoided by not buying products containing them. When an artificial food color is used, the product label must state it. The particular color that is used does not need to be specified, except for Yellow No. 5, which aspirin-sensitive people tend to be allergic to, along with about 10,000 other people in the United States. Unfortunately, there are cases when the desired (or needed) product is not available uncolored. Except in the case of drugs, this situation is becoming rarer, largely due to public pressure.

Regulatory Status

Food colors are regulated by the FDA. There are no restrictions on their use beyond good manufacturing practice. The use of Yellow No. 5 must be specified; otherwise food labels only need to say that artificial colors are used. Red dye No. 3 was recently banned in the United States from use in cosmetics and externally applied drugs, although existing stocks can be sold and used. The FDA plans to ban Red No. 3 from food shortly. The European Economic Community has banned the use of Red No. 40 and Green No. 3.

TABLE 29 Amount of Dye Used in the United States

Color	Tons/year (1984)
Red No. 3	120
Red No. 40	1315
Blue No. 1	130
Blue No. 2	50
Green No. 3	2
Yellow No. 5	810
Yellow No. 6	765
Total	3192

Technical Information

Although the amount of food dye ingested varies among individuals, the maximum intake is estimated to be 54 mg/day, whereas the average consumption is estimated to be 15 mg/day. Table 29 shows the number of tons of food dye used in the United States annually.

Further Reading

BLUMENTHAL, D. 1990. Red No. 3 and Other Colorful Controversies. *FDA Consumer* 24(4): 18–21.

The Public Citizen Health Research Group. 1985. Dyes in Your Food. *Health Letter* 1(1):2–3.

Formaldehyde

Other Names

Formalin; Methyl aldehyde

Trade Names

Lysoform; Morbicid; Paraform

Introduction

Formaldehyde ranks among the top 50 industrial chemicals produced in the United States each year in terms of weight. In 1985, some 5.7 billion pounds of formaldehyde were produced for an enormous variety of purposes. The chemical is used to make such diverse consumer products as molded plastic telephones, dinnerware, particle board, plywood, foam mattresses, building insulation, cosmetics, and drugs. It is used as a preservative, an embalming fluid, a *fumigant*, and a disinfectant. Moreover, it is a normal combustion product found in cigarette smoke, wood smoke, automobile exhaust, and emissions from incinerators and power plants. Formaldehyde is also a normal metabolic product of living cells. In short, both naturally occurring and man-made formaldehyde is found virtually everywhere—even in very unlikely places. A recent study from Europe reports that significant levels of formaldehyde were found in incubators used for premature infants.

Until recently, the toxic and irritant effects of formaldehyde were considered to be mainly a problem for workers directly exposed to the chemical. But an increased concern with energy conservation led to practices that increased the concentration of formaldehyde in indoor air. These included the move toward relatively airtight buildings and the use of urea–formaldehyde foam insulation (UFFI). Many construction materials emit appreciable amounts of formaldehyde gas (that is, they degas) for five or more years following manufacture. Consequently, as several studies of indoor air pollution have indicated, a significant segment of the public is exposed to formaldehyde at levels high enough to produce symptoms. There is evidence from numerous laboratory and *epidemiological* studies that formaldehyde causes cancer; other human health effects from long-term exposure are less certain.

Physical and Chemical Properties

Pure formaldehyde is a highly water soluble, colorless gas with a pungent odor and irritant properties. Generally sold in alcohol solutions, formaldehyde retains its odor and ability to irritate eyes and mucous membranes. Any biology student who has dissected a frog or a worm is familiar with formaldehyde in the form of the preservative formalin, a clear, watery solution having a characteristic pungent odor.

Exposure and Distribution

Virtually the entire population is exposed to formaldehyde because of its widespread distribution. The principal routes of human exposure are inhalation and skin absorption. The EPA estimates that as many as 27.7 million people living within a 12.5-mile radius of industries making or using formaldehyde may be exposed to excessive levels of the chemical. Building materials used in mobile homes and new conventional homes degas or release formaldehyde over a period of many years. The EPA estimates that over a 10-year period, as many as 7.8 million people living in mobile homes and another 6.3 million people living in conventional homes may be exposed to potentially harmful levels of the chemical. The amount of formaldehyde released from building materials increases as temperature increases, such as during the winter when indoor heaters are on and there is little ventilation. In the workplace, OSHA estimates that as many as 2.6 million full-time and part-time workers may be exposed to significant levels of formaldehyde.

Formaldehyde is found in a variety of

widely used consumer products, including toothpaste, particle board, vaccines, plywood, paper, shampoo, urea–formaldehyde foam insulation, plastics, permanent press fabrics, other textiles, paints, pigments, leather, and sealants. The extent of formaldehyde use in particle board and plywood alone is staggering. Both plywood and particle board are typically used in subflooring, countertops, cabinets, paneling, and furniture, and more than 90% of furniture made and sold in the United States is built with pressed wood products. In addition, formaldehyde is also a product of incomplete combustion and is thus found outdoors as well. In contrast to its fate in a closed building, however, it has a short *half-life* outdoors, as it is quickly degraded by exposure to the sun.

Health Effects

Formaldehyde is an irritant of the eyes at concentrations typical of outdoor air in Los Angeles. At levels that have been reported in various studies of indoor air pollution, it causes irritation of the upper respiratory system.

There has been considerable controversy over the long-term consequences of prolonged exposure to relatively low levels of formaldehyde—levels typically found in mobile homes or energy-conserving buildings. Nevertheless, the EPA has concluded, after much debate with the Formaldehyde Institute, that formaldehyde is a probable human carcinogen (group B_2) on the basis of experimental studies and human epidemiological studies. The epidemiological studies suggest an increased incidence of brain tumors, leukemia, and cirrhosis of the liver among professional workers. Laboratory studies indicate that formaldehyde causes nasal cancer in rats and that it appears to cause mutations in bacteria, yeasts, *Drosophila* (fruitflies), and mammalian and human cells. There is no clear evidence of reproductive effects. Some data indicate that the primary *metabolites* may be toxic to the nervous system, but those

data are too scanty to draw any conclusions as yet.

Acute exposure to formaldehyde can cause poisoning and is lethal at levels exceeding 100 ppm. Signs of poisoning include any of the following: abdominal pain, anxiety, irritation of nose and throat, depression of the central nervous system, coma, convulsions, diarrhea, headache, nausea, vomiting, and various respiratory problems, such as *bronchitis*, pneumonia, or *pulmonary edema*. Lower levels of exposure can cause *dermatitis*, cough, and decreased lung capacity. Classic symptoms of low-level formaldehyde exposure include runny nose, sore throat, sleeping difficulties, headache, fatigue, breathing difficulties, sinus irritation, chest pain, frequent nausea, and bronchitis. Symptoms have occurred at levels as low as 0.05 ppm—the level that has been proposed as the California indoor air quality standard.

Protection and Prevention

If formaldehyde is consumed, vomiting should be induced and large quantities of water should be given. Exposure via direct contact with eyes or skin should be treated by immediately irrigating the eyes and/or flushing the skin with water. Adequate ventilation and protective clothing for people working with the chemical are recommended to prevent intoxication. Application of surface barriers (such as paints, lacquers, and varnishes) to particle board or plywood can reduce the rate of formaldehyde degassing. Laboratory studies indicate that dehumidifiers can effectively reduce the level of formaldehyde in indoor air. Indoor humidity levels less than 35% should effectively reduce formaldehyde levels.

Consumers should be aware that the amount of formaldehyde emitted by building materials and certain other products varies (for example, medium density fiber board emits about three times more than particle board). Exterior grade plywood emits less formaldehyde than interior grade. And the

Swedish Glitsa hardwood floor finish is notorious for high formaldehyde emissions, but this finish is now banned in many areas. Exposure can be reduced by choosing products that emit less formaldehyde, maintaining adequate ventilation, and maintaining a relatively low humidity in homes in which formaldehyde-laden materials have been used (such as in new houses).

Regulatory Status

OSHA has put exposure standards into effect for the workplace, but those limits are many times higher than the lowest levels that produce effects or symptoms. Despite the recent recognition that a significant fraction of the general population is exposed to air concentrations of formaldehyde sufficiently high to produce eye or respiratory symptoms, there are no federal regulations governing public exposure to the substance. Three states are considering indoor standards that are much stricter—10 to 100 times lower—than federal workplace standards. Even those proposed tougher standards are higher than the threshold that affects the upper respiratory tract. The EPA has suggested allowable concentrations for water based on health considerations. The Department of Housing and Urban Development (HUD) has issued standards limiting formaldehyde in construction materials.

Achieving existing regulations has not been easy, despite a great deal of public concern, widespread exposure, and evidence of harmful effects. In February 1981, the National Toxicology Program concluded, on the basis of rat studies, that formaldehyde should be presumed to pose a risk of cancer to humans. Accordingly, EPA designated formaldehyde as a priority chemical for regulatory assessment, but a year later, it withdrew priority status in response to pressure from the formaldehyde industry. The Consumer Product Safety Commission voted to ban urea–formaldehyde products, following the lead of Canada and two states, Massachu-setts and Connecticut. Although the ban was overturned in court, production levels have dropped. In 1984, the EPA resumed its *Special Review* of formaldehyde and concluded in 1987 that it is a probable human carcinogen (group B_2; Chapter 3, Section B) and causes acute respiratory problems. The EPA says the general public is not at risk. It considers that only those 10 to 20 million people living in mobile homes or conventional homes with particle board or plywood building materials are exposed to significant levels, but not levels that warrant emergency action. Formaldehyde is listed as a *hazardous air pollutant* in the 1990 Clean Air Act, requiring the EPA to set emission standards. It is also on the EPA *community right-to-know* list.

The formaldehyde industry has consistently objected to proposed regulations in the workplace and in building materials. The industry's latest objection, as of December 1988, focused on an OSHA requirement that consumer products that release low levels (0.1 ppm) of formaldehyde carry cancer warning labels.

Technical Information

Chemical names: methylene oxide; methyl aldehyde

Chemical formula: CH_2O

Health effects at various air concentrations:

no effects reported	0–0.05 ppm
neurophysiological effects	0.05–1.05 ppm
odor threshold	0.05–1.0 ppm
eye irritation	0.05–2.0 ppm
upper respiratory irritation	0.10–25 ppm
lower airway and pulmonary effects	5.0–30 ppm
pulmonary edema, inflammation, pneumonia	50.0–100 ppm
death	100+ ppm

Typical ranges of measured concentrations:

ambient air	0.001–0.03 ppm

TABLE 30 Existing Government Standards, Recommendations, and State Proposals

	Standard	Status
Ambient air	0.01 ppm (maximum)	Recommended by AIHA
Indoor air	0.05 ppm	Proposed by California
	0.5 pm	Proposed by Minnesota
	0.4 ppm	Proposed by Wisconsin
Occupation air	3 ppm (TWA)	Promulgated by OSHA
	2 ppm (threshold)	Recommended by ACGIH
	1 ppm (30-min maximum)	Recommended by NIOSH
Water	42.4 μg/L	Suggested by EPA

cigarette smoke	0.4 mg/20 cigarettes/day
outdoor air (Los Angeles)	0.05–0.12 ppm
automotive exhausts	29–43 ppm
indoor air (degassing)	0.03–2.5 ppm

The status of government standards for regulating formaldehyde is shown in Table 30.

Further Reading

Report on the Consensus Workshop on Formaldehyde. 1984. Environmental Health Perspectives No. 58. December.

Fosetyl Al

Other Names

Phosetyl-Al; Aluminum-tris

Trade Name

Aliette

Introduction

One of the newest fungus fighters, fosetyl Al is actually not directly toxic to fungi, but rather it can prevent or cure plant diseases caused by a certain group of fungi. A *systemic organophosphate*, fosetyl Al protects the plant from fungal attack after being absorbed by roots or leaves and transported throughout the plant. The precise mechanism of its action is not yet understood, but it appears to trigger a defensive reaction in the affected plant that isolates the fungus and prevents its spread.

Because it is quite new, it has been subjected to more rigorous testing than the older pesticides still on the market. Although of low *acute toxicity*, fosetyl Al is registered for use only on pineapples (an application for use on citrus is pending). Its restricted use is largely because of quirks in the regulations and, paradoxically, because it has been so well studied. Studies provide clear evidence that fosetyl Al causes cancer in some animals and yet a National Academy of Sciences (NAS) study estimates a low risk and suggests that it might be a suitable replacement for more toxic or less well studied fungicides, such as **benomyl, captan,** and the **ethylenebisdithiocarbamates (EBDCs)**.

Fosetyl Al is effective in controlling downy mildew on vines, such as tomatoes and beans, and a number of other fungal pests on various fruits and vegetables, such as peppers, avocados, and citrus. Outside of the United States, fosetyl Al is used to protect rhododendrons and conifers.

Physical and Chemical Properties

Fosetyl Al contains aluminum. The colorless powder is slightly soluble in water, but essentially insoluble in organic solvents. It is stable under normal storage conditions, but it breaks down in either acid or alkaline solutions.

Exposure and Distribution

Because fosetyl Al is registered for use only on pineapples, not much of it is used. It is available alone or in combination with other fungicides, primarily **mancozeb** and **folpet,** acting *synergistically* with the latter. In plants, fosetyl Al is taken up rapidly and persists from four weeks to four months, depending on the species. Ultimately, it is broken down to a harmless compound.

Health Effects

There is a good data base on the tumor-producing potential of fosetyl Al. Studies show that very high dose levels (equivalent to 4% of the total diet) produce a significant increase in the incidence of kidney tumors. The pesticide is therefore classified as a tumor producer. A recent NAS report estimated that if fosetyl Al replaced the use of EBDCs on hops, the estimated risk of tumors from dietary exposure would be reduced substantially. The EPA has estimated the risk from fosetyl Al to be about 1 in 100 million. In contrast, the risk from the EBDCs (and their major metabolic product) has been estimated to be about 1 in 10,000 to 1 in 100,000.

Fosetyl Al is of moderate acute toxicity and low dermal toxicity, but it can cause irreversible eye damage. So far, animal tests reveal no evidence that it causes birth defects or mutations.

Protection and Prevention

Containers of this fungicide state that fosetyl Al may be hazardous to humans and domestic animals. The labels caution users not to apply the fungicide directly to bodies of water or wetlands and not to contaminate water by cleaning equipment where runoff can occur. Protective clothing and eyewear are indicated for people applying the pesticide. Field and other agricultural workers are warned to wait until the spray has dried before reentering fields and to wash the fungicide from the skin or eyes if contacted. Since fosetyl Al is registered for use only on pineapples, it is unlikely that consumers are exposed to high levels. Moreover, there is little evidence that residues of the fungicide remain on the fruit.

Environmental Effects

The available evidence suggests that the toxicity to honeybees, birds, and rainbow trout is low.

Regulatory Status

At present in the United States, the use of fosetyl Al is restricted to pineapples. A request for *tolerances* on hops was recently denied, and an application for use on citrus has been submitted.

Technical Information

Chemical name: aluminum tris(ethyl phosonate)
Chemical formulas: $C_6H_{18}AlO_9P_3$

Further Reading

National Academy of Sciences. 1987. *Regulating Pesticides*. Washington, D.C.: National Academy of Sciences Press.

Glyphosate

Trade Names

Roundup; Rodeo; Accord

Introduction

In nearly every nursery, supermarket, variety store, and hardware store—wherever plants and garden supplies are sold—you are likely to see row upon row of boldly displayed plastic spray bottles of the herbicide Roundup. In use since the mid-1970s, Roundup, or glyphosate, seems an especially attractive herbicide for several reasons. It is considered to be generally nontoxic or only slightly toxic to the vast majority of terrestrial and aquatic organisms tested, other than plants. Moreover, it is highly effective against a broad spectrum of weedy pest species. For example, glyphosate controls 76 out of 78 of the world's worst weeds. Some particularly hard-to-kill weeds are completely destroyed by this *systemic* herbicide. Successful applications include agriculture, vegetation control in non-crop areas (such as railroad right-of-ways and conifer plantations), and home gardening. It is registered for use on 134 different crops, including corn, wheat, barley, and soybeans, but its primary use is on hay and orchards. Finally, because of its behavior in soil and water and its degradability, glyphosate appears to pose little threat to the environment.

Physical and Chemical Properties

Glyphosate is formulated as a water-soluble liquid, but in its pure form it is a white crystalline solid with low water solubility. The pure form is insoluble in common organic solvents.

Exposure and Distribution

At present, about eight million pounds of glyphosate are used in the United States annually. In comparison, roughly eleven times more of the possibly more hazardous herbicide **alachlor** is applied. Glyphosate is applied as a liquid foliar spray using ground or aerial equipment. It is readily absorbed by the leaves and transported to the roots and growing shoots of the plant where it inhibits growth and sprouting. Effects are observed within two to seven days following application. Parts above ground turn yellow, wilt, and dry up; underground parts are also killed. Since glyphosate provides no residual weed control, it is often applied in combination with various other herbicides, such as **alachlor**, atrazine, and linuron.

The herbicide is generally considered to be immobile in soil because it is bound tightly to the soil particles, but some evidence suggests that it may leach under certain conditions. Because it is rapidly degraded by soil microorganisms, glyphosate shows little residual soil activity, although its *half-life* can range from a few days to a few months, depending on conditions. In water, degradation is slower than in soil.

Health Effects

To date, most animal (dog and rat) studies have indicated that glyphosate does not cause cancer. In some tests, however, a slight increase in benign kidney tumors in male mice at very high doses has been found. Additional studies are required before the carcinogenicity of glyphosate can be assessed. Tests for *mutations* have been negative, as have tests for birth defects in rats and rabbits. Other reproductive effects have not been observed.

Few published reports are available on the toxicity to mammals, but data supplied to the EPA by the manufacturer (as required by law) suggest a very low acute oral toxicity. Glyphosate is only slightly absorbed through the skin, so acute toxicity is low via that route. It is slightly toxic when inhaled. When injected directly into the body, glyphosate increases the body temperature and produces convulsions.

Protection and Prevention

Because glyphosate is so effective against so many species of plant, applicators must spray in such a way as to avoid drift to nontarget vegetation. Minute quantities can cause severe damage to most plants. As for all pesticides, consumers are cautioned to avoid direct contact with the skin and eyes, to wash or flush immediately if an accident occurs, to seek medical help if the herbicide is swallowed, and to avoid contaminating water bodies with the chemical. For one particular formulation of glyphosate called Accord, users are warned to use, mix, or store it only in stainless steel, aluminum, fiberglass, plastic, or plastic-lined containers. The product will react with unlined or galvanized steel and produce hydrogen gas, which is combustible.

Environmental Effects

In laboratory and field tests, glyphosate appears to be almost nontoxic or only slightly toxic to most nonplant species tested. Freshwater fish are relatively tolerant of the active ingredient alone, but certain additives in Roundup increase its toxicity. Similarly, glyphosate seems essentially nontoxic to the bird species that have been tested. Invertebrates, however, display a broad range of susceptibility, suggesting that glyphosate may be toxic to some species. The long-term effects of glyphosate on browsers such as deer is unknown, but must be considered since deer will eat treated forage. The most obvious effect of glyphosate on wild populations is the loss of desirable habitats following extensive spraying. Destruction of large areas of vegetation reduces or eliminates nesting sites, shelter, and food resources for birds and mice.

Regulatory Status

The use of glyphosate is generally restricted, and it is prohibited in areas specified by the

U.S. Fish and Wildlife Service where there are endangered species.

Technical Information

Chemical name: *N*-(phosphonomethyl)-glycine

Chemical formula: $C_3H_8NO_5P$

Government standards for food tolerances:

peanuts	0.1 ppm
asparagus, citrus, grapes	0.2 ppm
soybeans	6.0 ppm
fish	0.25 ppm

Heptachlor

Trade Name

Velsicol 104

Introduction

Heptachlor is an insecticide that works both on contact with the insect and as a stomach poison following ingestion. Isolated as a component of technical grade **chlordane**, another *organochlorine* insecticide, it was first registered for use in 1952. It was used in the control of malaria-carrying mosquitoes and has been used to control cotton insects, grasshoppers, soil insects, and some food crop pests. In certain parts of the world, heptachlor has also been used extensively to control termites in buildings, a practice that has resulted in high levels of human exposure. Today, its use is highly restricted in many countries, including the United States, the Soviet Union, Italy, Switzerland, and Japan. Currently, heptachlor is registered for the control of ants on pineapples in Hawaii and termites in other areas of the United States.

Despite restrictions on its use, heptachlor has been implicated in several incidents of contaminated dairy products in Hawaii, Oklahoma, Arkansas, and Missouri when dairy cows were fed fodder that had been treated with the pesticide. In Hawaii, for example, where pineapple plants are treated with heptachlor, the green tops of the plants called the chop are used as fodder for dairy cows after harvest of the pineapples. Legally, the chop can be used only after a prescribed interval following pesticide application to allow the heptachlor to break down. The contamination of dairy products suggested that either the waiting period was ignored or that it was not long enough.

Physical and Chemical Properties

The pure material is a white, crystalline solid with a mild camphor-like odor. It is essentially insoluble in water, but dissolves in kerosene and some other organic compounds. Heptachlor does not break down readily when exposed to light, moisture, air, or moderate heat, but it does break down in the presence of strong alkali.

Exposure and Distribution

Although heptachlor is not soluble in water, residues have been found in fish from various bodies of water. Heptachlor is taken up readily by living organisms and rapidly converted to heptachlor epoxide, which is highly *persistent* (resistant to decomposition) in living systems and in soils and water. Under moist environmental conditions, heptachlor reacts with water to produce the more stable and persistent heptachlor epoxide. In soils, residues of both heptachlor and its epoxide have been detected more than a dozen years after application.

As recently as 1986, about 500,000 pounds of heptachlor were used in California for termite control in residential buildings. As a result of recent use and persistence, some people are likely to be exposed to residues for years, although exposure levels for the general population are low. Trace amounts of the epoxide have been detected in the fat tissues of people around the world, due chiefly to past exposures. Relatively high levels of heptachlor epoxide have recently been detected in human breast-milk as a result of using animal fodder that contained residues.

Health Effects

In rats, heptachlor is of moderate *acute toxicity*, with female rats being more susceptible. Like other organochlorine compounds, heptachlor is toxic to the nervous system of mammals, causing excessive activity of the nervous system, tremors, and convulsions. It is readily absorbed by the skin, lungs, stomach, and intestinal tract.

The EPA has classified heptachlor as a probable human carcinogen (group B_2) on the basis of test results in rats and mice showing an increased incidence of certain kinds of cancers. In recent *epidemiological* studies in Hawaii, both heptachlor and heptachlor epoxide have been linked with an increase in the incidence of nerve cell tumors and tumors in children. Some scientists think that heptachlor probably plays a role in the development of cancer, even if it does not directly cause cancer.

Data regarding other long-term effects are less certain. In tests of moderate dose levels, heptachlor did not produce birth defects, but at high dose levels, both fertility and the survival of newborn pups were reduced. Some studies report changes in chromosomes associated with heptachlor exposure. Heptachlor epoxide is possibly more toxic than the parent compound, but the data are scanty.

Protection and Prevention

If heptachlor is ingested, immediate treatment should include inducing vomiting with water or salt solution. No oily substances or milk should be given. A physician should be contacted. If needed, the physician may give barbiturates and artificial respiration and oxygen. No epinephrine or stimulants should be given. Since the major current sources of exposure are buildings where heptachlor or chlordane have been used for termite control, residue levels should be checked in and around such structures. Moreover, the high levels of heptachlor and chlordane routinely detected in meat, dairy products, fish, and poultry should be reduced.

Environmental Effects

Several highly undesirable environmental effects have been observed. Following application of heptachlor to farms, fields, and forests, populations of nontarget species have been significantly reduced. Soil microorganisms are variously affected by the pesticide; some are very susceptible. Heptachlor is acutely toxic to aquatic organisms, including fish, invertebrates, and plants. Phytoplankton populations, for example, have been decimated following heptachlor entry to lakes, streams, and estuaries, where the toxicity is influenced by both the temperature and salinity. Evidence of effects on terrestrial organisms is scanty, but suggests that susceptibility varies among species. Bees and certain species of birds have been poisoned by heptachlor.

Regulatory Status

The use of heptachlor is highly restricted on the basis of its environmental effects and its potential to cause cancer. At present, cancellation of all uses of heptachlor is pending. It is listed as a *hazardous air pollutant* in the 1990 Clean Air Act and is on the *community right-to-know* list.

Technical Information

Chemical name: 1,4,5,6,7,8,8′-heptachloro–3a,4,7,7a-tetrahydro–4,7-methanoindene
Chemical formula: $C_{10}H_5Cl_7$
EPA food tolerances (heptachlor and heptachlor epoxide):
    cabbages, lettuce, snap beans: 0.1 mg/kg
    milk, meat, other vegetables: 0.0 mg/kg
WHO recommended level for drinking water: 0.1 µg/L
WHO acceptable daily intake: 0.0005 mg/kg
OSHA limit in workplace air: 0.5 mg/m³
Government criteria for maximum concentrations to which aquatic organisms can be exposed:

	brief exposure	*24-hour exposure*
salt water	0.52 µg/L	0.0038 µg/L
freshwater	0.053 µg/L	0.0036 µg/L

Further Reading

HAYES, W. J., JR. 1982. *Pesticides Studied in Man.* Baltimore, MD: Williams and Wilkins.
MERCIER, M. 1981. *Criteria (Dose/Effect Relationships) for Organochlorine Pesticides.* Oxford: Pergamon Press.
World Health Organization. 1984. *Environmental Health Criteria Report No. 38: Heptachlor.* Geneva.

Hydroquinone

Other Names

1,4-Benzenediol; *p*-dioxobenzene; arctuvin

Trade Names

Diak–5; Kodak D–76; Kodak DK–60a; Edwal Litho-F; Black and White Bleaching Cream; Eldoquin Cream; Esoterica Special

Introduction

Hydroquinone is a skin-bleaching agent, an artificial suntan agent, and an important ingredient in photographic developer. Its chronic toxicity has recently received scientific attention. Watch for new information on the toxic hazards of this chemical in the news.

Physical and Chemical Properties

Hydroquinone is a white, crystalline phenol that occurs naturally, but it is usually manufactured for human use. It combines readily with oxygen and becomes brown when exposed to air. It is generally stored and shipped for commercial use as a white or light tan powder in cardboard-fiber drums. Hydroquinone dust may be flammable.

Exposure and Distribution

The consumer or hobbyist can come into contact with hydroquinone either by using one of several skin-bleaching products, freckle removers, or suntan lotions, or by using a photographic developer containing the compound. People with dark skin are most likely to come into contact with cosmetics containing hydroquinone.

Health Effects

Ingestion of moderate amounts of hydroquinone (such as that contained in one or two cups of liquid photographic developer or skin-lightening cream) can cause ringing in the ears, nausea, dizziness, a sense of suffocation, increased respiratory rate, vomiting, pallor, muscle twitching, headache, difficulty in breathing, blue fingers, delirium, and collapse. The urine of exposed people turns green or brownish green. The adult oral lethal dose is estimated to be about a quart of liquid developer or skin-lightening cream (which contains 2 to 5 grams of hydroquinone). (A packet of dry developer mix formulated to make a quart of liquid developer contains 2 to 3 grams of hydroquinone.) Particles of hydroquinone dust in the eye cause immediate irritation and may lead to ulceration of the cornea. Repeated skin contact can cause *dermatitis*.

Prolonged exposure can lead to discoloration of the eyelids, clouded eye lenses, and eye color changes. Anemia and loss of skin pigmentation have also been associated with chronic exposure. The loss of skin pigmentation can be patchy in some individuals, particularly those with dark skin. Hydroquinone is also an active *allergen*, causing about 5% of people exposed to develop an allergic skin rash after repeated contact.

Hydroquinone has recently been found to cause bladder cancer in mice injected with the substance. In other tests, animals fed the chemical have developed aplastic *anemia* and atrophy of the liver, but no bladder cancer. Several short-term tests reveal that the compound may also be a *mutagen*. In addition, the offspring of female rats fed hydroquinone or injected with it exhibit birth defects. The health effects of hydroquinone are additive with other phenol compounds.

Protection and Prevention

Use photographic developer in a well-ventilated room. Mix with care to avoid getting dust from the dry mix in your eyes. Avoid skin contact by using protective gloves or tongs. Read the labels on skin bleaching or artificial tanning lotions and avoid those containing hydroquinone. If products containing hydroquinone are used, watch for signs of overuse, including dark urine, discoloration of the eyes, and ringing in the ears. People prone to allergies should use hydroquinone products with extra care.

Regulatory Status

Hydroquinone, being a phenol compound, is regulated with other phenols by the EPA. However, this status is likely to change as new evidence specific to hydroquinone is evaluated by the EPA. Hydroquinone is listed as a *hazardous air pollutant* in the 1990 Clean Air Act, requiring the EPA to set emission standards. It is also on the EPA *community right-to-know* list.

Technical Information

Chemical formula: $C_6H_3O_2$
Molecular weight: 107
Amount that affects eye pigment (in air):
  10–30 mg/m^3
Adult lethal dose (LD$_{50}$):
  ingested: 2g
  inhaled: 200 mg/m^3
OSHA limit in workplace air: 2 mg/m^3
EPA limit in drinking water (total phenols):
  0.001 ppm

Further Reading

SAX, N. I. 1988. Hydroquinone. *Dangerous Properties of Industrial Materials Report*, January/February, pp. 51–60.

Iodine-131

Other Names

^{131}I

Introduction

Iodine-131 is a *radioactive isotope* of the element iodine that is formed when uranium undergoes *fission* (see Chapter 15, Section D). The common nonradioactive form of iodine (^{127}I) is essential to good health because it plays a major role in the synthesis of thyroid hormones. Dietary supplements of nonradioactive iodine are often prescribed for thyroid deficiency, and radioactive iodine-131 is sometimes used to reduce overactivity in the thyroid (hyperthyroidism). Nuclear weapons testing and accidents at nuclear power facilities are the primary sources of iodine-131 in the environment. Because it decays relatively rapidly, the risk is greatly diminished a month or so after an accident.

Physical and Chemical Properties

Iodine-131 is a violet-colored, crystalline solid that is very *volatile*. It has a *half-life* of 8.1 days and decays by emitting a *beta particle*. When Iodine-131 is released into the atmosphere, it occasionally attaches to small naturally occurring *aerosol* particles, but it is more often bound chemically to hydrogen and oxygen or methane in gaseous form. It is soluble in rainwater, which accounts for its major pathway from the atmosphere to living organisms, and it concentrates very effectively in the thyroid gland.

Exposure and Distribution

Because of its half-life, iodine-131 would be nearly absent from the atmosphere and from *food chains* under natural conditions. Release of radioactive iodine into the atmosphere from nuclear weapons testing and nuclear power operations accounts for virtually all of the present-day exposure. The major pathway to humans is through the food chain; rain washes it out of the atmosphere onto grass, from which cows incorporate it into their milk. Dairy products such as cheese that have been stored for periods much longer than the half-life do not pose a problem. Milk, however, is usually stored for only a short time before consumption and is thus the major source. Leafy vegetables are another source of the isotope, for rain can wash it onto them. Iodine enters the bloodstream rapidly after ingestion. From there, about one-third of it ends up in the thyroid gland and two-thirds is excreted. Under normal nuclear power plant operation, about one-billionth of the iodine-131 produced in a reactor is released to the environment. Under normal operations, these plants result in a average radiation dose to humans that is negligibly small compared to background sources such as cosmic rays. In the early 1960s, however, nuclear weapons testing in the atmosphere resulted in annual doses to the thyroid that averaged, worldwide, a few percent of the total annual background radiation dose.

Several accidents at nuclear power facilities have also exposed people to significant doses. The accident at Three Mile Island, Pennsylvania, in 1979 released less than one-millionth of the total amount of iodine-131 produced from nuclear weapons testing in the atmosphere. In contrast, the 1986 accident at the Chernobyl power plant in the Soviet Union released in just a few days several percent of the amount produced from atmospheric testing. Following the Chernobyl accident, levels of radioactive iodine in milk in the United States increased sharply (see Technical Information section).

Health Effects

High levels of iodine-131 in the thyroid (such as might occur from nuclear warfare or proximity to a major nuclear reactor accident) result in complete destruction of the thyroid gland. Lower doses can induce thyroid cancer, the first symptom of which is a swelling in the front part of the neck. Thyroid cancer is treatable by surgical removal of the entire gland; thyroxine tablets will then be permanently required. At low doses, iodine-131 can also cause noncancerous excess thyroid activity, producing symptoms of hyperactivity, muscular spasms, and possibly heart palpitations and weight loss.

Protection and Prevention

Iodine-131 is one of the few radioactive substances for which protective measures are available and at least partially effective. By taking a large dose of ordinary nonradioactive iodine in the form of potassium iodide as soon as possible after knowing that exposure may occur or even right after exposure, iodine-131 is partially blocked from lodging in the thyroid. The National Council on Radiation Protection has suggested that public distribution of potassium iodide tablets may be warranted if radiation exposure to the thyroid is likely to exceed 0.1 gray (see Chapter 15, Section E). Considerable controversy still surrounds this advice, however, and as of this writing, no official policy is in effect to issue such tablets in the event of a major accident at a nuclear facility. It has been suggested that the nuclear power industry is resisting such a protective strategy because it would heighten public awareness of the possibility of a serious nuclear power plant accident.

An additional protective measure is to avoid ingestion of milk and leafy vegetables produced in the vicinity of a serious nuclear reactor accident during the month or two following the accident. Following this period of time, most of the radioactive iodine will have decayed.

Environmental Effects

One study (by DeSante and Geupel; see Further Reading) concluded that iodine-131 released from the Chernobyl accident caused a severe reduction in reproduction of certain land birds at the Point Reyes Bird Obser-

vatory in California. It will be difficult to confirm or rule out this claim until careful laboratory studies are carried out to assess the sensitivity of baby birds to the levels of radiation that the Point Reyes birds were likely to have received.

Regulatory Status

In the United States, the general restrictions on radiation exposure apply to radioactive iodine and can be found in Chapter 15, Section F.

Technical Information[3]

Iodine-131 decays by emitting a 0.81 million-electron-volt (MeV) beta particle. Nuclear weapons testing has resulted in a total of approximately 6×10^{20} becquerels of iodine-131 released to the environment. Because much of this material is released high in the atmosphere, the dose per becquerel from it, about 3×10^{-15} person-sieverts per becquerel, is less than that for releases from power plants. The total dose from weapons testing, 1.8×10^6 person-sieverts, corresponds to an average individual dose of about 5×10^{-4} sieverts.

Nuclear power plants produce about 10^{17} becquerels of iodine-131 per megawatt of produced electricity. Because of its relatively short half-life, the isotope is in equilibrium after a few weeks at 3×10^{15} becquerels per megawatt. In recent years, about 2×10^{13} becquerels of iodine-131 is released annually to the environment from normal power plant operation worldwide (about 7.5×10^4 megawatts per year), and 5×10^{11} becquerels per year is released from nuclear fuel reprocessing (at the Windscale plant in Great Britain). From such releases, the dose to people is about 10^{-11} person-sieverts per becquerel released, or a total of about 200 person-sieverts per year. Divided by the global population of

[3] For a discussion of the meaning of the units of radiation used below, see Chapter 15, Section E.

5×10^9 people, this amounts to a negligible dose per person per year.

Following the Chernobyl accident, the levels of iodine-131 in milk in the United States increased sharply. Prior to the accident, cow's milk typically contained less than a few hundredths of a becquerel of the isotope per quart. Over a two-week period following the accident, the levels rose to approximately 1 becquerel per quart, with levels in the northwestern United States reaching values about twice those in the southern and eastern regions. Even if a child ate or drank nothing but this contaminated milk during the period of iodine-131 increase, the increase in the annual *whole body dose* would have been far less than 1% of the normal background dose to that child.

Iodine-131 is absorbed readily in the blood from the *gastrointestinal tract* at a rate of about 5% per minute. Thirty percent of all iodine (and iodine-131) in blood ends up in the thyroid while the remainder is excreted from the body. Iodine-131 resides about four months in the thyroid before removal by natural flushing mechanisms. Since this is longer than the half-life of the isotope, decay rather than removal is what eventually reduces the dose. For each becquerel ingested, the dose to the thyroid is approximately 10^{-6} sieverts.

Further Reading

DeSante, D., and Geupel, G. R. 1987. Land Bird Productivity in Central Coastal California: The Relation to Annual Rainfall and a Reproductive Failure in 1986. *The Condor* 89:636–653.

National Council on Radiation Protection and Measurements. 1985. *Induction of Thyroid Cancer by Ionizing Radiation.* NCRP Report No. 80. Washington, D.C.

World Health Organization. 1983. *Environmental Health Criteria Report No. 25: Selected Radionuclides.* Geneva.

Laser Light

Other Names

Intense optical radiation; intense light sources (see also entry on **ultraviolet radiation**)

Introduction

Lasers are becoming a part of everyday life for more and more people each year. Lasers are critical components of compact disk players and top-of-the-line printers for home personal computers. They are increasingly used in medicine to perform eye surgery and are frequently encountered in scientific laboratories where they are an invaluable research tool. A laser is essentially just a light source of one single color that contains a great deal of energy in a small beam because the individual waves making up the beam are all moving in tandem and are packed tightly together. Ordinary light, such as from the sun or a flashlight, contains many colors, and the light waves are randomly jumbled together and spread out. Because waves in laser light are acting together, it can pack more of a wallop than ordinary light. The intense energy of laser light is what makes it so technologically useful, but it is also the source of concern over human health because this intense energy can damage living cells.

Physical and Chemical Properties

Laser light can be invisible if it is in the infrared or ultraviolet part of the spectrum, but most lasers in everyday use put out visible light (see Chapter 15, Section B). The rate of energy output from a laser is measured in watts, just like a light bulb. But a 100-watt laser focuses all its light energy into a very thin beam, unlike the light bulb whose energy is spread out. Thus, intensity of a laser is usually expressed in units of watts per square centimeter. For example, if a 1-watt laser produced a beam that was 0.1 centimeter in area, it would be rated at 10 watts per square centimeter. Lasers are usually encased in metal cylinders; its identification as a laser and its intensity are usually clearly labeled.

Exposure and Distribution

Despite occasional public fears, the everyday environment is not polluted by stray laser beams. The lasers in such home appliances as laser printers and compact disk players pose no threat to human health under normal use because the laser beams in these appliances are entirely confined within a protective housing. Of slightly more concern are laser light shows and the use of devices such as laser screen pointers that deliberately cast an external beam. Hospitals and scientific laboratories are the major places where the most serious exposure is possible. But in all these applications, exposure will be so low as to pose no threat as long as safety rules are followed.

Health Effects

The greatest danger is to the eye. Temporary vision impairment, permanent retinal injury, or cataracts can result from a direct hit to the eye from a laser beam. Exposure of the skin on any part of the body to laser light can also cause immediate harm, ranging from a minor skin reddening to severe blistering burns. Skin cancers (including *melanoma*) can result long after the exposure. Some ingested chemical substances are thought to increase the sensitivity of the skin to intense light: these include some oral contraceptives, diuretics, sweeteners, antibiotics, laxatives, and tranquilizers. (See a doctor for more specific information.) Very powerful lasers (for example, 100 watts per square centimeter, which are not the type found in home appliances) can cause severe damage from exposures as short as a thousandth of a second. Damaging exposure to weak lasers (for example, 1 watt per square centimeter) takes a second or so. (For more information on the risk of different intensities of laser light, see Regulatory Status section.) At a fixed intensity, or watt-age, ultraviolet lasers are more hazardous than visible ones and visible ones are more hazardous than infrared ones, although even infrared lasers can cause cataracts.

Protection and Prevention

Following an intense accidental exposure to the eye, an eye examination should be done immediately. (The entry on **ultraviolet radiation** also gives general guidelines for reducing skin and eye exposures.) In laboratories and other places where relatively powerful lasers might be easily accessible, read labels carefully before handling equipment. Avoid playing with lasers; they are not toys.

Regulatory Status

Lasers are grouped into classes by the Department of Health and Human Services. General safety guidelines have been created for each class. Lasers rated at less than 1 microwatt of total power output (class 1 lasers) are generally sufficiently weak that their health risk is not a concern; most home appliances with lasers fall into this category. Between 1 microwatt and 1 milliwatt (class 2), lasers can cause harm if their output is in the ultraviolet part of the spectrum and if exposure is lengthy. Between 1 milliwatt and 0.5 watt (class 3), eye injury can result even from short exposures, but skin injury is unlikely. Above 0.5 watt (class 4), severe injury can occur to any part of the body, but particularly to the eyes. Detailed guidelines covering use of lasers in each of these classes are available from manufacturers.

Further Reading

World Health Organization. 1982. *Environmental Health Criteria Report No. 23: Lasers and Optical Radiation*. Geneva.

Lead

Introduction

Lead is a common industrial metal that has become widespread in air, water, soil, and food. It causes severe health effects even at relatively low levels in the body, including often irreversible brain damage and injury to the blood-forming systems.

Lead is a naturally occurring chemical element. It was first mined over 5000 years ago when it was discovered that small quantities of silver could be extracted from lead ore. The ancient civilizations of Phoenicia, Egypt, Greece, India, and China used lead for vessels, roofs, water ducts, utensils, ornaments, and weights, and the Romans used lead extensively in the transport of water and the storage of wine and food. Lead poisoning from these sources has been implicated in the decline of the early Greek and Roman civilizations. To this day, lead glazes on ceramic pottery and lead in antique pewter pose a hazard. The use of lead as an antiknock additive in gasoline in this country has created a contamination problem of global proportions. Background concentrations of lead in even remote regions are believed to be three to five orders of magnitude greater than in prehistoric times. This vast increase in environmental lead has raised the measured blood concentrations of lead in some people close to the point of clinical symptoms. The addition of lead-based pigments to paints has caused the poisonings of thousands of preschool age children who have inadvertently eaten chips and flakes of or dust from these paints eroded from old buildings.

Physical and Chemical Properties

Lead is a soft, gray-white metal. It is slightly *soluble* in water and is transported mainly through the atmosphere. Lead behaves like calcium in the body and accumulates in bone. At times of calcium deficiency or greater calcium requirements, such as during pregnancy, lead can be mobilized from bone and enter the bloodstream, where it creates elevated levels in the blood. There are no known physiological requirements for lead.

Exposure and Distribution

The main source of adult human exposure is food, which is believed to account for over 60% of blood levels; air inhalation accounts for approximately 30% and water for 10%. In food, canned goods contribute approximately one-fifth and unprocessed food approximately four-fifths of the lead to the diet. Lead gets into foods by crops absorbing it from the soil, dry fallout from the air onto leaves, absorption from cooking water, contamination during processing, solder from cans, and leaching from storage materials.

For preschool age children, soil, dust, and lead-based paints are also significant sources of exposure. Children of this age spend a great deal of time on the ground, placing their fingers in their mouths, and tasting and swallowing nonfood objects. The ingestion of chips and flakes of leaded paint in this manner remains a major source of childhood lead poisoning in many inner urban areas of the United States today.

The major uses of lead in the United States are in storage batteries (72%), gasoline additives and other chemicals (13%), ammunition (shot and bullets, 4%), solder (2%), and other uses (9%). World production exceeds three million tons per year.

Lead is released into the environment primarily through the air by the burning of gasoline and solid wastes; from the atmosphere it is deposited onto soils, plants, and water. (Lead storage batteries, the largest use category, tend to be recycled.) Fortunately, emissions of lead into the air have declined dramatically in recent years because of progressive restrictions on the lead content of gasoline and the increasing use of unleaded gasoline. Since 1976, the year of peak emissions, lead releases have declined more than 94% from all sources and more than 97%

from vehicles. A smaller but corresponding decrease of 89% in lead air concentrations has been reported over the same period. Just between the years 1985 and 1986, lead emissions declined 59% and outdoor air levels declined 35%. These are impressive numbers that ultimately will translate into improved health of the population, particularly inner city groups.

Except in the immediate vicinity of mining, smelting, and manufacturing facilities, where concentrations are locally high, outdoor lead levels increase from rural to urban locations, as shown in Table 31. Drinking water concentrations are typically low, but most measurements have been taken at treatment plants, not at points of use. Leaded pipe and solder in pipe joints in water distribution systems and home plumbing can release lead. Recent evidence indicates that drinking water is a more important source of lead intake than previously believed and may account for up to 40% of lead exposure in some instances.

Health Effects

Lead affects the human nervous system, the production of blood cells, kidneys, reproductive system, and behavior. At the typical levels to which individuals are normally exposed, the blood and nervous systems are primarily affected. The symptoms of lead poisoning, unless it is acute, are often vague and nonspecific and may mimic other conditions. Symptoms include pallor, vomiting, abdominal pain, constipation, listlessness, stupor, loss of appetite, irritability, and loss of muscular coordination. The risks of lead poisoning are greatest in children and in pregnant women. Children are at high risk because of their potentially greater ingestion of lead particles and because harmful effects begin at lower blood lead levels. Pregnant women are at high risk because lead can cross the placenta and damage the developing fetal nervous system; lead can also induce miscarriage.

The margin of safety between measured blood lead levels and the levels causing clinical symptoms is remarkably small. Surveys of lead in the blood of children show typical concentrations already above the level at which changes in blood enzymes occur. Only a factor of two or three separates the blood lead level in many children and the level necessary to cause anemia and the onset of mental losses. This situation is undoubtedly caused by the vast increase in environmental lead in the last two centuries. Humans did not evolve under conditions of this much lead and are not adapted to it. Table 32 shows various groups of people and their typical blood lead levels, and Table 33 lists the health effects that occur at various blood lead levels.

Protection and Prevention

Foods should be washed prior to cooking or eating. Hands, particularly those of young children, should be washed before meals. Older ceramic pottery and antique pewter should not be used for food consumption. Most modern glazes, pewter, and food cans made in the United States are lead free. Nevertheless, be wary of imported pottery and food cans. (See Sources for Home Testing Equipment.) Water standing overnight in pipes should be flushed at the tap for 3 minutes prior to its use in cooking or drinking. Flaking lead-based paint should be removed by a professional; intact lead paint on buildings should be maintained by occasionally painting over with lead-free coatings. Joggers and cyclists should exercise away from traffic and should avoid peak driving hours.

Cases of suspected lead poisoning should be immediately diagnosed. If confirmed, chelation therapy is performed in which chemicals are administered that bind lead in the blood and allow it to be excreted in urine.

Regulatory Status

Lead is one of six air pollutants for which the EPA is required to set outdoor ambient air quality standards for protection of human health and to review their adequacy peri-

TABLE 31 Lead Concentrations in Various Environments

Medium	Range of Typical Concentrations
Air	
Natural, prehistoric	$0.00001-0.0001\ \mu g/m^3$
Rural or remote	$0.008-0.01\ \mu g/m^3$
Urban	$0.1-10\ \mu g/m^3$
Near lead smelter	$0.1-75\ \mu g/m^3$
Near urban freeway	$8.2-18\ \mu g/m^3$
Maximum permissible level	$1.5\ \mu g/m^3$
Water	
Drinking	$<1-20$ ppb
Maximum permissible level	20 ppb
Food	$0.01-10$ ppm

TABLE 32 Blood Lead Levels for Various Groups of People

Population	Blood Lead Concentration (μg/100 mL)
Rural children	7–11
Urban children	9–33
Adults	15–22
Children near smelter	35–68

TABLE 33 Health Effects at Various Blood Lead Levels

Health Effect	Blood Lead Concentration (μg/100 mL)
Level of concern for fetal effects	10–15
Blood enzyme changes	15–20
IQ deficiencies in children	<25
Clinical anemia, children	40
Clinical anemia, adults	50
Reproductive effects in adults	50
Mental losses (writing and speech problems and mental retardation)	50–60
Irreversible brain damage	100

odically, making adjustments as necessary. Currently about 1.6 million people live in U.S. counties that are in violation of the federal standard. As lead has been removed from gasoline, emissions to the air have dropped dramatically: 93% between 1979 and 1988. (The air quality standards for lead are given in the Technical Information Section.)

Drinking water concentrations are also regulated by the EPA, which has recently reduced the permissible level. The Consumer Product Safety Commission (CPSC) has banned toys and other articles for use by children, as well as consumer furniture, that have paint with a lead content greater than 0.06%. The FDA is studying ways to reduce the lead content of foods.

Technical Information

Chemical symbol: Pb
Atomic number: 46

Atomic weight: 106
Government standards:
National Ambient Air Quality Standard, maximum quarterly average: 1.5 μg/m³
National Drinking Water Standard, maximum contaminant level: 20 μg/L (20 ppb)
Gasoline, allowable lead content: 0.10 g/gal
Paint, allowable lead content: 0.06%

Further Reading

Agency for Toxic Substances and Disease Registry. 1988. *Toxicological Profile for Lead*. Washington, D.C.

Environmental Protection Agency. 1977. *Air Quality Criteria for Lead*. EPA–600/8–77–017. Washington, D.C.: Office of Research and Development.

National Research Council. 1980. *Lead in the Human Environment*. Washington, D.C.: National Academy Press.

Lindane

Other Names

Hexachlorocyclohexane (HCH); often incorrectly called benzene hexachloride (BHC)

Trade Names

Agronexit; Lindafor; Gamma BHC; Kwell (shampoo)

Introduction

For a time, lindane was a popular household *fumigant*, effective against flies and cockroaches, until it was found to be hazardous to people and pets. Lindane was commercially produced in the United States between 1945 and 1976 and is now imported in an undisclosed amount. It is actually only one component—the insecticidally active component—of the commercially available product properly called hexachlorocyclohexane (or HCH). Pure or essentially pure lindane is also available, but it is relatively more expensive than the mixture and impractical for large-scale use.

Discussions of lindane can be confusing. First, the names lindane and hexachlorocyclohexane (HCH) are often used interchangeably when referring to the insecticide. Commercial preparations of the insecticide generally consist of a mixture of hexachlorocyclohexane *isomers*, one of which is the gamma isomer, or lindane. Lindane is the insecticidally active isomer and may be present in the pesticide product in relatively small amounts. Of the other isomers of HCH, the beta isomer appears to be most important biologically. Adding to the confusion is the problem that HCH has been misnamed and is commonly referred to as benzene hexachloride (acronym BHC).

Used primarily in agriculture on fruit, nut, and vegetable crops, HCH has proven especially effective against grasshoppers, cotton insects, and rice pests. Additional uses include the treatment of hardwood logs and lumber, the control of head lice (in prescription shampoo), and the fumigation of stored grain products. It is also effective in controlling the mosquitoes that transmit malaria, but has been used to a far lesser extent than **DDT**.

Like most other *organochlorines*, HCH/lindane is highly *persistent* (resistant to physical, chemical, and biological breakdown) in soils and water. Presumably as a consequence of its persistence, residues have been detected on corn, for which use HCH/lindane is not registered. But widespread use of HCH on crops has been impractical since it imparts an off taste to some edible crops, especially potatoes. Because of its persistence and toxicity, it has been certified by the EPA as a toxic waste constituent.

Physical and Chemical Properties

HCH is a mixture of isomers, with the proportion of the lindane isomer being about 12%. Purified HCH is a colorless, crystalline solid that is only very slightly soluble in water. The commercial or technical grade (containing impurities) is an off-white to brownish powder with a characteristic penetrating, musty odor. The purified form has only a slight odor. HCH resists chemical breakdown when exposed to heat, light, and oxygen.

Exposure and Distribution

Available as dusts, sprays, and aerosols, HCH was used in large quantities in the United States until fairly recently. Since most uses have been canceled, it is estimated that only about 200,000 pounds of HCH are now used annually. Before the EPA cut back use of HCH/lindane, approximately 480,000 workers were occupationally exposed.

HCH can be absorbed from the digestive system, lungs, and skin. The lindane component is rapidly metabolized and excreted, but another isomer of HCH is not as readily broken down. Instead, it is stored in the fat, persists for years, and is more toxic to mammals than lindane. Studies show that over 30 times

more of this beta isomer is stored than lindane. Nevertheless, it is gradually lost from tissues; the National Human Adipose Tissue Survey reveals that the level of this component has declined steadily since 1970.

Quite persistent in the environment, HCH/lindane is apparently taken up by plants from previously treated soils and can be transferred through the *food chain*, as are other organochlorines. Consumption of contaminated food is the major route of exposure to the general public. Major dietary sources include eggs, milk and other dairy products, and to a lesser extent, seafood. Generally, the residue levels are low and declining.

Health Effects

HCH/lindane is of moderate to high *acute toxicity*. Compared to related insecticides, it is less toxic than **aldrin** and **dieldrin** and slightly more toxic than **DDT**, **heptachlor**, and **chlordane**. Linked to several accidental human deaths, lindane, like other organochlorines, is toxic to the nervous systems of insects and mammals. Signs of poisoning include headache, weakness, diarrhea, dizziness, increased blood pressure, decreased heart rate, tremors, convulsions, and physical collapse. Lindane poisoning is distinguishable from DDT poisoning in two respects: (1) the progress of poisoning is typically more rapid than with DDT, and (2) victims show no sign of the early excessive irritability associated with DDT poisoning.

The EPA classifies lindane as a possible human carcinogen (group C) on the basis of limited test data (see Table 5 in Chapter 3). Some studies found liver tumors in mice; other forms of HCH also produced tumors. Studies on rats and dogs are considered inadequate to assess lindane's ability to cause cancer. A variety of chronic ill effects are associated with HCH/lindane. In humans, these include bone marrow changes and aplastic anemia at exposure levels associated with normal use. Liver and kidney damage and various reproductive effects, including birth defects, reduced fertility and litter size, and increased fetal death, have been observed in rats. There is also some evidence that lindane affects the immune system and causes mutations in human cell cultures.

Protection and Prevention

Poisoning victims who have ingested the insecticide should be induced to vomit using Ipecac syrup or water. No milk or oily fluids should be given. In cases of skin or eye contamination, the insecticide should be flushed away with water. Contaminated clothing should be removed. A physician should be contacted. Phenobarbitol may be prescribed to counter the increased blood pressure, while atropine may be prescribed, as needed, for the decreased heart rate.

It is uncertain whether HCH/lindane residues can be removed from fresh fruits and vegetables by washing or peeling since it seems to be taken up by plants. As a rule, however, it is a good idea to wash or peel fresh produce. Cooking and canning seem to reduce the amount of residues left.

Environmental Effects

Typical of organochlorines, HCH accumulates in the fatty tissues of many species, is taken up by plants, and concentrates in the food chain. Fish and other aquatic organisms are particularly efficient at taking up the pesticide from the surrounding water. HCH is highly toxic to various species of fish and moderately toxic to some bird species that have been tested.

Technical Information

Chemical name: 1,2,3,4,5,6-hexachlorocyclohexane
Chemical formula: $C_6H_6Cl_6$
Residue levels in human fat (1970): 0.37 ppm
(1983): 0.10 ppm
Acute toxicity in rats based on lethal dose (LD_{50}):
    oral: 100–300 mg/kg
    dermal: 100 mg/kg

Acute toxicity in fish based on lethal dose (LD_{50}):
    0.003–0.01 ppm
Comparative toxicity ranking of related organochlorine insecticides in order of decreasing toxicity, based on the LD_{50} of rats: aldrin > dieldrin > lindane > heptachlor > DDT > chlordane
OSHA limit in workplace air: 0.5 mg/m³

Further Reading

MOTT, L., and SNYDER, K. 1987. *Pesticide Alert.* San Francisco: Sierra Club Books.
National Academy of Sciences. 1987. *Regulating Pesticides in Food.* Washington, D.C.: National Academy Press.

Malathion

Trade Name

Cythion

Introduction

Malathion, introduced in 1950, is an insecticide and *acaricide*, commonly used against mosquitoes, flies, household insects, human head and body lice, animal ticks and fleas, and sucking and chewing insects on fruits and vegetables. Considered one of the safest of the *organophosphates*, it is used extensively by the World Health Organization for malarial control programs and for the control of a recent massive outbreak of locusts in North Africa. Although malathion itself is fairly safe, most commercial products contain impurities, many of which are more toxic than the parent compound or which interact with malathion to enhance its toxicity. Moreover, improper storage, such as at temperatures greater than 100°F, can result in the formation of highly toxic impurities.

Physical and Chemical Properties

Pure malathion is a clear, colorless to amber-colored liquid that dissolves slightly in water. The technical grade is a brown liquid with a garlic-like odor. It is rapidly broken down under wet conditions at a pH greater than 7.0 or less than 5.0. Malathion is incompatible for use with alkaline pesticides.

Exposure and Distribution

About three million pounds of malathion are applied annually in the United States, mostly as sprays and dusts. It is a very common household insecticide. Residues of most organophosphates, including malathion, break down in about four weeks.

Health Effects

There is no evidence that malathion causes *mutations*, but some evidence suggests birth defects in mammals, and it produces a characteristic deformity in chickens. At high doses, malathion reduces the size of rat litters and decreases the survival rate of the young. Like other organophosphates and the *carbamates*, malathion inhibits *cholinesterase*, the *enzyme* that functions in the transmission of nerve signals (see Chapter 14, Section B). Moreover, in chickens it produces yet another effect on the nervous system, an irreversible inability to coordinate muscular movements, which evidently does not occur in humans. Unlike other organophosphate pesticides, malathion is rendered nontoxic when it is metabolized.

This pesticide, when manufactured and stored properly, is only slightly toxic to rats. Studies indicate, however, that humans are more susceptible than rats. And there are numerous reports of occupationally related poisonings. Treatment of poisoning depends on the level of severity, but artificial respiration and the administration of oxygen may be required. Atropine is usually given, followed by the drug pralidoxime chloride, if necessary. In general the skin, eyes, and stomach (depending on the route of entry) should be thoroughly flushed.

In studies using rats, the toxic impurities in malathion caused delayed effects and, ultimately, death. These impurities evidently inhibit the enzymes that normally function to metabolize malathion and other organophosphates. Malathion and certain other pesticides interact in such a way that the toxic effects are enhanced. Malathion interacts in this manner with several other organophosphates, possibly the **pyrethroid** insecticides, and some carbamate pesticides. In general, however, interactions between organophosphates and chlorinated hydrocarbon pesticides such as DDT do not appear to produce significantly different toxicities.

Protection and Prevention

Although malathion is not a *systemic* insecticide (that is, it acts only on the surface of the plant), there is some indication that it may be absorbed into the peel of fruits and vegetables. Washing with a small amount of detergent then rinsing well may be more effective at reducing the residues than rinsing alone. Cooking and heat processing may also reduce the residues, but residues tend to concentrate in dried fruits. The toxic agent of malathion and most other organophosphates can be neutralized by treating with alkali. This is an effective treatment for industrial effluents and wastes.

Environmental Effects

Malathion is moderately toxic to freshwater fish and invertebrates. Overall, it is considerably less toxic to aquatic organisms than **parathion** or chlorpyrifos, but more toxic than either **dichlorvos** or **diazinon**.

Regulatory Status

Because it is considered relatively safe, malathion is available to householders. Its use is not restricted, although the labels on containers caution people to store it properly, dispose of water–malathion solutions immediately after use, prevent contamination of streams and lakes by following directions for disposal, and avoid direct contact with the product.

Technical Information

Chemical names: $O,O,$-dimethyl-(S)-(1,2-dicarbethoxyethyl)phosphorodithioate or O,O-dimethyldithiophosphate of diethyl-mercaptosuccinate
Chemical formula: $C_{10}H_{19}O_6PS_2$
Toxicity in rats based on lethal dose (LD_{50}):
 oral: 885 mg/kg
 dermal: 4000 mg/kg
OSHA limit in workplace air: 15 mg/m^3
EPA food tolerances (examples):
 cabbage, broccoli, kale, lettuce: 8 ppm

Further Reading

HAYES, W. J., JR. 1982. *Pesticides Studied in Man*. Baltimore, MD: Williams and Wilkins.
World Health Organization. 1984. *Environmental Health Criteria No. 63: Organophosphate Pesticides*. Geneva.

Mercury

Other Name

Quicksilver

Introduction

Mercury, the silvery-white liquid metal used in thermometers, is a potent *neurotoxin*, capable of causing severe brain damage in developing fetuses and mild tremors and emotional disturbances in exposed adults. While not as dangerous as **lead** (the other major metal that causes nervous system damage) in causing widespread harm, mercury has been responsible for numerous poisoning episodes in the past. The expression "mad as a hatter" comes from mental disorders that occurred in hat workers caused by the mercury once used to process felt for hats (a use that no longer exists). Seafood is the largest source of present-day exposure because mercury accumulates in aquatic animals and reaches significant levels at the tops of both salt water and freshwater *food chains*.

Physical and Chemical Properties

Mercury is a naturally occurring metallic element and is commonly encountered as a heavy, silvery-white liquid. It is the only metal that is liquid at room temperature. Liquid mercury evaporates readily, so whenever liquid mercury is open to the air (for example, when a thermometer breaks and spills its contents or a bottle breaks in a laboratory or dental office), there can be a relatively high concentration of mercury vapor in the air. Mercury vapor is more hazardous than liquid mercury because it can be inhaled and is easily absorbed into the bloodstream.

In addition to pure mercury (vapor and liquid), compounds of mercury can also be harmful. *Inorganic* compounds used in paints as antimildew agents and in batteries are not highly toxic themselves, but are easily converted by bacteria to the far more hazardous *organic* forms, of which methylmercury is the best known and most important. Methylmercury is rapidly accumulated by fish and concentrates along aquatic food chains, reaching high levels at the top predators through the process of *biomagnification* (see further discussion in Environmental Effects section). Methylmercury is also rapidly absorbed by people who eat such fish and can readily pass through the placenta of pregnant women, exposing developing fetuses, and through the *blood–brain barrier* into the brain.

Exposure and Distribution

The exposure to mercury depends on its form, with mercury vapor and methylmercury being the most likely forms since they are nearly completely absorbed into the body. Methylmercury in fish and fish products is by far the largest source of mercury exposure (94%), followed by breathing mercury vapor from the air (6%). Drinking water makes a negligible contribution. These figures are averages for people not exposed at the workplace.

Above average exposures to mercury vapor are confined primarily to occupations where mercury is used. Of special importance are women of child-bearing age who work as dentists or dental assistants and may be exposed to mercury vapor in preparing dental fillings containing mercury metal amalgams. Such individuals may be exposed to above average levels of mercury vapor on a daily basis. Because the developing fetus is especially vulnerable, pregnant dental workers are of most concern. There is little evidence, however, that finished fillings in people's teeth release mercury vapor in sufficient quantities to cause health effects. People living with workers (such as dental workers and thermometer manufacturers) who are occupationally exposed may also experience higher than average exposures to mercury vapor because of mercury metal brought home on hands, hair, and clothes worn at the workplace.

People who receive above average exposures to methylmercury are mainly those who eat large amounts of fish. The EPA states that those who eat more than 30 pounds of fish per year are in the high risk group. Freshwater fish tend to have slightly higher levels than marine species. Pike, trout, and bass are the freshwater varieties tending to have the highest concentrations; shrimp, snapper, and halibut are the marine species most frequently consumed having the highest levels.

Geographically, mercury tends to be distributed in the vicinity of manufacturers using it, as well as near mines, smelters, municipal solid waste incinerators, and fossil-fueled power plants, since mercury is a trace contaminant of ores and fuels. Mercury is used in the manufacture of electrical equipment (56%), including small batteries, mercury cells in smoke detectors, and mercury lamps and switches; in the production of chlorine and caustic soda (12%); as an antimildew agent in paints (10%); in industrial and control instruments (6%); and in other products (16%). Workers in any of these industries and people living in the vicinity of these plants may be exposed to above average mercury concentrations. Total mercury consumption in the United States was 2000 tons in 1986.

Small batteries can be a hazard for children if swallowed not only because of choking, but also because the battery cover can dissolve in stomach acid, releasing the mercury within. There have been two reported cases of swallowed mercury batteries, both with successful outcomes. In one, the battery was successfully removed by physicians; in the other, it was passed in the stools.

Health Effects

The toxic effects of mercury depend on its chemical form. Inhaled mercury vapor, mainly a hazard to workers exposed on the job, primarily damages the nervous system. Memory losses, tremors, emotional instability (anxiety and irritability), insomnia, and loss of appetite characterize milder exposures. Introversion appears to be the most prominent personality trait in affected people. At moderate exposures, more significant mental disorders and motor disturbances, as well as kidney damage, are seen. Short-term exposures to high levels of mercury vapor may lead to lung damage and death. The milder effects of mercury vapor appear to reverse after exposure has stopped, with the muscular disorders improving sooner than the mental ones. Mercury vapor passes through the placenta to the fetus, but there is little reported information on prenatal effects in exposed pregnant women. Evidence does show a higher rate of spontaneous abortions and other complications of pregnancy in pregnant workers exposed to mercury vapor such as in dental offices.

Methylmercury is the form to which most people are exposed. It has dramatic effects on the nervous system, particularly in the developing fetus and in small children. The mildest cases of poisoning show nonspecific symptoms, such as malaise, blurred vision, and pins-and-needles tingling. Symptoms usually appear after a *latency period* of a few weeks to months during chronic low-level exposures or following acute high-level exposure. More severe cases show constriction of vision, diminished hearing, speech disorders, and shaky movements and unsteady gaits. The most severe cases show mental derangement and coma, with death the frequent outcome.

Prenatal and early childhood are the most sensitive stages to methylmercury poisoning because the brain is developing rapidly at these times. If exposure to a pregnant woman is mild, there may be only delayed achievement of development milestones and modest neurological abnormalities in the baby. More severe exposure can result in dramatic effects on development, including abnormal placement of brain structures and gross impairment of motor and mental development (such as severe cerebral palsy, generalized spasticity, incontinence, blindness, and poor or nonexistent language development). The effects are irreversible. Two major incidents of methylmercury poisoning occurred in Japan in the areas of Minamata Bay and the Niigata River, and one occurred in rural Iraq. In Japan, industrial effluents contaminated fish, a main component of the diet; in Iraq, contaminated grain was used to make bread that was subsequently eaten.

Inorganic mercury compounds are not highly toxic because they are not well absorbed and do not easily penetrate the blood–brain or placental barriers. Consumption of several grams of mercury compounds can cause death by kidney failure, and smaller doses over longer times can lead to kidney and nerve damage. Cancer has not been associated with mercury in the laboratory or in human studies. Laboratory studies show that methylmercury is a weak *mutagen*.

In summary, several major groups are at risk for mercury exposure. One is workers, especially women of child-bearing age, who are exposed to mercury vapor on the job. In particular, this group includes female dental assistants and women in the thermometer and scientific apparatus manufacturing industries where calibration of instruments often involves use of liquid mercury. Other groups at risk include pregnant women, young children, and people who consume two or more times the national average of 15 pounds of fish per year.

Protection and Prevention

Workers using mercury on the job should pay careful attention to all safety requirements and regulations and should promptly clean up spilled mercury. Pregnant workers should avoid areas where mercury is in use. People who frequently eat fish and other seafood should pay special attention to reports of high levels of mercury in local fish and should reduce their consumption of those varieties accordingly. The federal government sets action limits that prevent fish containing mercury above certain levels from entering the food supply. Actions that are taken are usually reported in the local news media.

Environmental Effects

Two main environmental processes result in heightened exposures to humans. Inorganic mercury discharges by industry are converted by bacteria in freshwater and seawater and in sediments to organic methylmercury. Methylmercury is rapidly taken up by fish and stored in fish muscle. Through biomagnification, fish low in the aquatic food chain are eaten by fish at higher levels, causing the methylmercury to reach progressively higher concentrations in fish tissue. When people eat fish at the tops of food chains, such as swordfish, pike, and trout, they receive methylmercury at much greater concentrations than are present in the water the fish came from. In fact, this is the main mechanism of mercury exposure for most people. The second environmental process relates to acid rain and the increasing acidification of surface waters that it causes. The more acidic conditions shift the organic mercury to forms that are more readily absorbed by fish (dimethyl- to monomethylmercury), thus raising the levels in fish to which humans are ultimately exposed. If acidification of surface waters continues, this process will become increasingly important.

Mercury is toxic to fish and other aquatic organisms. Freshwater species are more vulnerable than marine species because **selenium** in seawater provides partial protection against mercury's effects. Rainbow trout appears to be the most sensitive fish species and *Daphnia magna* the most sensitive invertebrate; various species of algae are also affected. Terrestrial organisms are generally not exposed to levels of mercury that are harmful.

Regulatory Status

Mercury concentrations in water are regulated by the EPA, in food by the FDA, and in workplace air by OSHA. If mercury concentrations in fish reach a certain "action level," the FDA prohibits fishing for those species. Mercury is listed as a *hazardous air pollutant* in the 1990 Clean Air Act, requiring the EPA to set emission standards. It is also on the EPA *community right-to-know* list.

Technical Information

Chemical symbol: Hg
Atomic number: 80
Atomic weight: 200.5
Density: 13.6 g/cm^3
Primary drinking water standard: 0.002 mg/L (2 ppb)
FDA action level: 1.00 µg/g (1 mg/kg)
OSHA limit in workplace air: 0.1 mg/m^3

Further Reading

CLARKSON, T. W. 1983. Methylmercury Toxicity to the Mature and Developing Nervous System *in* SARKAR, B., ed. *Biological Aspects of Metals and Metal-Related Diseases.* New York: Raven Press.

Environmental Protection Agency. 1984. *Mercury Health Effects Update—Health Issue Assessment.* EPA–600/8–84–019F. Washington, D.C.

———. 1981. *An Exposure and Risk Assessment for Mercury.* EPA–440/4–85–011. Washington, D.C.

Methyl Ethyl Ketone

Other Names

MEK; 2-butanone; methyl acetone; ethyl methyl ketone; butanone

Introduction

Methyl ethyl ketone, or MEK, is a popular industrial solvent. It is used to make lacquers and varnishes, plastics, lubricating oils, and artificial leather. It is also used during the manufacture of drugs and cosmetics. Some furniture finish strippers and specialty adhesive products (such as fishing rod cement and china cement) also incorporate MEK.

Physical and Chemical Properties

Methyl ethyl ketone is a colorless, volatile liquid with a sharp, mint-like smell that resembles acetone. It mixes equally well with water and oils. It can explode when heated or exposed to flame.

Exposure and Distribution

About 300,000 tons of MEK are manufactured in the United States each year. More than three million workers are regularly exposed to MEK vapors. Consumer exposure is negligible, although the solvent is used in a small group of adhesives and furniture finish strippers. The acetone-like odor of MEK can be smelled before any acute ill effects are likely to be felt. Low levels of MEK are known to migrate into water from polyvinyl chloride (PVC) water supply pipes.

Health Effects

Methyl ethyl ketone is irritating to the eyes, mucous membranes, and skin. Headache and throat irritation are reported among people exposed to concentrations near the maximum level allowed in the workplace. At higher levels, workers complain of numbness in the fingers and arms and sometimes the legs.

Dermatitis is sometimes reported following prolonged exposure to MEK vapors.

Easily absorbed into the body from the lungs and skin, MEK is removed from the body during exhaling and in the urine. Absorbed MEK causes lethargy among exposed laboratory animals, but this symptom is generally not seen in humans. However, people who experience low-level chronic exposure to MEK fumes tend to show decreased memory and slowed reaction time. The chronic toxicity of MEK is not well understood. No good studies exist with which to evaluate its cancer-causing potential. Birth defects were reported in one study in which mice inhaled MEK fumes during pregnancy. However, this study has not been duplicated. Exposure to MEK increases the toxicity of several solvents, including methyl *n*-butyl ketone, ethyl butyl ketone, *n*-hexane, 2,5-hexanedione, **carbon tetrachloride**, and **chloroform**.

Protection and Prevention

Methyl ethyl ketone fumes are most likely to be encountered in the workplace. Request a *Material Safety Data Sheet (MSDS)* whenever working with solvents. If one is not available, contact the local department of public health. MEK fumes can also be encountered at home during the use of certain furniture finish strippers and adhesives. Unfortunately, the ingredient list on products likely to contain MEK often states only that ketones are present, without specifying which ketone. Since the class of chemicals known as ketones includes the less toxic **acetone**, any product giving off an acetone-like smell should be used with care and plenty of ventilation.

Environmental Effects

When MEK is spilled, it evaporates quickly into the atmosphere where it is easily broken down. However, MEK does dissolve in water, so that spills on land are capable of traveling through the soil to groundwater.

Regulatory Status

Vapor concentrations in the workplace are regulated by OSHA. MEK is listed as a *hazardous air pollutant* in the 1990 Clean Air Act, requiring the EPA to set emission standards. It is on the EPA *community right-to-know* list.

Technical Information

Chemical formula: C_4H_8O
Molecular weight: 72
Amount produced in the United States:
  300,000 tons/year
Odor threshold in air: 0.25–25 ppm
Health effects thresholds in air:
  eye irritation: 100 ppm
  dermatitis: 300 to 600 ppm
  lethal level: 3000 ppm
OSHA limit in workplace air: 200 ppm
EPA reportable spill quantity: 5000 pounds

Further Reading

YANG, RAYMOND. 1986. The Toxicity of Methyl Ethyl Ketone. *Residue Reviews*, vol. 97. New York: Springer–Verlag.

Methylene Chloride

Other Names

Dichloromethane; methane dichloride; methylene bichloride

Trade Names

Aerothene; NM; Narkotil; Solaestine; Somethine

Introduction

Methylene chloride is the most common chemical used to remove paint. Anyone who has tried to remove dried paint with a chemical paint remover has probably come into contact with it. Its toxicity is complicated because it decomposes into **carbon monoxide** in the body, and the toxic effects felt by an individual are most likely caused by carbon monoxide in the blood rather than the chemical itself. In turn, individual susceptibility to carbon monoxide intoxication depends on body weight, smoking habits, and breathing rate. Methylene chloride is also found as a residue in chemically decaffeinated coffee, as it has replaced **trichloroethylene** as the decaffeinating solvent.

Some hairspray formulations contain methylene chloride. It is also used as an aerosol propellant and an inert ingredient in fumigants, pesticides, and industrial cleaning solutions, as well as in shoe polish, fabric waterproofing, fire extinguishers, air deodorizers, and spot removers.

Physical and Chemical Properties

Methylene chloride is a colorless, *volatile* liquid. Its sweet chloroform-like odor is pleasant. It can be quite dangerous when heated, as it emits the toxic gas phosgene. It is nonflammable.

Exposure and Distribution

Methylene chloride is widely used by consumers. Domestic production is estimated to be over 300,000 tons annually, about 30% of which is used in paint strippers and removers. Aerosol finishes are a second major source, accounting for an additional 20% of the methylene chloride used. About 80% of the methylene chloride manufactured each year is released into the atmosphere immediately following its use. But it degrades quickly in the air, so that accumulation throughout the atmosphere is unlikely. Methylene chloride is a common pollutant of urban air, and wells can become contaminated with the chemical as a result of spills or leaking storage tanks.

Health Effects

The major route of exposure is through inhalation. Methylene chloride is readily absorbed once inside the lungs. Uptake is directly proportional to exposure concentration and time. Uptake increases with exercise and the amount of body fat present in the exposed individual. Absorbed methylene chloride is distributed throughout the body and easily crosses the *blood–brain barrier* and the placenta. It can also be found in the breast milk of exposed women. Absorption through the skin and *gastrointestinal tract* is slow. Such routes of exposure are unlikely to contribute much to a total dose received because the chemical burns on contact with skin. Once inside the body, methylene chloride is rapidly converted to carbon monoxide, although it can also be stored in body fat. *Carboxyhemoglobin* levels can remain high for many hours following exposure because of delayed conversion of methylene chloride from fat stores.

Liver changes have been found following exposure to high doses in mice. People exposed to high levels of methylene chloride show decreased manual performance and attention lapses. Heart arrhythmias and death have been ascribed to excessively high levels of the solvent in air. At high levels, methylene chloride is irritating to the eyes and respiratory tract. At such levels, the exposed person also becomes sleepy and may experience nausea. Warning signs of overexposure include headache, fatigue, giddiness, irritability, and numbness in the extremities. Damage to the liver and central nervous system is also possible as a result of chronic exposure to the solvent.

Methylene chloride may cause cancer. National Toxicology Program inhalation bioassay tests found "clear evidence of *carcinogenicity*" in female rats and "some evidence of carcinogenicity" in male rats, causing liver and lung cancers. It has also been shown to be a *mutagen* in some strains of mice, but not in humans. The EPA classifies methylene chloride as a probable human carcinogen (a B_2 substance according to the classification of Table 5 in Chapter 3).

Protection and Prevention

Exposure to methylene chloride can be avoided by using alternative methods of removing paint, such as a heat gun and a scraping knife. (But be careful when removing paint that may contain lead, as the high heat produced by the heat gun will vaporize the lead in the paint, allowing it to be inhaled, and scraping may produce lead-containing dust.) Use all chemical paint removers with plenty of ventilation. Air concentrations of methylene chloride in excess of those allowed in industry can be reached within 2 hours in a basement shop or a closed garage.

Try to buy hairsprays and aerosol products that do not contain methylene chloride, although it may be difficult to determine if methylene chloride is an ingredient in these products. Use water-processed decaffeinated coffee in place of regular decaffeinated coffee. Avoid water-proofing chemicals, particularly aerosol types. If methylene chloride is used at work, ask for a *Material Safety Data Sheet (MSDS)*. It should provide information about methylene chloride toxicity and exposure routes and will suggest protective measures.

Environmental Effects

Methylene chloride stays in the groundwater for many years. It is removed from surface water via evaporation, which cannot happen from groundwater. In addition, it does not undergo any degradation as a result of microbial activity. It also does not stick well to soil particles and thus travels freely; allowing it to move great distances in an aquifer following its release into soil.

Regulatory Status

Methylene chloride is regulated by OSHA, the EPA, and the FDA. It is listed as a *hazardous air pollutant* in the 1990 Clean Air Act, requiring the EPA to set emission standards. It is on the *community right-to-know* list.

Technical Information

Chemical formula: CH_2Cl_2
Molecular weight: 85
OSHA limit in workplace air: 100 ppm
EPA standard for drinking water: 0.150 ppm
FDA standards for foods:
   spice extracts: 30 ppm
   decaffeinated coffee: 10 ppm
   brewing hops: 220 ppm

Further Reading

Agency for Toxic Substances and Disease Registry. 1988. *Toxicological Profile for Methylene Chloride*. Washington, D.C.: U.S. Public Health Service.

Microwave and Radio Frequency Radiation

Other Names

Radio waves; RF radiation

Introduction

Both microwave radiation and radio frequency radiation are each a part of the *electromagnetic spectrum* (see Chapter 15, Section B). Microwave radiation is increasingly being used for heating and cooking foods quickly and is also used in telecommunications, satellite tracking, and industrial welding processes. Radio frequency (RF) radiation is used to transmit radio, television, and radar signals.

Physical and Chemical Properties

The human eye cannot detect microwave and RF radiation directly because the *wavelengths* of these kinds of radiation are far longer than those of visible light (or equivalently, their *frequencies* are far lower). Microwave radiation of sufficient intensity striking a person can be detected directly by the warmth it creates. The RF radiation used for radio and television transmission can pass around large objects, such as buildings, but the higher frequency RF radiation, such as that used for radar transmission, is blocked by small metallic objects.

Exposure and Distribution

The major source of human exposure to microwaves is microwave ovens in the home or office. Even from normal use of such ovens, exposures vary by as much as a factor of 100, with actual exposures depending on the amount of leakage from the appliance. RF radiation exposure is mainly a potential problem for people living near radar installations, radio or television transmitters, or other telecommunications facilities. Human exposure from man-made sources of both microwave and RF radiation far exceeds that from natural sources.

Health Effects

Microwave and RF radiation can cause health damage by direct heating of tissue, which can result in damage ranging from mild burns to the death of isolated patches of tissue, hemmorrhaging, and even death. Thermal damage to the eyes from microwave radiation can result in cataracts. Microwave and RF radiation can also cause nonthermal effects, such as virus activation, interference with enzyme synthesis or cell division, damage to the nervous and immune systems, changes in cardiac rhythm, and possibly mutations and birth defects. Surveys conducted among people receiving excessive industrial exposures indicate that the most common symptoms of excessive exposure are headaches, fatigue, dizziness, confusion, and insomnia. Test animals exhibit changes in conditioned reflex behavior at high doses. (See Table 34 in Technical Information section for more quantitative information on health risks.)

Protection and Prevention

Older microwave ovens may be leaky, whereas models now being sold are subjected to more rigorous standards. A poor fitting door is a clear sign that you should replace the unit. For more information on safe brands, consult the *Consumers Guide* put out each year by the Consumers Union. If possible, avoid spending large amounts of time near RF radiation transmitters. Fortunately, there is little risk one-half mile away from a large transmitting facility.

Regulatory Status

The U.S. Code of Federal Regulations (1970) restricts leakage from microwave ovens (see Table 34 in Technical Information section). In the United States, exposures to the general public from telecommunications are unregulated.

TABLE 34 Sources, Effects, and Permissible Levels of Microwave Radiation

Sources	Intensity (mW/cm^2)
Natural background	10^{-3}
Typical RF radiation intensity 0.5 mile from large transmitting facilities	0.01
Range of exposures from home microwave ovens	0.005–0.1
Exposure in worst 1% of U.S. area from telecommunication facilities	Greater than 0.1
Exposure in worst 0.01% of U.S. area from telecommunications facilities	Greater than 10

Effects	Minimum Intensity to Cause Effect (mW/cm^2)
Possible effect on cardiac rhythm	0.1
Possible burning of tissue	1
Possible damage to nervous tissue and immune system from long-term exposure	1
Severe burns likely	100
Death of test animals in the laboratory from long-term exposure	100
Cataracts possible from short-term exposure	200

Regulations and Standards	Intensity (mW/cm^2)
WHO's suggested occupational exposure limit	0.1
U.S. microwave standard for intensity 5 cm (2 in.) from oven surface	1
Soviet Union's microwave exposure standards:	
20 minutes per day	1
10 hours per day	0.01

Technical Information

Microwave radiation wavelengths range from 1 millimeter to 1 meter, with corresponding frequencies of 3×10^{11} to 3×10^8 cycles per second. RF radiation wavelengths range from 1 meter to 3 kilometers, with corresponding frequencies of 3×10^8 to 1×10^5 cycles per second.

The intensity of microwave and RF radiation is usually expressed in units of milliwatts per square centimeter (mW/cm^2). Table 34 gives the most important numbers characterizing sources and effects. Intensities refer to both RF and microwave radiation unless otherwise specified.

Further Reading

World Health Organization. 1981. *Environmental Health Criteria Report No. 16: Radiofrequency and Microwaves.* Geneva.

Mineral Fibers (Nonasbestos)

Other Names

Glass wool; rock wool; fiberglass; mineral dust

Introduction

Materials manufactured from mineral fibers are commonly used for heat insulation in buildings. Fiberglass bonded with epoxy resin is also used in the construction of boat shells and other rigid structures. A very small quantity is used in the manufacture of fireproof drapery material. When mineral fibers are bonded into rigid structures or formed into cloth, practically no harmful human contact can occur. When used as insulation, however, loose fibers can come into contact with skin or be inhaled, and in these cases, the possibility of toxic risk arises. Home insulation usually consists of panels of fluffy, fibrous material attached to heavy paper and is purchased in rolls. In some houses, however, loose mineral fibers are blown between the inner and outer walls. In either case, loose fibers can become airborne, or one's skin can come into direct contact with the fibers during installation or removal of the insulation. (**Asbestos** is a particular type of mineral fiber that is treated as a separate entry in Part II because it is far more hazardous than the minerals discussed here.)

Physical and Chemical Properties

Mineral fibers are generally gray to yellowish in color. They are composed primarily of the element silica (SiO_2), the building of glass and the most common constituent in rock. Mineral fibers can vary in length from a tiny fraction of an inch to several inches; their thickness ranges from roughly that of a human hair to about one-hundredth of that thickness.

Exposure and Distribution

Nearly ten million tons of mineral fiber were produced worldwide in 1988, and production is increasing at a rate of about 3% per year. About 80% of commercially available mineral fiber is produced from glass, while most of the remainder is made from various types of rocks. In clean outdoor air, the background concentration of mineral fibers is about one fiber per cubic foot of air. In homes with mineral fiber insulation that is not being installed or removed, the indoor air typically has a mineral fiber concentration that is ten times the background level.

Health Effects

Upon direct contact with skin, mineral fibers can cause a mild irritation and itching. Eye irritation can also occur, although normal watering of the eye should remove the foreign material. Mineral fiber derived from glass (that is, glass wool) poses little or no risk to the respiratory system. Rock wool is of more concern and may be implicated in respiratory disease and possibly lung cancer after prolonged and heavy exposures such as can occur in mines or in factories manufacturing rock wool products. Normal household installation of nonasbestos mineral fiber insulation appears to pose very little respiratory risk and is not considered to be a cause of cancer.

Protection and Prevention

To be entirely safe, wear a dust mask when installing or removing mineral fiber installation (and never attempt to install or remove asbestos insulation). If you discover loose mineral fibers in your home (flaking off pipe insulation, for example) and are unsure if they are asbestos or not, you can perform this simple test: place the fibers in water and if they do not dissolve, they could be (but are not necessarily) asbestos and should be examined by a professional. To avoid prolonged skin irritation after contact with mineral fibers, shower thoroughly.

Regulatory Status

No regulations currently exist for indoor air except in the workplace, where mineral fibers alone are not regulated, but dust levels (which include mineral fibers) are. The current OSHA standard for total dust concentrations in the workplace are set at about 1000 times the highest levels currently encountered in ordinary homes.

Technical Information

OSHA air levels for workplace dust (<1 μm in diameter):
respirable dust: 5 mg/m³
total dust: 15 mg/m³

Further Reading

World Health Organization. 1988. *Environmental Health Criteria Report No. 77: Man-made Mineral Fibers*. Geneva.

Monosodium Glutamate (MSG)

Trade Name

Accent

Introduction

Monosodium glutamate, or MSG, is a natural salt found in low concentrations in seaweed, soy beans, and sugar beets. Refined MSG is used to enhance the flavor of certain foods, particularly red meat, poultry, and fish. It is widely used for that purpose by the processed food industry and in Asian restaurants, particularly Chinese and Japanese. The most common processed foods to be seasoned with MSG are meat products (such as gravies, bouillons, soups, and precooked packaged dinners), condiments, pickles, candy, and baked goods.

Physical and Chemical Properties

Monosodium glutamate is the sodium salt of the amino acid glutamate. It is a white powder with a salty taste.

Exposure and Distribution

It can be encountered by almost anyone who eats processed food or eats out in Asian restaurants. Most of the health complaints associated with MSG have come from people who have eaten at Chinese restaurants. Soups and foods coated with a liquid sauce often contain the highest concentrations of MSG of all foods. The rice used to make Japanese sushi can also contain relatively high concentrations of MSG.

Health Effects

In susceptible people, MSG has been known to cause a tight feeling in the face and head, headache, chest pain, dizziness, sweating, and numbness. This malady is known as "Chinese restaurant syndrome" because it was first associated with eating Chinese food. We now know that MSG is the cause of these symptoms. It appears that a certain (but as yet undefined) subgroup of the population is particularly susceptible to discomfort due to eating MSG. The FDA estimates that approximately 4% of the population in the United States will have occasional negative reactions to MSG in food, and about 2% will react to it regularly.

The discomfort, however, may be a symptom of a far more serious problem. MSG is known to significantly raise glutamate levels in the blood. In monkeys, raised glutamate levels can produce brain damage in the area of the brain that controls thirst, hunger, body temperature, and other automatic nervous system activity. However, this finding is still subject to debate. Some researchers think that the nerve degeneration associated with diseases such as Huntington's, Parkinson's, and Alzheimer's may be due to abnormal glutamate *metabolism*. But it is not clear that high glutamate levels in humans cause brain damage similar to that observed in monkeys, or whether glutamate circulating in the blood contributes to the progression of degenerative diseases, such as those just mentioned, in susceptible people. In addition, glutamate levels in the blood tend to be much lower when MSG is eaten with food, rather than administered alone. (Animal studies usually give MSG dissolved in water, with no food.)

Nevertheless, John Olney, a leading researcher who has spent over 20 years studying various aspects of glutamate toxicity, is convinced that MSG does indeed harm some people. He is particularly concerned about infants and children. Olney has found that infant animals are much more susceptible to brain damage caused by glutamate than are adult animals, leading him to conclude that human infants and children are also at risk from MSG added to food. Olney also argues that children are at risk from the artificial sweetener **aspartame** because it contains the amino acid aspartate that excites the brain in a similar fashion to glutamate. The FDA does not find adequate support in the scientific literature to accept Olney's conclusions.

Protection and Prevention

When MSG is added to packaged foods, the labels are required to list the ingredient. By shopping carefully, it should be fairly easy to avoid the substance. Pay particular attention to soups, bouillons, gravy mixes, and other products that contain poultry, fish, and meat or their flavors. Avoiding MSG at restaurants is much more difficult since the menu is unlikely to state that the food contains the flavor enhancer. Some Asian restaurants now cater to people who want to avoid MSG by prominently displaying that they do not use the substance. Unless it is explicitly stated otherwise, it should be assumed that Asian food served in restaurants contains MSG. Asian restaurants are not the only eating establishments where MSG is likely to be found, however. Many inexpensive and fast-food restaurants use packaged mixes, dry soup bases, and other convenience foods that contain MSG. Chinese restaurant syndrome is more frequently reported among people who drink alcoholic beverages during their meal.

Regulatory Status

Monosodium glutamate is considered safe by the FDA. No regulations are available to guide or restrict use of the substance. Grocery products that contain MSG must list it on the ingredient label.

Further Reading

BARINAGA, MARCIA. 1990. Amino Acids: How Much Excitement Is Too Much. *Science*. 247:20–22.

OLNEY, J. W. 1982. The Toxic Effects of Glutamate and Related Compounds in the Retina and the Brain. *Retina* 2:341–359.

Naphthalene

Other Names

Naphthalin; naphthene; tar camphor; white tar; moth balls

Introduction

Naphthalene is probably best known as moth balls or moth flakes. Its musty smell is familiar to most people. It is used in the home in carpet cleaners, typewriter correction fluid, adhesives, and toilet bowl deodorizers. Naphthalene is particularly toxic to children.

Physical and Chemical Properties

Naphthalene is a white, crystalline solid at room temperature, although it is sometimes brown. It has an easily recognized musty smell. It melts if left in the sun, and vaporizes easily in a warm room. Pure naphthalene can be explosive at high concentrations.

Exposure and Distribution

Inhalation is the most common route of chronic exposure both in the home and in industrial settings. Naphthalene is most toxic, however, when accidentally ingested or upon prolonged skin contact. Naphthalene used in the home as moth balls or flakes and as a toilet bowl deodorizer is a common household poison. It is used industrially as a raw material with which to make other chemicals, including dyes, synthetic resins, **carbon black**, solvents, lubricants, and fuels.

Health Effects

Naphthalene is irritating to the eyes upon exposure in the air. Nausea, vomiting, and disorientation may occur following prolonged inhalation of the chemical. Accidentally swallowed naphthalene can also cause nausea, vomiting, and disorientation. Prolonged exposure to naphthalene can alter kidney function and may cause cataracts to form.

Naphthalene on the skin may cause allergic reactions characterized by *dermatitis*.

Absorbed naphthalene can cause delayed disruption of the red blood cells in sensitive people. In addition to the more typical symptoms of exposure, people who are sensitive to naphthalene complain of headache, confusion, either excitement or malaise, profuse sweating, and irritation of the bladder. Infants are particularly susceptible to harm from naphthalene poisoning, as are people with a glucose–6-phosphate dehydrogenase (G6PD) deficiency (afflicting 100 million people worldwide).

Protection and Prevention

Moths can be repelled using natural substances rather than moth balls. Store wool in a cedar chest or cedar-lined closet, or tuck bay leaves between stored wool articles. Not only will the stored wool smell nicer, but a poison will have been eliminated from the closet. Scrub toilets (outside as well as inside) often, and ventilate the bathroom to control odors rather than masking them with toxics.

Environmental Effects

Naphthalene accumulates in lake and stream sediments. Sediment concentrations can be more than 100 times higher than concentrations measured in the overlying water. Naphthalene is also known to *bioaccumulate* in aquatic organisms.

Regulatory Status

Human exposure to naphthalene is regulated only by OSHA. The EPA regulates naphthalene concentration in water only to the extent that aquatic life is protected.

Technical Information

Chemical symbol: $C_{10}H_8$
Amount produced in the United States:
  300,000 tons/year

Background concentrations:

- urban air: 0.00035 μg/m³
- rural air: 0.00006 μg/m³
- urban water: 2 μg/L
- drinking water: 1.4 μg/L

Typical industrial exposures:

- naphthalene industries: 1,000 mg/m³
- coke oven workers: 1,120 μg/m³
- aluminum reduction
  plant workers: 0.3 mg/m³

OSHA limit in workplace air: 50 mg/m³
Lethal level in air: 2.5 gram/m³

Further Reading

GOSSELIN, R. E., SMITH, R. P., and HODGE, H. C. 1984. *Clinical Toxicology of Commercial Products*, 5th edition. Baltimore, MD: Williams and Wilkins.

Nickel

Introduction

Nickel is a naturally occurring silvery metal that is used in a wide variety of consumer and industrial products. It also occurs naturally in foods. The most important effect of nickel in the general population is a skin reaction called nickel contact dermatitis. Nickel refinery dust can cause lung, throat, and nasal cancer in workers exposed to it. Nickel in food and water is not believed to be hazardous; in fact, there is some evidence that small amounts of nickel may be required for good health. Nevertheless, because nickel is *carcinogenic* under some circumstances, its potential for causing cancer by ingestion is uncertain.

Physical and Chemical Properties

The element nickel occurs in ores in the earth's crust and is mined and smelted to produce nickel metal and other nickel compounds. Nickel metal is a hard, silvery solid with a high melting point; it does not easily dissolve in either water or organic solvents, and it does not burn. Other nickel compounds vary in their chemical and physical properties. The two most important compounds from a health perspective are nickel subsulfide and nickel carbonyl, both found in nickel refineries. Nickel carbonyl, a volatile liquid, is the most acutely toxic nickel compound known, causing both immediate poisoning and delayed lung effects. It is a hazard only within nickel refineries, however, because it degrades in minutes to harmless end products. Nickel subsulfide, in contrast, is a long-lasting component of nickel refinery dust that causes lung cancer (it is discussed further in Health Effects section).

Exposure and Distribution

The greatest exposure to nickel for the average person comes from food (approximately 90% of total intake), but ingested nickel is not believed to present a health hazard, mainly because humans have evolved efficient ways to prevent nickel absorption from the *gastrointestinal tract*. Exposures that cause the greatest harm are skin contact with nickel-containing products by people who are sensitive to it and inhalation of nickel compounds by workers in various industries. Nickel also occurs in tobacco and therefore in tobacco smoke; it is breathed both by smokers and others nearby. The form of nickel in tobacco smoke may be the hazardous nickel carbonyl.

Because nickel is used in coins and in hundreds of consumer products (including buttons, zippers, jewelry, stainless steel kitchen utensils, appliances, faucets, and pipes), it is difficult not to come in contact with it. For those who are sensitive, either because of a family history of skin reactions or because of sensitization at an early age, handling nickel coins or products can bring on nickel contact dermatitis (see Health Effects section). Beauticians can also be highly exposed because of nickel in hairsprays and shampoos. Among industrial workers, those with greatest exposures include nickel refining and fabricating workers, stainless steel makers, welders, electroplates, battery makers, jewelers, spray painters, paint makers, and varnish makers. An estimated 250,000 workers are exposed to nickel on the job.

Nickel is widespread in the environment because it is a natural elemental substance and because it is produced through human activities. The greatest concentrations occur in the air, soil, and water in the vicinity of nickel-producing facilities, metal refineries, and municipal solid waste incinerators. Since 1985, there have been no operating nickel producers in the United States, but the deposits in soils from prior years of operation represent a continuing source of nickel exposure.

Health Effects

Cancers of the lung, nasal passages, and possibly the larynx (voice box) are the most serious effects of nickel exposure, but these are probably limited to occupational exposures. Workers in the nickel refining industry who are exposed to nickel subsulfide—a component of nickel refinery dust—show increased rates of these cancers. There are no nickel refining plants in the United States today. Nickel-plating workers and welders exposed to various nickel compounds have developed allergic lung reactions, such as *asthma*; loss of the sense of smell; and severe nasal injuries, such as perforated septa and chronic sinus infections. Increased susceptibility to respiratory infections is also possible, as shown by experiments conducted on animals. The EPA concludes on the basis of exposure levels that these effects are probably limited to workplace exposure.

Animal studies have provided compelling evidence that nickel causes cancer, but only limited evidence from human studies exists. Based on all information, the EPA and the International Agency for Research on Cancer (IARC) conclude that nickel subsulfide causes cancer in humans. The IARC further indicates that other forms of nickel probably cause human cancer. The EPA ranks nickel subsulfide, nickel carbonyl, and nickel refinery dust as human carcinogens (class A substances, according to Table 5 in Chapter 3).

Nickel contact dermatitis, a form of skin eczema or rash, is the most common health effect among the general public. An estimated 2.5 to 5% of the population is sensitive to nickel. The rash is characterized by redness, itching, and small blisters. Women are more sensitive than men, perhaps because of greater exposure to nickel-containing household items. Contact with such commonplace objects as coins, jewelry, tools, cooking utensils, stainless steel kitchen appliances, and clothing fasteners can bring on the reaction. A family history of nickel sensitivity and early exposure to nickel items (for example, pierced earrings in teenage girls) are risk factors for the condition. Medical implants such as artificial joints also can cause a reaction among sensitive individuals. Relatively high levels of nickel in the diet can aggravate the condition, while nickel-restricted diets may improve it.

Acute nickel poisoning is only a problem if large quantities of nickel compounds are swallowed (several thousand times the average daily dose) or if exposure to nickel carbonyl in nickel refineries is excessive. Developmental and reproductive effects have been shown in animal tests at very high levels of exposure, but no human effects have been demonstrated. Similarly, genetic effects have been demonstrated in experimental animals and bacteria, but not directly in humans. The fact that nickel compounds produce cancer, however, indicates their potential to affect genetic material (*DNA*).

Protection and Prevention

People who are sensitive to nickel and develop skin reactions should reduce their contact to nickel-containing items, such as stainless steel, jewelry, kitchen implements, buttons, zippers, and so on. Use of cosmetics that contain nickel as shown on ingredient labels should also be discontinued. Lowering the amount of nickel consumed in foods may also help reduce skin reactions. This can be done by lowering the consumption of those foods highest in nickel content, as shown in Table 35 in the Technical Information section.

Relatively high levels of nickel are found in the vicinity of metal smelters, municipal solid waste incinerators, and (now defunct) nickel refineries. Children should not be allowed to play nearby or downwind of such facilities.

Environmental Effects

In general, nickel presents few environmental problems. Water concentrations are usually below the levels that cause toxicity to aquatic organisms. Only infrequently and for short periods of time have higher concentrations been measured. These have tended to be in the highly industrialized Ohio River basin and North Atlantic river systems. Freshwater algae and invertebrates are more sensitive than freshwater fish, which in turn are more sensitive than saltwater species. Nickel will accumulate in aquatic food chains, and *biomagnification factors* ranging as high as 2000–40,000 in algae and 40 in freshwater fish have been reported. Plant life in the vicinity of metal smelters and nickel refineries is often damaged or destroyed, but nickel is only one of many substances released from such factories and it is not clear how much of the impact is caused by nickel itself.

Regulatory Status

Federal regulations limit the concentration of nickel in workplace air and require that state and federal emergency planning and response centers be notified when more than 1 pound of nickel or other nickel compounds are accidentally released.

Various health advisory figures are also published, indicating levels below which safety is assumed (see Technical Information section). Nickel is listed as a *hazardous air pollutant* in the 1990 Clean Air Act, requiring the EPA to set emission standards. It is also on the EPA *community right-to-know* list. The FDA considers nickel to be *generally recognized as safe (GRAS)* as a direct human food ingredient.

Technical Information

Chemical symbol: Ni
Atomic number: 28
Atomic weight: 58.7
Average daily intake from all sources: 120 to 520 µg
OSHA limit in workplace air: 1 mg/m^3
EPA water advisory limits:
  adjusted acceptable daily intake (AADI): 0.35 mg/L (0.35 ppm)
  10-day health advisory (child): 1.0 mg/L (1 ppm)
  10-day health advisory (adult): 3.5 mg/L (3.5 ppm)

TABLE 35 Nickel Concentrations in Typical Environments and Foods

Medium	Concentration
Air	
Rural	1–20 ng/m^3
Urban	10–60 ng/m^3
Heavily industrialized areas	>100 ng/m^3
Near major nickel facility	2000 ng/m^3 (maximum measured)
Water	
Surface freshwater	15–20 μg/L (15–20 ppb)
Groundwater	3–4430 μg/L (<50 μg/L is typical)
Drinking water	<10 μg/L
Seawater	0.1–0.5 μg/L
Soils	
Agricultural	5–500 μg/g (5–500 ppm) (50 μg/g is typical)
Nonagricultural	4–80 μg/g
Near metal refineries	<24,000 μg/g
Foods[a]	
Grains, vegetables, fruits	0.02–2.7 μg/g (0.02–2.7 ppm)
Meats	0.06–0.4 μg/g
Seafoods	0.02–20 μg/g
Cow's milk	<100 μg/L (<100 ppb)
Breast milk	20–500 μg/L

[a] Foods with concentrations greater than 1 ppm include oatmeal, wheat bran, dried beans, soya products, hazelnuts, peanuts, sunflower seeds, licorice, cocoa, and dark chocolate.

ambient water quality criterion:

632 μg/L (632 ppb)

Typical concentrations of nickel in various environments and foods are given in Table 35.

Further Reading

Agency for Toxic Substances and Disease Registry. 1988. *Toxicological Profile for Nickel.* ATSDR/TP–88/19. Washington, D.C.: U.S. Public Health Service.

Environmental Protection Agency. 1986. *Health Assessment Document for Nickel and Nickel Compounds.* EPA/600/8–83/012FF. Washington, D.C.

National Academy of Sciences. 1975. *Nickel.* Washington, D.C.: National Research Council, Committee on Medical and Biological Effects of Environmental Pollutants.

Nicotine

Other Names

1-Methyl–2-(3-pyridyl)pyrrolidine; tetrahydronicotyrine; Black Leaf

Introduction

Nicotine is a powerful drug and insecticide found naturally in tobacco leaves. Tobacco infusions were first used as an insecticide in 1690. Although rarely used as an insecticide today, nicotine is still considered potent and effective even when compared to modern synthetic insecticides. Nicotine is sometimes used during leather tanning and as an animal tranquilizer. Nicotine is the *active ingredient* in cigarettes, although as discussed in Chapter 5, Section B, many other toxic chemicals result when tobacco is burned. Nicotine is also found in a variety of antismoking lozenges, gums, and pills.

Physical and Chemical Properties

Pure nicotine is a pale yellow, oily liquid with a slightly fishy smell. It turns brown upon exposure to air or light. It is chemically related to such drugs as **caffeine**, cocaine, morphine, quinine, and strychnine.

Exposure and Distribution

Tobacco is the most common source of exposure to nicotine. People who smoke, chew tobacco, handle tobacco leaves, or use nicotine-based insecticides can receive high doses of nicotine. Although present in second-hand cigarette smoke, the amount of nicotine received by people who breathe smoky air is less than that received by smokers. Small children who eat tobacco can receive significant doses of nicotine. People can also be exposed when nicotine solutions are sprayed on vegetable crops shortly before harvest.

Health Effects

Nicotine is a potent and rapidly acting poison. It is easily absorbed into the body following inhalation, swallowing, and skin contact. Nicotine can be absorbed into the body from green tobacco leaves, giving rise to an illness known as green tobacco sickness. This sickness causes pallor, vomiting, and severe cramps which diminish after exposure to the green leaves stops.

Small doses of nicotine can cause nausea, vomiting, diarrhea, headache, sweating, salivation, dizziness, and neurological stimulation. Large doses of nicotine cause convulsions and irregular heartbeat. Large doses can also lead to death in only a few minutes, but it is difficult to get lethal amounts of nicotine into the body from exposure to tobacco because people who receive massive doses of tobacco usually become too sick to continue the exposure. Nevertheless, it is possible for small children to receive fatal doses of nicotine as a result of eating cigarettes or other products that contain nicotine. Regular smokers develop tolerance to the effects of nicotine, and regular drinkers tend to eliminate nicotine from their bodies faster than nondrinkers do. Nicotine is known to cause birth defects in mice, but this effect has not been proven for people.

Protection and Prevention

All tobacco products should be avoided. Small children should not be allowed access to tobacco. Eating tobacco can be fatal to small children; seek medical attention quickly if children eat tobacco or nicotine-containing products. Use nicotine-based insecticides with extreme caution.

Regulatory Status

OSHA regulates skin contact with nicotine in the workplace. Smoking is now banned on all domestic flights in the United States and in most workplaces and all public buildings in some states.

Technical Information

Amount in average cigarette: 15–25 mg
Amount inhaled from one cigarette: <3 mg
Total dose from one small cigar: 1–4.5 mg
Average nicotine blood levels in smokers: <0.003 mg/100 mL blood
Fatal concentration in blood: 1 mg/100 mL blood

Further Reading

GOSSELIN, R. E., SMITH, R. P., HODGE, H. C. 1984. *Clinical Toxicology of Commercial Products*, 5th edition. Baltimore, MD: Williams and Wilkins.

Nitrates, Nitrites, and Nitrosamines

Introduction

Nitrates and nitrites are salts that are added to cured foods for protection against botulism. Nitrates also occur naturally in certain water supplies and have a major use as inorganic fertilizers. Nitrates are converted to nitrites in the human body, where excessive levels can cause a condition in which blood loses its normal ability to transfer oxygen. This condition can be fatal in infants. Nitrites also react in the stomach with other food components to form nitrosamines, which are extremely potent carcinogens. Because nitrates, nitrites, and nitrosamines form an interrelated hazard, they are treated here as a group rather than separately.

Salting has been used to preserve the aesthetic and healthful qualities of meat and fish for more than 3000 years. Nitrates are added to salting mixtures both to preserve the color of food and to prevent the growth of the bacterium responsible for producing the foodborne disease known as botulism. Botulism is generally regarded as the most serious life-threatening foodborne disease caused by microorganisms. The disease is caused by a toxin released into food contaminated with the bacterium *Clostridium botulinum*. The toxin affects the nervous system, eventually causing paralysis. An average of 40 cases per year have been reported in the United States over the last decade, of which 5 per year have been fatal. Symptoms usually develop 18 to 36 hours after ingestion, but the induction period can be as short as 2 hours or as long as 14 days. Symptoms begin with *gastrointestinal* disturbances, such as nausea, diarrhea, and vomiting, followed by neurological symptoms of dizziness, blurred vision, respiratory impairment, and progressive muscular paralysis.

In the 1920s and 1930s, scientists discovered that nitrites, not nitrates, are responsible for preventing the growth of *Clostridium botulinum* and that nitrates added to food are converted to nitrites by the action of normally occurring nonharmful food bacteria. Nitrates act solely as a source of nitrites. With that understanding, it became possible to reduce the levels of nitrates added to foods. Some nitrates, however, are still added because nitrites break down as food is stored, and the nitrates serve to replace the lost nitrites.

Physical and Chemical Properties

Nitrates are the chemically stable form of *inorganic* nitrogen in natural water. Nitrites and **ammonia** (the other major inorganic form of nitrogen) are readily converted to nitrates by natural *organic* processes. Nitrosamines are generally stable compounds that only slowly decompose when exposed to light. There are no easy ways to recognize the presence of nitrates, nitrites, or nitrosamines in foods, except by reading ingredient labels.

The major use of nitrates is in inorganic fertilizers; other uses include explosives and glassmaking. Nitrites are manufactured primarily for use in food preservation. Approximately 700 tons of nitrites are added to the 4 million tons of cured meats (ham, bacon, frankfurters, bologna, and sausage) and cured fish consumed in the United States each year.

Exposure and Distribution

Nitrates are part of the natural cycle of living things, formed by the normal breakdown of *organic matter* and taken up by plants as they grow. Under certain conditions, nitrates can accumulate in the environment, as when natural uptake is slower than breakdown. In these situations, excess nitrate accumulates in the soil and can wash into lakes and streams or percolate into groundwater, causing naturally elevated concentrations.

Human actions also greatly affect the presence of nitrates. Nitrogen fertilizers applied to agricultural lands and wastes from farm animals and feedlots often dramatically raise nitrate levels in farming areas. Well waters in these areas, for example, often contain high levels of nitrates owing to fertilizer use. Urban industrial and municipal water discharges frequently raise water nitrate levels within certain regions. Also, air pollution is now believed to be responsible for a significant rise in nitrates in the nation's rivers, particularly in the Midwest and East, as a result of the conversion of emitted *nitric oxides* to nitrates in the atmosphere and their subsequent raining down over broad areas of the country. Nitrate levels in public drinking water supplies are regulated. It is estimated that fewer than 1% of people served by such systems receive water in excess of the permitted limit of 10 milligrams per liter. (Representative concentrations of nitrates in various media are listed in the Technical Information section.)

Because nitrates are a natural food for plants, all vegetation contains them, including crops grown for food and tobacco. Surprisingly, by far the greatest exposure to nitrates for the typical person comes from vegetables. Vegetables provide an estimated 87% of all nitrate consumption to the average American eating a typical diet; fruits and juices contribute 6%, water 3%, and cured meats 2%. These proportions will be different for people who live where drinking water nitrate levels are higher than average, for people who consume a diet high in cured meats, and for vegetarians (for whom nitrates from vegetables can be close to 100% of their total nitrate intake). Vegetables with the highest nitrate levels include beets, celery, lettuce, parsley, radishes, rhubarb, spinach, and turnip greens.

Nitrites, in contrast to nitrates, are not found naturally in the environment at significant levels (Table 36). However, nitrites are formed from nitrates by the action of bacteria. As vegetables are stored, for example, their nitrate levels go down and their nitrite levels go up. The most important source of nitrites to humans is the production of nitrites from

TABLE 36 Nitrate and Nitrite Concentrations[a] in Various Media

Source	Nitrates	Nitrites
Cured meats	40 mg/kg	10 mg/kg
Fresh meats	10 mg/kg	1 mg/kg
Vegetables	12–6600 mg/kg	0.2–4 mg/kg
Fruits	20 mg/kg	0
Baked goods and cereals	12 mg/kg	2.6 mg/kg
Milk and milk products	0.5 mg/L	0
Water	1.3 mg/L	0

[a] Concentrations are in weight of ion per unit of medium.

Data from National Academy of Sciences. 1981. *The Health Effects of Nitrates, Nitrites, and N-Nitroso Compounds.* Washington, D.C.

nitrates by bacteria within the human body, a natural process that is quite interesting.

Nitrates (mainly from vegetables) are digested and then absorbed from the *gastrointestinal tract*. About one-fourth of the absorbed nitrates are transported in the blood to the salivary glands where they are released in saliva. Approximately one-fifth of the released nitrates are converted to nitrites by bacteria in the mouth and then swallowed. The net result is that 5% of ingested nitrates are converted to more hazardous nitrites, and the exposure occurs not when foods are first swallowed, but a few minutes later in nitrite-containing saliva. Because vegetables are the main source of nitrates to the body, they are also the main source of nitrites via the conversion pathway just described. For an average American adult, vegetables contribute 72% of the total nitrite exposure, cured meats 9%, baked goods and cereals 7%, fruits and juices 5%, fresh meats 2%, and water 2% (Table 37).

Nitrosamines are a class of complex organic molecules formed by the chemical reaction of nitrites and the nitrogen-containing (amine) groups of certain proteins. The reaction takes place in the human stomach from swallowed nitrites and food proteins. Nitrosamines are also formed when foods containing both nitrites and proteins, such as bacon, are cooked and when tobacco is burned. Nitrosamines can also be found already formed in beer (from malt), in certain cosmetics and drugs, in car interiors (where cured leather releases them into the air), and in the work environment of certain industries (Table 38).

Scientists now believe that production of nitrosamines in the stomach accounts for about half of the average human exposure, with nitrosamines already formed from other sources accounting for the other half. This pattern varies greatly, however, depending on smoking habits, diet, water nitrate levels, and occupation. Smokers, for example, receive roughly eight times more exposure to nitrosamines than do nonsmokers. Diet is a particularly important factor, because vegetables contain inhibitors to the formation of nitrosamines, in addition to being the main source of nitrites. Vitamin C is the best known inhibitor, but vitamin E and other antioxidants also are effective. A diet rich in vegetables that contain vitamin C will moderate exposure to nitrosamines, whereas most cured meats, high-nitrate water, and other such sources generally do not contain these protective ingredients. (For a further discussion, see Protection and Prevention section.)

A sense of the relative importance of various sources of nitrosamines, depending on dietary and other patterns, is shown in Table 39. What should be noted in this table is the percentage contribution within each dietary or lifestyle category and the relative differences of total exposures among categories. The absolute magnitudes of estimated exposures for each category are highly depen-

TABLE 37 Exposure to Nitrates and Nitrites for Average U.S. Adult (in milligrams per person per day)

Source of Exposure	Dietary Nitrite	Dietary Nitrate	Salivary Nitrite	Total Nitrite	Contribution of Nitrite from Each Source (%)
Cured meats	0.30	1.2	0.06	0.36	9
Fresh meats	0.06	0.6	0.03	0.09	2
Vegetables	0.12	65	3.0	3.1	72
Fruits and juices	0.1	4.3	0.20	0.21	5
Baked goods and cereals	0.26	1.2	.06	0.32	7
Milk and milk products	0.01	0.2	0.01	0.02	<1
Water	0.01	2	0.09	0.10	2
Total	0.77	75	3.5	4.2	

Data from National Academy of Sciences. 1981. *The Health Effects of Nitrates, Nitrites, and N-Nitroso Compounds*. Washington, D.C.

TABLE 38 Concentrations of Nitrosamines in Various Media

Source of Exposure	Nitrosamine[a]	Exposure Route	Concentration
Cigarette smoking	NDEA	Inhalation	1.0 ng/cig
	NEMA	Inhalation	0.5 ng/cig
	NDMA	Inhalation	0.5 ng/cig
	NPYR	Inhalation	6.5 ng/cig
	NDELA	Inhalation	7 ng/cig
	NNN	Inhalation	24 ng/cig
	NAT	Inhalation	310 ng/cig
	NNK	Inhalation	150 ng/cig
Automobile interiors	NDMA	Inhalation	1.0 μg/m^3 (new cars)
	NMOR	Inhalation	
	NDEA	Inhalation	0.34 μg/m^3 (avg. all cars)
Beer	NDMA	Ingestion	1.0 μg/L
Cosmetics	NDELA	Dermal	11 mg/kg
Cured meat (cooked bacon)	NPYR	Ingestion	5 μg/kg

[a]The abbreviations given stand for different complex chemical forms of nitrosamines.

Adapted from National Academy of Sciences. 1981. *The Health Effects of Nitrates, Nitrites, and N-Nitroso Compounds*. Washington, D.C.

TABLE 39 Exposure to Nitrosamines (micrograms per person per day)

Source of Exposure	Average Diet, Nonsmoker		Average Diet, Smoker		High Cured Meat Diet		Vegetarian, No Beer		Nitrate-rich Water, No Beer, Nonsmoker	
Diet	1.3	(54%)	1.3	(7%)	2.0	(55%)	12	(95%)	14	(95%)
Cosmetics	0.41	(17%)	0.41	(2%)	0.41	(11%)	0.41	(3%)	0.41	(3%)
Beer	0.34	(14%)	0.34	(2%)	0.34	(9%)	0		0	
Bacon	0.17	(7%)	0.17	(1%)	0.68	(19%)	0		0.17	(1%)
Car interiors	0.20	(8%)	0.20	(1%)	0.20	(6%)	0.20	(2%)	0.20	(1%)
Tobacco smoke	0		17	(87%)	0		0		0	
Total exposure	2.4	(100%)	19	(100%)	3.6	(100%)	13	(100%)	15	(100%)

Adapted from National Academy of Sciences. 1981. *The Health Effects of Nitrates, Nitrites, and N-Nitroso Compounds* (Table 10-9). Washington, D.C.

dent on assumptions and should not be relied on without consulting the original National Academy of Sciences report.

Health Effects

The two health effects of concern are *methemoglobinemia* caused by nitrites and cancer caused by nitrosamines; nitrates themselves are not particularly harmful. Methemoglobinemia is a condition in which normal blood *hemoglobin* (the oxygen-carrying protein) is converted to methemoglobin, a form in which oxygen is not effectively transported. Normal blood contains about 1% methemoglobin. Nitrites absorbed through the *gastrointestinal tract* will react with hemoglobin and raise this level. When blood methemoglobin levels reach 10%, such symptoms as blueness of skin appear; at 20% blood methemoglobin, oxygen to the brain is reduced; and when methemoglobin levels reach 60%, stupor, coma, and death occur. Most cases of methemoglobinemia have been the result of consumption of well waters high in nitrates (>100 milligrams per liter), which are then converted to nitrites within the body.

Virtually all fatalities from methemoglobinemia have occurred in infants. Infants are particularly at risk for several reasons: (1) the infant stomach is less acidic than the adult stomach, permitting bacterial conversion of virtually 100% of ingested nitrates to nitrites within the stomach; (2) infant hemoglobin is more susceptible to conversion to methemoglobin; and (3) infants consume ten times more water per body weight than do adults. The worst situation occurs when infant formula is reconstituted with water high in nitrates. In this case, practically all of a baby's nourishment is a source of nitrates. Other groups at increased risk include pregnant women, whose normal blood methemoglobin levels rise to a peak of around 10% at the thirtieth week; cancer patients, whose hemoglobin is especially sensitive; and other people with reduced stomach acidity, such as those being treated for ulcers. All of these

groups are unusually sensitive to nitrite induction of methemoglobinemia. Except in infants, however, methemoglobinemia is generally not fatal and can be treated with no lasting effects.

Nitrosamines have been implicated in stomach cancer and cancers of the esophagus and nasal passages. The human statistical evidence for cancer production is strong, showing positive associations of cancer with the substances that form nitrosamines, but it is not yet deemed conclusive. The laboratory evidence, however, is quite compelling. Of over 300 N-nitroso compounds tested (a group that includes nitrosamines), more than 90% were found to be *carcinogenic,* and they were found to be carcinogenic in every species tested. Moreover, it has been shown that humans are capable of converting nitrosamines to the metabolic intermediate capable of altering *DNA,* the genetic material. On the strength of this evidence, the International Agency for Research on Cancer (IARC) considers nitrosamines to "probably" cause cancer in humans. The Cancer Assessment Group of the EPA has placed various nitrosamines in the top third among 54 chemicals ranked for potency in producing cancer.

Cigarette smoking adds yet another component to the nitrosamine hazard. Not only are nitrosamines and other cancer-causing tars present in tobacco smoke, but cyanide occurs as well. Cyanide is converted by bacteria in saliva to the thiocyanate ion, which accelerates the formation of nitrosamines in the stomach when swallowed.

Protection and Prevention

The most effective protection against methemoglobinemia is avoiding water high in nitrates. Infant formulas, in particular, should not be reconstituted with such water. In cases where only water high in nitrates is available, infants should be breastfed or bottled water should be used to make up the formula. Public water supply systems are required to maintain nitrates at safe levels and to issue warnings if levels become dangerous. Attention should be paid to such notices. People obtaining their water from private wells should have the water tested periodically. Should methemoglobinemia occur, it can be effectively treated with the antidote methylene blue; when treated, there are no lasting effects.

Protection from nitrosamines involves three strategies: dietary reduction of foods and water containing added nitrates and nitrites, an increase in the consumption of fruits and vegetables rich in vitamin C and other antioxidants, and the elimination of smoking. Vitamin C is found in citrus fruits and juices, berries, peaches, melons, green and leafy vegetables, tomatoes, green peppers, and sweet potatoes. Vitamin C (also known as ascorbic acid or ascorbate) is now added to some brands of cured meats and to bacon to counter the effects of the added nitrates. Check the labels of different brands for this ingredient. Vitamin E is another antioxidant that is found in whole-grain cereals, wheat germ, soybeans, broccoli, brussel sprouts, leafy greens, spinach, and vegetable oils.

It is important to note that to be effective, vitamin C must be present in the stomach at the same time that the nitrosamine-forming reaction is taking place, that is, while the nitrites and proteins are present. It will not work to take vitamin C supplements once a day to protect against nitrosamine formation. Instead, foods rich in vitamin C should be added to the daily diet. If a meal is consumed in which it is known that a high level of nitrates or nitrites is present (such as bacon or frankfurters), it would be prudent to serve a citrus juice or other food rich in vitamin C with it.

Regulatory Status

The level of nitrate in drinking water is limited by the EPA. No regulations exist for nitrites or nitrosamines in water. Workplace exposures to nitrosamines in air are recommended by the National Institute of Occupational Safety and Health (NIOSH).

Technical Information

Chemical formulas:
  nitrate: NO_3
  nitrite: NO_2
Maximum permitted level of nitrate in drinking water:
  10 mg/L (10 ppm)

Further Reading

Environmental Protection Agency. 1985. *Drinking Water Criteria Document for Nitrates/Nitrites, Final Draft*. TR–540–59D. Washington, D.C.: Office of Drinking Water.

National Research Council. 1981. *The Health Effects of Nitrate, Nitrite, and N-Nitroso Compounds*. National Academy of Sciences. Washington, D.C.

World Health Organization. 1978. *Nitrates, Nitrites, and N-Nitroso Compounds*. Geneva.

Nitrogen Oxides

Other Names

Nitrogen dioxide; oxides of nitrogen; nitric oxide

Introduction

Nitrogen oxides are a group of air pollutants formed during the combustion of fuels and in subsequent chemical reactions in the atmosphere. The two main nitrogen oxides are nitrogen dioxide and nitric oxide. Together they are sometimes referred to by the term NOX (pronounced "knocks"). They cause health and environmental harm directly, and they stimulate the formation of **ozone** at the earth's surface, which causes further damage. Dissolved in the water of fog, rain, and snow, nitrogen dioxide turns to nitric acid, causing ecological damage in the form of acid rain.

Physical and Chemical Properties

Nitrogen dioxide is a yellowish brown gas that gives smog its characteristic brownish color. It is produced by the *photochemical reaction* in air of nitric oxide, the oxide of nitrogen actually released when fuels burn. Nitrogen dioxide is a chemically very reactive compound called an *oxidant,* which means it has the ability to strip electrons away from other molecules. This property is important for two reasons. First, it makes nitrogen dioxide biologically harmful. Second, it causes it to be a catalyst for the production of ozone from *volatile organic compounds* (VOCs) in the presence of sunlight. Nitrogen dioxide also reacts with water vapor in the atmosphere and with other substances to produce nitric acid and acid *particulates.*

Exposure and Distribution

The most significant outdoor exposure to nitrogen oxides occurs in polluted urban air. The concentration rises during the morning hours from about 6 to 9 A.M. when auto exhaust is greatest and sunlight is present for the photochemical reactions to proceed. Peak urban levels are hundreds of times greater than in clean rural areas, with cities such as Los Angeles several times higher still, as shown in the following table. Even in areas that meet current air pollution regulations based on annual average conditions, short-term peaks (1-hour averages) can be quite high on many days out of the year. (Table 40). These exposure peaks are important because new research is showing that repeated short-term exposures to higher concentrations can be more damaging than long-term exposures to lower levels. The greatest build-up of nitrogen oxides occurs during *atmospheric inversions,* when overlying stagnant air traps pollutants below it (see Chapter 9, Section A).

Indoor air pollution is also a significant source of nitrogen dioxide exposure (see Chapter 5, Section C). Homes with gas ranges have higher levels than homes equipped with electric ranges. Houses with unvented heating appliances, such as kerosene heaters, contain the highest concentrations. Inside air is more polluted in winter than in summer because of additional space heating and because doors and windows are closed, thus reducing ventilation.

The major sources of nitrogen oxides are fossil fuel fired electric power plants and factories (55%) and transportation (41%). Emissions have remained steady over the latest five years for which figures are available (1984 to 1986). On a national scale, average measured air quality has improved less than 1% over the same period. However, various regions were reporting higher levels at the end of the period than at the beginning. The Los Angeles area is the only region that regularly exceeds the annual nitrogen dioxide standard.

Health Effects

Nitrogen dioxide, the most toxic oxide of nitrogen, is a deep lung irritant that damages the delicate cells lining the lungs. Unlike

TABLE 40 Outdoor Air Concentrations of Nitrogen Oxides

Region	Concentration (ppm)
Remote areas	0.001
Inhabited nonmetropolitan areas	0.01
Urban areas	
National annual average	0.029
Highest cities, annual average	0.060
Repeated short-term peaks (1-hour)	0.06–0.5

upper respiratory irritants (such as **ammonia**), which mark their presence by causing coughing and mucous congestion, nitrogen dioxide is largely symptomless except at the highest concentrations. The acute danger comes about 5 to 72 hours later when a progressive *inflammation* sets in, leading to *pulmonary edema*; death can result. Ambient air rarely reaches levels at which such acute effects occur, although occupational exposures sometimes do. Farmworkers, for example, have succumbed to the levels present in grain silos, a condition called silo fillers' disease.

Studies in animals show that lower level, longer term exposures cause changes in lung structure and function resembling *emphysema* and chronic *bronchitis*. Children living in homes equipped with gas stoves show higher rates of respiratory infections (common colds) and reduced lung functions compared with children in homes with electric ranges. The higher rate of infection appears to be due both to the reduced ability of damaged lining cells to clear inhaled bacteria and viruses and to damage to the immune system cells that fight infection. *Asthmatics* and people with chronic bronchitis may be particularly sensitive to the repeated peak exposures commonly seen in urban air. Some of the effects of nitrogen dioxide and the concentrations at which they occur are shown in Table 41.

Protection and Prevention

Adequate ventilation of home appliances can reduce indoor exposures. Fans above gas stove tops should be used whenever cooking is done. (This is advisable for cooking with electric ranges, too, to vent other pollutants such as **nitrosamines** formed when food cooks.) Water heater and furnace flues should be maintained and vented away from the house. Doorways leading from a garage to the interior of a house should be closed whenever a car motor is running. Exercise should be curtailed during rush hours and during periods of atmospheric inversions when nitrogen oxide levels can be significantly higher than usual (see Chapter 9, Section A). Immediate removal from exposure is indicated if any respiratory or neurological symptoms (such as headache or dizziness) develop.

Environmental Effects

Severe ecological effects are produced by nitrogen oxides. The worst harm appears to be caused by nitric acid, the end-product of nitrogen dioxide chemical reactions in the air. Acidification and loss of buffering capacity of freshwaters in Canada, New England, and mountainous regions of the western United States has occurred, with consequent declines in populations of fish and other species. Acid rain in concert with stresses produced by ozone, heat, and drought are leading to declining forests in numerous regions of the East. In sensitive estuaries and coastal regions along the eastern seaboard, nitrogen pollution from fertilizer runoff, sewage, and atmospheric deposition may be stimulating production of unwanted plants and organisms and damaging commercially valu-

TABLE 41 Some Health Effects of Nitrogen Dioxide Exposure

Effect	Concentration (ppm)
Airway resistance increases in chronic bronchitics	1.6 (3-minute exposure)
Symptoms in asthmatics (nasal discharge, headaches, dizziness, and labored breathing)	0.5 (2-hour exposure)
Infections in young children	0.15–0.30 (repeated peak exposures)

able fish and shellfish. The long-term consequences of these changes are not known.

Regulatory Status

The EPA sets outdoor air quality standards to protect human health and to prevent damage to plants and other items affecting human welfare (such as visibility). The standards are subject to periodic review and revision as necessary. Currently, 8.3 million people live in counties in violation of the standard for protection of health, which is based on the average nitrogen dioxide concentration over a year. Recent research indicates that short-term peak levels of nitrogen dioxide may be just as important in causing health effects as long-term exposures to lower levels. But this new information has not yet been incorporated into federal standards. Occupational exposures are regulated by limiting the concentration in workplace air.

The 1990 amendments to the Clean Air Act require emissions of nitrogen oxides in the year 2000 be reduced by 2.5 million tons per year below the levels projected for that year.

Technical Information

Chemical formulas:
nitrogen dioxide: NO_2
nitric oxide: NO
nitrogen oxides: NO_x
National Ambient Air Quality Standards for NO_2:
    primary (protection of human health)
        (annual average): 0.053 ppm
        (100 $\mu g/m^3$)

    secondary (protection of welfare): same as
      primary standard
OSHA limit in workplace air: 25 ppm
(30 mg/m^3)

Further Reading

Environmental Protection Agency. 1982. *Review of the National Ambient Air Quality Standards for Nitrogen Oxides: Assessment of Scientific and Technical Information.* EPA-450/5-82-002. Washington, D.C.

National Research Council. 1977. *Nitrogen Oxides.* Washington, D.C.: Committee on Medical and Biological Effects of Environmental Pollutants, National Academy of Sciences.

Noise

Introduction

While by no means the most lethal of environmental pollutants, noise is arguably the most widespread. Contamination of the everyday environment with loud noise is to some extent a result of twentieth-century developments in transportation and electronics, but even in the early stages of the industrial revolution, the whine of the steam engine and the clanging of metals posed a hazard to factory workers. And the stress that comes from the inability to escape from incessant human voices has probably been with us since our evolutionary beginnings.

Noise is a necessary means of communication, as in speech, music, theater applause, clock alarms, fire engine sirens, a tea kettle's whistling, or a baby's cries. It is also an unavoidable and useless by-product of many activities, as in the clanging of steam pipes and the racket of factory equipment. Of course, one person's communication is another's racket, for the noise in a factory might serve to warn an unsuspecting visitor against stepping too close to a dangerous machine.

Physical and Chemical Properties

We hear sounds when vibrations in the air stimulate the nerve endings in the inner ear. The vibrations in the air are created by the object making the noise. In some cases, such as the plucking of a violin string, it is easy to see what starts the air vibrating—the moving string vibrates the air back and forth directly. In less obvious cases, such as the squeal of a car's brakes, the air is set to vibrating by the alternating slipping and sticking of the brake pad against the wheel drum. Noises can differ in their pitch and in their loudness. The more rapid the vibrations in the air, the higher the pitch; the greater the amount of air moved in each vibration, the louder the noise.

Exposure and Distribution

The loudness of sound is measured on the decibel scale. Some typical values of decibels for common sounds are listed in the following table.

Sound	Decibel Level
Limit of normal human perception	0
Rustle of leaves	10
Whisper	25
Typical conversation indoors	60
Typical vacuum cleaner	85
Typical gas lawnmower (as heard by operator)	95
Unmuffled motorcycle (as heard by operator)	110
Jetliner (taking off 200 feet away), discotheque, or rock concert	120

The perceived loudness approximately doubles when the noise level is increased by 10 decibels. The higher the pitch of the sound, the louder it has to be for us to hear it.

Health Effects

Noise can cause health problems ranging from annoyance and sleeplessness to intense pain, stomach ulcers, hearing loss, and total deafness. In addition to direct stress on the ears, the body responds to excess noise by increasing the heart rate and blood pressure. At the chemical level, noise stimulates the body's production of the hormone ACTH (a pituitary secretion that in turn stimulates the adrenal gland's production of steroids, causing elevated blood sugar levels). Loudness levels associated with different types of health hazards are shown in Table 42.

Temporary or permanent deafness can result from brief but intense exposures to noise. Temporary or permanent hearing loss can result from prolonged exposures to even moderate noise levels. Hearing loss usually occurs at a pitch that is slightly higher than that of the noise causing the damage and is due to damage to the auditory nerves themselves rather than to the physical structures in the

TABLE 42 Loudness Levels of Hazardous Noises

Symptom	Lowest Decibel Level That Can Cause Symptom
Difficulty falling asleep	35
Increased heart rate and blood pressure; awakening from sleep	70
Discomfort, stress, annoyance	80
Temporary hearing loss from prolonged exposure	85
Pain threshold	110
Extreme pain; permanent deafness if prolonged	135

ear that transmit sound to the nerves. The extent of hearing loss is often measured in decibels; for example, a loss of 10 decibels means that the lowest noise level that can be heard is 10 decibels higher (that is, louder) than it was before the loss. In a study of industrial metal workers, a loss of 25 decibels was associated with prolonged exposure to 95 decibels of factory noise. Steady noise appears to do less permanent damage than sudden bursts of noise of the same loudness.

Protection and Prevention

It is best to control noise pollution at the source by turning down the stereo, fixing the noisy car engine, and so on. But often it is impossible to control a source, and in such circumstances the use of ear protection (plugs or muffs) may be the only recourse. Rooms can also be soundproofed with acoustical tile, most easily done if the need can be anticipated during home or workplace construction.

Environmental Effects

Noise scares wild animals and degrades their habitat. Wildlife refuges can exist near noisy airports, as in Jamaica Bay, New York, but the result is undesirable for both the wildlife and the people coming to enjoy the refuge. The intrusion of noise from motorized vehicles in the wilderness, such as all-terrain vehicles in the desert and snowmobiles in the forest during winter, is a growing problem in the world and particularly in the United States. While the effects of noise in the wilderness are difficult to measure, noise is certainly a major psychological hazard to people who treasure the chance to enjoy the sounds of nature.

Regulatory Status

Many nations have set industrial standards to control noise exposures to workers. The maximum allowable daily average exposure in most nations is typically set at 85 decibels. In the United States, the current OSHA standard limits the permissible exposure of all governmental and nongovernmental workers to 90 decibels for 8 hours per day. In addition, OSHA requires that for every 5 decibels above 90, the exposure time must be cut in half. Thus, exposure to 95 decibels must be limited to 4 hours, exposure to 100 decibels must be limited to 2 hours, and so forth. Also, sudden bursts of noise must be limited to 140 decibels. In recent years, cases of violations of these standards have numbered in the thousands. As measured by the number of citations and penalties associated with its noise standard, this is one of the most vigorously enforced of all of OSHA's regulations. Nevertheless, the OSHA standards have been strongly criticized both by the EPA and by citizens' environmental groups as being too lenient. They have argued that an 8-hour noise limit of 75 decibels in the workplace is warranted by available scientific evidence and that although such a tight standard might be economically impractical, at the very least the standard should be tightened from 90 down to 85 decibels. Such a change in the rules governing noise levels in the workplace is now pending.

In addition to the regulation of workplace noise levels, the Noise Control Act of 1972 sets forth goals to protect all U.S. residents from excess noise and empowers the EPA to set noise limits on commercial products and to work with the Federal Aviation Administration to regulate airplane noise. Most of the progress in noise reduction stemming from this legislation has been in the design and operation of aircraft, although current regulations permit the extremely noisy supersonic Concorde airliner to use some U.S. airports. Progress in regulating the noise emissions from trucks, buses, motorcycles, power lawn mowers, and other commercial products responsible for much of the noise the public experiences outside the workplace has not been particularly impressive in the 1980s.

Technical Information

While the decibel scale is the common one used to express noise levels in the environment, the actual physical intensity of sound is measured in units of watts per square meter. This is a measure of the intensity of the energy flow associated with the sound wave. Every tenfold increase in the physical intensity of the sound corresponds to an addition of 10 to the decibel value of the loudness. For example, a sound intensity of 1 milliwatt (one-thousandth of a watt) per square meter corresponds to 90 decibels, while 10 milliwatts per square meter corresponds to 100 decibels.

Further Reading

ARBUCKLE, J. G., and others. 1987. *Environmental Law Handbook,* 9th edition. Rockville, MD: Government Institutes, Inc.
World Health Organization. 1980. *Environmental Health Criterion Report No. 12: Noise.* Geneva.

Oxalic Acid

Other Names

Oxalic acid dihydrate; ethane dioic acid

Trade Names

ZUD Heavy Duty Household Cleaner; White Bear metal polish

Introduction

Oxalic acid is used as an industrial metal cleaner and is found in some heavy duty household cleaners and metal-polishing compounds. Oxalic acid is used by a wide variety of industries as a bleaching agent; to remove paint, rust, varnish, and ink stains; and as a metal polish. It is also used by dentists to harden plastic molds. Some freckle and skin-bleaching cosmetics contain oxalic acid. Rhubarb leaves also contain oxalic acid, which accounts for their toxicity. Very low nontoxic concentrations of oxalic acid are also found in spinach and other edible greens.

Physical and Chemical Properties

Oxalic acid is a white, odorless powder, although it is often used in liquid form. Once inside the body, some *halogenated* compounds are metabolized into oxalic acid.

Exposure and Distribution

Oxalic acid is used by a variety of industries, but there is little recent information available on how many workers may be exposed to the chemical. People who work with dentists or the dentists themselves may also be exposed to oxalic acid. Some heavy duty household cleaners and polishes use oxalic acid. The label will usually identify it as the active ingredient.

Health Effects

Swallowing strong oxalic acid results in corrosion of the mouth, esophagus, and stomach. Vomiting, burning abdominal pain, collapse, and sometimes convulsions follow ingestion of small amounts of pure oxalic acid. Death may come quickly.

Oxalic acid is caustic on the skin. Cracking and fissuring of the skin and development of slow-healing ulcers are common responses to repeated skin contact. The skin may also turn bluish, and the fingernails may become brittle and yellow. Contact with oxalic acid solutions can also cause tingling, burning, and soreness of the skin. Splashes in the eye cause reversible surface damage.

Oxalic vapors can be inhaled when hot mixtures containing the acid are used. If such vapors are inhaled, inflammation of the upper respiratory tract is possible. Inhalation of oxalic acid dust can also cause irritation to the upper respiratory tract and eyes, ulceration of mucous membranes of the nose and throat, *gastrointestinal* disturbances, gradual loss of weight, increasing weakness, headache, irritability, and nervousness.

The target organ for absorbed oxalic acid is the kidney. Kidney effects are attributed to the removal of calcium from the blood. The kidney becomes clogged with insoluble calcium oxalate, which causes kidney stone formation. Oxalate stone formation is promoted by large quantities of vitamin C in the body.

Protection and Prevention

Avoid direct contact with strong oxalic acid solutions or powder whenever possible. Workers suspecting that oxalic acid is used in the workplace should request a *Material Safety Data Sheet (MSDS)*, which should describe the form of the chemical used and how to avoid exposure. Use consumer formulations containing oxalic acid with care, and use rubber gloves when possible. Spinach and other edible greens are safe, as are rhubarb stalks in moderation. Never eat rhubarb leaves.

Regulatory Status

Oxalic acid is regulated by OSHA. Since the toxicity of oxalic acid is fairly well under-stood, no adjustment to its regulatory status is expected.

Technical Information

Chemical formula: $C_2H_2O_4$
Molecular weight: 90
OSHA limit in workplace air: 1 mg/m^3

Further Reading

PROCTOR, NICK H., HUGHES, JAMES P., FISCHMAN, MICHAEL L. 1988. *Chemical Hazards of the Workplace*, 2d edition. Philadelphia: J. B. Lippincott.

Ozone and Other Photochemical Oxidants

Other Names

Smog; photochemical smog; oxidant

Introduction

Ozone, the major ingredient in smog, produces some of the worst air pollution conditions in this country. In the upper atmosphere, ozone absorbs harmful **ultraviolet radiation**, protecting humans from skin cancer. Its depletion there by human activities may lead to increased skin cancers (see Chapter 11, Section B). In the lower atmosphere where people breathe and plants grow, however, ozone causes serious health effects and significant damage to forests and crops.

Physical and Chemical Properties

Ozone is not released directly into the air. It is formed in the atmosphere by the chemical reaction of *volatile organic compounds* (VOCs) and **nitrogen dioxide** (together known as precursors) in the presence of sunlight. Because sunlight is required, the reaction is called a *photochemical reaction* and the product of the reaction is called photochemical air pollution, photochemical smog, or just plain *smog*. Elevated temperatures stimulate the reaction, which is why ozone conditions tend to be worse in the summer. The yellowish brown color of smog comes from nitrogen dioxide.

While ordinary oxygen contains two oxygen atoms (O_2), ozone is a gas composed of three oxygen atoms (O_3). It is called an *oxidant* and causes its toxic effects because it readily strips away electrons from other molecules (oxidation), starting chain reactions and disrupting key structures within cells.

Other oxidants are also created during the photochemical reactions that produce ozone. While they make up a much smaller proportion of the mixture called smog, many are more irritating than ozone and are responsible for some of the eye and nose irritation suffered during very smoggy conditions. The most important of these other oxidants are peroxyacetyl nitrate (PAN), nitrogen dioxide, hydrogen peroxide, nitric and nitrous acids, and formic acid. Because all oxidant concentrations tend to rise and fall together, only the ozone level is usually reported as an indicator of total oxidant concentrations.

Exposure and Distribution

The worst conditions of ozone exposure occur during *atmospheric inversions*, in which pollutants are trapped and build up beneath an overlying layer of stagnant warm air (see Chapter 9, Section A). Generally ozone is at its lowest level at sunrise; as precursor emissions from morning traffic build up and as the sun shines and temperatures rise, so do ozone levels. The peak concentrations occur in the late morning and early afternoon. Because oxidants are not released directly but often take several hours to form, the precursors have time to move with the prevailing winds. Frequently, oxidant levels are highest in rural areas downwind from the major urban centers where the precursors are emitted.

Ozone is a truly national problem. Over half of the 89 largest urban areas in the United States exceed the primary standard for the protection of human health, with many of the rest barely meeting the standard. More than 110 million people live in counties in violation of the standard. The worst regions are characterized by enormous emissions of precursors and by hot and sunny climates. They include California and the Texas Gulf Coast year round and the northeast corridor and the Chicago–Milwaukee area in summer. From 1984 to 1988, the national ozone levels increased 9%. The figures fluctuate greatly with weather conditions, however. For example, 1988 ozone levels were the highest of the decade because of unusually hot weather.

Precursor emissions come from a wide variety of sources, which makes their control extremely difficult. Automobiles, gas stations, power plants, dry cleaners, paint shops, chemical manufacturing plants, oil refineries, and other businesses using solvents all release VOCs. Nitrogen oxides are released by automobiles and stationary sources of fuel combustion (factories and power plants). Table 43 shows the proportion of precursor emissions from various sources on a national basis.

The latest available data indicate that emissions of VOCs decreased by 8% and emissions of nitrogen dioxide did not change at all over the 5-year period from 1984 through 1988, a relatively insignificant decline considering the magnitude of the problem.

Health Effects

The symptoms of ozone (oxidant) exposure in polluted urban air include chest pain, coughing, wheezing, lung and nasal congestion, labored breathing, sore throat, nausea, faster breathing, and eye and nose irritation. These symptoms show up at ozone levels only slightly higher than the national standard for health protection, a level that some areas reach regularly. Laboratory studies on human volunteers also show that typical ozone exposures combined with only intermittent exercise reduces the normal functioning of healthy lungs in both adults and children, preventing them from being able to inhale deeply.

A major question is whether the respiratory effects due to exposure are reversible when exposure ceases or if they persist, causing permanent damage. One study of children exposed to ozone levels typically reached during summer months showed that lung changes persisted for many days after the ozone episode passed. In experimental animals, permanent lung structure damage is caused by ozone levels typical of smoggy conditions, if the exposure lasts for several weeks. *Inflammation* occurs, causing injury

TABLE 43 Sources of Oxidant Precursors

Source	Percentage of Precursor Emissions
Transportation	39
Stationary fuel combustion	32
Industrial processes	22
Nonindustrial organic solvent use	4
Other sources	3

to the specialized cells lining the respiratory tract. Those cells are replaced by useless scar tissue, a process described as premature aging of the lungs. Other health effects reported include an increase in *asthma* attacks, increased risk of infections because of damage to cells lining the airways, and reductions in heart and circulatory function and aerobic fitness. Data from animal studies suggest further systemic damage is possible, including effects on the central nervous system, liver, blood, and endocrine system.

The groups in the population at greatest risk are those with preexisting respiratory diseases, including asthmatics, people with *chronic obstructive pulmonary disease,* and "responders" in the general population (people unusually sensitive to ozone). Such people number as many as 20 to 30 million in the major urban areas where ozone levels are at least 25% above the current health standard.

Protection and Prevention

Because increased breathing brings more oxidants in contact with the respiratory system, exercise should not be performed during severe smog episodes or at the smoggiest times of the day. People with respiratory diseases should curtail even moderate exertion during these periods. Air quality districts frequently announce smog alerts and suggest restricted activities; such notices should be heeded. No treatments other than reducing exposure can be recommended at this time.

Reducing ozone levels requires reducing emissions of the precursors responsible for ozone formation. Individuals can and should participate by reducing unnecessary driving, buying fuel-efficient vehicles, keeping them properly tuned, and avoiding spills of gasoline during refueling. Water-based paints can be used instead of oil- or solvent-based paints, and oil-based items should be properly disposed of. Tightly sealing household solvents and reducing their use by using water-based products also helps.

Environmental Effects

Ozone and other oxidants severely damage crops, forests, and man-made materials. The main damage to plants is to the foliage, with secondary effects on growth and yield. Yield losses on major cash crops such as soybeans, peanuts, corn, and wheat frequently exceed 10%, and losses to tomatoes, beans, and snapbeans are higher than 20%. Cash values of such losses are estimated at several billion dollars per year.

Significant damage to forest trees occurs at ambient ozone levels. In the San Bernardino National Forest of southern California, ponderosa and jeffrey pines suffer foliar injury, premature leaf drop, decreased photosynthetic activity, curtailed growth, and an increase in fatal infestation of bark beetles. Evidence is accumulating that air pollution, in combination with natural stresses such as drought, is severely damaging forests throughout the eastern United States. Spruce and fir trees along the crest of the Appalachian Mountains and sugar maples in New England are declining. Ozone is partly responsible for the reduced growth rate of commercial yellow pines in the Southeast. Other organisms and ecosystem processes, such as lichens and nutrient cycling, are also affected.

Oxidants damage materials as well as living things. They cause cracking of plastics and rubber (as in tires) and degradation and fading of textile fibers and dyes.

Regulatory Status

Ozone is one of the air pollutants for which the EPA is required to periodically review and revise air quality standards. Since the last review in 1985, accumulated evidence indicates that exposure to ozone at the current standard is likely to cause harm in at least some portions of the population. But rather than setting a new, more stringent standard, the emphasis adopted in the Clean Air Act amendments is to attain compliance with the existing one. Occupational exposures to ozone are regulated by limiting the concentration in workplace air.

Technical Information

Chemical formula of ozone: O_3
National Ambient Air Quality Standards:
  primary (protective of human health), maximum daily 1-hour average: 0.12 ppm (0.235 mg/m^3)
  secondary (protection of welfare): same as primary standard
OSHA limit in workplace air: 0.1 ppm (0.2 mg/m^3)

Further Reading

Environmental Protection Agency. 1986. *Air Quality Criteria for Ozone and Other Photochemical Oxidants*. EPA–600/8–84–020F. Washington, D.C.
———. 1986. *Ozone in the Lower Atmosphere: A Threat to Health and Welfare*. OPA–86–010. Washington, D.C.
National Research Council. 1977. *Ozone and Other Photochemical Oxidants*. Washington, D.C.: National Academy of Sciences, Committee on Medical and Biological Effects of Environmental Pollutants.

Paraquat

Trade Names

Orthoparaquat; Ortho Spotweed and Grass-killer; Gramoxone

Introduction

Since it was first introduced in 1962, paraquat has gained notoriety as the herbicide of choice in federally sponsored efforts to eradicate marijuana (or pot) plants. From 1970 until 1978, marijuana fields in Mexico, prime sources of the weed, were heavily sprayed—with the help of the United States government. U.S. involvement was curtailed when health officials reported a link between irreversible lung damage and smoking marijuana cigarettes contaminated with paraquat. Nevertheless, state and federal agencies have sprayed or proposed to spray marijuana plots from Florida to California on private and public lands. Increasingly, though, drug eradication efforts have turned to another less toxic herbicide: **glyphosate**. Paraquat, however, continues to be a popular agricultural herbicide.

Physical and Chemical Properties

Paraquat is a white, crystalline solid that is insoluble in hydrocarbons, but very soluble in water. It does not break down readily in acid solutions, but does in alkaline solutions. The herbicidal and toxicological properties of paraquat depend on the formation of the *ionic* form. This is what causes cell death.

Exposure and Distribution

Paraquat is an effective nonselective herbicide used in 130 countries around the world to control weeds in rice, soybeans, coffee, bananas, citrus, apples, plums, rubber, potatoes, sunflowers, and pineapples. Its primary nonagricultural use is to control weeds along roadsides. About 2.8 million pounds of paraquat were sprayed on U.S. crops in 1987—a significant drop from the 4 million pounds sprayed annually on cotton, wheat, corn, soybeans, fruit trees, and grape vines through the mid-1980s. Sloppy manufacturing methods in many countries produce impurities in paraquat that are more toxic than the parent compound. The herbicide is not very volatile, so the concentration in the air is generally low after spraying. It does not tend to accumulate in animal tissues or transfer to milk. In soils, paraquat *adsorbs* strongly to clay and minerals and is therefore inactivated. As a result, it degrades very slowly. But when exposed to sunlight, paraquat breaks down rapidly to less toxic products. Although very soluble in water, it is not thought to be a serious contaminant of water supplies because of its adsorption to vegetation and sediments.

Health Effects

On the basis of studies to date, the EPA has classified paraquat as a possible carcinogen (group C; see Chapter 3, Section B). There is some evidence that it is a weak *mutagen*. Some studies show that the herbicide is toxic to developing embryos, but only at doses that would also kill the mother. It does not appear to cause birth defects or other significant reproductive problems.

Paraquat, however, is highly toxic in concentrated form and can lead to death when ingested and to irreversible lung damage when inhaled in cigarette smoke. Use of dilute spray mixes, however, are thought to pose little health hazard. Paraquat poisoning following ingestion, injection, or inhalation results in edema of the lungs because the lungs selectively take up the herbicide from the blood. The edema is accompanied by bleeding and often *fibrosis*. Both the liver and kidneys are also damaged after exposure to high concentrations of paraquat. It is highly irritating to the linings of the respiratory and digestive tracts. Effects range from nosebleeds and vomiting to ulceration of the mouth and perforation of the esophagus. It can cause *dermatitis* on contact with the skin.

Protection and Prevention

To prevent accidental poisonings, the manufacturer has colored the herbicide solution brown, added a skunk-like odor, and included an ingredient that induces vomiting in anyone who swallows it. Since paraquat is very water soluble, it can be washed off the skin or from the eyes readily.

There is no specific effective treatment for paraquat poisoning. Stomach pumping and cleansing with salt solutions work in some cases. Treatment often focuses on increasing urinary output since paraquat is excreted in the urine. Blood transfusions have been successful in some cases. Because concentrated paraquat is so toxic, factory and agricultural workers using or handling the herbicide must use caution and wear protective clothing, goggles, and respirators.

Environmental Effects

Paraquat does not appear to be directly toxic to fish, but it may kill fish indirectly. The herbicide kills aquatic plants, which then decay, using up oxygen in the water. Some fish species such as trout are particularly susceptible to low oxygen levels. Fish kills resulting from depletion of oxygen in the water are generally a short-term, localized effect from which the population can recover. Birds appear to be less affected by paraquat than mammals. Studies of bird populations in England indicate no adverse effects in areas with high paraquat use. Used at normal recommended rates, paraquat has no apparent effect on soil organisms.

Technical Information

Chemical names: 1,1′-dimethyl-4,4′-bipyridyl, 1,1′-dimethyl-4,4′-bypyridinium dichloride, or (bis)methyl
Chemical formula: $C_{12}H_{14}N_2 + Cl^-$ or CH_3^-
OSHA limit in workplace air: 0.1 mg/m^3

Further Reading

HAYES, W. J. 1982. *Pesticides Studied in Man.* Baltimore, MD: Williams and Wilkins.

Parathion and Methyl-Parathion

Trade Name

Phoskil

Introduction

In use for decades almost entirely in agriculture, on field crops, in greenhouses, and in nurseries, parathion (technically, ethyl-parathion) and methyl-parathion have been the most widely used *organophosphates* in the world. They are highly effective against a broad spectrum of chewing and sucking insect pests: aphids, mites, moths, beetles, leaf hoppers, and leaf miners. In the United States, parathion is applied to nearly 100 food crops as well as to cotton.

Because parathion has a high *acute toxicity* to mammals through both oral and dermal exposure, it is the chief cause of accidental poisonings among crop workers. Consequently, many countries have prohibited or severely restricted its use. Methyl-parathion, however, has the advantage of being somewhat less toxic to humans and domestic animals; it is also more effective against insects and is therefore a suitable replacement. Neither form of parathion is available for use by the homeowner.

Although the residual life of methyl-parathion is shorter than that of parathion, residues of both have been found on various fresh domestic produce, including broccoli, carrots, cantaloupes, cherries, oranges, peaches, and strawberries. One characteristic of parathion that is both an advantage and a disadvantage is that it is more resistant to breakdown than some other organophosphate insecticides (such as **malathion**) so the residues in soils and on crops persist longer. This means that fewer applications are needed but that the highly toxic residues remain a threat to fieldworkers longer.

Physical and Chemical Properties

In its pure form, parathion is a yellowish liquid, while in its less pure form, it is a dark brown liquid with a garlic-like odor. It is practically insoluble in water and resists breakdown under neutral and acidic conditions. Even slightly acidic soils will extend the normal breakdown time manyfold. Unlike the parent compound, the breakdown product of parathion is quite soluble in water. Methyl-parathion is a white, crystalline powder that dissolves slightly in water and is broken down under *alkaline* conditions more quickly than parathion.

Exposure and Distribution

Domestically, about 7 million pounds of parathion are applied annually to food and fiber crops, chiefly as sprays, while some 11 million pounds of methyl-parathion are sprayed primarily on cotton. There is enormous regional variation in the amount of parathion used. In temperate regions, for example, one or two applications may suffice for a growing season, whereas in hot, humid areas as many as fifty applications have been reported for a single growing season.

Although parathion is a *contact* insecticide (it is absorbed through an insect's outer surface), it is more *persistent* in the environment than first believed. Unlike many other contact pesticides, it is apparently taken up by the plant and remains intact in plant tissue for as long as 70 days. The principal route for the breakdown of parathion in the environment is a reaction with water, which yields generally nontoxic water-soluble forms. Under certain conditions, however, particularly hot, dry conditions, the insecticide combines with oxygen, which results in a breakdown product that is considerably more toxic than the parent compound and that remains on the plant surface longer than does parathion. Both the unexpectedly long persistence of parathion and its metabolism to a more toxic product in the environment suggest that human exposure may be significant. A recent report by the Natural Resources Defense Council indicates that young children may be exposed to excessively high levels of residues of both parathion and methyl-parathion.

In 1976, the National Institute of Occupational Safety and Health estimated that about 250,000 factory workers and field-workers were exposed to parathion and another 150,000 workers were exposed to methyl-parathion annually. Generally, it is thought that exposure of factory workers during normal manufacture of the pesticide is probably negligible since the process takes place in closed vessels. Farmworkers, including mixers, applicators, and fieldhands, however, are exposed to much higher levels. Because the principal route of exposure is through the skin and because residues of parathion or the more toxic breakdown product remain on the plant surfaces for a long time following application, parathion poses a serious threat to fieldworkers returning to fields after treatment.

Health Effects

Parathion is extremely acutely toxic to mammals when ingested or absorbed through the skin, although toxicity varies among species. Even at very low doses, it is a potent inhibitor of the enzyme *cholinesterase,* which is critical in the transmission of nerve signals. This insecticide also causes another kind of nerve damage that leads to delayed paralysis from which recovery is generally slow and seldom complete in adults. Children and young animals appear to be less affected by this nerve damage. Parathion has been used frequently by people for intentional poisonings. In rats, there is evidence that toxicity varies between the sexes and among laboratory strains and that protein deficiency increases susceptibility.

In people, absorption through the skin can result in severe poisoning up to several days following exposure, which is characteristic of crop worker poisoning. Respiratory exposure to fine dusts and aerosols may be extremely hazardous. Symptoms of parathion poisoning include headache, dizziness, restlessness, confusion, convulsions, abnormally slow or speeded up heart activity, increased sweating, and increased salivation. Death is caused by respiratory failure due to a combination of inhibition of the respiratory center of the brain and paralysis of the respiratory muscles.

The EPA has classified parathion as a possible human carcinogen (group C; see Chapter 3, Section B) on the basis of some evidence from animal tests. There is scanty information about parathion's ability to cause *mutations*, little or no evidence that it causes birth defects, but some indication that it impairs reproduction in mice and birds. Single high doses of parathion by animals result in increased embryo deaths and reabsorption of embryos. Depression of the immune system has been observed in several species at dose levels associated with other toxic effects.

Protection and Prevention

Protective clothing and equipment, routine medical examinations, and medical monitoring are recommended for workers exposed to the insecticide. Treatment for exposure depends on the severity of poisoning and is essentially the same for all organophosphates. First aid should focus on decontamination: washing and flushing the skin and eyes and inducing vomiting if the insecticide is swallowed. A physician should be contacted immediately. Atropine is given, usually in conjunction with an oxime such as pralidoxime (which relieves the paralysis of the respiratory muscles). Artificial respiration and oxygen are given as needed.

Industrial effluents and wastes containing parathion or certain other organophosphates can be rendered nontoxic by treating them with alkali. Because residues of the pesticide remain primarily on the surface of fruits and vegetables, washing and peeling may reduce the levels, as may cooking and heating.

Environmental Effects

Like certain of the *carbamate* pesticides, parathion is quite toxic to honeybees. One form of the chemical, however, is highly selective against most insects, but considerably less toxic to honeybees than parathion itself. Like many other organophosphates, parathion is strongly toxic to a variety of aquatic organisms, particularly invertebrates such as *Daphnia*. It is considerably more toxic to freshwater fish species than **malathion** and **dichlorvos**, but much less toxic than chlorpyrifos, which is one of the most toxic organophosphates to aquatic organisms. Massive fish kills have been associated with accidental spills or leaks of parathion and other organophosphates into bodies of water.

In laboratory studies, when parathion was administered to quail in combination with the insecticide DDE (the primary *metabolite* of **DDT**), an additive effect was observed; the dual exposure resulted in greater mortality than exposure to a single compound.

Regulatory Status

Because parathion poses a substantial threat to fieldworkers reentering fields following spraying, there have been numerous state and federal attempts to regulate the reentry periods to reduce the threat. To date, there is little agreement on the optimal reentry period because of regional and weather-related variations in breakdown products and variations in the length of time the residues persist. Consequently, significant differences exist in prescribed reentry times, with California laws being considerably more stringent than those of the federal government (see Chapter 17, Section D). Parathion is listed as a *hazardous air pollutant* in the 1990 Clean Air Act, requiring the EPA to set emission standards. It is also on the EPA *community right-to-know* list.

Technical Information

Chemical name of parathion: O,O-diethyl O-(p-nitrophenyl)phosphorothioate
Chemical formula: $C_{10}H_{14}NO_5PS$
Comparative toxicity in rats based on the lethal dose (LD_{50}):

	parathion	*methyl-parathion*
oral	3 mg/kg	14 mg/kg
dermal	5 mg/kg	67 mg/kg

No observed effects level in humans:
0.05 mg/kg

Government standards:
NIOSH recommended limit: 0.05 mg/m^3
OSHA limit in workplace air: 0.11 mg/m^3
EPA water quality criterion for aquatic life: 0.013 μg/L

Further Reading

SEWELL, B., and WHYATT, R. 1989. *Intolerable Risk: Pesticides in Our Children's Food*. New York: Natural Resources Defense Council.

World Health Organization. 1984. *Environmental Health Criteria No. 63: Parathion*. Geneva.

Particulate Matter

Other Names

Particulates; total suspended particulates; TSP

Introduction

Particulate matter is a general term used to describe a variety of substances that exist as distinct particles, either liquid droplets or solid matter. Particulate matter can be considered among the most dangerous of air pollutants because it includes such cancer-causing materials as **asbestos** and tobacco smoke and because it almost always makes the effects of gaseous pollutants (such as **sulfur dioxide**) worse.

Physical and Chemical Properties

It is difficult to generalize about the properties of particulate matter because it includes such a wide variety of substances, arising from an assortment of activities. Two size classifications are generally referred to: fine particulates that are smaller than 2.5 *microns* (about 0.0001 inch) and larger, coarse material. Fine particulates tend to arise from combustion sources and from the transformation of gaseous pollutants in the atmosphere. Sulfur dioxide gas, for example, rapidly turns into fine sulfate particulates after its release from power plants and smelters. Fine particulates are usually more dangerous than the coarser ones because they can be inhaled deeper into the lungs, lodging there, and damaging the delicate tissues involved in gas exchange. Fine material also provides more total surface area (for a given weight of matter) for chemical reactions to occur and to which toxic substances (such as **trace metals**) may stick. Fine particles can remain in the air for weeks or months and therefore can travel great distances from their source.

Coarse particulate matter tends to arise from mining, construction activity, natural fires, and windblown dust. It settles out of the atmosphere faster than do fine particulates and therefore is primarily a hazard closer to where it originates.

Particulate matter used to be called "total suspended particulates" (TSP) because instruments used to measure it would collect essentially all of the material floating in air. In recognition of the more hazardous nature of fine particulates, new equipment favors the collection of smaller particles, giving a more accurate estimate of the portion most likely to cause harm. Unfortunately, most health effects information is still based on the earlier method of collection, so it will take some time before new research carefully documents the concentrations at which the finer material does damage.

Exposure and Distribution

Children are the most exposed group in the population. Recent research shows that children inhale particulates deeper into their lungs than do adults. Children also tend to spend more time outdoors where particulate pollution can be higher than indoors (although in households with smokers this may not be true), and they tend to be more active, thus breathing faster and deeper. As with other types of air pollution, exposures are greatest in urban areas and around major point sources of pollution (such as factories, power plants, and smelters).

Table 44 shows the percentage contribution to total particulate emissions made by each major source in 1988. Care should be used in evaluating these percentages, however, because they are based on the older "total" method of measurement and because the industrial emissions often occur in areas that are relatively unpopulated. Transportation sources probably account for a greater portion of the fine particulate matter inhaled by a majority of the population than these percentages would suggest.

In 1988, a total of 7 million tons of total suspended particulates was emitted to the atmosphere. From 1984 to 1986, a 7% reduc-

TABLE 44 Sources of Particulate Emissions (1988)

Source	Percentage of Total Emissions
Industrial processes	38
Stationary fuel combustion	25
Transportation	20
Other sources	17

tion in emissions took place. Air quality, as measured by total suspended particulates, improved less than 1% over this same period. A total of 26 million people live in counties in violation of the national standard for protection of human health. The worst areas tend to be in the industrial Midwest and the arid West, although violations of the national standard occur in all parts of the country.

Health Effects

The health effects of particulate pollution include an aggravation of *bronchitis* in adults and children with preexisting respiratory illness, small but significant changes in lung functioning in children, and immediate additional deaths of the elderly and of people with preexisting heart or lung disease if pollution levels are high enough. *Asthmatics* and others with allergies may react, especially to sulfate particulates. At current levels of particulate pollution, the severity and frequency of symptoms increase with any increase in particulate matter. These are the short-term results of elevated levels of particulates.

Long-term exposure to particulate matter causes damage to lung tissues, which contributes to chronic respiratory disease, cancer, and premature illness and death. Children in areas of higher particulate pollution have more colds, coughs, and other symptoms than do children in less polluted areas. Particulate matter from industrial sources contribute to relatively high lung cancer rates, particularly around smelters. Symptoms of *chronic obstructive pulmonary disease* are correlated with particulate levels, and death rates have been related to total sulfate and particulate pollution.

Protection and Prevention

Tobacco smoke is the greatest source of particulate exposure for smokers and possibly for people who live or work with smokers. Eliminating this source of pollution is perhaps the only measure immediately within the control of individuals. Close proximity to point sources of pollution for long periods of time should be avoided. Children's playgrounds and ball fields should not be located downwind of major factories, power plants, or smelters. When the air is of unusually poor quality, such as during periods of atmospheric inversions, outdoor exercise and other strenuous activities should be curtailed. Exhaust fans should be used when cooking.

Environmental Effects

Particles cause soiling of fabrics, buildings, and statuary, as well as loss of visibility and damage to structures and materials. Some of the most severe ecological effects of air pollution come from the conversion of gaseous **sulfur dioxide** and **nitrogen oxide** emissions to acid particulates, which later fall to Earth either as acid rain or snow or as dry particulates. These acids are changing the chemistry of freshwaters in much of the Northeast, Canada, and the mountainous regions of the West. They are also dissolving metals from soils, which later wash into streams, and in combination with ozone, contribute to the dieback of forests in many regions of the country. Particles in the atmosphere can also alter the climate because they block sunlight.

Regulatory Status

The EPA recently changed the standard for measuring particulate air pollution to better reflect the hazard of the smaller particles. The older standard was based on total suspended particulates, while the new standard (in effect since 1987) covers mainly particles smaller than 10 microns in diameter. A 24-hour standard is imposed to restrict short-term peaks in particulate concentrations, and a lower annual standard is meant to keep the *background level* in check. As noted previously, however, 26 million people live in counties in violation of the standards. The EPA is required by law to periodically review, and revise if necessary, the particulate standards.

Technical Information

New definition of particulate matter: discrete matter with an effective aerodynamic diameter less than or equal to a nominal 10 μm (abbreviated PM_{10})

National ambient air quality standards:
Primary (protection of human health):
24-hour average, 1 expected exceedance per year: 150 μg/m^3
annual average, no allowable exceedances: 50 μg/m^3
Secondary (protection of human welfare): same as primary standards

Further Reading

Environmental Protection Agency. 1987. Revisions to the National Ambient Air Quality Standards for Particulate Matter. *Federal Register* 52(126):24,634–24,669.

———. 1986. *Second Addendum to Air Quality Criteria for Particulate Matter and Sulfur Oxides (1982): Assessment of Newly Available Health Effects Information.* EPA–600/8–86–020A. Washington, D.C.

PCBs and PBBs

Other Names

Polychlorinated biphenyls (PCBs) and poly-brominated biphenyls (PBBs)

Trade Names

Arachlors; Arochurs; Kanechlors; Firemaster FF-1

Introduction

Four decades after their introduction to the world market, the organochlorine compounds called the PCBs were linked to extensive global contamination and serious human illness. By the late 1960s, significant levels of PCBs were being detected in air, soil, water, sediments, fish and other wildlife, and human tissues throughout the world. More alarming to the public was the major human poisoning incident that occurred in Japan in 1968. People who had consumed cooking oil that had been contaminated with PCBs during the manufacturing process showed signs of chemical poisoning. Some became seriously ill and some died.

As the name implies, polychlorinated biphenyls (PCBs) belong to a class of compounds containing a variable number of chlorines. Toxicity varies with the degree of chlorination and the actual position of the chlorine atoms on the basic structure. Theoretically, more than 200 different *isomers* or forms of PCBs are possible, although commercial mixtures are generally made up of 40 to 70 PCB compounds. In addition, most commercial PCB products contain chlorinated **naphthalene** and chlorinated dibenzofurans.

Because of their low flammability, PCBs have been used extensively for insulating and cooling electrical equipment, such as transformers and capacitors, and in hydraulic fluids and lubricants. In such applications, the flow of PCBs to the environment is restricted. Widespread environmental distribution of PCBs, however, has occurred from their use as plasticizers, in inks and dyes, as part of pesticide preparations, in adhesives, as protective surface coatings for wood, and in carbonless-copy paper.

At the height of production (around 1970), about 85 million pounds of PCBs were produced annually in the United States. Following disclosure that PCBs *persisted* in the environment, accumulated in the *food chain*, and posed a hazard to human health, U.S. manufacturers voluntarily stopped sales of the chemicals for those uses that could be expected to leak PCBs to the environment. Until recently, however, PCBs have continued to be used in closed systems, such as electrical capacitors and transformers—despite numerous accidental leaks from electrical equipment and the incidental release of **dioxin** and dibenzofurans following incomplete combustion of PCBs.

Polybrominated biphenyls (PBBs) differ from PCBs in that bromine atoms, rather than chlorine atoms, are attached to the basic structure. The two related chemicals share the property of low flammability and have therefore been used in similar ways. PBBs have been used chiefly as fire retardants and, secondarily, in plastic parts that are subject to heating, such as televisions, radios, business machines, typewriters, and even handtools. PBBs, like PCBs, have been headline news. In one well-publicized incident, substantial amounts of animal feed contaminated with the PBB hexabromophenyl (Firemaster) were fed to livestock. Dairy cattle, beef cattle, chickens, and eggs had been contaminated and the products consumed before the mistake was discovered. About 1.5 million chickens and 23,000 dairy cattle had to be destroyed.

Physical and Chemical Properties

The physical appearance of PCBs ranges from oily liquids to white, crystalline solids to hard, noncrystalline resins. Typical mixtures occur as light straw-colored liquids with an aromatic odor. PBBs typically exist in solid form and decompose at temperatures greater than 600°F. Both PBBs and PCBs are generally resistant to breakdown by light, heat, and air and are not soluble in water.

Exposure and Distribution

Polychlorinated biphenyls and related organochlorines, such as **DDT** and **dioxin**, are the most widely distributed and persistent chemicals known. Although manufacture and leaky uses of PCBs were curtailed in the mid-1970s, significant reservoirs of PCBs remain in soils, sediments, water, waste disposal sites, and existing electrical capacitors and transformers. Consequently, the compounds are taken up from soils and sediments by organisms and transferred through the food chain, released accidentally from existing electrical equipment, and allowed to escape to the atmosphere when improperly incinerated (that is, at temperatures insufficiently high to destroy them).

The North Atlantic Ocean is the dominant sink for PCBs, accounting for 50 to 80% of the PCBs in the environment. The major continental reservoir is the freshwater sediments in the United States. Particularly high levels of PCBs have been detected in numerous places throughout the Great Lakes. PCBs have even been found in the sediments on the bottom of a remote wilderness lake, apparently as a result of atmospheric deposition. Because of their persistence and continuing inadvertent release, PCBs threaten commercial and/or sport fishing in many major U.S. rivers and lakes. For example, as a result of contamination, commercial fishing for striped bass and five other species of fish was prohibited in New York's Hudson River. Health advisories have been issued to limit the consumption of fish taken by sport fishermen in many industrialized areas around the country. A recent report by the National Wildlife Federation concluded that eating certain popular species of fish from Lake Michigan poses human health risks.

Although resistant to breakdown, PCBs can be slowly decomposed by soil bacteria. The length of time required depends on the degree of chlorination. Certain PCBs react to **ultraviolet light** in a way that produces new forms that are considerably more toxic than the parent compounds. PCBs can be absorbed by the digestive tract, skin, and lungs. Monitoring indicates that nearly everyone has been exposed to PCBs, typically through consumption of water or contaminated foods, especially fish and possibly waterfowl. Poultry, eggs, and milk have been contaminated in the past. Certain segments of the population have been exposed or run the risk of exposure from faulty or leaky electrical equipment, such as office building air conditioning systems, or from low-temperature incineration of wastes containing PCBs as might occur when PCB-containing wastes are unwittingly handled by municipal disposal companies.

Health Effects

PCBs are considered highly toxic, but the toxicity varies from one commercial product to another depending on the extent of chlorination of the mixture. In general, the greater the chlorination, the greater the toxicity. Symptoms associated with PCB poisoning include *chloracne* (as with **dioxin** poisoning), increased pigmentation of fingernails and gums, changes in the immune system, and respiratory distress. Also, acute and chronic exposure can cause irritation of the eyes, nose, and throat, as well as liver damage, jaundice, nausea, vomiting, abdominal pain, and gray-brown discoloration of the skin.

Laboratory studies show that PCBs produce a variety of unwanted effects in diverse test animals. PCBs can cross the placenta and are toxic to the embryo, causing numerous adverse reproductive effects, particularly increased stillbirths, spontaneous abortions, and fetal absorptions. They also affect survival of weanlings in rodents, monkeys, and mink. In addition, following exposure to PCBs, the immune system of rodents is suppressed; chickens exhibit changes in the liver and edema in the young; and skin lesions are produced in several species of animals besides humans, including primates, horses, and cattle.

On the basis of animal tests, PCBs are classified as probable human carcinogens (group B_2; see Chapter 3, Section B). NIOSH regards PCBs as occupational carcinogens. Rodent tests indicate that PCBs cause liver cancer and possibly stomach cancer, perhaps as a result of interactions with **nitrosamines**. Moreover, in humans, there is some evidence of increased incidence of melanoma among men exposed to Arachlor 1254, a tradename for a certain mixture of PCBs. Also, an unexplained association exists between high PCB levels in the blood and both elevated cholesterol levels and elevated blood pressure.

Studies indicate that PBBs produce an array of health effects (including liver cancer in rodents) similar to those of PCBs, but that exposure is much less likely since PBBs have been used in far smaller quantities and distributed more locally.

Protection and Prevention

The primary means of protection is to avoid eating fish (or waterfowl) that are contaminated with PCBs. State wildlife agencies or fish and game agencies monitor PCB levels in food fish species and issue warnings about consumption, which should be heeded. Because PCBs cross the placenta, pregnant women are advised to be especially careful to avoid contaminated fish. Workers involved in the cleanup of accidental leaks and spills of PCBs are required to wear special protective clothing, eye covering, and respirators. Anyone exposed to PCBs should flush contaminants from the skin or eyes and should contact a physician immediately.

A key element in protecting the public and the environment from exposure to PCBs (and PBBs) is to get rid of existing stocks—in sediments, at hazardous waste sites, and in electrical equipment. But disposal or destruc-

tion of PCBs and similar organochlorines is tricky. Although a few chemical waste disposal facilities have been approved for their disposal, there is serious concern about the likelihood of preventing future groundwater and soil contamination from these sites. Certain physical and chemical treatments can effectively decompose or destroy PCBs, but these methods are generally expensive and thus impractical for large volumes or dilute concentrations of PCBs. The preferred method of dealing with PCBs is high-temperature (2000 to 3000°F) incineration with excess oxygen, which can achieve virtually complete destruction. Unfortunately, even in very efficient incinerators, some unwanted by-products may be produced, particularly dioxin and dibenzofurans. So the *bottom ash* and *fly ash* from smokestacks with scrubbers that remove chlorine-containing compounds must be treated as hazardous wastes.

Environmental Effects

Numerous studies show that some kinds of phytoplankton are highly sensitive to PCBs (and other organochlorines). The degree of sensitivity varies with certain physical conditions, such as the intensity of light. The primary effect is a reduction in growth of sensitive species, which permits resistant species to become dominant. The long-term effects of such changes are uncertain, but may have significant impacts on those organisms that depend on phytoplankton as a food source.

Because PCBs are as persistent and widespread in the environment as DDT, their potential impact on a variety of nontarget species has been well studied. While PCB residues have been found in the tissue of adult birds (for example, ospreys and bald eagles) and in their nonsurviving eggs, PCBs are not directly correlated with eggshell thinning and consequent breakage. Instead, it appears that PCBs may significantly enhance the effect of DDE, the primary breakdown product of DDT. Recent wildlife studies on several species of birds and fish in the Great Lakes region suggest a link between elevated tissue levels of chlorinated hydrocarbons, including PCBs, and a diverse array of effects. These range from hormonal and behavioral changes to tumors, suppression of the immune system, and abnormal development of the young.

Regulatory Status

Beginning in the mid-1970s, a series of EPA regulations has restricted the manufacture, import, export, use, transportation, and disposal of PCBs. Similarly, PBBs are no longer commercially manufactured or distributed. Current law requires that many, but not all, existing PCB-containing electrical transformers be retired by October 1990. In response to reports that PCB wastes have been improperly handled, Congress has been grappling with a set of proposals intended to ensure adequate and safe disposal of remaining PCB stocks. PCBs are listed as *hazardous air pollutants* in the 1990 Clean Air Act.

Technical Information

Chemical name: chlorodiphenyl (PCBs)
Chemical formula:
  PCBs, composition 54% chlorine:
    $C_{12}H_5Cl_5$
  PCBs, composition 42% chlorine:
    $C_{12}H_7Cl_3$
Concentrations found at contaminated sites:
  surface waters near waste sites: 8.5–6100 ppb
  sediments near waste sites: 66,500–550,000 ppb
  fish near waste sites: 15–730 ppm
  soil near waste sites: 0.1–3,500 ppm
Concentrations found in flue gas effluents from incinerators:
  9.4–234$\mu g/m^3$
Concentrations found in human blood:
  1–348 ppb
Residues found in osprey eggs:
  1970: 9.8 ppm
  1979: 8.6 ppm

OSHA limits in workplace air:
  for mixtures with 54% chlorine:
    0.5 mg/m^3
  for mixtures with 42% chlorine:
    1 mg/m^3
NIOSH recommended limit for both compounds: 1.0 $\mu g/m^3$

Further Reading

BARTEL, D. B. 1981. *PCBs, Papermaking, and the Fox River.* Chicago: CBE Environmental Review, Citizens for a Better Environment.

COBURN, T. E., DAVIDSON, A., GREEN, S. N., HODGE, R. A., JACKSON, C. I., and LIROFF, R. A. 1990. *Great Lakes: Great Legacy?* Washington, D.C.: Conservation Foundation.

Environmental Health Perspectives. 1985. Vol. 59, February (entire issue).

National Research Council. 1979. *Polychlorinated Biphenyls.* Washington, D.C.: National Academy of Sciences.

World Health Organization. 1976. *Environmental Health Criteria No. 2: Polychlorinated Biphenyls and Triphenyls.* Geneva.

Plutonium

Other Names

^{239}Pu; ^{238}Pu; ^{240}Pu

Introduction

Plutonium (Pu) surely must rank among the most widely publicized toxic substances. Sometimes referred to as the most toxic substance known, its name conjures up images of terrorists, nuclear bombs, and leaking nuclear waste stockpiles. Our concern over this substance derives from its copious production in nuclear power plants, its very long lifetime in the environment, its extraordinary ability to cause cancer when lodged in lung tissue, and its common use as the power source for nuclear weapons. Breeder reactors, which generate nuclear fuels faster than they burn them, would contain even larger quantities of plutonium than conventional reactors; such reactors are in commercial use in France and the Soviet Union, but not in the United States.

Releases of plutonium to the environment figured prominently in several major nuclear accidents that have occurred in the past few decades. Among these were a series of fires and leaks at the Rocky Flats plutonium fabrication plant in Colorado (with the most serious accident occurring in 1957); the crash of an airplane with nuclear weapons aboard at Thule, Greenland, in 1968; and a major fire at Great Britain's Windscale fuel reprocessing plant in 1957. These accidents have produced localized increases in environmental plutonium that far exceed that from other sources. Nevertheless, on a global basis, over a thousand times more plutonium has entered the environment from nuclear weapons testing than from all accidents and routine reactor operations combined.

Several other radioactive elements, including americium (Am), neptunium (Np), and californium (Cf), are associated chemically and physically with plutonium and are among the elements that are produced artificially. Americium is almost as potent a *carcinogen* as plutonium. It is produced from the decay of plutonium-239 and has been used in smoke detectors as a source of *alpha particles* (in such detectors, an electrical signal rings a buzzer when a stream of alpha particles is interrupted because they are absorbed by smoke). We will refer occasionally to americium in our discussion.

Physical and Chemical Properties

Plutonium oxide, the most common form of plutonium in the environment, is a nonvolatile, relatively insoluble solid. Plutonium-239, the most hazardous of the plutonium isotopes, decays by alpha particle emission and has a *half-life* of 24,000 years. Americium-241, the most hazardous form of that element, also decays by alpha emission, with a half-life of 432 years. It is more water soluble than plutonium.

Exposure and Distribution

Plutonium occurs naturally only in incredibly minute quantities (perhaps a few pounds of it in all of the Earth's crust). But plutonium is produced copiously in normally operating nuclear reactors from the common isotopic form of uranium, uranium-238, which constitutes over 90% of uranium fuel. In a typical 1000-megawatt nuclear power plant, about 450 pounds of plutonium are produced each year. (For comparison, a small nuclear bomb requires about 20 pounds of plutonium.) Under routine operating conditions, only a trace amount of that plutonium is released to the environment. Weapons testing, in contrast, has released about 8000 pounds of plutonium to the atmosphere, most of which has been deposited on the ground all around the world.

Several isotopes of plutonium exist, all of which pose some health hazard, but the one of greatest concern is plutonium-239. One reason is that plutonium-239 is ideal for making nuclear weapons. Moreover, it emits alpha particles (which are the most dangerous of the particles of radiation), and it has a very long half-life, which means that it is a potent source of radiation in the environment for many thousands of years.

Inhalation of windblown dust on which plutonium has been deposited is the most frequently encountered pathway by which plutonium enters the human respiratory system. Once inhaled, a large fraction of plutonium on fine dust particles lodges in tiny crevices in the lung, where alpha particles from its decay can cause intense damage. Plutonium can move from the respiratory tract to the liver and skeleton, where liver and bone cancers can result. Americium, being more soluble than plutonium, is more rapidly spread throughout the body. Because alpha particles have very little penetrating power, skin contact with plutonium is not as serious as inhalation or ingestion of the substance.

Health Effects

There is little question about the type of damage caused by exposure to plutonium; lung, bone, and liver cancer and leukemia are the most frequently occurring serious results of exposure. The magnitude of the risk at small doses is less certain, however. Estimates of the dose needed to cause lung cancer differ by as much as a factor of a thousand. At the high end of the range, many tens of thousands of cancers worldwide may have been caused by atmospheric testing of nuclear weapons. At the low end, the risk to the public may have been negligible. Even those who accept the low risk estimate, however, agree that up to 30 deaths from cancer resulted from the fire at Britain's Windscale plutonium production plant, which exposed the general population living nearby the plant, as well as plant workers.

Believers of either of the extreme estimates will not be easy to convince that the other extreme is correct. In such an uncertain situation, it is tempting for those not polarized on the issue to assume that the truth lies somewhere in the middle. But this may not be the case: the true risk may actually be one or the other of the extreme views.

Protection and Prevention

Once plutonium has been inhaled, there is nothing that medical science can do to reduce the risk of lung cancer. It would be prudent to keep away from the sites of accidents where plutonium levels in the surrounding soils are much higher than average.

Regulatory Status

In the United States, the general restrictions on radiation exposure apply to radioactive strontium and can be found in Chapter 15, Section F. Plutonium is listed as a *hazardous air pollutant* in the 1990 Clean Air Act.

Technical Information[4]

Plutonium-239 decays with a half-life of 24,400 years to uranium-235 by emitting a 5.15 million-electron-volt alpha particle. Weapons testing released about 1.5×10^{16} becquerels of plutonium, most of which has by now been dispersed worldwide. About 60% of this is ^{239}Pu (85% by mass, 60% by *activity*) and most of the remainder is ^{240}Pu. Nuclear power plants produce about 1.2×10^{12} becquerels of ^{239}Pu per megawatt of electricity produced. Of this, more than half *fissions* in the reactor and contributes to the generation of electricity; only trace amounts are released in normal operations.

The Rocky Flats leak released 2×10^{11} becquerels of plutonium, of which about half went off site. An accident at the Mound Laboratory in Ohio released 4×10^{11} becquerels of plutonium. The airplane crash at Thule, Greenland, resulted in the release of 9×10^{11} becquerels, and the recent reentry and burnup of a spacecraft over the Indian Ocean dispersed about 5×10^{11} becquerels. Each

[4]For a discussion of the meaning of the units of radiation used below, see Chapter 15, Section E.

smoke detector using americium as an alpha source contains about 1×10^5 becquerels of ^{241}Am. The collective dose per unit of released activity for plutonium and americium is about 1×10^{-9} person-sieverts per becquerel released. The absorbed dose to the lung per unit of inhaled intake of ^{239}Pu is approximately 3.2×10^{-4} sieverts per becquerel. Doses per unit intake to the liver and bone-lining cells are of the same magnitude.

At the low end of the range of uncertainty, the lung cancer risk from inhaled ^{239}Pu is estimated to be one case of cancer for every 300 person-sieverts absorbed by the lung. At the high end, the estimated risk is roughly 100 times as great. Every microgram of ^{239}Pu inhaled into the lung results in a lung dose of approximately 1 sievert, and hence if the higher risk estimate is correct, the inhalation of merely a few micrograms of plutonium is sufficient to cause lung cancer. Even with the lower risk estimate, less than a milligram, suffices.

Further Reading

GOFMAN, J. W. 1981. *Radiation and Human Health.* San Francisco: Sierra Club Books.

National Council on Radiation Protection and Measurements. 1975. *Alpha Emitting Particles in Lungs: NCRP Report No. 46.* Washington, D.C.

World Health Organization. 1983. *Environmental Health Criteria Report No. 23: Selected Radionuclides.* Geneva.

Pyrethroids
(Pyrethrum and Permethrin)

Other Name

Pyrethrins

Trade Names

Permethrin; Ambush; Pounce

Introduction

Two species of daisy-like chrysanthemums naturally produce the pyrethroid substance pyrethrum, whose insecticidal properties have been known and used for centuries. Earliest records of pyrethrum use to kill insects date from about 1800 in parts of Asia. During the Napoleonic wars, ground chrysanthemum flowers were used to control lice.

Pyrethrum today remains a very popular insecticide with home gardeners and farmers practicing alternative agriculture (see Chapter 14, Section F). Although pyrethrum is a highly effective, rapidly acting *contact* (or knock-down) insecticide against a broad spectrum of flying insects, it has some drawbacks that limit its use. First, pyrethrum degrades very quickly, losing its insecticidal ability, once it is exposed to sunlight. As a result, some insects are able to recover from the knock-down effects. To bolster pyrethrum's effect, the insecticide is commonly formulated with a *synergist* (a chemical that enhances the activity of the insecticide, but is not itself insecticidal). Second, pyrethrum is relatively more expensive than many synthetic pesticides. The costs of growing the pyrethrum flowers, extracting the active components, and combining them with a synergist all add up. As a result of its expense and instability to sunlight, the naturally occurring insecticide has not been used in conventional agriculture. Finally, while pyrethrum is a natural pesticide, it is not entirely benign (as discussed under the sections on Health Effects and Environmental Effects).

In recent years, several synthetic pyrethroid-like insecticides such as permethrin have been developed and have become the fastest growing sector of the insecticide market. They can be used at very low rates of application and are therefore cheaper to use than pyrethrum and many other synthetic insecticides. Permethrin, available since 1978, resists breakdown in sunlight; is effective against most agricultural pests, particularly leaf- and fruit-eating beetles and moths; and controls cockroaches and other crawling insects, external animal parasites, and biting flies. Despite the relatively small amounts of permethrin applied, some pests have developed *resistance* to it.

Physical and Chemical Properties

Pyrethrum extracts are thick liquids. Although insoluble in water, they are soluble in organic solvents and oils. They do, however, break down readily in water. The natural extracts are unstable in the presence of light, moisture, and air; stored powders lose about 20% of their potency in a year.

In its pure form, the synthetic pyrethroid, permethrin, is a solid that melts at temperatures above 100°F. In its less pure form, permethrin is a yellow-brown liquid that crystallizes slightly at room temperature. It is barely soluble in water, but dissolves readily in most organic solvents. Permethrin is considerably more resistant to decomposition in sunlight than pyrethrum due to the addition of chlorine.

Exposure and Distribution

Pyrethrum is available for home use and is widely used by home gardeners to eliminate a variety of insect pests. Because it breaks down rapidly under most environmental conditions, residues are not likely to remain in soils, in water, or on fruits and vegetables. Synthetic permethrin lasts longer in the environment than does pyrethrum, but is used at very low application rates. Although it is used on more than 40 vegetable crops, only

500,000 pounds of permethrin are applied annually. In contrast, five times that amount of **azinophos-methyl** and about seven million pounds of **parathion** are used annually.

Health Effects

Long considered to be among the safest insecticide to humans and domestic animals, pyrethrum is nevertheless of low to moderate *acute toxicity* to mammals, depending on the route of entry. It can be absorbed by the intestinal tract, where it is readily converted to nontoxic products. In fact, it has been used in some parts of the world to treat people for intestinal worms. Studies of rats indicate that exposure to moderate, repeated doses can lead to changes in the liver. Toxic effects that have been observed in test animals suggest that the pyrethroids affect the nervous system much the same way **DDT** does, producing diarrhea, convulsions, paralysis, and death by respiratory failure.

The EPA classifies permethrin as a possible human carcinogen (group C; see Chapter 3, Section B) on the basis of animal studies in which mice developed tumors at high dose levels. The EPA concluded that at expected exposure levels, however, the cancer-causing potential of permethrin is extremely low. Observed toxicity in people generally seems to be the result of an allergic response following repeated skin exposures, or possibly inhalation, rather than direct toxicity of the material. Allergic responses range from mild to severe skin rashes to sneezing and other respiratory problems, such as *asthma*, sinusitis, and *bronchitis*. Apparently, pyrethrum powder from ground-up flowers produces an allergic response more readily than the commercially prepared liquid extracts.

Protection and Prevention

Antihistamines have proven effective in treating pyrethrum allergies in people. If pyrethrum is ingested and produces nervous system responses, phenobarbital may be prescribed by the physician. People using and handling any pesticide should exercise caution, read the directions on the label, and avoid inhalation or skin contact. Residues of pyrethroids on fresh produce can be reduced or eliminated by washing with a liquid dishwashing detergent and rinsing with water or peeling.

Environmental Effects

Neither the naturally occurring pyrethrum nor the synthetic permethrin has been associated with well-publicized, major environmental problems of the sort that made DDT infamous. Nevertheless, the cultivation of pyrethrum-bearing flowers may be contributing indirectly to the extinction of the endangered mountain gorilla of east-central Africa. Most of the world's supply of commercial pyrethrum comes from central and eastern Africa. In that region, land that is used for cultivating chrysanthemum flowers—a very important cash crop—is unavailable for other purposes, such as growing food or providing habitat for other species. In crowded Rwanda where flower production is intensive and economic incentives to grow the flowers are severe, farmers have been clearing new patches of land within the Virunga Volcanoes National Park. The park (and adjacent areas in Zaire and Uganda) is the last territory of the 240 or so remaining endangered mountain gorillas. Park boundaries, and thus gorilla habitat, have been steadily shrinking under the onslaught.

Regulatory Status

Pyrethrum products and permethrin are general use pesticides, which means that they are not restricted in use. Because permethrin residues tend to accumulate in processed foods, there are no *tolerances* for certain crops.

Technical Information

Naturally occurring pyrethrum actually consists of six different but related compounds, collectively called pyrethrins. These are ex-

tracted primarily from the two species of commercially grown chrysanthemum that contain sufficiently high levels of the chemicals to be used for insecticide production. The concentration of pyrethrins varies geographically and within strains. Flowers from Kenya, for example, contain 1.3 to 3.0% pyrethrins, while Japanese flowers average about 1.0% and Yugoslavian flowers contain less than 1.0%.

Chemical names:
  pyrethrum: pyrethrins I and II; cinerins I and II; jasmolins I and II
  permethrin: *m*-phenoxybenzyl(*cis, trans*-3-(2,2-dichlorovinyl)-2,2-dimethylcyclopropanecarboxylate
Chemical formulas (examples):
  pyrethrin I: $C_{21}H_{28}O_3$
  jasmolin II: $C_{22}H_{30}O_5$
  permethrin: $C_{21}H_{20}Cl_2O_3$

Further Reading

MATSUMURA, F. 1985. *Toxicology of Insecticides.* New York: Plenum Press.

Radon

Other Name

^{222}Rn

Introduction

In terms of how many cases of cancer it is estimated to cause each year, radon (Rn) is among the most dangerous of toxic substances in the United States. Unlike many other toxics described in this Guide, its major sources are natural; where we live and how we design our dwellings determine the dose we receive. Radon contributes to the problem of indoor air pollution; outdoors it is sufficiently diluted by the atmosphere to pose a far lower hazard. Radon is a radioactive gas produced by the decay of radioactive radium in the earth's crust. When radon decays in the home, it produces a sequence of *decay products* that are also radioactive; the phrase "radon hazard" actually refers to the health risk from all of the radioactive elements in the sequence.

Physical and Chemical Properties

Radon itself is an odorless, colorless, chemically nonreactive gas. It and its decay products, called radon daughters, are present in the environment in quantities too small to be detected directly by the senses; radiation detectors are needed to determine the level of their presence. Radon and its daughters often find their way into the lung either as gases or attached to fine *particulates*. In the lung, two of the radon daughters are particularly hazardous (see Technical Information section) because they emit *alpha particles* when they decay. Such particles can cause intense damage to the lining of the inner recesses of the lungs.

Exposure and Distribution

For the average person, the major source of exposure is from indoor air, although miners working underground at some locations are also at risk. Radon usually enters the home from the soil beneath the foundation; well water used for domestic supply can also be a source. The rate at which radon emanates from soil varies from place to place by a factor of a thousand or more. In some parts of the United States, such as the region where New York, Pennsylvania, and New Jersey come together (northeast of Reading, Pennsylvania), the radon source is particularly large because of high radium concentrations in underlying bedrock. More work is needed to map out all the "hot spots" in the United States. Based on a study of 552 homes in the United States, indoor radon levels are often 100 times greater than those outdoors. They are higher in winter than in summer because ventilation of indoor air is lowest in cold weather.

Health Effects

Lung cancer is the primary threat from radon. Animal studies and data on cancer incidence among uranium and other miners suggest that in an average home in the United States, an individual has about a 1-in-300 chance of developing lung cancer in his or her lifetime from indoor radon. Expressed differently, the best estimate is that about 10% of all cases of lung cancer in the United States are caused by indoor radon. This statistic must be qualified because smokers are more susceptible to cancer from radon than are nonsmokers. It is estimated that each year in the United States, radon exposure plays a role in causing roughly between 2000 and 20,000 deaths from lung cancer, but that about 75% of these deaths are caused by the combination of radon exposure and smoking. Based on the 552-home study, there are about one million homes in the United States where the chances of developing lung cancer from radon are at least as great as 1 in 40 over a lifetime.

Protection and Prevention

In the section on Sources for Home Testing Equipment at the back of the book, we tell how to get a home monitoring kit or expert help to determine the level of radon in your home. Several options are available for those whose homes have high radon levels. The basements or crawl spaces of most houses have slightly lower air pressure than does the soil beneath, and this speeds the rate at which radon gas can enter the house through the foundation. One remedial step is to install pipes to the outdoors that ventilate the soil beneath the house. Another is to pressurize the basement or crawl space slightly by means of an air blower. Increasing the rate of ventilation in indoor living spaces is effective because it helps to flush out the radon. The extra ventilation can also increase heating bills significantly in winter, but that can be prevented by installing a heat exchanger in the ventilator (which removes the heat from the outgoing warm air and deposits it in the incoming cold air). Sealing cracks in the foundation and basement floor has not been shown to be an effective way to reduce the inflow of radon.

In the future, maps of the United States showing regions where the radon problem is most likely to be severe will be available. Using these maps, people with mobility can, if they choose, avoid living in regions where the risk is high. Finally, smokers who want to greatly reduce the risk of radon-caused lung cancer should quit smoking.

Regulatory Status

The National Council for Radiation Protection and Measurement (NCRP) has set a guideline for the maximum radiation level in indoor air at a value of about 5.5 times higher than that found in the average U.S. home. This guideline is probably exceeded in several million homes. OSHA and the Bonneville Power Administration recommend maximum exposures about two-thirds as great as that of the NCRP. The EPA has not taken a regulatory approach and has not issued standards to protect the public against the radon threat. In 1986, however, the EPA and the Depart-

ment of Health and Human Services (HHS) jointly issued guidelines advising the public about the need for action. (These action guidelines are summarized in the Technical Information section.)

Technical Information[5]

The radon isotope of concern is radon-222 or ^{222}Rn. It has a half-life of 3.8 days. The daughters of radon that are of greatest concern are two polonium isotopes (^{218}Po and ^{214}Po). Both of these isotopes decay by emitting an alpha particle. In the study of 552 houses, the measured radioactivity ranged from 4 to 8000 becquerels per cubic meter (Bq/m^3). The study suggested that in an average house in the United States, the concentration of indoor radon and its daughters produces a radioactivity level of about 55 Bq/m^3 and that in about one million homes the level probably exceeds 300 Bq/m^3.

In the United States, the unit of picocurie per liter (pCi/L) or of working level (WL) is usually used instead of becquerels per cubic meter to express indoor radon levels. The relationship among these three units are as follows:

1 pCi/L = 37 Bq/m^3 = 0.005 WL

1 WL = 200 pCi/L = 7400 Bq/m^3

1 Bq/m^3 = 0.027 pCi/L = 1.35 × 10^{-4}WL

In the average U.S. home, the radon level is about 1.5 pCi/L or 0.0075 WL.

Table 45 gives estimates prepared by the EPA and HHS of the risk of dying from lung cancer as a result of radon exposure. These data are the basis for their guidelines. These risk estimates apply to the average person—the risk for a smoker is higher and the risk for a nonsmoker is lower. The 1986 EPA and HHS guidelines are given in Table 46.

[5]For a discussion of the meaning of the units of radiation used below, see Chapter 15, Section E.

TABLE 45 Lung Cancer Risk and Radon Exposure

pCi/L	Estimated Number of Lung Cancer Deaths per 1000 People[a]
200	440–770
100	270–630
40	120–380
20	60–210
10	30–120
4	13–50
2	7–30
1	3–13
0.2	1–3

[a]These values are based on the assumption that an entire lifetime is spent at these levels.

Further Reading

Environmental Protection Agency. 1986. *A Citizen's Guide to Radon.* Washington, D.C.: Department of Health and Human Services.

National Council on Radiation Protection. 1984. *Evaluation of Occupational and Environmental Exposures to Radon and Radon Daughters in the United States.* Report No. 78. Bethesda, MD.

NAZAROFF, W. W., and NERO, A. V., eds. 1988. *Radon and Its Decay Products in Indoor Air.* New York: John Wiley.

NERO, A. V. 1988. Controlling Indoor Air Pollution. *Scientific American* 258:42.

TABLE 46 EPA and HHS Radon Guidelines

Radon Level pCi/L	WL	Suggested Reduction Level	Time Frame for Taking Action
200+	1+	Relocate or reduce levels drastically	Within several weeks
20–200	0.1–1	Reduce levels as far below 20 pCi/L as possible	Within several months
4–20	0.02–0.1	Lower levels to 4 pCi/L or below	Within a few years, but sooner at the upper end of range

Saccharin

Other Names

Sodium saccharin; 1,2-benzisothiazolin-3-one 1,1-dioxide

Trade Name

Sweet-N-Low

Introduction

The name saccharin is derived from the Latin word *saccharun*, meaning sugar. This artificial sweetener was discovered by accident in 1878, and it is the only sugar substitute to be used continuously for over 80 years. The health effects of saccharin were called into question almost from the beginning. First criticized because it offered no food value, now it is the object of considerable controversy regarding its potential to cause cancer.

Only about 80% of the saccharin produced in the United States is used for sweetening. Most of the rest is used in the nickel-electroplating industry to create a brighter finish.

Physical and Chemical Properties

Pure saccharin is a white powder that is often odorless, but can have a faint aromatic odor. It easily dissolves in warm water, but it is destroyed by high heat. Saccharin is about 400 times sweeter than sugar.

Exposure and Distribution

Saccharin is used in a wide variety of artificially sweetened foods and beverages, most commonly soft drinks, processed fruits, chewing gum, gelatin desserts, and commercial sauces. It is also available in powdered or liquid form as a tabletop sweetener. Nearly all commercial brands of toothpaste are sweetened with saccharin. Many mouthwashes, lipsticks, and drugs are also sweetened with it. While more **aspartame** is used in foods today than saccharin, many cosmetics and drugs are still formulated with saccharin.

Health Effects

Saccharin has been studied extensively for harmful health effects using many different kinds of laboratory animals. For the most part, saccharin has not been found to cause cancer. Statistically significant tumors in the bladder were found only in the male offspring of rats whose mothers were fed saccharin and who received saccharin themselves from birth. Many researchers now think that saccharin may promote the growth of tumors that already exist, rather than help create them. Evidence from short-term tests indicates that saccharin does not cause cell mutations. Several studies following groups of people who use saccharin regularly have failed to detect a link between the sweetener and cancer.

Nevertheless, uncertainties remain regarding its safety. The urine of mice fed saccharin has been shown to be *mutagenic*. In addition, some researchers believe that impurities associated with the manufacture of saccharin may be cancer causing. Some researchers believe that children, especially those under 10 years of age, may be at special risk from saccharin consumption because of the long time required for most cancers to develop. Others are concerned about pregnant women consuming saccharin, given the increased risk of cancer reported among rats who were exposed to saccharin before and after birth.

Protection and Prevention

While exposure to saccharin is voluntary, most people are not aware that almost every brand of commercial toothpaste is sweetened with saccharin. Many drugs are also formulated with saccharin, but these are relatively easy to avoid. The label usually indicates which sweetener, if any, is used, or you can ask the pharmacist. Saccharin exposure from toothpaste, mouthwash, and lipstick may be more difficult to avoid. This information is seldom on the label.

Concerned parents should monitor what their children eat and drink. There is no need for most children to use saccharin. Try to avoid exposure via pediatric drugs and toothpastes as well. Pediatric drugs that contain saccharin say so on the label. But toothpastes that do not contain the sweetener are difficult to find.

Regulatory Status

In 1977, the FDA banned the use of saccharin from foods. However, strong consumer protest forced the FDA to reconsider this ruling. Today, saccharin use is restricted by the FDA. It is not a *GRAS* substance, so specific guidelines must be followed by manufacturers so that average daily consumer doses are unlikely to exceed certain thresholds. Saccharin is on the EPA *community right-to-know* list.

Technical Information

Chemical symbol: $C_7H_5NO_3S$
Molecular weight: 183
FDA restrictions on use:

beverages:	12 mg/fl. oz.
processed foods:	30 mg/serving
tabletop sweetener:	20 mg/teaspoon of sugar substituted

Further Reading

CONCON, JOSE M. 1988. *Food Toxicology, Part B: Contaminants and Additives*. New York: Marcel Dekker.

VANDER, ARTHUR J. 1981. Saccharin, Cancer, and the Delaney Amendment, in *Nutrition, Stress, and Toxic Chemicals*. Ann Arbor: University of Michigan Press.

Selenium

Introduction

Selenium is a metallic element required in small amounts for human health, but which in large quantities can be toxic. Very few cases of selenium poisoning in humans have been reported, and those are mainly from regions of the world where selenium reaches high levels in the soil. Selenium poisoning is more of a problem for farm animals and birdlife than for people. In the San Joaquin Valley of California, drainage from selenium-rich agricultural soils has polluted wildlife preserves, causing hundreds of deaths and deformities among ducks and other waterfowl. Farm families whose drinking water comes from wells nearby may also be at heightened risk.

Physical and Chemical Properties

Selenium has properties of both metals and nonmetals and is properly classified as a metalloid. Its many commercial uses depend on its unusual ability to produce an electric current when light shines on it. For this reason, it finds widespread use in photoelectric cells, light meters, photocopying machines, and other electrical components. It is used in trace quantities to decolorize the greenish tint in glass caused by iron impurities, and in large amounts to create the ruby-red color of traffic lights, automotive tail lights, and other warning signals.

Exposure and Distribution

The primary exposure to selenium is from food; typically, about two-thirds of dietary selenium comes from meat, fish, and dairy products and the rest from cereal products, especially bread. The average intake per person in the United States ranges from 50 to 200 micrograms per day, which is considered sufficient to prevent deficiency symptoms yet low enough to be safe. Drinking water contributes only a small fraction of daily intake.

Selenium is widely distributed geologically. Sedimentary rocks, from which many agricultural soils are derived, and phosphate rocks, the source of phosphate fertilizers, contain relatively high concentrations. This explains how selenium enters the food supply. Animals obtain selenium in their feed or forage and retain it in their bodies for their own needs. People then consume animal products containing selenium. Because animals maintain fairly constant levels of selenium, everyone obtains roughly the same intake from meats, poultry, and dairy foods. Grain and cereal concentrations, however, more closely reflect the selenium content of the soils in which they are grown. People eating breads and other grain products in selenium-rich areas tend to have higher daily intakes compared to people eating grains grown in selenium-poor regions. The regions of North America having the highest soil selenium levels, and therefore the highest levels in locally produced grains, are parts of Canada, South Dakota, Wyoming, Montana, North Dakota, Nebraska, Kansas, Colorado, Utah, Arizona, and New Mexico. Low soil levels occur in the Pacific Northwest, the northeastern United States, and the South Atlantic seaboard.

Selenium occurs in drinking water only as a minor constituent. Surface waters rarely contain toxic concentrations. Although well waters from areas with selenium-rich bedrock contain variable concentrations, the vast majority of wells tested are far below the federal drinking water standard. Selenium also occurs in coal and crude oil and therefore in emissions from power plants and factories using such fuels.

Health Effects

Selenium is required for human nutrition. It is part of an *enzyme* (glutathione peroxidase) that protects cells from *oxidation*, a damaging chemical reaction. Selenium is therefore considered to be an *antioxidant*. Selenium deficiency is rare, but it has been observed among children and pregnant women in the Chinese region of Keshan (Keshan disease), where a type of congestive heart failure was successfully treated with selenium supplements. Other widespread cases of selenium deficiency have not been reported, probably because most diets contain adequate amounts to protect health. Selenium has been shown to reduce the toxicity of **cadmium**, inorganic and methyl **mercury**, thallium, and silver by altering the way these metals react in the body.

An anticancer role has been proposed for selenium based on both laboratory experiments and some human population studies. Animals fed selenium supplements show reduced rates of skin and liver tumors when exposed to certain cancer-causing substances. Human populations living in areas with relatively high soil selenium levels show lower rates for various cancers, including those of the breast, digestive tract, lung, and lymph glands. At this time, however, the studies are not extensive enough to permit a consensus that selenium protects against cancer. This is presently an area of active research. Similarly, some studies indicate that selenium may help reduce cardiovascular diseases, such as high blood pressure and coronary artery disease. Again, additional research is required before a scientific consensus can emerge. The Department of Agriculture recommends an adequate and safe intake of selenium in the range of 100 to 200 micrograms per day.

Selenium toxicity is more of a problem for farm animals than for people (see Environmental Effects section). There have been relatively few clear-cut examples of human selenium poisoning. In one such instance in the Peoples' Republic of China in the early 1960s, approximately 100 villagers showed signs of chronic selenium poisoning. Loss of hair and fingernails was the most common sign, with disorders of the skin, nervous system, and teeth also reported. Selenium entered the local food supply from soils that had been contaminated by weathered coal of a very high selenium content. In other regions with high selenium levels in the soil, including the Great Plains area of the United States, vague symptoms have been reported, including anorexia, indigestion, general pallor, and malnutrition. Other more obvious conditions of bad teeth, yellowish discoloration of the skin, diseased fingernails, and other skin disorders have also been described. Several studies, however, could not determine selenium to be the cause of these conditions.

Acute poisoning by selenium is rare, but has been observed. Within a few hours of eating nuts grown in a very high selenium area of Venezuela, people reported nausea, vomiting, and diarrhea. Several weeks after the initial episode, hair loss and fingernail changes occurred, but satisfactory recoveries were made.

Environmental Effects

Selenium intoxication of farm animals is a well-known condition, the result of grazing on plants that accumulate selenium from soils rich in the substance. Death can result from acute overexposure, but is rarely seen because the animals tend to avoid overconsumption of such plants if other forage is available. Chronic ingestion over periods of weeks or months can produce two conditions: the blind staggers and alkali disease. In the former, affected animals have impaired vision; they wander, stumble, and eventually succumb to respiratory failure. In the latter, signs include liver cirrhosis, hoof malformations, loss of hair, and emaciation. There is no treatment; the only remedy is to remove the animals from the selenium-rich soils.

Drainage of irrigation water from agriculture soils rich in selenium has polluted both groundwater and surface water in the Central Valley of California. Billions of gallons of water are used each year to irrigate crops in this area. The water percolates through the soils, picking up selenium on its way. Upon reaching the hardpack clays several feet underground, the excess water moves horizontally, arriving at sloughs and canals that channel the water to reservoirs and streams. Many of these reservoirs have been set aside as bird and wildlife refuges. The Kesterson Wildlife Preserve has suffered the most damage, with very high selenium levels in the water and hundreds of cases of deaths and fetal malformations in ducks and other waterfowl. How dangerous the well waters are in this area is currently uncertain, but families living in the area are understandably concerned.

Protection and Prevention

At the present time, no serious human maladies in the United States have been linked either to selenium poisoning or to selenium deficiency. Normal well-balanced diets provide adequate selenium intake, and no evidence suggests that selenium supplements are beneficial. Vague symptoms have been reported in selenium-rich areas, but are not definitely linked to selenium consumption. People living in such regions where the symptoms just described occur may want to have their well waters tested and to consume less locally produced grains and cereal products.

Regulatory Status

The EPA has set a maximum level for selenium in drinking water (maximum contaminant level) and a water quality criteria level for the protection of aquatic life. No ambient air or food standards have been set for the general public; however, occupational exposure to selenium in factory air is regulated. Selenium is listed as a *hazardous air pollutant* in the 1990 Clean Air Act, requiring the EPA to set emission standards. It is on the EPA *community right-to-know* list.

Technical Information

Chemical symbol: Se
Atomic number: 34
Atomic weight: 79

Department of Agriculture recommended daily allowance: 100–200 mg/day

Federal drinking water limit (maximum contaminant level): 10 μg/L (10 ppb)

EPA water quality criterion for protection of aquatic life: 1 μg/L (1 ppb)

OSHA limit in workplace air: 0.2 mg/m³

Further Reading

National Academy of Sciences. 1983. *Selenium in Nutrition*, revised edition. Washington, D.C.: National Research Council, National Academy Press.

Sodium Hydroxide

Other Names

Lye; caustic soda; white caustic; soda lye

Trade Names

Drano; Liquid Drano; Liquid Plumber; Easy Off

Introduction

Sodium hydroxide is a strong, *caustic* substance often called lye. It is frequently found in drainpipe and oven cleaners. Other strongly corrosive materials also go by the name of lye (including potassium hydroxide, sodium and potassium carbonates, oxides, and peroxides). The damage caused by all of these substances is similar to that of sodium hydroxide.

Physical and Chemical Properties

A strongly *alkaline* substance that is soapy or slippery to the touch, sodium hydroxide usually takes the form of a white solid (pellets, flakes, lumps, or sticks) or a liquid solution (generally 45 to 75% sodium hydroxide in water). The solid form readily absorbs moisture from the air and is called *deliquescent* because it appears to be melting as the absorption takes place. The solid also dissolves rapidly in water with the release of a great deal of heat. Liquid sodium hydroxide is quite slippery, creating a serious slip hazard when spilled.

Sodium hydroxide does not burn, but it will react with many metals to release hydrogen gas, which may then form an explosive mixture. Some of the more common reactive metals are aluminum, tin, zinc, copper, bronze, and brass. Because it is a strong base, sodium hydroxide reacts with all acids in a neutralizing reaction that releases heat. For reasons discussed in the Protection and Prevention section, however, it is generally not recommended to neutralize swallowed sodium hydroxide by giving acid (such as vinegar).

Exposure and Distribution

The most common household exposures are to drain cleaners and oven cleaner pads. Drano is the best known product for opening clogged drains and contains a high concentration of lye; some drain cleaners are 100% lye. Thoughtless adult action is responsible for most childhood poisonings. As noted by Gosselin and others (see Further Reading), "most of the reported cases of poisoning have resulted from the careless practice of leaving lye solutions in beverage containers within the reach of a thirsty child." Oven cleaner pads can cause injury if the sodium hydroxide concentration is greater than 5%.

Exposure to children may also result from their swallowing small alkaline batteries used in calculators, hearing aids, and cameras. Such batteries contain sodium hydroxide solutions as strong as 45% and can dissolve in contact with stomach acid. In the homes of diabetics, urine sugar reagent tablets (for example, Clinitest) also present a swallowing hazard to children because of their high content of anhydrous sodium hydroxide.

An estimated 150,000 workers may be exposed on the job. Sodium hydroxide is produced in large quantities (11 million tons in 1985 in the United States) and is used in a wide variety of products. About half is used within the chemical industry, 25% in the paper and pulp industry, and most of the remainder in cleaning products and petroleum and natural gas processing.

Health Effects

Sodium hydroxide causes severe corrosive damage to the eyes, skin, *mucous membranes,* and alimentary canal (mouth, throat, esophagus, and stomach). It acts just like a cleaning agent by dissolving the fats and proteins on the surfaces of cells and resulting in the continuous disintegration of attached tissues.

Damage to the eye is probably the severest injury, caused most frequently by contact with the liquid or with dust particles. Injury can be immediate; as little as 2 seconds have been observed between exposure and development of symptoms. Complete blindness results in many cases, with partial blindness, burns of the cornea, sticking of the eyelid to the eyeball, and other severe effects reported in most other instances. Blindness was reported in a majority of experimental animals exposed to dilute solutions (2%) for as little as 1 minute.

Skin effects range from redness and swelling to destruction of the entire outer skin layers, depending on the duration of contact and the strength of the solution. Damage to healthy skin has been reported following contact for 1 hour to solutions as weak as 0.12%. Contact with the scalp may cause baldness.

Breathing sodium hydroxide dust or mist leads in mild cases to irritation of the mucous membranes of the nose, causing sneezing, and in severe cases to damage of the upper respiratory tract and lungs (*chemical pneumonitis*). Healthy volunteers exposed to spray from oven cleaner developed respiratory tract irritation in 2 to 15 minutes.

Swallowing sodium hydroxide causes violent pain in the esophagus and stomach, accompanied by severe corrosion of the lips, mouth, throat, and tongue. The form ingested determines the location and severity of the injury, liquid sodium hydroxide being more dangerous than the solid form. Solids tend to adhere to and damage the mouth, throat, and upper esophagus, while liquids travel all the way to the stomach, affecting the entire esophagus, stomach, and small intestine. Death can occur from extensive *gastrointestinal* injury following liquid ingestion, although more often severe narrowing of the esophagus results (esophageal stricture). Swallowing lye often leads to complications with a risk for early death, including shock, pneumonia, perforation of the esophagus, and hemorrhage.

No significant cancer, mutation, or birth defect actions have been established for sodium hydroxide. Cancer of the esophagus is more common in people who have swallowed lye, but this appears to be due to the tissue repair process, not to the chemical itself. Exposure to concentrations that do not cause tissue destruction are not associated with higher rates of esophageal cancer. The EPA considers the evidence to be inadequate to rank sodium hydroxide on the basis of its *carcinogenic* hazard.

Protection and Prevention

Eye contact is the severest problem and must be treated without hesitation. Flushing with copious amounts of water for 5 to 10 minutes followed by prompt medical attention is the proper course of action. Splashes to the skin should also be treated by thorough rinsing and removal of contaminated clothing. If lye is swallowed, contact the nearest poison control center for instructions. There is debate about whether or not to neutralize the lye by administering dilute acid (such as vinegar) or milk. The problem is that the heat released on neutralization may cause further damage. Some authorities remain unconvinced that this is a problem and recommend neutralization. Speak with a poison control center or physician before administering dilute acid or milk.

Protection involves wearing protective clothing (goggles or glasses, long sleeves, and gloves) when using household products containing sodium hydroxide. All instructions found on product packages should be followed, and adequate ventilation should be maintained. Spills create a serious slip hazard and should be wiped up thoroughly. Risk of exposure can be avoided by using available oven and drainpipe cleaners that do not use caustic substances for their action.

Environmental Effects

No significant environmental effects have been reported, although major spills could cause local damage. Airborne emissions from factories using sodium hydroxide are neutralized in the air in close proximity to the plants.

Regulatory Status

Workplace limitations on the sodium hydroxide concentration in air are set in most industrialized countries. Interestingly, the standard in the Soviet Union is much stricter than that in countries in western Europe and the United States. (The U.S. standard is given in the Technical Information section.)

Sodium hydroxide affects water quality by influencing the *acidity* or *pH* of the water. No specific standard for sodium hydroxide is set, but the EPA has recommended a range of pH values for protection of various categories of aquatic life and for human drinking water. It is on the EPA *community right-to-know* list.

Technical Information

Chemical formula: NaOH
Molecular weight: 40.01
pH of 0.05% solution: about 12
pH of 0.5% solution: about 13
pH of 5% solution: about 14
Water quality criteria for pH:
 to protect freshwater aquatic life:
  pH 6.5–9.0
 to protect saltwater aquatic life:
  pH 6.5–8.5
 to protect human drinking water:
  pH 5–9
OSHA limit in workplace air: 2 mg/m^3

Further Reading

Environmental Protection Agency. 1988. *Summary Review of the Health Effects Associated with Sodium Hydroxide.* EPA/600/8-88-081. Springfield, VA: Department of Commerce, National Technical Information Service.

GOSSELIN, R. E., SMITH, R. P., and HODGE, H. C., eds. 1984. Lye, in *Clinical Toxicology of Commercial Products.* 5th edition. Baltimore, MD: Williams and Wilkins.

Strontium-90

Other Name

^{90}Sr

Introduction

Strontium-90 is a *radioactive isotope* of the element strontium (Sr), a substance that is chemically much like calcium. Thus, this isotope tends to concentrate in bone, where it can induce bone cancer. The major source has been atmospheric testing of nuclear weapons. Under routine operations, nuclear power plants release a negligible quantity to the environment, but accidents such as the one at Chernobyl in the Soviet Union can result in hazardous releases of the isotope. Another radioactive isotope, strontium-89, is also produced in nuclear reactors and in nuclear weapons tests. It is of less concern than strontium-90 only because it has a shorter *half-life*.

Physical and Chemical Properties

Strontium-90 emits *beta particles* and has a half-life of 28 years. Strontium-89 also decays by beta emission, but has only a 52-day half-life. Strontium is a white, water-soluble solid. Because of its chemical similarity to calcium, it is incorporated within the body in the same places as calcium. Mother's milk and bone tissue are two such places. Because bone is such a long-lasting substance, strontium can be retained in the body for many years.

Exposure and Distribution

Nuclear weapons testing and nuclear power production are the major sources of radioactive strontium in the environment, but weapons testing has resulted in nearly a million times more release than from power plants. Strontium released to the atmosphere enters the *food chain* primarily as a result of its deposition onto soil and subsequent uptake by plants. Several percent of the strontium-90 deposited on a cow pasture, for example, will generally be taken up by cows and be incorporated into milk. Because strontium moves very slowly downward through soil to below the root zone and because of its long half-life, a contaminated plot of land will remain a hazard for many years. Typically, only a small fraction of uptake of radioactive strontium by humans is through drinking water or fish and other aquatic foods. Because infants retain in their bodies a much larger fraction of the strontium they ingest than do adults, they are especially at risk.

Health Effects

The major health hazard associated with ingestion of radioactive strontium is bone cancer, although leukemia and other bone-related cancers resulting from irradiation of the bone marrow can also be induced. The first symptom of bone cancer is generally a lump on a bone; subsequent symptoms include weakening and breakage of the bone. For the average person not living near a serious nuclear power plant accident nor having been involved in the monitoring of nuclear weapons tests, the risk of cancer from radioactive strontium is miniscule—possibly less than one in a billion.

Protection and Prevention

Because of the long half-life of strontium-90, the substance can appear in foods such as milk long after a release to the environment from a nuclear reactor accident. Thus, unlike the case for **iodine-131**, the option of waiting a month or two after an accident before drinking fresh milk offers only short-term protection from strontium-90. Also, no substance is available that will effectively block radioactive strontium from reaching bone tissue, as will nonradioactive iodine for iodine-131.

Regulatory Status

In the United States, the general restrictions on radiation exposure apply to strontium-90 and strontium-89 and can be found in Chapter 15, Section F.

Technical Information[6]

Strontium-90 decays by emitting a beta particle with maximum energy of 0.59 million electron volts and has a half-life of 28 years. Strontium-89 decays by emitting a beta particle with maximum energy of 1.5 million electron volts and has a half-life of 52 days.

From nuclear weapons testing, approximately 4×10^{15} becquerels of strontium-90 are released per megaton. Thus, about 8×10^{17} becquerels have been released to date from surface and atmospheric testing. Under normal operations, nuclear reactors release to the environment less than one-millionth of the strontium-90 they produce. To date, the industry has released only about 1×10^{-6} as much of the isotope to the environment as has resulted from nuclear weapons testing. Nuclear reprocessing has resulted in releases about one-tenth as great as that from the rest of the nuclear fuel cycle.

For every becquerel deposited per square meter globally, the average lifetime individual dose to bone is about 4×10^{-7} sieverts. For every becquerel per cubic meter in air, the average inhaled dose to bone is about 1.3×10^{-7} sieverts per day. The global collective dose to humans per unit of radiation released is about 1×10^{-11} person-sieverts per becquerel released. Hence, the average individual dose from all environmental releases of radioactive strontium has been about 2×10^{-3} sieverts, with nearly all of this resulting from nuclear weapons testing. (For a discussion of the health implications of this, see Chapter 15, Section G.)

[6] For a discussion of the meaning of the units of radiation used below, see Chapter 15, Section E.

Further Reading

World Health Organization. 1983. *Environmental Health Criteria Report No. 25: Selected Radionuclides.* Geneva.

Styrene

Other Names

Cinnamene; cinnamol; phenylethylene; styrene monomer; vinylbenzene

Introduction

Spurred by dwindling supplies of natural rubber during World War II, the United States developed styrene–butadiene rubber to keep the nation's automobiles, trucks, and tanks rolling. Today, styrene is one of the most widely used chemicals in the United States. Some 3.6 million tons of it were manufactured in 1986, making it one of the top 20 chemicals that the United States produces. Plastics made from styrene are used in countless consumer products: automobile tires, PVC pipe, adhesives, photographic film, copy paper and toner, ink, auto parts, plastic food wrap, styrofoam cups and trays, combs, cushions, eyeglass lenses, bottles, boxes, jars, and kitchen utensils. Unfortunately, this widely used chemical can have harmful effects on human health and the environment.

Physical and Chemical Properties

Pure styrene is a colorless, oily liquid with a sweet, penetrating odor. At room temperature, the vapors are heavier than air and the liquid is lighter than water. Styrene does not dissolve easily in water. Pure styrene is heated to make plastic in a process called polymerization. Unfortunately, styrene does not need to get very hot before it starts to solidify. So to keep the styrene liquid during shipping and storage, manufacturers add stabilizing chemicals to the liquid styrene. One of these stabilizers is **hydroquinone**. It is thought by some researchers that allergic reactions to styrene products are due to the hydroquinone additive rather than to the styrene itself. The plastics made from styrene range from clear and rigid to multicolored and impact resistant. Styrene-containing plastics include acryonitrile–butadiene–styrene (ABS), styrene–acrylonitrile (SAN), polystyrene foam (Styrofoam®), and styrene–butadiene copolymers (synthetic rubber).

Exposure and Distribution

Most pure styrene is manufactured in Texas and Louisiana, but the chemical is used all over the United States by both large and small manufacturers. People are most likely to come into contact with pure styrene vapors at work. The National Institute of Occupational Safety and Health (NIOSH) estimates that 30,000 workers in the United States are regularly exposed to pure styrene at work, and an additional 300,000 use mixtures containing styrene.

People who do not work with styrene can be exposed to it in outdoor air. Highest nonoccupational exposures to styrene are likely downwind from plants that make styrene-containing products. Indoor air can also be contaminated with small amounts of styrene resulting from *volatilization* from plastic and plastic foam products used in the home. Styrene vapor is also associated with adhesives, asphalt, carpet backing, cushions, gasoline and other petroleum products, jet inks, photographic film, putty, PVC pipe, and copier paper and toner. There is some evidence that styrene can migrate from packaging material into food stored in styrene containers. Food and water stored in refrigerators with plastic interiors can contain styrene, as can commercial hickory wood smoke flavor and cigarette smoke. Styrene can also be found in some rivers receiving industrial effluent.

Health Effects

Styrene can be readily absorbed through the skin, respiratory system, and *gastrointestinal tract*. Styrene tends to accumulate in fatty tissues. *Acute exposure* to styrene vapor is irritating and damaging to the eyes and mucous membranes. High doses of styrene can cause dizziness, narcosis, and death due to respiratory system paralysis. Acute exposure is also associated with suppressed estrogen production in females and high-frequency hearing loss.

Data reported in the scientific literature indicate that styrene may be a *carcinogen*. The EPA classifies it as a group C carcinogen (see Chapter 3, Section B), meaning that the evidence is limited for both animals and humans. When inhaled everyday by laboratory animals, styrene causes an increase in breast tumors, lung tumors, and leukemias. However, no cancers are reported when styrene is ingested or injected. Early *epidemiological* studies following workers that were chronically exposed to styrene indicate that styrene may be responsible for some leukemias and lymph node cancers in humans, but recent studies do not support this hypothesis. Styrene was shown to be *mutagenic* in bacterial tests following metabolic activation. But no chromosomal aberrations have been found among exposed workers.

Protection and Prevention

Immediately dangerous levels of styrene vapor are rarely encountered outside the workplace. If styrene is used at work, request a *Material Safety Data Sheet (MSDS)* to get more information about products and processes in which exposure is likely and to learn more about recommended protective measures.

The low-level exposures encountered by the average person are harder to detect and therefore to avoid. In general, exposure to styrene vapor can be reduced by avoiding plastics and plastic foams, including plastic food wraps, foamed plastic insulated cups, plastic beverage bottles, and foam beds and cushions.

Environmental Effects

Styrene plastics degrade slowly in the environment. In many ways, disposal of solid styrene products is a larger environmental problem than are styrene vapors or liquid emissions. The sheer volume of solid waste that is disposed of daily is staggering. Plastics and foam products are thought to represent 5% by weight of our solid wastes. This percentage is deceptively small because plastics are relatively lightweight. Since plastics do not degrade in landfills, they tend to accumulate rather than disappear following disposal.

Regulatory Status

Styrene is regulated by OSHA, the EPA, and the FDA. Styrene is subject to EPA *community right-to-know* reporting (see Chapter 17, Section G). It is also listed as a *hazardous air pollutant* in the 1990 Clean Air Act. The FDA regulates the chemical because styrene tends to migrate from packaging material into food.

Technical Information

Chemical formula: C_8H_8
Molecular weight: 104.1
OSHA limit in workplace air: 430 mg/m^3 (50 ppm)
EPA limit in drinking water: 0.14 mg/L

Further Reading

National Institute for Occupational Health and Safety. 1983. *Criteria for a Recommended Standard: Occupational Exposure to Styrene*. Department of Health and Human Services Document No. 83-119. Washington, D.C.: U.S. Government Printing Office.

Sulfites

Other Names

Sulfur dioxide; potassium bisulfite; potassium metabisulfite; sodium bisulfite; sodium metabisulfite; sodium sulfite; sulfiting agents

Introduction

Sulfites are a group of food preservatives permitted for use to retard the spoilage and discoloration of numerous foods and beverages. In the early 1980s, the FDA began receiving reports of adverse reactions following the consumption of various foods containing sulfites, notably fresh fruits and vegetables served at restaurant salad bars. Most of the reactions were breathing difficulties among people with *asthma*. As of December 1987, the FDA had received approximately 1400 complaints from consumers, including reports of 26 deaths. Upon investigation, the FDA concluded that 17 of the deaths may have been caused by sulfites in food. Since that time, the FDA has required that any packaged food containing detectable quantities of sulfites, whether added or naturally present, must list the presence of sulfites on the ingredient label. Foods that are sold in bulk or served in restaurants (and thus have no labels) are no longer permitted to contain sulfites. The only exceptions are grapes and potatoes, which are currently being reviewed and require labels on the grocery shelf.

Physical and Chemical Properties

Sulfites are added to foods for a variety of reasons: to prevent browning of freshly cut fruits and vegetables when exposed to air, to control the growth of bacteria and molds, to prevent the breakdown of various oils that would lead to off flavors, and to whiten potatoes. There is no way to discern by sight, smell, or taste whether or not food contains sulfite. The only exception would be if sulfur dioxide were present at high enough levels to

be smelled, but food with that much sulfur dioxide would probably not be served.

Sulfur dioxide is the active ingredient to which the various other sulfites are converted within treated food. Sulfur dioxide is also a major air pollutant and is described more fully under its own entry in Part II.

Exposure and Distribution

Sulfites are used in a wide variety of foods. The ones with the highest levels have been dried fruits, dehydrated vegetables, dehydrated potatoes, wine, and restaurant salads and potatoes. The last two uses are no longer permitted. The list of other foods that may contain sulfites is extensive: baked goods and baking mixes, alcoholic and nonalcoholic beverges, coffee and tea, condiments and relishes, dairy product substitutes, fresh and prepared fish and shellfish, fresh and processed fruits and fruit juices, fresh and processed vegetables and vegetable juices, gelatins, grain products, gravies and sauces, jams and jellies, nuts and nut products, snack foods, soups and soup mixes, sugar and sweet sauces, toppings, and syrups. This list contains all categories of foods in which the use of sulfites has been identified, but it is not meant to imply that all foods within these categories necessarily contain sulfites. Its purpose is simply to flag products for which consumers may wish to consult ingredient labels, since labeling of sulfites on all packaged products is now required.

Sulfites are also used to preserve certain prescription medications and drugs that are given intravenously. Sensitive individuals may react to either of these applications. Wine always contains sulfites because the yeasts that ferment the grapes unavoidably produce it. Sulfur dioxide may be applied to wine barrels and grapes to control the growth of molds and other microorganisms. Sulfur dioxide is also a major air pollutant, with its highest concentrations found near electric power plants that burn fossil fuels and near smelters.

Health Effects

In people who are sensitive, mainly asthmatics, sulfites produce a variety of symptoms often involving the respiratory system. The symptoms range in severity from mild discomfort to life-threatening episodes and death. They include narrowing of the airways (bronchoconstriction), wheezing, difficulty in breathing, nausea, stomach cramps, diarrhea, hives, generalized itching and swelling, tingling sensations, flushing, lowered blood pressure, blueness of the skin, shock, and loss of consciousness.

Reaction to sulfites occurs mainly among asthmatics, who suffer an allergic-like respiratory reaction to various foods, air pollutants, and other environmental and emotional stresses. It is estimated that up to 10% of the asthmatic population may react to sulfites, particularly asthmatics who require steroids for their condition. This estimate implies that as many as one million asthmatics may be at risk in the United States.

Nonasthmatics have also reported reactions to restaurant meals containing sulfites, and these reactions have been confirmed by clinical studies. It is now recognized that people without asthma can be sensitive to sulfites, but there is no information to estimate what fraction of the general population may be sensitive; the fraction is presumed to be far lower than the 10% estimate for asthmatics.

Long-term exposure to sulfur dioxide as an air pollutant can lead to respiratory disease, which is discussed at greater length under the sulfur dioxide entry. Studies of chronic exposure to other sulfites have not demonstrated health effects, although the studies have been criticized. No evidence of cancer has been reported, although some laboratory test systems show that free sulfite (not bound to food) can cause mutations of genetic material.

Protection and Prevention

All packaged foods now require labels that indicate the presence of sulfites if they are added for any reason or are naturally present in detectable quantities. People who suspect that they may be sensitive (because they are asthmatic, allergic to other substances, or have a family history of allergies) should read ingredient labels to avoid consumption of foods containing sulfites. Moreover, they should be aware that some restaurants may not obey the regulations discussed below under Regulatory Status.

Regulatory Status

The *generally recognized as safe (GRAS)* status of sulfites, allowing their use in food without mention, was revoked by the FDA as of August 8, 1987. Sulfites are still permitted to be used, but only when foods containing them have labels that indicate the presence of sulfites to potential consumers. Foods sold in bulk or served in restaurants are not allowed to contain detectable levels of sulfites, with the exception of canned, frozen, or dehydrated potatoes. This last exception is currently under review. Sulfur dioxide as an air pollutant is regulated by EPA standards (see its entry).

Technical Information

Chemical formulas:
  sulfur dioxide: SO_2
  potassium bisulfite: $KHSO_3$
  potassium sulfite: $K_2S_2O_5$
  sodium bisulfite: $NaHSO_3$
  sodium sulfite: $Na_2S_2O_5$
  sodium metabisulfite: Na_2SO_3
Limit above which bulk foods may not be sold or served: 10 ppm

Further Reading

Food and Drug Administration. 1987. Sulfiting Agents: Proposal To Revoke GRAS Status for Use on "Fresh" Potatoes Served or Sold Unpackaged and Unlabeled to Consumers. *Federal Register* 52(237):46,968–46,978.

———. 1986. Food Labeling: Declaration of Sulfiting Agents. *Federal Register* 51(131):25,012–25,020.

———. 1985. Sulfiting Agents: Proposal To Revoke GRAS Status for Use on Fruits and Vegetables Intended To Be Served or Sold Raw to Consumers. *Federal Register* 50(157):32,830–32,837.

TAYLOR, S. L., HIGLEY, N. A., and BUSH, R. K. 1986. Sulfites in Foods: Uses, Analytical Methods, Residues, Fate, Exposure Assessment, Metabolism, Toxicity, and Hypersensitivity. *Advances in Food Research* 30:1–76.

Sulfur Dioxide and Sulfates

Other Names

Sulfur oxides; sulfiting agents

Introduction

Sulfur dioxide and some of its reaction products, such as sulfates, are responsible for some of the worst air pollution episodes in this century. The famous London fogs of the 1950s contained a mixture of sulfur dioxide and smoke. Thousands died during these events and numerous others were hospitalized for respiratory disease. The word *smog* actually was coined to describe the debilitating mixture of smoke and fog, which was a combination of sulfur dioxide and **particulate matter** suspended in water droplets. Today the term smog generally refers to *photochemical* air pollution, of which **ozone** is the main component.

Sulfur dioxide has been used for thousands of years as a *fumigant* for grapes and wine barrels and as a preservative, bleach, and steeping agent for grapes, apricots, and other fruits and vegetables. It prevents formation of **nitrosamines** in beer. It is one of a group of preservatives known as **sulfiting agents** permitted for use in foods and is the active ingredient responsible for the allergic-like reaction in *asthmatics* and others who consume such foods (see the entry on **sulfites**).

Physical and Chemical Properties

Sulfur dioxide is a colorless gas. At high concentrations it has a pungent, irritating odor. In the atmosphere it readily reacts with **oxidants** or particles to form sulfates and sulfuric acid particles, both of which are more hazardous than the original sulfur dioxide (except to asthmatics). Sulfuric acid is the main component of acid rain (see Chapter 11, Section C), which causes widespread environmental damage.

Exposure and Distribution

The greatest exposures occur in the vicinity of electric power plants that burn coal and near factories that process metal ores other than iron (nonferrous smelters). Emissions are highest at older facilities without modern pollution controls. The greater the distance away from the smokestack, the greater the transformation to the more hazardous sulfate forms. The plume of pollution tends to disperse with greater distances, however, so the area of most significant human exposure tends to be within 15 miles of a plant or factory.

The main sources of sulfur dioxide are fuel burning and metal ore processing. Sulfur is an impurity in fossil fuels (especially coal) and in many ores. When fuels are burned and ores roasted to extract their metal content in a process called smelting, sulfur dioxide is produced. Stationary fuel combustion (power plants and other factories) accounts for 79% of emissions, smelting for 17%, and transportation for 4%. For the nation as a whole, electric utilities generate two-thirds of all emissions.

Emissions in the United States have decreased 17% between 1979 and 1988 as a result of the installation of "scrubbers" (flue gas desulfurization controls) at coal-fired power plants and a reduction in the average sulfur content of fuels burned. More recently, the decrease in emissions has leveled off; between 1984 and 1988, emissions declined only 4%. Total sulfur dioxide releases for 1988 are estimated at 22.8 million tons. By comparison, natural sources in the United States release an estimated 5 to 6 million tons per year, approximately one-fourth of the human contribution.

The air in regions remote from major sources contains the least sulfur dioxide. In urban areas, the concentrations are typically ten times greater than in remote areas. Also, in the vicinity of industrial sources with inadequate controls, the levels are sometimes nearly 1000 times greater for periods of one hour, as Table 47 shows.

TABLE 47 Sulfur Dioxide Concentrations in Various Locations

Location	Concentration (ppm)
Remote areas	<0.004
Polluted urban areas	>0.03
Near industrial sources with inadequate controls	
24-hour average	0.40
3-hour average	1.4
1-hour average	2.3

Most monitoring stations report no violations of the national standard for protection of health. Approximately 1.7 million people live in the 2% of U.S. counties that are in violation. Pittsburgh, Pennsylvania, and the region around the Great Lakes report the highest concentrations. For the nation as a whole, sulfur dioxide levels in outdoor air dropped 30% between 1979 and 1988. The improvement leveled off, however, between 1984 and 1988, reflecting the smaller emission reductions during that period.

Health Effects

Short-term exposure to sulfur dioxide causes constriction of the airways in asthmatics and other sensitive individuals. The most recent research shows that even 5- to 10-minute exposures to peak levels currently occurring around power plants, smelters, and smaller sources within cities are sufficient to trigger asthmatic attacks. There are approximately 10 million diagnosed asthmatics in the United States and another 20 million sensitive individuals. The EPA estimates that about 100,000 asthmatics live close enough to power plants to experience exposures high enough to trigger asthmatic attacks at least once per year. The EPA does not expect all these people to react severely, however.

Chronic exposure to sulfur dioxide causes a thickening of the mucus layer of the trachea, similar to *chronic bronchitis*. Sufficient thickening covers and inactivates the beating hair-like *cilia* lining the upper airways, which normally remove infectious agents and other minute foreign particles. Recent studies indicate an increase in respiratory illness associated with chronic exposure to sulfur dioxide, sulfate, and particulate pollution at today's levels. In one such study, 10,000 elementary schoolchildren were examined in St. Louis, Missouri, and several cities in Ohio and Tennessee. Children in the more polluted areas had significantly higher incidences of coughing, bronchitis, and lower respiratory infections compared with children in the less polluted cities. A combination of factors appears to be at work. **Particulates** and sulfur dioxide react to form more hazardous acid sulfate particles; the particles are inhaled more deeply into the lungs than sulfur dioxide gas and lodge there; and children tend to be more active, breathing through their mouths and bypassing the filtering mechanisms of the nasal passages. In another study, nondrinking, nonsmoking Mormons living in California were found to have significantly more symptoms of *chronic obstructive pulmonary disease* (cough, wheezing, shortness of breath, and emphysema) with longer and greater exposures to ambient sulfur dioxide and particulate pollution. Death rates have also been correlated with levels of sulfate and particulate pollution.

Exercise increases the severity of reaction to sulfur dioxide and sulfate particulates, both because more rapid breathing takes in more total pollutants and because mouth breathing is favored during vigorous activity, causing the nasal filtering mechanisms to be bypassed. Fog stimulates the conversion of sulfur dioxide to acid sulfate *aerosols,* which, like particulates, are more deeply inhaled and more dangerous than sulfur dioxide gas. The health effects of sulfur dioxide are summarized in Table 48.

Protection and Prevention

Avoiding polluted conditions is the surest way to prevent exposures to sulfur dioxide. Exercise and other strenuous outdoor activities should be curtailed if the air is of poor quality, such as during *atmospheric inversions.* Asthmatics in particular, as well as others with allergies and respiratory conditions, should not exercise in the vicinity of power plants and other industrial sources of air pollution. Asthma attacks can usually be treated with drugs that widen the airways (bronchodilators).

Long-term solutions to sulfur dioxide pollution include the following: (1) conservation of electricity (something individuals can do immediately), (2) development of solar-powered electricity generation and increased use of renewable power sources (such as wind and water) to replace fossil fuel burning, (3) use of low-sulfur coals by power plants, and (4) installation of additional pollution control equipment in existing power plants and industrial facilities.

Environmental Effects

Sulfur dioxide damages plants directly, causing leaf injury and discoloration. Lichens, mosses, and tree seedlings are especially vulnerable. The most severe damage is caused by the conversion of sulfur dioxide to sulfuric acid in the atmosphere and its subsequent deposition as acid rain, snow, and dry acid particles. Freshwater lakes in large regions of Canada, the northeastern United States, and mountainous regions of the West are becoming acidified because of acid rain. Forested regions of the East also are succumbing to the combined stresses of acidity, ozone pollution, heat, and drought. Such effects on ecosystems may eventually alter rates of soil formation and erosion, change the composition of the atmosphere, alter regional climates, and disrupt the balance of animal species in forests. Sulfuric acid is believed to account for 60% of the acid in acid deposition (see Chapter 11, Section C).

Sulfur dioxide has been associated with corrosion of steel and other metals, degradation of **zinc** and other protective coatings, and deterioration of building materials (concrete and limestone), as well as deterioration

TABLE 48 Health Effects at Various Concentrations of Sulfur Dioxide

Effect	Concentration (ppm)
Lung function changes in resting asthmatics	1–2
Lung function changes in asthmatics with light to moderate exercise	0.6–0.75
Lung function changes in asthmatics with moderate to heavy exercise	0.4–0.6
No effects in free-breathing asthmatics at light exercise and insignificant effects at moderate exercise	0.1–0.3

of paper, leather goods, works of historical interest, and certain textiles.

Regulatory Status

The EPA sets limits on the concentration of sulfur dioxide in the *ambient* (outdoor) air. States are then required to enforce the limits. There is a 24-hour maximum limit to guard against peak concentrations and a lower annual average limit to control background levels. In a recent action, the EPA decided not to impose an additional 1-hour limit in spite of the evidence that asthmatics and other sensitive individuals respond to 5- to 10-minute bursts of sulfur dioxide pollution. A secondary standard is also set for the protection of *welfare* (visibility, buildings, and environmental damage). The EPA is required to review the adequacy of the standards periodically and revise them as new evidence warrants.

The 1990 amendments to the Clean Air Act require emissions of sulfur dioxide be reduced by 10 million tons per year by the year 2000. Ninety percent of the reduction is to come from utilities and the rest from other sources.

Technical Information

Chemical formulas:
sulfur dioxide: SO_2
sulfur oxides: SO_x
National ambient air quality standards:
Primary (protection of health), annual
average: 80 $\mu g/m^3$ (0.03 ppm)
Primary, 24-hour average:
365 $\mu g/m^3$ (0.14 ppm)

Secondary (protection of welfare), 3-hour average: 1300 $\mu g/m^3$ (0.50 ppm)

Two studies have been conducted to estimate the effect on death rates of elevated sulfate levels in urban air. A Brookhaven National Laboratory study found that for every $\mu g/m^3$ of sulfate in the air, about 30 people out of a million exposed to that air can be expected to die each year because of the sulfate. A National Academy of Science study concluded that only about 2 of the million would die. Both studies recognized large uncertainties in the analysis.

Further Reading

Environmental Protection Agency. 1988. Proposed Decision Not To Revise the National Ambient Air Quality Standards for Sulfur Oxides (Sulfur Dioxide). *Federal Register* 53(80): 14,926–14,952.

———. 1982. *Review of the National Ambient Air Quality Standards for Sulfur Oxides: Assessment of Scientific and Technical Information.* EPA–450/5–82–007. North Carolina: Research Triangle Park.

National Research Council. 1978. *Sulfur Oxides.* Washington, D.C.: Committee on Sulfur Oxides, National Academy of Sciences.

For 2,4-D, see page 281.

2,4,5-T

Trade Names

Estron Brush Killer; Weedar 2,4,5-T

Introduction

The herbicide 2,4,5-T gained notoriety as a result of the extensive use of Agent Orange, which is a 50:50 mix of **2,4-D** and 2,4,5-T, to defoliate trees and destroy crops during the Vietnam War. Initially, objections to the use of Agent Orange were based largely on its potential environmental impact, but published findings in 1969 indicated a link between 2,4,5-T and birth defects, particularly cleft palate, and focused attention on human health effects. Other reports revealed that 2,4,5-T was contaminated with highly toxic **dioxins**, particularly TCDD.

Since the war, many veterans and Vietnamese citizens have blamed 2,4,5-T and the associated dioxins for a large number of health problems. But despite a tremendous *epidemiological* effort to determine the long-term health effects of Agent Orange, the 2,4,5-T component, and the contaminant TCDD on veterans of the Vietnam War and citizens of South Vietnam, the data still are inconclusive.

The herbicidal activity of 2,4,5-T has been known since the mid-1940s. Like 2,4-D, another phenoxy acid weed-killer, 2,4,5-T is readily taken up by roots or absorbed through leaves and transported to other parts of the plant. It is relatively selective in its action against broad-leaved plants and more effective against woody species than 2,4-D.

Physical and Chemical Properties

The compound 2,4,5-T is produced in several different forms: as an acid, a salt, or an ester (a compound formed by the combination of an acid and an alcohol), each of which has slightly different properties. The pure acid is a white, crystalline solid that is slightly soluble in water. The salt formed with certain metals is water soluble, but is not soluble in petroleum oils. Conversely, another form is petroleum soluble, but not water soluble. People report a metallic taste lasting for a few hours following ingestion.

Exposure and Distribution

Use of 2,4,5-T had been widespread in the United States for brush clearing and for roadside and right-of-way maintenance until it was curtailed in the early 1970s following public concern about health effects. The U.S. military sprayed about 11 million gallons of Agent Orange over 3.6 million acres of South Vietnam between 1965 and 1970.

The herbicide breaks down fairly rapidly in soils; its *half-life* ranges from a few weeks to four months at most. In the form used in Agent Orange, 2,4,5-T degrades more slowly than 2,4-D. Aerial spraying is the most common method of application—a factor that influences breakdown rates. With aerial spraying, the vegetation intercepts as much as 75% of the herbicide (and the TCDD contaminant), resulting in even faster breakdown and *volatization* than in soils. 2,4,5-T is readily taken up by mammals, but does not *bioaccumulate*. In factories, most of the reported occupational illnesses have been traced to TCDD. Long-term occupational exposure has not produced any consistent signs of toxicity.

Health Effects

In terms of *chronic* effects, 2,4,5-T does not seem to cause cancer or mutations, although the contaminant TCDD has been positive in some tests. Fetal toxicity and birth defects, especially cleft palate, have been reported for 2,4,5-T in mice and for TCDD in mice and hamsters. Early work did not determine whether 2,4,5-T itself was the culprit or whether the observed effects were caused by low levels of TCDD. Subsequent studies have shown that 2,4,5-T produces similar effects in the absence of any detectable contaminant. Most of the tests using rats and monkeys show no evidence that 2,4,5-T causes birth defects.

This herbicide is of moderate *acute toxicity*. The signs of poisoning are similar to those for 2,4-D and include a range of disturbances of the nervous system, such as muscular weakness, depression, paralysis, and coma, as well as loss of appetite, loss of weight, and vomiting. 2,4,5-T also produces a mild spasticity in dogs. At high doses, 2,4,5-T is toxic to the kidneys. Low doses, however, are excreted quite rapidly, and chronic low doses are tolerated fairly well since there is no cumulative effect.

Protection and Prevention

Following public outcry about the possible effects of the herbicide, stringent restrictions on 2,4,5-T use were imposed to prevent contamination of aquatic systems and the destruction of nontarget plant species and habitats. TCDD is released to the atmosphere when vegetation treated with 2,4,5-T is burned at ordinary combustion temperatures. Consequently, recent concern has focused on proposals to incinerate existing stocks of the now-suspended pesticide.

Environmental Effects

The herbicide is toxic to many species, but it is more acutely toxic to aquatic than to terrestrial organisms. Of greater concern is a secondary effect—devastating habitat modification—that results from the widespread use of herbicides. The destruction of both target and nontarget plant species as a consequence of aerial drift from the target site can have a serious impact on animal species that use the affected vegetation for food, shelter, or nesting sites.

Regulatory Status

In a rare move, the EPA has issued emergency suspension orders for 2,4,5-T; it has taken similar action on a pesticide in only three other instances. The decision to sus-

pend the herbicide was based on the EPA's judgment that exposure to 2,4,5-T created an immediate and unreasonable health risk for people. The herbicide is no longer produced or used in the United States, and existing stocks are being destroyed.

Technical Information

Chemical name: 2,4,5-trichlorophenoxy acetic acid

Chemical formula: $C_8H_5O_3Cl_3$

OSHA limit in workplace air: $10mg/m^3$

EPA water quality criterion for human health: $10\mu g/L$

Further Reading

American Farm Bureau Federation. 1979. *Scientific Dispute Resolution Conference on 2,4,5-T.* Park Ridge, Illinois.

Committee on the Effects of Herbicides in Vietnam. 1974. *The Effects of Herbicides in South Vietnam: Part A, Summary and Conclusions.* Washington, D.C.: National Academy of Sciences.

HAYES, W. J., Jr. 1982. *Pesticides Studied in Man.* Baltimore, MD: Williams and Wilkins.

Tetrachloroethylene

Other Names

PCE; carbon dichloride; perchloroethylene; PERC; 1,1,2,2-tetrachloroethylene

Trade Names

Fedal-Un; Perclene; PerSec; Nema; Tetlen; Tetracap; Dee Solv; Dow-Per; Dow-clene; Percosolv; Perklone

Introduction

Tetrachloroethylene, or PCE, is the most widely used dry-cleaning chemical in the United States. Dry cleaning accounts for half of the nearly 300,000 tons of PCE used in the United States annually. Carried home from the cleaners on clothing, it is a common indoor air pollutant. It can be purchased as a spot remover, rug and upholstery cleaner, and paint stripper. About one-fourth of the PCE manufactured is used to make CFC-113. It is also used extensively for textile processing during the manufacture of clothing and other goods made with fabric. PCE is used industrially to remove grease and dirt from metal.

Physical and Chemical Properties

PCE is a colorless, heavy liquid with a sweet, chloroform-like odor. It is relatively insoluble in water and volatile but not flammable. These properties make it easy to work with both in industrial settings and retail dry-cleaning establishments.

Exposure and Distribution

Tetrachloroethylene can be found in the air almost everywhere, but especially in urban areas. Since over 90% of emissions are to the air, the highest outdoor levels of the solvent are in the vicinity of dry cleaners. The U.S. Census Bureau estimates that 26,000 of these businesses exist in this country. Air concentrations of the solvent near dry cleaners can be 40 times that of average city air. PCE is also a common indoor air pollutant. It is carried into homes on freshly dry-cleaned clothing, draperies, and upholstery.

This chemical has also been detected in the drinking water of several U.S. cities. Most cities report very low concentrations of PCE in drinking water, but some highly industrialized cities in the Ohio River basin have reported levels that significantly exceed EPA drinking water standards. Elevated concentrations of the solvent have also been found in cities using vinyl-coated asbestos–cement pipes. PCE is used in the manufacture of these pipes, and it is thought that the solvent leaches into the water carried by the pipes. Researchers have found extremely high levels of PCE in the water stored in unflushed coated pipes. Vinyl-coated asbestos–cement pipes are used in parts of the northeastern United States in response to concerns that water carried in uncoated pipes could contain asbestos fibers.

Spilled PCE that makes its way into groundwater is remarkably *persistent*. It does not degrade or evaporate. Thus, proper disposal of PCE residues is important. Yet, the fact that PCE is used in so many small businesses across the country makes ensuring proper disposal of waste products difficult for local officials.

Recently published research indicates that butter purchased from stores located adjacent to dry cleaners may have PCE levels higher than butter purchased at stores more than two doors removed from such operations. It is likely that other fatty foods stored at shops adjacent to dry cleaners may be similarly contaminated.

Health Effects

Liver, kidney, and central nervous system effects have been observed in people exposed to PCE in the workplace. Inhalation is the most important route by which PCE enters the body. Uptake is proportional to exposure level and increases with exercise. Drinking water contamination is also of concern because PCE is rapidly and almost completely absorbed following ingestion. Limited absorption may also occur through the skin via direct contact with the solvent. PCE tends to accumulate in body fat. Most PCE is removed from the body via exhaled air from the lungs.

People exposed to high levels of PCE vapor experience eye irritation, lightheadedness, confusion, and respiratory depression. These are generally short-term effects, and careful studies have failed to show any permanent neurological or behavioral problems that could be specifically attributed to accidental or chronic exposures. Liver and kidney damage has been found in laboratory mice subjected to *chronic exposures* to PCE. Temporary liver damage in humans is associated with short-term exposure high enough to cause lightheadedness. The level of exposure at which permanent damage to liver and kidneys might occur in humans is unclear.

Until recently, evidence of PCE's ability to cause cancer was limited. This is changing, however. Inhalation studies are now showing that PCE is capable of causing cancer in mice and rats. As a result, the EPA has reclassified PCE as a probable human carcinogen (class B_1), up from its former B_2 classification (see Chapter 3, Section B). With thousands of people exposed to PCE daily at dry-cleaning businesses, it would seem that human health effects from daily exposure would be obvious. Unfortunately, human exposure data are confused by exposure to other potentially cancer-causing chemicals used at these businesses.

Animal tests do not indicate that it is a *mutagen*. However, some commercial preparations have elicited weak positive responses in the *Ames test*. These positive findings may be explained by the presence of mutagenic contaminants or stabilizers in the commercial preparations.

It is not known whether PCE exposure can cause birth defects in humans. Observed changes primarily reflect delayed development and are considered reversible. But these conclusions are based on a very small number of studies. PCE can be transferred to infants via breast milk. Potential health effects to infants receiving PCE-contaminated breast milk are unknown.

Protection and Prevention

Most doses of PCE result from vapor inhalation. Workers in dry-cleaning establishments receive the highest doses, but people living next door to or above such businesses can also receive significant doses. Thus, it is prudent to avoid living in close proximity to a dry-cleaning business.

Dry-cleaned clothing is a source of indoor PCE exposure. This problem is easily avoided by purchasing clothing that does not require frequent dry cleaning. Sometimes dry cleaning is suggested for clothing that is delicate or fragile. Ironically, dry-cleaning solvents wear out fabric faster than does water cleaning. When clothing does need to be dry-cleaned, make sure that the freshly cleaned fabric is thoroughly dry and aired outside for at least six hours before hanging inside the house. Open a car window when carrying freshly cleaned clothes home from the dry cleaner. Pay particular attention to airing dry-cleaned sleeping bags for several days before use. Better yet, avoid having them dry cleaned. An unfortunate number of deaths have resulted from the use of sleeping bags that have not been thoroughly aired to remove the solvent prior to their use.

Solvent recycling is practiced by many dry-cleaning firms, but virtually no recycling is practiced at coin-operated dry cleaners. Therefore, coin-operated dry-cleaning machines emit twice as much PCE into the atmosphere per garment than do commercial machines. So use commercial laundries when dry cleaning is required. Also consider shopping at grocery stores that are not located adjacent to dry cleaners.

Environmental Effects

About 90% of the PCE produced ends up in the air. These emissions contribute to *photo-*

chemical *smog* in urban areas. PCE has been found to be moderately toxic for aquatic organisms. Normal levels of the chemical in industrial areas probably do not pose a significant risk to wildlife.

Regulatory Status

The EPA now regulates PCE in drinking water. Moreover, the 1990 amendments to the Clean Air Act list PCE as a *hazardous air pollutant,* requiring the EPA to set emission standards. PCE is also regulated by OSHA. It is on the EPA *community right-to-know* list. PCE was the first chemical to be classified as a *carcinogen* by the Consumer Product Safety Commission, but this action was later withdrawn.

Technical Information

Chemical formula: $C_2 Cl_4$
Molecular weight: 166
Odor threshold (in water): 300 µg/L
OSHA limit in workplace air: 50 ppm
EPA limit in drinking water: 0.001 ppm

Further Reading

Agency for Toxic Substances and Disease Registry. 1988. *Toxicological Profile for Tetrachloroethylene.* Washington, D.C.: U.S. Public Health Service.
Environmental Protection Agency. 1985. *Health Assessment Document for Tetrachloroethylene.* EPA/600/8–82/005f. Cincinnati, OH: Center for Environmental Research.

Toluene

Other Names

Methylbenzene; methylbenzol; phenylmethane; toluol

Introduction

As the United States phases hazardous **lead** compounds out of gasoline, refiners have been adding increasing amounts of toluene and other *aromatic hydrocarbons* (particularly **benzene**) to improve gasoline octane ratings and antiknock performance. Ironically, refiners first separate toluene from petroleum, its major source, and then later mix it back into the refined gasoline. Refineries, automobiles, trucks, and petroleum-burning engines disperse significant amounts of the compound into the atmosphere each day. Two factors drive the continuing search for new toluene applications. First, refineries currently produce huge surpluses of the chemical as a by-product. Second, toluene can be used as a substitute for its more toxic relative, benzene. Besides being a gasoline additive, toluene has applications as a strong solvent for model glues, paints, inks, resins, and adhesives, and it is used in the manufacture of detergents, dyes, lacquers, linoleum, perfumes, pharmaceuticals, **saccharin**, and TNT.

Physical and Chemical Properties

An organic compound distilled from crude oil, toluene shares many characteristics with other oil-derived aromatics such as benzene, **styrene**, and **xylene**. Pure toluene is a colorless, noncorrosive, highly volatile liquid (like rubbing alcohol) with a pungent odor much like that of benzene. In water, it is insoluble and will float on the surface. The vapors are heavier than air and are readily ignitable, which is why it is a useful additive in gasoline. When mixed with *oxidants* or strong *acids,* toluene may explode like its product, TNT.

Exposure and Distribution

The United States produces about three million tons of toluene each year, which is about one-third of the world's total. The most extensive public exposure to toluene results from atmospheric contamination. Exhaust from cars, trucks, and planes, along with oil and fuel spills and evaporation from gas tanks and carburetors, release toluene vapors into the air. However, catalytic converters can remove up to 95% of the compound in vehicle exhaust if the converter is properly installed and functioning. Because of its low water solubility, toluene in the atmosphere is not appreciably removed by rain and thus it can travel long distances downwind from its source. Nevertheless, levels of toluene in the air around gas stations are higher than those likely to be encountered elsewhere by the public. This is particularly a problem at gas stations where nozzles lack vapor barriers. Because of the standard petroleum industry practice of disposing of a small fraction of toluene wastes into rivers, lakes, and oceans, toluene is now found in Gulf Coast waters adjacent to the major U.S. petrochemical manufacturing area at concentrations that far exceed natural *background levels*. Cigarette smoking is another source of toluene exposure, both to the smoker and the passive bystander. Exposure to toluene also results from the use of oil-based paints and inks, resins, and solvent-based glues.

Health Effects

Evidence on whether toluene causes cancer is inconclusive at present, but other types of health damage are well documented. Contact with toluene liquid irritates and dries out skin by removing underlying fat. Toluene vapors are an irritant, especially to the eyes. Upon inhalation, the vapors aggravate the respiratory tract, depress the central nervous system, and damage the liver and kidneys. The early symptoms of toluene exposure can include some combination of the following: fatigue, weakness, confusion, euphoria, dizziness, headaches, dilated pupils, insomnia, extreme light sensitivity, and skin irritation. Intentional sniffing of model glue, which is composed mainly of toluene, can cause malfunctions of the nerves that control movement and irregular heart rate; in some cases, it may lead to death. Long-term exposure to toluene may lead to kidney and liver damage. Exposure of pregnant women to toluene has been associated with damage to the unborn child. Interestingly, ethyl alcohol (the alcohol in beer, wine, and liquor) causes most of the toluene in a person's body to migrate to the blood, resulting in increased exposure to vital organs such as the brain (see Chapter 7, Section B).

Protection and Prevention

Any action that decreases the burning or spilling of gasoline and other petroleum-derived products will decrease the public's exposure to toluene. Wise practices include using fuel-efficient cars, sharing rides, and taking mass transit where available. In addition, care should be taken at gas stations not to overfill the tank. Laws requiring vehicle inspection and gas pump vapor barriers should be supported. Using substitutes for oil-based paints and solvents containing toluene will also reduce the amount of toluene in the air and water. Not only do water-based products generally perform as well as their oil-based counterparts, but they are also less toxic and easier to clean up. Sometimes a little "elbow grease" can make paint strippers or other commercial solvents unnecessary.

Much of the hazardous waste in this country's landfills comes from discarded household products. Instead of throwing away old paint cans, oil, or gasoline, people should take such wastes to a waste oil reclaimer, a solvent recycler, or an industrial waste handler; look for these in the yellow pages. In addition, some county solid waste authorities organize hazardous waste "roundups" as a service for the public. OSHA requires industries using large amounts of toluene to provide workers with a well-ventilated work area, protective clothing, and goggles.

If accidental exposure to the skin occurs, wash promptly with soap. If toluene gets into the eyes, flush with water immediately. Upon inhalation of toluene, get to fresh air quickly. If toluene is swallowed, do not induce vomiting, as that would increase the risk of aspiring resuspended liquid droplets. Get medical attention promptly in any of these cases, except minor skin contact or routine inhalation.

Environmental Effects

In the urban atmosphere, toluene helps to form **ozone** and contributes to the problem of *photochemical smog*. Natural plant and animal populations are likely to be at risk from industrial and vehicle-related releases of toluene because natural levels are very low in comparison. Indeed, people have used petroleum to kill aquatic plants because of the toxic effects of toluene and other aromatic hydrocarbons. Because toluene is volatile, much of the substance released to water soon passes into the atmosphere, but some *adsorbs* to sediments where it can cause long-term exposures to aquatic life.

Regulatory Status

The EPA decided not to restrict toluene emissions to the atmosphere based on the assumption that typical outdoor concentrations will probably not harm human life. But now toluene is listed as a *hazardous air pollutant* under the Clean Air Act of 1990, requiring the EPA to set emission standards. The EPA does recommend upper limits for freshwater and saltwater concentrations as guidelines. The Resource Conservation and Recovery Act prohibits land disposal of toluene, and OSHA restricts workplace levels of the substance. Toluene is on the *community right-to-know* list.

Technical Information

Chemical formula: $C_6H_6CH_3$
Clean Water Act (1977): toluene is one of 129 priority pollutants
Safe Drinking Water Act, maximum contaminant level: 2 mg/m^3
OSHA limit in workplace air: 375 mg/m^3
Superfund reportable quantity for a spill: 1000 lbs

Further Reading

HALEY, T. J. 1987. Toluene. *Dangerous Properties of Industrial Chemicals Report* 7(5):2–14.

Trichloroethane

Other Names

1,1,1-Trichloroethane; TCA; methyl chloroform; chloroethane; methyltrichloromethane

Trade Names

Aerothene TT; Chlorotene; Chlorothane; Alpha-T; Inhibisol

Introduction

Trichloroethane, or TCA, is one of the most commonly used solvents in the United States. It is used in such products as drain cleaners, shoe polish, spot removers, insecticides, and printing inks. TCA is sometimes used as an aerosol propellant. Industry relies on this chemical for cleaning and degreasing electric motors, generators, semiconductors, and high vacuum equipment. It is particularly effective at removing waxes, oil, and grease. It is also used as a coolant to combat the frictional heat created during the drilling and tapping of metals. **Vinylidene chloride** is made using TCA.

Physical and Chemical Properties

Trichloroethane is a colorless, nonflammable liquid with a sweet odor. It evaporates easily at room temperature. TCA is soluble in **acetone, benzene,** and **carbon tetrachloride.**

Exposure and Distribution

It is estimated that about one-fourth of all industries use TCA during some manufacturing and/or cleaning process. It is widely used because it is generally believed to be the least toxic of the chlorinated solvents. TCA is also widely used in consumer products and in many art and craft supplies. TCA may be found in well water taken from wells located near industrial areas. Low levels are also known to migrate from polyvinyl chloride (PVC) pipes into drinking water. Outdoor air in highly urbanized areas is also contaminated with low levels of TCA.

Health Effects

Trichloroethane is rapidly absorbed through the lungs and *gastrointestinal tract*. It can also be absorbed through the skin. TCA is not considered to be highly toxic because a large dose is needed to elicit adverse health effects. It is eliminated from the body rapidly and unchanged. Nevertheless, workers have died in incidents in which TCA exposure occurred in enclosed spaces. At high levels, TCA causes central nervous system depression, irregular heartbeat, loss of balance and coordination, and pulmonary edema. Of these problems, irregular heartbeat and edema are the most serious. TCA can be easily smelled at levels that cause these problems, and mild eye irritation and dizziness might also be felt before the more severe symptoms set in.

Long-term problems associated with inhaling high levels are few. Six-month exposures at levels that cause eye irritation can cause fatty and enlarged livers in laboratory animals, but this condition is reversible. Limited *epidemiological* studies have not revealed human liver dysfunction resulting from long-term exposure to TCA.

Trichloroethane does not appear to cause cancer or birth defects. Unfortunately, studies completed to date are inadequate to eliminate the possibility that TCA causes cancer. Two closely related chemicals, **chloroform** and 1,1,2-trichloroethane, do cause cancer when high doses are administered to test animals. One test revealed that TCA may be a weak *mutagen*. At extremely high doses administered to pregnant rats, exposed fetuses showed decreased weight gain and delayed kidney development, but these changes disappeared when exposure stopped.

Protection and Prevention

Toxic levels of TCA are generally not found in the air or water and only rarely at the workplace. In water, TCA can be smelled and tasted at levels that are far below the smallest dose required to affect the health of any laboratory animal. Drinking water standards are set based on the smell and taste threshold, thus tap water that contains trace amounts of TCA is probably safe. Concentrations found in outdoor air are also far below levels likely to cause health problems.

Workers who suspect that they are exposed to excessive levels of TCA should request a *Material Safety Data Sheet* from their supervisors. If it is unavailable, contact the local department of health or OSHA office.

Environmental Effects

Trichloroethane is known to contribute to depletion of stratospheric ozone (see Chapter 11, Section B). It is a less potent depleter than are the **CFCs**, but the chemical is of concern to scientists because so much of it is routinely released into the atmosphere. TCA is very persistent in soil and groundwater.

Regulatory Status

Trichloroethane is regulated by OSHA. Moreover, TCA is listed as a *hazardous air pollutant* in the 1990 Clean Air Act, requiring the EPA to set emission standards. TCA production will be phased out by 2002 because of its ozone-depleting characteristics. It is on the *community right-to-know* list.

Technical Information

Chemical formula: $H_3C_2Cl_3$
Molecular weight: 132
Amount released into the air from industry: 250,000 tons/year
Occurrence:
air, near production sites: 0.02–2 ppb
air, in highly urbanized areas: 1 ppb
water, in highly contaminated wells: 3g/L
water, in dirty municipal systems: 0.8–142 ppb
food, in everyday foodstuffs: 10 ppb

Government regulations:
OSHA limit in workplace air: 350 ppm
EPA limit in drinking water: 350 ppm

Further Reading

International Agency for Research on Cancer. 1979. *IARC Monographs on the Evaluation of the Carcinogenic Risk of Chemicals to Humans: Some Halogenated Hydrocarbons*, vol. 20. Lyon, France.

Trichloroethylene

Other Names

TCE; trichloroethene; ethylene trichloride; 1-chloro–2,2-dichloroethylene; 1,1-dichloro–2-chloroethylene; 1,1,2-trichloroethylene; TRI

Trade Names

Tri-clene; Dow-Tri; Germalgene; Westrosol; Flock-Flip; Permachlor

Introduction

Trichloroethylene, or TCE, is one of the most frequently found toxic chemicals in water in the United States. The EPA estimates that about 38% of cities that rely on groundwater for municipal supplies show average TCE contamination above the EPA drinking water quality criteria. TCE is a solvent that was first synthesized in 1864 and became commercially available in 1908 in Austria and England. Not until the 1940s did it become widely used in the United States.

Physical and Chemical Properties

Trichloroethylene is a colorless, volatile, nonflammable liquid with a characteristic sweet odor. Some people compare the odor to that of chloroform. It is soluble in water and highly soluble in organic solvents. TCE decomposes to form phosgene and hydrogen chloride.

Exposure and Distribution

Trichloroethylene is produced in Michigan and Pennsylvania, then shipped around the United States by rail and truck. Production of TCE in the United States is presently under 100,000 tons annually and has been declining since 1983. Almost all of the solvent is used industrially for metal degreasing. The remainder is used in a wide variety of products, including dyes, printing inks, typewriter correction fluid, spot removers, rug cleaners, and disinfectants. It is used in the manufacture of polyvinyl chloride, varnishes, adhesives, paints, and lacquers. TCE is also a common *inert ingredient* used to carry the active ingredient in *fungicides* and insecticides.

There is a move away from using TCE in consumer products as its toxicity becomes better understood. TCE was once used as a dry-cleaning solvent, a *fumigant,* and as an general anesthetic, but these uses have been discontinued. **Tetrachloroethylene** is now the prevalent dry-cleaning solvent. TCE was also once used to decaffeinate coffee, but is now being replaced by **methylene chloride**.

Most of the TCE produced eventually ends up in the environment. It is widely distributed in the air, water, and soil of most industrialized nations. TCE released into the atmosphere breaks down in a matter of days. Nevertheless, it is widely detected in the air in urban and industrial areas, indicating that it is constantly being released. A significant amount finds its way into groundwater. TCE is the most frequently detected contaminant of groundwater, probably due to past disposal practices. It poses a particular problem in groundwater because it degrades very slowly. TCE spilled in a lake or stream disappears (into the atmosphere) in a few weeks, whereas TCE released into groundwater can take months or even years to degrade. Moreover, TCE is often broken down by microbes found in soil and groundwater, resulting in the formation of **vinylidene chloride** (a suspected human carcinogen) and **vinyl chloride** (a known human carcinogen). TCE that was disposed of in landfills is another major concern because decomposing TCE is a more important source of vinyl chloride in landfills than is plastics decomposition.

TCE has also been detected in low concentrations in food such as beverages, dairy products, fruits, vegetables, edible oils and fats, and marine fish.

Health Effects

Trichloroethylene is easily absorbed when inhaled. Data on oral absorption are limited, but it appears to be poorly absorbed from the stomach. Once in the bloodstream, TCE is distributed throughout the body, with the highest concentrations found in the fat, kidneys, liver, lungs, adrenal glands, and brain. TCE and its by-products are excreted via the urine, exhaled air, and to a lesser degree, the sweat, feces, and saliva.

Trichloroethylene is a narcotic at high doses. It produces headache, dizziness, and sleepiness following inhalation. At significant doses, the mucous membranes, eyes, and respiratory tract become irritated. Nausea, convulsions, and irregular heartbeat may also occur. Liver and kidney damage occur when extremely high concentrations are inhaled, even for short periods. Death by cardiac arrest is also possible at extremely high concentrations. Although potentially fatal doses of TCE are not likely to be encountered even in a contaminated workplace, fatal doses are possible when TCE is deliberately inhaled by people wanting a "high."

The chronic effects of TCE exposure in humans include fatigue, headache, irritability, memory loss, transient euphoria, and depression. Intolerance to alcohol may also be experienced. Cirrhosis of the liver may occur when TCE is inhaled over extended periods.

Trichloroethylene may cause cancer. Studies of humans exposed to TCE are inconclusive, but rats and mice exposed to TCE have an increased incidence of liver and lung cancers. It is considered a probable human carcinogen (group B_2; see Chapter 3, Section B) by the EPA. TCE does not cause birth defects, but it easily crosses the placenta. Measurable amounts of TCE have been found in the fetus within 2 minutes following maternal exposure.

Protection and Prevention

Avoid buying products that contain TCE. These include some spot removers, carpet cleaners, and typewriter correction fluid (except those that are water based). If you rely on untreated well water for drinking and you live in an urban or industrial area, you may want to have the water tested. TCE is known to contaminate water wells close to refineries, metal processing plants, chemical manufacturers, military bases, and electroplating operations. If TCE is used at your workplace, request a *Material Safety Data Sheet*. It should explain the hazards associated with its use and suggest measures to avoid overexposure.

Environmental Effects

Trichloroethylene *bioconcentrates* to a limited degree in marine organisms, but the chemical clears from exposed fish quickly after the source of TCE is removed. TCE is directly toxic to freshwater and saltwater organisms. *Benthic* organisms are the most vulnerable to TCE spills, as the chemical smothers them.

Regulatory Status

Trichloroethylene is regulated by OSHA, the EPA, and the FDA. The EPA regulates its concentrations in drinking water at levels that take cancer into consideration. TCE is listed as a *hazardous air pollutant* in the 1990 Clean Air Act, requiring the EPA to set emission standards. The FDA has proposed regulations that prohibit the use of TCE in the processing of food and drugs. Today, TCE residues are allowed in decaffeinated coffee and spice extracts. Occupational and *ambient* exposure limits are often higher in the United States than limits set in other countries. Therefore, adjustments to current regulations are likely. TCE is on the *community right-to-know* list.

Technical Information

Chemical formula: C_2HCl_3
Molecular weight: 131.4

Amount produced in the United States:
98,000 tons/year
Estimated amount released into environment: 91,000 tons/year
Air concentration in urban areas: 0.5 ppb
(3 μg/m^3)
Odor thresholds:
air: 2.5–900 mg/m^3 (0.5–160 ppm)
water: 0.5 mg/L
Government regulations:
OSHA limit in workplace air: 50 ppm
EPA limit in drinking water: 0.005 mg/L
FDA limits:
decaffeinated ground coffee: 25 ppm
decaffeinated instant coffee: 10 ppm
spice extracts: 30 ppm

Further Reading

Agency for Toxic Substances and Disease Registry. 1987. *Toxicological Profile for Trichloroethylene*. Washington, D.C.: U.S. Public Health Service.

World Health Organization. 1985. *Environmental Health Criteria Report No. 50: Trichloroethylene*. Geneva.

TRIS

Other Names

Tris(2,3-dibromopropyl)-phosphate;
1-propanol-2,3-dibromophosphate

Trade Names

Fyrol HB 32; FireMaster LV-T 23P;
Flammex AP; Bromkal P 67–6HP; ES 685;
3PBR; Zetofex ZN; Tris-BP

Introduction

TRIS is the common name for the fire-retardant chemical tris(2,3-dibromopropyl)-phosphate. TRIS was heavily used in the 1970s after the Consumer Product Safety Commission (CPSC) promulgated regulations setting fire safety standards for fabrics. Children's sleepwear was of particular concern. Shortly after the widespread use of TRIS began, the *toxicological* data began to surface. It was found to have cancer-causing properties, yet the chemical was not banned for use as a flame retardant in children's sleepwear for some ten years after this was discovered. And only then was it banned after the CPSC was sued by the Natural Resources Defense Council.

TRIS provides a fascinating case study of how good regulations can foster deleterious outcomes. Almost everyone can support the notion of fire-retardant sleepwear. But the use of TRIS to produce such sleepwear posed a greater health risk to children than the risk posed by fire. The catch is that fire retardants toxicologically safe enough to apply to children's clothing may not exist. Nevertheless, manufacturers are forced to use whatever is available to comply with the law.

The fire safe sleepwear law is still on the books. Manufacturers now use acrylic fabrics that do not need chemicals applied to them to comply with fire safety regulations. This is why parents cannot buy all-cotton pajamas for their children. Cotton cannot pass the fire safety tests without the application of a flame-retarding chemical.

Physical and Chemical Properties

TRIS is a clear liquid compound originally designed to be applied to polyester and acetate fabrics to slow their rate of burning. The active element in TRIS is bromine, an element with well-known flame-retarding properties. TRIS is a formulation designed to ease the application and the staying power of bromine in fabric while maintaining the fabric's strength and aesthetic qualities. (Bromine itself is a smelly brown ooze.) TRIS is often contaminated with 2,3-dibromopropane, another chemical suspected of causing cancer.

Exposure and Distribution

TRIS was banned for use in children's sleepwear in 1977. At the time of the ban, it is estimated that 50 to 60 million children wore TRIS-treated garments. Although the chemical was banned for use in children's clothing, TRIS-treated garments remain warehoused. Owners sell them as industrial rags. However, from time to time, these garments make their way into the marketplace. (They are expensive to warehouse, yet too valuable to destroy.) Thus, TRIS remains a danger to children. In addition, the chemical is still used as a flame retardant in polyurethane foam, car seat cushions, and other consumer products.

Health Effects

TRIS causes cancer in laboratory animals. Studies in mice suggest that the liver, kidney, lung, and stomach may be affected, while only the kidney is affected in rats. TRIS also causes *mutations* in some bacteria tested using the *Ames test*. Some of the mutations found can be passed on from generation to generation of bacteria. Reproductive effects have also been demonstrated. TRIS is reported to cause testicular shrinkage and to reduce female reproductive capacity in laboratory animals.

Protection and Prevention

Avoid hand-me-down childrens' pajamas made during the 1970s. Do not buy unlabeled sleepwear because you may be purchasing some of the warehoused garments. (The labels were required to be cut out prior to warehousing.) In general, garments labeled "flame resistant" are untreated and therefore harmless, whereas garments labeled "flame retardant" may be chemically treated.

Regulatory Status

TRIS is banned from use on fabrics that people are likely to come into direct contact with. It is still allowed to render furniture filling, car seat cushions, and other stuffing material fireproof.

Technical Information

Chemical formula: $(BrC_3H_5O)_5PO$
Molecular weight: 698

Further Reading

ABELSON, P. H. 1977. The Tris Controversy. *Science* 197:4299.
BLUM, A., and AMES, B. N. 1977. Flame-Retardant Additives as Possible Cancer Hazards. *Science* 195:17.

Tritium

Other Names

T; ^{3}H; heavy hydrogen; tritiated water

Introduction

Tritium is a *radioactive* form of hydrogen. It is one of the fuels used in nuclear fusion weapons and may someday be a major fuel for providing electricity from fusion power plants (see Chapter 15, Section D). Tritium is produced naturally in the upper atmosphere when *cosmic rays* strike air molecules. It is also produced in the atmosphere during above-ground explosions of nuclear weapons. Other man-made sources include nuclear reactors used by the military to produce tritium for nuclear weapons and by power companies for electricity generation.

Tritium has had only minor nonmilitary commercial use so far; it has been used to make luminous dials and as a source of unfailing light for safety signs (by placing tritium inside a phosphor-coated glass tube). Because tritium has the same chemical properties as ordinary hydrogen but differs in that it emits a detectable signal when it radioactively *decays*, it is used by biologists as a tracer to study the movement of hydrogen-containing substances in organisms. If fusion power technology becomes feasible, the associated rate of release of tritium into the environment could far exceed the present release rate. The tritium fuel for fusion power plants would likely be produced by bombarding the element lithium with neutrons in a fission reactor.

Physical and Chemical Properties

Tritium is a colorless, odorless gas. Like ordinary hydrogen, it reacts readily with oxygen to form water. Because tritium is heavier than hydrogen, this tritiated water is sometimes called "heavy water," but it should not be confused with another more common type of heavy water that results when a heavy nonradioactive form of hydrogen, called deuterium, combines with oxygen. Pure tritiated water would be about 22% denser than ordinary water and would be detectable by weight, but water that contains enough tritium to be harmful need not contain sufficient tritium to be noticeably denser than ordinary water.

Tritium has a *half-life* of 12.3 years, and it decays to harmless helium and a *beta particle*. Because half of any quantity of tritium will decay in 12.3 years, over three-fourths of the tritium produced during the atmospheric nuclear weapons testing in the 1950s and early 1960s is now decayed and poses no threat.

Exposure and Distribution

Most of the tritium released from nuclear explosions and nuclear reactors is in the form of tritiated water. In vapor form, this water can be dispersed rapidly. Tritium in liquid water can fall as rain and enter streams, lakes, groundwater, and oceans. Gaseous tritium can enter the human body by inhalation, ingestion, or absorption through the skin; tritium in the form of water enters by direct ingestion of drinking water and food. When tritium is taken up by plants or animals, it enters the *food chain*. Fortunately, within a month or two following ingestion of tritium, most of it is excreted from an animal's body. Thus, the level in the human body does not build up the same way that isotopes such as **strontium-90** and **iodine-131** do. Because hydrogen is found throughout the body and is biologically reactive, tritium tends to be uniformly distributed throughout body fluids within about an hour of ingestion. The radiation from tritium can only penetrate a few ten-thousandths of an inch (2 or 3 microns) into tissue, which is less than the depth of sensitive basal skin cells, so decay of tritium outside the body is relatively harmless.

Since the 1950s, fallout from atmospheric weapons testing has resulted in a tenfold increase over *background levels* in the amount of tritium present in the environment. The single largest U.S. source of environmental tritium has been the Savannah River reactor in Georgia (now shut down), where tritium was produced for military purposes. Each year this single reactor released to the environment about the same amount of tritium as is produced naturally by cosmic rays. The annual production of tritium from all the world's nuclear power generation is about twice that from cosmic rays, but under normal operations only about 4% of this man-made tritium is released to the environment. Most of that released tritium is found in the cooling water, but about 10% is released into the atmosphere in gaseous form. Presently, about half the total environmental release from nuclear power production results from *fuel reprocessing*, but that is because there is only one major fuel reprocessing plant in operation today (at Windscale in Great Britain). If fuel reprocessing becomes more widespread, significantly larger releases can be expected. Commercial applications of tritium lead to an annual release to the environment that is only about one-thousandth of the natural background production rate.

Current world-averaged environmental levels of tritium from both natural and man-made sources are sufficiently low that a typical person receives from tritium only about one hundred-thousandth as much radiation as is received from all other sources (see Chapter 15, Section F). The health risk from tritium is thus negligible for the average person. But for those living near or working in a tritium production plant or a fuel reprocessing facility, the risk of accidental releases is a serious health threat. Only a nuclear war or a major reactor accident is likely to expose a large population to hazardous levels of tritium.

Health Effects

Because tritium does not preferentially concentrate in any particular organ (in contrast to many other radioactive substances), the symptoms and health risks of radiation poisoning by tritium are typical of those from whole body exposures to radiation from any source. (These are described in Chapter 15, Section G.)

Protection and Prevention

No antidotes or other first-aid practices are available. People severely radiated with tritium must seek professional medical care. The only practical way to minimize exposure is to choose not to live near a tritium production plant or a nuclear fuel reprocessing facility.

Regulatory Status

In the United States, the general restrictions on radiation exposure apply to tritium and can be found in Chapter 15, Section F.

Technical Information[7]

The chemical symbol for hydrogen is H, but tritium (^{3}H) is sometimes denoted by T even though it is an isotope of hydrogen. Tritium decays with a half-life of 12.3 years to an isotope of helium (^{3}He) by emitting an electron with a maximum energy of 18 KeV (kilo-electron-volts).

The natural production rate of tritium from cosmic ray bombardment of the atmosphere is 7.2×10^{16} becquerels per year. Nuclear weapons testing has produced a total of about 2.4×10^{20} becquerels of tritium. Nuclear power plants produce tritium at the rate of about 7×10^{11} becquerels per megawatt-year of electricity produced. (A megawatt-year is the amount of energy that a 1-megawatt power plant produces in 1 year or the amount that a more typically-sized 1000-megawatt plant produces in one-thousandth of a year.) Properly functioning new plants release to the environment about 3×10^{10} becquerels per megawatt-year, and prop-

[7]For a discussion of the meaning of the units of radiation used below, see Chapter 15, Section E.

erly functioning old power plants release tritium at about 10 times that rate.

Of the current quantity of tritium in the environment, about 3×10^{16} becquerels are the result of nuclear power plant operations, 3×10^{19} becquerels the result of nuclear weapons testing, and about 1×10^{18} becquerels of natural origin. The average worldwide concentration of tritium in freshwater is about 0.5 becquerels per liter. The dose to people per unit of released tritium is estimated to be 7×10^{-15} person-sieverts per becquerel released. Hence, the individual radiation dose from tritium released from nuclear power operations currently averages about 1×10^{-8} sieverts per year. (For a discussion of the health implications of this, see Chapter 15, Section G.)

Further Reading

National Council on Radiation Protection and Measurements. 1979. *Tritium and Other Radionuclide Labeled Organic Compounds Incorporated in Genetic Material.* NCRP Report no. 63. Washington, D.C.

World Health Organization. 1983. *Environmental Health Criteria Report No. 25: Selected Radionuclides.* Geneva.

Ultrasound

Other Name

High-frequency sound

Introduction

Ultrasound is noise that is too high pitched for humans to hear. New household gadgets that use ultrasound and increasing applications of ultrasound in medicine are exposing more and more people to it. As with radioactivity, some of our exposure to ultrasound brings substantial benefits that cannot be gained without it, while other exposures are unnecessary. Our understanding of the hazards of exposure is primitive, but it appears prudent to avoid unnecessarily high levels of exposure.

The common dog whistle produces ultrasound, which dogs can hear but not people. There are also less well known uses in a host of other consumer and workplace devices, including some types of automatic rangefinders on cameras, television remote controls, garage door openers, burglar alarms, and equipment for monitoring the flow of fluids. Ultrasound is also used increasingly in medicine, particularly to examine the position and shape of the human fetus throughout pregnancy, a practice that is now routine in the United States. Another new and potentially important medical application is to break up kidney stones so they can be passed relatively painlessly.

Physical and Chemical Properties

Sound is characterized by frequency, or pitch, and intensity. For sound that can be heard, intensity is another name for loudness, but whether or not the sound can be heard, intensity is a measure of the energy carried by the sound. Sound that is higher in frequency than the limit of normal human hearing is called ultrasound. This limit is approximately 20,000 cycles per second, or about one and a half octaves above the highest note on the piano keyboard. Because sound waves possess energy, when high-intensity ultrasound is absorbed by any material object such as the human body, the energy of the wave can heat the object and even deform the material. The more intense the sound, the greater the heating and deformation.

Exposure and Distribution

Bats emit ultrasound for navigation, but with that exception, levels of ultrasound in the natural environment are negligible. Human exposures vary tremendously depending on how much one uses the household devices previously listed and on how much medical exposure one gets. For many children born in the past few years in the industrialized countries, most of their exposure to ultrasound is likely to have been the dose absorbed during ultrasound diagnostics before birth (*in utero*).

Health Effects

Symptoms of exposure to ultrasound at intensities greater than that encountered from household devices include irritability, headaches, nausea, persistent ringing in the ear, pain from localized heating of tissue, and altered blood sugar levels. There is some evidence that high-intensity ultrasound can also retard bone growth, trigger muscular contractions, and alter thyroid activity. The biological hazards of ultrasound appear to be *synergistic* with those of *X-rays*; in other words, the total damage from ultrasound and X-rays applied together is greater than the sum of the damages from the two applied separately. At levels normally encountered in the household, no convincing evidence for health damage exists. Some recent research, however, suggests that the diagnostic application of ultrasound for human fetal examinations might result in reduced birthweights.

Protection and Prevention

The preliminary results on effects of fetal exposure indicate that more research is needed and suggest the need both to avoid unnecessary ultrasound examinations and to develop medical equipment that produces the minimum necessary intensity of ultrasound for the purpose. In the workplace, sound barriers can greatly reduce occupational exposures to all types of noise, including ultrasound. Household devices such as burglar alarms using ultrasound should be turned off when not in use.

Environmental Effects

The possibility exists that ultrasound in the home does psychological harm to household pets. Outdoor intensities are too low to cause concern over effects on wild populations.

Regulatory Status

The Soviet Union, Canada, and Japan have set industrial exposure guidelines for ultrasound. In addition, Japan limits fetal exposures to a value that is near the upper end of the range normally used in the United States. In the United States, only the U.S. Air Force has set guidelines (see Technical Information).

Technical Information

The intensity of ultrasound is usually expressed either on a decibel scale or in units of watts per square centimeter (W/cm^2). (In the entry on **noise**, the relationship between these units is explained.) The frequency of sound is expressed in units of cycles per second, or hertz. A frequency of 20,000 cycles per second can be denoted in several equivalent ways: 20,000 cps, 20,000 hertz (Hz), or 20 kilohertz (kHz).

The threshold for people to feel pain from heat generated by absorbed sound waves is $3 \ W/cm^2$. The lethal threshold for people is $100 \ W/cm^2$. The Japanese restrict fetal diagnostic exposures to $10 \ mW/cm^2$. In the frequency range near or above 20 kHz, the intensity guideline is set at 110 decibels, which corresponds to $0.1 \ mW/cm^2$. The U.S. Air

Force limits its workers' exposure to ultrasound to 85 decibels, or about 0.3 μW/cm².

Further Reading

Department of National Health and Welfare. 1980. *Guidelines for the Safe Use of Ultrasound. Part I: Medical and Paramedical Applications. Safety Code–23.* Publication 80-EHD–59. Ottawa, Canada.

World Health Organization. 1982. *Environmental Health Criteria Report No. 22: Ultrasound.* Geneva.

Ultraviolet Radiation

Other Names

Ultraviolet light; UV; UV radiation; short wavelength radiation

Introduction

The sun is the primary source of natural light and warmth on earth, but it is also the source of harmful ultraviolet radiation. Ultraviolet radiation is much like visible light except that it is at a different *wavelength* and is thus invisible to the eye and more damaging to biological tissue. Both are different parts of the *electromagnetic spectrum*. Fortunately, much of the ultraviolet radiation beamed by the sun at earth never reaches us because it is absorbed in the upper atmosphere by the ozone layer (see Chapter 11, Section B). Ultraviolet radiation has important uses in research and medicine and industry, notably for sterilization of biological samples, treatment of skin diseases, and heat-treating materials during manufacturing. Most important, exposure to the sun's ultraviolet radiation permits the human body to manufacture vitamin D; deficiency of this vitamin can result in rickets in children. Direct exposure to sunlight for only a few minutes per day in summer and about one-half hour per day in winter is all that is needed to produced an adequate amount of vitamin D.

Physical and Chemical Properties

Ultraviolet radiation cannot be detected directly by the senses until it has caused damage and pain. It can penetrate light clothing and many commercial suntan lotions. The glass in a window blocks much of the sun's ultraviolet radiation, but not enough to ensure complete safety. Ultraviolet radiation and ordinary visible light differ in the size of the wavelengths; ultraviolet radiation is made up of shorter wavelengths, which makes it more damaging to cells and other objects it strikes.

Exposure and Distribution

The most commonly occurring exposures result from time spent in full sunlight, although accidental laboratory and industrial exposures occur as well. Snow reflects both visible and ultraviolet radiation, so especially severe burns from ultraviolet radiation can occur on sunny days in winter when exposure occurs from the sun directly and by reflection off snow. Despite the increase in exposure associated with snow, however, the overall risk of skin cancer caused by ultraviolet radiation is greatest near the equator. This is because here the radiation intensity is greatest and the ozone layer is thinnest. A move of about 8° of latitude closer to the equator, say from Chicago to Atlanta, causes the skin cancer risk from ultraviolet radiation to approximately double. Also, exposures are greater at higher elevations, even ignoring the snow effect, but this is usually not a problem except for mountain climbers.

Health Effects

Light-skinned people are most at risk. Damage can range from mild sunburn to premature aging of the skin to cancer. Both the readily treatable basal cell and squamous cell skin cancers and the more life-threatening skin melanoma can result. Temporary loss of vision can result from direct exposure to the eyes, as occurs in snow blindness. More permanent damage, including the formation of cataracts or damage to the retina, occurs less frequently. It is believed that repeated, separate incidents of severe sunburn are more likely to cause skin cancer than the same total amount of ultraviolet radiation received more gradually over time without severe sunburn occurring.

Protection and Prevention

A wide-brimmed hat is probably the single best form of protection, but it is often not adequate. Wear good dark sunglasses that provide UV protection outdoors in bright conditions. The effectiveness against ultraviolet radiation of many sunglasses is now labeled. Because ultraviolet radiation penetrates light clothing such as T-shirts, a heavy, dark shirt is advised when hiking in snow, particularly in spring and summer when sunlight is more intense. Sun lotions or sun screens vary tremendously in their effectiveness; they are rated by an index denoted SPF, or sun protection factor. SPF values above 18 are considered to provide adquate protection against most ultraviolet radiation exposure. However, for some activities, such as high-elevation skiing, and for children with fair skin, even higher SPFs are recommended. Recently, some dermatologists have warned that the UV-A (see Technical Information) portion of the ultraviolet radiation spectrum may be more harmful than hitherto thought and that the SPF index does not provide a measure of protection against the threat. Be aware that some brands of sun lotion wash off more easily than others as a result of swimming or sweating; water-proof brands are now available. People spending a great deal of time outdoors in sunny weather should be especially conscientious about having regular medical exams to check for skin cancers. Deliberate sunbathing and tanning should be avoided; temporary cosmetic effects will be paid for with severely wrinkled skin in later life and a higher chance of cancer.

Environmental Effects

Ultraviolet radiation can probably damage any living species that is exposed to it. If exposure increases because of stratospheric ozone depletion, we can expect to see major ecological effects. Little research on this has been carried out, however, so detailed predictions of damage are unavailable. Ultraviolet radiation can damage many plastics, making them brittle. It also initiates chemical reactions in the atmosphere that produce some of the most worrisome air pollutants, such as **ozone** in urban air (not to be confused with stratospheric ozone).

Regulatory Status

Exposure to man-made sources of ultraviolet radiation are regulated by the same standards that apply to other forms of radiation (see Chapter 15, Section F). The World Health Organization recommends that exposure to tropical sun without sun screen or protective clothing should be limited to one hour per day between 10 A.M. and 2 P.M.

Technical Information

Ultraviolet radiation has a wavelength between 100 and 400 nanometers (nm) (a nanometer is one-billionth of a meter). In this range, three types of ultraviolet radiation are distinguished: UV-A, UV-B, and UV-C. These have wavelengths in the range of 400 to 320 nm, 320 to 280 nm, and 280 to 100 nm, respectively. UV-B and the longer wavelength end of the UV-C spectrum have long been considered the most threatening types. This is because UV-B has shorter wavelengths than UV-A (and therefore is capable of inflicting more damage to biological tissue) and because nearly all of the shorter wavelength UV-C is blocked by the ozone layer. New evidence, however, has suggested that the risks of UV-A have been underestimated; more information on this should be forthcoming over the next few years.

Further Reading

World Health Organization. 1979. *Environmental Health Criteria Report No. 14: UV Radiation.* Geneva.

Vinyl Chloride

Other Names

Vinyl chloride monomer; VCM; chloroethylene; chloroethane; monochloroethylene; ethylene monochloride; monochloroethane; Vinyl C monomer

Trade Name

Trovidur

Introduction

Vinyl chloride is a widely produced chemical that is primarily used to make polyvinyl chloride resin, which is the raw ingredient of polyvinyl chloride (PVC) plastic. It is sometimes used to make the solvent **trichloroethane**. Before its cancer-causing properties were recognized, it was also used as an aerosol propellant, a refrigerant, an ingredient in drugs and cosmetics, and an anesthetic, but these uses have been abandoned.

Physical and Chemical Properties

Vinyl chloride is a colorless gas with a characteristic "plastic" odor. It is about twice as heavy as air, so that when the gas is released into the atmosphere, it tends to sink. There are no known natural sources of vinyl chloride.

Exposure and Distribution

Vinyl chloride is widely distributed throughout the industrialized world. The highest outdoor air concentrations are usually found near vinyl chloride manufacturing plants and near industrial sites that work with polyvinyl chloride plastics. Residents in the Houston, Texas, area are the most likely group to be exposed as a result of industrial activity because 40% of U.S. production capacity is located in that area.

Vinyl chloride can also be found in some municipal drinking waters and in a variety of foods and beverages, including alcoholic drinks, vinegar, oil, butter, and mineral water. The source for this vinyl chloride contamination is believed to be PVC pipes and plastic packaging. Other sources of vinyl chloride exposure include new automobile interiors, tobacco products, and marijuana cigarettes. Concentrations found in foods and beverages are usually quite low; it is estimated that the average person ingests less than 100 micrograms of vinyl chloride per day. Inhalation of contaminated air is considered to be the most significant route of exposure for the general public. Occupational exposure is likely anywhere vinyl chloride or PVC plastics are made or used during a manufacturing process.

Health Effects

Vinyl chloride can cause cancer in people following both inhalation and ingestion. It is known to cause liver, brain, and central nervous system cancers in people, and it may also cause human lung cancer, leukemia, and lymphoma. Vinyl chloride is a *mutagen* both to animal and human cells, reinforcing the *epidemiological* evidence that vinyl chloride causes cancer. Vinyl chloride may also be responsible for birth defects among children of parents who live near vinyl chloride and polyvinyl chloride plastic plants.

Chronic exposure to vinyl chloride also causes liver damage and a bone loss disorder known as acroosteolysis, which affects the fingers. Circulatory changes have also been recorded among humans exposed to vinyl chloride for long periods. Symptoms of acute exposure to the chemical include feelings of intoxication, dizziness, lightheadedness, nausea, abdominal pain, slow response time, weakness, and headache. Symptoms of overexposure rapidly disappear when vinyl chloride exposure is stopped. Deep anesthesia and death are possible following prolonged exposure to high concentrations.

Protection and Prevention

It is probably impossible to avoid exposure to vinyl chloride when it comes from outdoor air, but people can take steps to limit their exposure from other sources. Probably the most important step is to avoid storing foods in PVC containers. These containers are not allowed to be sold for the purpose of food storage, but they are available for other purposes. Therefore, heed the warning labels if they state that the container is not recommended for food storage. Do not drink liquids that have been mixed or stored in plastic pails or garbage cans (as is sometimes the case at large gatherings). Ventilate new cars well before sitting in them. Do this by opening the doors for a few minutes after the car has been sitting in the sun or leaving the windows partially open while driving until that "new car smell" is no longer noticeable.

Regulatory Status

Vinyl chloride emissions and workroom concentrations are strictly regulated by the government. The FDA has set maximum contamination levels for foods, drugs, and cosmetics. Vinyl chloride is on the EPA *community right-to-know* list. It is also listed as a *hazardous air pollutant* in the 1990 Clean Air Act.

Technical Information

Chemical formula: C_2H_3Cl
Molecular weight: 62.5
Typical concentrations:
    air, near vinyl chloride manufacturing
      plants (average): 8–8000 $\mu g/M^3$
    food, maximum concentrations:
      alcohol beverages: 2.1 mg/kg
      vinegar: 9.4 mg/kg
      edible oils: 0.05–14.8 mg/kg
      butter: 0.05 mg/kg
    water, average highest concentrations:
      10 $\mu g/L$
OSHA limit in workplace air: 1 ppm

Further Reading

Agency for Toxic Substances and Disease Registry. 1988. *Toxicological Profile for Vinyl Chloride*. Washington, D.C.: U.S. Public Health Service.

Vinylidene Chloride

Other Names

1,1-dichloroethylene; VDC; *asym*-dichloro-ethylene; 1,1-dichloroethane; 1,1-DCE

Introduction

Vinylidene chloride is an important chemical ingredient used during the manufacture of plastics used for food packaging, including some commercial plastic food wraps. It is also used to make modacrylic fiber. Vinylidene chloride plastics are also used in many solvent-based resin and glue products. Most vinylidene chloride is made from 1,1,2-trichloroethane.

Physical and Chemical Properties

Vinylidene chloride is a clear liquid with a sweet odor. It mixes easily in water, **acetone**, and **benzene**. It is a highly flammable chemical.

Exposure and Distribution

About 70,000 tons of vinylidene chloride are manufactured in the United States annually. Although most exposure occurs in factories where vinylidene chloride is made or where products containing it are produced or stocked, consumers can come into contact with the chemical via outdoor air, water, and some foods. Factories that manufacture vinylidene chloride typically emit about 150 tons per year of the substance into the air. Consequently, people who live near these factories may be exposed to trace amounts in outdoor air. Some tap water is contaminated with very small amounts of the substance. Trace amounts have been found in potato chips packed in bags coated with vinylidene chloride plastics. Taken as a whole, however, consumer exposure to vinylidene chloride is believed to be quite low.

Health Effects

In humans, vinylidene chloride is highly irritating to the eyes and skin, but it is most dangerous when inhaled. Breathing high concentrations can cause depression of the central nervous system, including unconciousness. Chronic inhalation of small quantities of vinylidene chloride can produce liver and kidney damage.

Vinylidene chloride exposure has been linked to various cancers among exposed laboratory mice. Evidence of its cancer-causing properties has been inconclusive in experiments using rats and negative in Chinese hamsters. However, experiments in which rats were exposed from birth, rather than as adults only, found that vinylidene chloride caused cancer. Vinylidene chloride is a *mutagen* in some, but not all, short-term tests. The chemical does not appear to cause birth defects in laboratory animals, but it does cross the placenta and is toxic to the unborn fetus. Unfortunately, most studies describing vinylidene chloride exposure and toxicity are 10 to 20 years old.

Protection and Prevention

People who are exposed to vinylidene chloride at work should use protective gear when it is recommended. Pregnant women should try to avoid all workplace exposure. Request a *Material Safety Data Sheet* whenever vinylidene chloride exposure is suspected. Consumer exposure can be limited by avoiding the use of plastic food wraps to cover food.

Regulatory Status

Vinylidene chloride exposure in the workplace is regulated by OSHA. It is listed as a *hazardous air pollutant* in the 1990 Clean Air Act, requiring the EPA to set emission standards. The chemical is on the EPA *community right-to-know* list.

Technical Information

Chemical formula: $C_2H_2Cl_2$
Molecular weight: 97
OSHA limit in workplace air: 5 ppm
Amount produced in the United States:
  70,000 tons/year
Lethal dose (LD_{50}):
  in fasting rats: 500–2500 ppm
  in nourished rats: 10,000–15,000 ppm

Further Reading

PROCTOR, NICK H., HUGHES, JAMES P., and FISCHMAN, MICHAEL L. 1988. *Chemical Hazards of the Workplace*. Philadelphia: J.B. Lippincott.

Warfarin

Trade Names

Arthrombine-K; Dethmore; Panwartin

Introduction

The *rodenticide* warfarin belongs to a family of chemicals called coumarins that are used in medicine to prevent blood clotting. In fact, warfarin was used in 1955 to treat President Eisenhower. The anticoagulant properties of warfarin and related compounds were originally discovered when cattle that had eaten improperly cured cattle fodder (spoiled sweet clover) developed a bleeding disorder. To determine the cause of the problem, the fodder was chemically analyzed, and the causative agent, warfarin, was isolated in 1939. It was synthesized in 1940 and used in medical field trials in 1942. Used successfully since 1950 as a rodenticide, primarily to poison rats, warfarin inhibits blood clotting and damages small blood vessels, which causes internal bleeding.

To be effective as a rodenticide, several repeated doses of the chemical must be ingested over a period of days, thus weakening the rodents gradually. Available for household use, warfarin is considered relatively safe because accidental ingestion of a single dose is unlikely to produce serious illness. Other kinds of rodenticides could be fatal if ingested and are therefore not safe for household use. Warfarin has proven successful because rats do not exhibit bait shyness; that is, they continue to feed on poisoned baits. One problem with continued and extensive use of warfarin is that *resistance* to the poison has developed in many rat populations.

Physical and Chemical Properties

Warfarin occurs as colorless, tasteless crystals. It is practically insoluble in water, but it is easily converted to a water-soluble form. The pesticide is readily soluble in acetone.

Exposure and Distribution

Warfarin is available as a dust to use in rodent holes and runs and as a powder to mix with suitable protein-rich baits. It also comes ready-to-use in prepared baits. The primary method of delivery of warfarin prevents the escape of appreciable quantities to the environment. But children and domestic animals could find and eat the baits.

Health Effects

Accidental human poisonings have occurred, but treatment has successfully reversed the effects. Symptoms of poisoning include increased pallor, weakness, and hematomas (a tumor or swelling containing blood). In general, warfarin and other coumarins are relatively free of unwanted side-effects, although occasional *gastrointestinal* disturbances, *dermatitis*, and loss of white blood cells have been reported. Moreover, a high incidence of birth defects is associated with the administration of warfarin to pregnant women. The chemical interacts with other chemicals in various ways. For example, its activity is enhanced by the drug disulfiram, but phenobarbital and certain pesticides (such as **lindane**) interfere with its effect.

Both people and rats exhibit varying susceptibilities to warfarin, ranging from an increased susceptibility to total genetic resistance. In people, the underlying mechanism of resistance is unclear, but in rats, one form of resistance is based on an ability to metabolize the chemical.

Protection and Prevention

Children, domestic pets, and wildlife can be poisoned by warfarin baits. If the poison is used, it should be placed in or near rodent nests, holes, or trails in such a manner as to avoid inadvertent poisonings. Anyone using this or any other pesticide should read the label on the container and follow the directions carefully.

Warfarin is far safer than certain other poisons, such as compound 1080 (sodium fluoroacetate), which are used to kill warm-blooded animals. (Because the controversial compound 1080 is extremely hazardous to humans, domestic animals, and other wildlife, its use has been suspended.) An alternative to chemical poisons is the use of traps. Ultrasonic devices can be used effectively against backyard gophers, and some people recommend flooding the holes and tunnels of gophers and other burrowing pests. Another alternative is to share our planet with other creatures.

Environmental Effects

The major environmental concern is accidental poisonings of wildlife, particularly endangered species. Although the need for repeated ingestion of the poison decreases the likelihood of unwanted deaths, evidence of species variability in susceptibility urges caution. Another concern is that because of the development of resistance in some strains of rats, other considerably more toxic poisons will begin to replace warfarin.

Regulatory Status

Use of warfarin is not restricted and is therefore available for household use.

Technical Information

Chemical name: 3-(a-acetonylbenzyl)–4-hydroxycoumarin
Chemical formula: $C_{19}H_{16}O$

Further Reading

HAYES, W. J. 1982. *Pesticides Studied in Man.* Baltimore, MD: Williams and Wilkins.

Xylene

Other Names

Xylole; ksylen; dimethylbenzene; xiloli; *m*-xylene; *o*-xylene; *p*-xylene

Introduction

Xylene is widely used in industry and consumer products. It is a petrochemical building block used by the chemical industry to make a myriad of other chemicals including *solvents*, plastics, and pharmaceuticals. Xylene is also commonly used by itself as a solvent and as an *inert* base for many pesticide formulations. In the home, xylene can be found in a variety of common products, including paint, paint remover, nail polish, air fresheners, degreasing cleaners, lacquers, glues, and marketing pens.

Physical and Chemical Properties

Xylene is a clear, aromatic liquid that is highly flammable when exposed to an open flame or excessive heat.

Exposure and Distribution

Large numbers of people are likely to be exposed to xylene fumes. Over 600,000 tons of the chemical are released into the air each year during industrial processing, making it one of the more common outdoor air pollutants in urban and industrialized areas. People can also come into contact with xylene fumes at home whenever products that contain the chemical are used. People who work in industries that make use of solvents and metal cleaners or that manufacture chemicals are also likely to come into contact with it.

Health Effects

Xylene is the most acutely toxic of the common *aromatic hydrocarbons*, a group of petrochemicals that include **benzene** and **toluene**. Most fatal poisonings are the result of breathing xylene vapors. Ingestion is rare, but when it does occur, it can lead to severe respiratory illness because inhalation of small amounts of xylene is likely to accompany ingestion.

High concentrations of xylene in the air can cause irritation to the eyes and nose, coughing, hoarseness, and even pulmonary edema. Continued inhalation at levels that cause irritation leads to symptoms that resemble drunkenness, including slowed reaction time, poor balance, and central nervous system depression or agitation, followed by unconsciousness, tremors, and restlessness. Death is usually caused by respiratory arrest, but sometimes the heart stops beating.

Simultaneous exposure to alcoholic beverages and xylene can be dangerous. It is possible for workers to receive such simultaneous exposures when they drink after leaving a workplace contaminated with xylene because the chemical is stored in body fat and then released over a period of hours into the bloodstream. Women and overweight men tend to excrete xylene more slowly than do thin men.

When xylene is spilled onto the skin, a skin condition characterized by redness and small blisters results. Repeated exposure to levels that are only slightly irritating may lead to kidney damage. Exposure to high levels of xylene in the air by pregnant laboratory rats causes slowed fetal development. Xylene does not appear to cause cancer.

Protection and Prevention

Exposure to low levels of xylene in outdoor air is unavoidable. For the average person, the highest and potentially most dangerous exposures are likely when oil-based paints are used in enclosed spaces. Oil-based paint (and paint removers) should always be used with good ventilation. Better yet, use water-based products whenever possible. People who suspect that xylene is used at their workplace should request a *Material Safety Data Sheet (MSDS)*, which should list the products and processes in which xylene exposure is likely and suggest protective measures. If xylene or xylene-based products are swallowed, seek medical attention immediately. Do not induce vomiting because this will increase the risk of inhaling liquid xylene.

Environmental Effects

Xylene emissions contribute to the formation of urban *smog*.

Regulatory Status

Xylene concentrations in workplace air are regulated by OSHA. It is listed as a *hazardous air pollutant* in the 1990 Clean Air Act, requiring the EPA to set emission standards. The chemical is also on the EPA *community right-to-know* list.

Technical Information

Chemical formula: $C_6H_4(CH_3)_2$
Molecular weight: 106
OSHA limit in workplace air: 100 ppm
Immediately dangerous to life or health level: 1000 ppm
Odor threshold (air): 1 ppm

Further Reading

PROCTOR, NICK H., HUGHES, JAMES P., and FISCHMAN, MICHAEL L. 1988. *Chemical Hazards of the Workplace*. Philadelphia: J.B. Lippincott.

Zinc

Other Names

Chinese white; flowers of zinc; philosopher's wool; zinc white; zincite

Introduction

Zinc is a naturally occurring trace element required for human health. Although there are more reports of adverse effects from zinc deficiency than from zinc overload, compounds of zinc can be toxic if inhaled and will cause stomach distress if too much is ingested. Excessive consumption of zinc by taking too many mineral supplements should by avoided because of the possibility of cardiovascular problems.

Physical and Chemical Properties

Pure zinc is a relatively soft, bluish-white metal. It readily combines with other metals to form alloys, the most important of which is galvanized steel. Zinc combines with copper to form brass and with copper and tin to make bronze.

Zinc oxide is the most important zinc compound and is used in the vulcanizing of rubber, in photocopying papers, and in the treatment of burns, infections, and skin diseases. It is an odorless, tasteless, white or yellowish-white powder.

Zinc chloride is a primary ingredient in smoke bombs used by the military for screening purposes and crowd dispersal and occasionally in fire-fighting exercises by both military and civilian services. Breathing this smoke has caused severe lung damage and death in several cases.

Exposure and Distribution

Exposure to zinc occurs mainly from food and less importantly from water. Average dietary intake ranges from 7 to 16 milligrams per day, which means that intake is often lower than the Recommended Dietary Allowances (15 milligrams per day for men and 12 milligrams per day for women). Zinc tends to be supplied with protein. The best sources are meat, fish, poultry, dairy products, cereals, and grains. Dietary supplements (vitamin pills) usually contain zinc and can increase exposures to 75 milligrams per day. Overconsumption of vitamin pills can lead to high-level exposures.

Environmental concentrations of zinc are highest near zinc mines and smelters, iron and steel foundries, electroplating shops, and city streets (owing to tire wear). Workers in these industries and welders are exposed to the highest levels of zinc, usually in the form of zinc oxide fumes.

Health Effects

Zinc is required for human health, and most of the health effects literature concerns zinc deficiency rather than zinc overload. Nevertheless, overconsumption of zinc may impair heart function, and a balance must be struck between preventing deficiency and avoiding overload.

First, let's look at zinc deficiency. Zinc is required for all animal and plant life; it is the second most common metal found in human tissues (after iron). More than 20 zinc metalloenzymes (*enzymes* containing metals) have been identified, and over 100 enzymes require zinc for maximum function. Zinc plays a role in the *metabolism* of proteins and nucleic acids and is essential for the synthesis of the genetic material *DNA*. The most severe effects of zinc deficiency occur in children and include dwarfism and delayed sexual maturation. Less severe effects are loss of appetite, decreased sense of taste and smell, slow wound healing, rough and dry skin, and mental lethargy. Chronic, severe, and untreated zinc deficiency can be fatal.

In contrast, too much zinc can result in a condition called zinc toxicosis. Overconsumption of zinc leads to stomach distress, cramps, nausea, vomiting, and diarrhea. Most reported cases have resulted from eating or drinking foods stored or cooked in galvanized metal containers or from consuming too many vitamin supplements (two or three capsules per day, each containing 50 milligrams of zinc). Because the body rids itself efficiently of zinc through the *gastrointestinal system*, there is little risk of long-term buildup. Some experimental studies on human subjects, however, have shown that daily exposure to 150 milligrams of zinc over a period of several weeks has led to a reduction in high-density lipoprotein cholesterol levels and an increase in low-density lipoprotein cholesterol levels. Such changes may increase the risk of heart disease, indicating the danger of taking too many zinc supplements. Chronic, high-level zinc consumption may affect the immune system as well.

Workers exposed to zinc oxide fumes on the job can develop a condition known as metal fume fever, a general term applied to disorders associated with breathing fumes of metals heated above their melting points. The symptoms of zinc metal fume fever include rapid breathing, shivering, fever, sweating, chest and leg pain, and weakness. Symptoms usually abate within one or two days, but it is not known whether long-term lung damage may result. Zinc chloride is the primary ingredient in smoke bombs. It can cause severe lung damage and death if breathed in confined spaces. Milder exposures have not been found to cause lasting effects.

Zinc is not associated with cancer or mutations in humans. Only limited experimental evidence is available for laboratory animals. Such evidence shows that zinc may indirectly affect tumor formation either as a growth promoter or as an inhibitor. The EPA classifies zinc as a Group D substance, meaning that inadequate evidence exists to evaluate its cancer potential (see Chapter 3, Section B).

Protection and Prevention

To prevent the overconsumption of zinc, foods and drinks should not be stored or prepared in galvanized metal containers. Excessive use of vitamin supplements should be eliminated. To ensure the adequate consumption of zinc, the Recommended Dietary Allowances (RDAs) established by the National Academy of Sciences should be followed.

Environmental Effects

Zinc is more of a hazard to aquatic organisms than to humans. In areas around smelters and mine runoff, plant growth is depressed and aquatic life and waterfowl are impaired. Tens of thousands of fish have been killed from zinc pollution. The effects of zinc are greater in soft water than in hard water.

Regulatory Status

The EPA limits the drinking water concentration of zinc based on the taste considerations, not health effects. Water quality criteria have been established for the protection of aquatic life. OSHA limits the concentration of zinc fumes in the workplace.

Technical Information

Chemical symbol: Zn
Atomic number: 30
Atomic weight: 65.38
Density: 7.14 g/cc
Recommended Dietary Allowance (RDAs):
  men: 15 mg/day
  women: 12 mg/day
  children, preadolescent: 10 mg/day
        ½ to 1 year: 5 mg/day
        birth to 6 months: 3 mg/day
  pregnant women: 20 mg/day
  lactating women: 25 mg/day
Secondary drinking water standard (taste):
  5 mg/L (5 ppm)
Permissible level in bottled water:
  5.0 mg/L (5 ppm)
Ambient water quality criteria (protection of aquatic life):
    freshwater, 24-hour average, total recoverable zinc: 47 µg/L (47 ppb)
    saltwater, 24-hour average, not to exceed 170 µ/L at any time: 58 µg/L (58 ppb)
OSHA limits in workplace air:
  zinc chloride fume: 1 mg/m^3
  zinc oxide fume: 5 mg/m^3

Further Reading

Agency for Toxic Substances and Disease Registry. 1989. *Toxicological Profile for Zinc.* ATSDR/TP–89/25. Washington, D.C.: U.S. Public Health Service.

Environmental Protection Agency. 1980. *An Exposure and Risk Assessment for Zinc.* EPA–440/4–81–016. Washington, D.C.: Office of Water Regulations and Standards.

National Research Council. 1979. *Zinc.* Baltimore, M.D.: University Park Press, Committee on Medical and Biologic Effects of Environmental Pollutants, National Academy of Sciences.

Glossary

acaricide a poison specifically used to kill mites and ticks (sometimes called a *miticide*)

acceptable daily intake (ADI) the maximum dose of a substance that can be consumed daily without posing a significant lifetime risk

acid (acidity) a corrosive chemical that in high concentrations can cause burns or other tissue damage; technically, a hydrogen ion donor

action level the concentration of a chemical in food, air, or water that initiates regulatory action

active ingredients the components of a commercial pesticide preparation that actually kill the pest; more generally, the substances in consumer chemical products that do the advertised job

activity the number of nuclear decays per unit time in a sample of a radioactive substance

acute effect an effect occurring shortly (usually within 24 hours) after an acute exposure

acute exposure a short exposure to a toxic; technically, exposure for 14 days or less

acute toxicity (acute poisoning) the toxic or poisoning effect that occurs shortly after an acute exposure

adsorption attachment of a gas, liquid, or dissolved substance to a solid surface, such as soil particles

aerosol a suspension of extremely small liquid or solid particles in air

alcohol dehydrogenase (ADH) an enzyme that breaks down alcohol (ethanol) in the body

aliphatic hydrocarbon organic compounds with carbon-to-carbon linkages that form chain-like structures

alkaline basic (opposite of acidic); the ability to neutralize an acid

allergen a substance that causes an allergic reaction

allergic (allergy) extreme reaction to specific substances, whether inhaled, ingested, injected, or by skin contact; the reaction varies with the tissue affected

alpha particle (alpha ray) the nucleus of a helium atom, comprised of two protons and two neutrons

alveoli the tiny sacs or spaces deep in the lungs where the actual exchange of gases (oxygen up-take and carbon dioxide release) between the air and blood occur

Alzheimer's disease a progressive brain disease of the middle-aged and elderly; symptoms are loss of memory, changes in personality, loss of control over bodily functions, impaired reasoning ability, and disorientation; the cause is unknown and there are currently no treatments

ambient surrounding, as in the phrase "the ambient air"

Ames test a relatively rapid and inexpensive screening procedure to determine if a substance causes mutations

anemia a reduction of oxygen-carrying hemoglobin in the blood

aneurysm a balloon-like swelling in the wall of an artery

antacid a drug that neutralizes the hydrochloric acid secreted in the digestive juices of the stomach

anthropogenic resulting from human activities

antibodies blood proteins made in response to the appearance of certain types of foreign substances in the body that attack and render harmless these substances

antioxidant a chemical that reduces or protects against certain destructive chemical reactions known as oxidations

aquifer a natural underground supply of water, usually found permeating porous rock

aromatic hydrocarbons volatile organic compounds bearing a structural resemblance to benzene, containing a high ratio of carbon to hydrogen atoms, and possessing a fragrant aroma

arteriosclerosis an imprecise term for several diseases of the arteries; most often used mistakenly to mean atherosclerosis

asbestosis a lung disease (pneumoconiosis) caused by inhaling asbestos fibers

Aspergillus flavus a species of mold that produces the very toxic substance aflatoxin

asthma a condition characterized by attacks of spasms of the small muscles encircling the airways and release of excessive mucus that plugs them, leading to difficulties in breathing; attacks may be triggered by exposure to numerous sub-

439

stances, either breathed or swallowed, as well as by exertion, emotions, or infections

atherosclerosis a progressive disease of aging in which fatty deposits and scar tissue form on the inner walls of arteries, leading to their narrowing and weakening and eventually limiting blood flow

atmospheric inversion a condition of the lower atmosphere in which the normal rate of reduction of temperature with increasing altitude is reduced; because the normal rising of air currents is prevented, pollutants can build up in a stagnant air layer right above the ground

atomic number the number of protons in the nucleus of an atom, used to uniquely identify an element

atomic weight the number of protons and neutrons in the nucleus of an atom

avicide a poison used to kill birds

background level the level of a substance that is present from all sources of human activity and from all natural sources, but not including the amount from a specified source (such as a nuclear accident or a smokestack release)

background risk the underlying chance of contracting a disease or dying without exposure to a specific substance; the risk due to natural causes alone

bactericide a chemical used to kill bacteria (such as a disinfectant)

barbiturate a drug that depresses the activity of the central nervous system

base (basic) a chemical that, in high enough concentration, can burn and destroy tissue by disrupting chemical bonds between molecules; technically, a base is a hydrogen ion acceptor; a base and an acid are chemical opposites and can neutralize each other

becquerel a unit of activity of radiation; the mass of a radioactive substance that decays at the rate of one atom per second

benthic deep or bottom; benthic organisms are those that live in the mud or other bottom material of lakes, streams, and marine ecosystems

beta decay the disintegration of a radioactive substance in a process that is accompanied by the emission of a beta particle

beta particle (beta ray) an electron that is given off by an unstable radioactive isotope

bioactivate a metabolic process by which a nontoxic chemical is made toxic once inside the body

biocide a chemical that kills various life forms

bioconcentrate (biomagnify; bioaccumulate) the ability of a plant or animal to bring a substance to a higher concentration in its own tissue than is found in its food supply or surrounding air, water, and soil.

biodegradable capable of being decomposed by microorganisms

biomagnification (bioconcentration) the progressive increase in concentration of a substance along a food chain because of the ability of some or all of the individual organisms in the food chain to concentrate the substance

biomagnification factor (bioconcentration factor) the ratio of the concentration of a substance in an organism to that typical of its environment or to that in its food supply

blood–brain barrier the set of membranes surrounding the brain that prevents the passage of harmful substances from the blood to the brain

bottom ash residue from burning that falls through the grates in an incinerator firebox and is collected below

broad spectrum pesticide one that is effective against a wide variety of very different pest species

bronchitis inflammation of the air passages in the respiratory system

cancer potency slope a measure of the increase in cancer risk resulting from an increase in dose; it is determined by assuming that the dose-response relation is linear for any dose between zero (no response) and the lowest dose that tests show causes cancer in laboratory animals

carbamate a group of synthetic pesticides made up of carbon, hydrogen, oxygen, and nitrogen

carboxyhemoglobin (COHb) a substance formed when carbon monoxide combines with red blood cells, which reduces the ability of blood to carry oxygen to the body's tissues

carcinogen a substance capable of causing cancer (carcinogenicity is the ability to cause cancer)

cardiopulmonary having to do with the heart and lungs

catalyst a substance that expedites a chemical reaction (or other process), but is itself not consumed in the process

caustic able to irritate, burn, and destroy tissue

ceiling value (CL) a concentration of a substance that should not be exceeded, even instantaneously

centimeter a unit of length in the metric system that is equal to about 0.4 inch

chemical intermediary a chemical used to make another chemical

chemical pneumonitis inflammation of the walls of the air exchange spaces (alveoli) of the lung caused by inhalation of foreign substances

chloracne a skin disease resembling acne

chloramines gases formed by the reaction of chlorine-containing substances with ammonia; they are able to penetrate to the deep portions of the lung (alveoli) where tissue damage is caused

cholinesterase a crucial enzyme that is involved in the transmission of signals from one nerve fiber to another

chronic bronchitis a condition of excessive mucus secretion and narrowing of the airways, accompanied by cough and breathing difficulties; it is associated with smoking, air pollution, and emphysema and is one of the chronic obstructive pulmonary diseases

chronic effect a disease of gradual onset and long duration; the term does not imply anything about the severity of the disease

chronic exposure an exposure at low concentration but of long duration, typically months or years; technically, an exposure of more than one year

chronic obstructive pulmonary disease (COPD) a group of several lung diseases, often indistinguishable except at autopsy, including chronic bronchitis, small airway disease, and emphysema; the main symptom is breathlessness, sometimes accompanied by a phlegmatic cough, and it is associated with smoking, a wide variety of occupational exposures, and air pollution

chronic toxicity (chronic poisoning) the toxic or poisoning effect of a series of small doses given over a relatively long period of time

cilia small, hairlike projections lining the upper respiratory tract; their rhythmic beating helps to bring dust and other foreign matter up the throat where they are swallowed or coughed out

co-distill the evaporation of a substance along with the liquid in which it is dissolved

coliform bacteria the common microorganism *Escherichia coli* (or *E. coli*) that inhabits the intestinal tracts of humans and other animals; in the gut, the bacteria do not cause disease, but a high coliform count (that is, a large concentration of the bacteria) in drinking water supplies or aquatic ecosystems is often an indicator of pollution

community right-to-know programs informa-tional programs designed to reduce the risk of toxics based on the assumption that an informed public will make the appropriate personal and political decisions that promote health. These programs typically require inventories of hazardous substances found in local businesses and establish procedures for emergency response planning and public education about toxics.

concentration the ratio of the amount of a substance to the amount of the medium it is mixed in; concentrations are usually measured in such units as milligrams per liter (mg/L), milliliters per liter (mL/L), micrograms per cubic meter ($\mu g/m^3$), or parts per million (ppm)

contact (or knockdown) insecticide one that kills or immobilizes insects on contact

cosmic rays particles of radiation that emanate from beyond the earth

criteria data about pollutants compiled from scientific findings and used to set enforceable standards or regulations

curie a unit of radioactivity equal to 37 billion becquerels

daughter in nuclear physics, the isotope formed when a radioactive isotope decays

decay in nuclear physics, the spontaneous breakup of an isotope; also called radioactive decay

decay products all of the particles formed when a radioactive isotope decays; includes the daughter plus particles of radiation

deliquescent able to dissolve in water absorbed from the air, giving the appearance of melting

dementia a persistent disorder of mental processes caused by brain disease; symptoms are losses of memory, personality changes, impaired reasoning ability, disorientation, and deterioration in personal care

dermatitis inflammation of the skin caused by an external agent; the skin is red, itchy, and small blisters may form

detoxification any process in which a toxic is either changed into a harmless form or is removed from the body

DMSO dimethyl sulfoxide; an industrial cleaner that is also used under medical supervision to treat skin inflammation or to improve absorption of drugs applied to the skin

DNA abbreviation for deoxyribonucleic acid, the chemical that makes up genes

dose–response curve (dose–response relation) a graph of relationship between the dose (amount of a toxic substance to which an organism is exposed) and the response (amount of damage that each dose causes); in a typical experiment to determine a dose–response curve, many test animals are exposed to various doses and the amount of damage is taken to be the percentage of animals that come down with a particular disease

dry deposition the settling to the earth's surface of atmospheric aerosol or particulates in dry form, as opposed to their descent in rain or snow

electromagnetic spectrum a continuous sequence of forms of energy that includes X-rays, light waves, heat, and radiowaves; the energy is generated by objects with electric charge, such as electrons, and is transmitted as a wave form whose wavelength determines the specific portion (or energy form) of the spectrum

electrons the very light, negatively charged particles that encircle the nuclei of atoms; the carrier of electrical current in wires and other conductors; the source of the electrical forces that bind molecules

electron volt (eV) a unit used to describe the energy of particles of radiation and equal to about 1/30 of the amount of energy needed to ionize an atom; compared to everyday energies, an electron volt is an incredibly small amount: roughly a trillionth of a trillionth as much as that required to boil a pot of water

element one of the basic building blocks of matter, distinguished from one another by their atomic number

emphysema a lung disease in which the walls of the air sacs (alveoli) are enlarged and damaged, resulting in reduced oxygen exchange and producing breathlessness as the main symptom; one of the chronic obstructive pulmonary diseases caused by tobacco smoke, occupational exposures, and general air pollution

Environmental Protection Agency (EPA) the agency within the executive branch of the federal government charged with setting environmental standards and regulations and enforcing environmental laws

enzyme a chemical produced (or synthesized) by living cells that initiates or accelerates a chemical reaction but is not itself altered by the reaction; enzymes play a crucial role in all of the basic chemical reactions that go on in living organisms

epidemiology the scientific study of the pattern of disease in a population; often epidemiologists seek to determine the causes of disease by looking for a pattern of overlap between those who get a particular disease and those who are exposed to some particular factor, such as an air pollutant, in their environment

fibrosis thickening and scarring of connective tissue, usually the result of injury or inflammation

fission in physics, the splitting of the nucleus of a heavy element to yield energy (in the form of particles of radiation) plus two lighter nuclei that together weigh slightly less than the original one

fission fragments the lighter nuclei produced in the process of fission

fly ash the solid residue from burning that rises out of the firebox; it may be either captured in pollution control devices or released out of the smokestack (*see also* bottom ash)

Food and Drug Administration (FDA) the primary federal agency concerned with the protection of consumer food, drugs, and cosmetics

food chain a hierarchy of the organisms in an ecosystem, organized according to who eats whom

frequency the number of times an event repeats in a fixed time interval; for example, in wave motion, the number of times per second that the peak of the wave passes by a fixed reference point

fuel reprocessing the extraction and purification of useful fissionable material from the radioactive waste produced in a nuclear power plant

fumigant a pesticide that is dispersed as a gas or smoke, often used to disinfect interior spaces

fungicide a chemical designed to kill molds, mildew, and fungi

fusion the joining of the nuclei of two light elements to create energy (in the form of particles of radiation) plus a third element that weighs slightly less than the sum of the first two

gamma rays massless packets of energy associated with the short wavelength, high-energy portion of the electromagnetic spectrum; more energetic than X-rays

gastrointestinal (GI) tract the lower portion of the digestive system, including the stomach and the small and large intestines

gene pool the collection of genes in a population and thus an indicator of the variety of individuals that is possible in future generations

generally recognized as safe (GRAS) food additives that are deemed safe often on the basis of a long history of use rather than rigorous testing

genes segments of DNA that contain the instructions by which the body makes its own molecules; all information about the inherited characteristics of an organism are contained in its genes

gram a metric system unit of mass, equivalent to about 1/28 of an ounce

gray a unit used to describe the amount of energy that radiation deposits in tissue

half-life the time it takes for a quantity to decrease by half; often used to describe how long radioactive isotopes take to disintegrate or pesticides take to break down; halogenated means that a chemical contains one or more halogen atoms

halogens any of the elements bromine, chlorine, fluorine, iodine, astatine

hazardous air pollutants locally (rather than widely) dispersed air pollutants that can cause serious illness or death; regulations exist for arsenic, asbestos, benzene, beryllium, some coke over emissions, mercury, radioactive substances, and vinyl chloride

hemoglobin the protein in blood cells that transports oxygen; it is responsible for the red color of blood

hepatic relating to the liver

herbicide a chemical that kills plants

hydrocarbon a substance that contains a preponderance of hydrogen and carbon atoms, usually of biological origin

hydrosphere all of the water on earth, including surface water, groundwater, glaciers, and water vapor in the atmosphere

hypertension high blood pressure

hypochlorite the active ingredient in bleach

immediately dangerous to life or health (IDLH) the maximum concentration of a toxic for which a 30-minute exposure will not impair ability to escape from the exposure and will not cause irreversible health damage

immune system the body's defense mechanisms against foreign substances, including white blood cells and proteins called antibodies

inert unable to react; stable

inert ingredients components of a chemical product that do not contribute to its efficacy

inflammation the immediate defensive reaction of tissue to injury; it may involve pain, heat, redness, swelling, and the loss of function of the affected part

inorganic not of biological origin; generally a substance without significant carbon content

insecticide a chemical that kills insects

integrated pest management (IPM) a method of pest control that employs a carefully chosen mix of management techniques, with an emphasis on maintaining healthy plants, encouraging natural enemies of the pests, and judicious use of chemical pesticides

intermediate exposure a technical term for exposure to a chemical for a duration between 15 and 365 days

in utero occurring within the uterus

in vitro in isolation from a living organism; artificially maintained, as in a test tube

in vivo within a living organism

ionize to remove or add one or more electrons from an atom or a molecule

ionizing radiation radiation that is capable of ionizing atoms or molecules

ions atoms or molecules that have lost or gained electrons so that they are electrically charged

irritant a material that causes local stress to tissue; typical symptoms include itching, rash, watering eyes, skin thickening, and local minor swelling

isomer one of two or more chemical compounds having the same number of atoms of the same elements in the molecule, but differing in the structural arrangement of the atoms

isotope a particular form of an element; all isotopes of a given element have the same number of protons in their nuclei but differ from one another in the number of neutrons and therefore in atomic weight

juvenile hormone naturally or synthetically produced chemical that regulates insect growth by preventing continued development

kidneys the pair of organs responsible for filtering the blood to remove waste products of metabolism (mainly urea) (*see* renal)

kidney dialysis the filtering of blood in an external machine when the kidneys have failed

kilogram a metric system unit of mass equal to 1000 grams or about 2.2 pounds

latency period the time between exposure to a toxic and the development of discernible effects

LC$_{50}$ the concentration of a toxic substance that kills 50% of the organisms exposed to it; sometimes a time period for exposure to that concentration is specified, as in LC$_{50}$: 7 days

LD$_{50}$ the dose of a toxic substance that kills 50% of the organisms exposed to it; a time period is often specified

leach to dissolve and move substances through soil with percolating water

lesion an abnormal change in the structure of tissue due to injury or disease

linear hypothesis an assumption about how cells or organisms respond to exposure to a toxic; usually thought to be the most conservative model, it assumes that any exposure carries a risk and that the risk is in direct proportion to the duration and degree of the exposure

liter a metric system unit of volume, equal to about 1.06 quarts

lowest observed effect level (LOEL) the lowest dose of a toxic that causes some effect; most testing of toxics is concerned with whether adverse effects occur, so the term lowest observed adverse effect level (LOAEL) is sometimes used instead

lye any of several highly corrosive substances capable of causing caustic burns; lye usually refers to sodium hydroxide

Material Safety Data Sheet (MSDS) a reference form required by OSHA listing certain types of hazardous chemicals found in the workplace and describing precautionary measures

megaton a unit of energy used to describe the energy yield of nuclear weapons, approximately equal to that released by a million tons of TNT

melanoma an often fatal type of skin cancer that can spread quickly to other parts of the body

metabolism all of the biochemical reactions taking place within a cell or an organism; one very important role of metabolism is the breaking down of complex organic compounds to liberate energy and/or create the building blocks used to make other compounds

metabolite (metabolic product) a chemical product of metabolism

meter a metric system unit of length approximately equal to 39.4 inches, slightly over a yard

methemoglobinemia a disease in which blood hemoglobin is converted to a form (methemoglobin) that cannot transport oxygen; the severity of symptoms (fatigue, headache, dizziness, and blue skin) depends on the fraction of hemoglobin affected

micron a metric system unit of length equal to one millionth of a meter or about the diameter of a typical bacterium

microsomal ethanol oxidizing system (MEOS) a set of enzymes that break down alcohol in the body

mole a unit used to express the quantity of a chemical; for example, if a substance has a molecular weight of 50, then a mole of that substance weighs 50 grams; also, Avogadro's number (6.02×10^{23}) of molecules of a substance

molecular weight sum of the atomic weights of all the atoms in a molecule of the substance

moles per liter a unit often used to express the concentration of a dissolved substance in water

monoculture in agriculture, a system of planting vast areas with a single crop such as wheat or cotton

mucous membranes the mucus-secreting lining of many passageways in the body, including the nasal sinuses, respiratory tract, and gastrointestinal tract

mucus a viscous fluid secreted internally by the body that acts as a protective barrier for the surfaces of membranes, as a lubricant, and as a carrier of enzymes

mutagen an external agent able to cause a mutation; various chemicals, forms of radiation, and viruses are mutagens (mutagenicity is the ability to cause mutations)

mutation a change in the genetic material (DNA) of cells; the change can be spontaneous or externally caused, and if it occurs in a developing sex cell (sperm or egg), the mutation may be passed on to the offspring

nasal septum the piece of cartilage that divides the nose into left and right nostrils

natural background level the level of a substance that would occur naturally in the environment if humans were not present

nematicide a poison used specifically to eliminate roundworms

neuritis a disease of the peripheral nerves involving inflammation

neurotoxicity (neurotoxins) the occurrence of adverse effects on the nervous system following exposure to certain chemicals; such chemicals are called neurotoxins

neutral in chemistry, neither acidic nor basic; a pH near 7

neutrons electrically neutral particles that, along with protons, make up the nucleus of an atom

nitric oxides a general term for several air pollutants containing nitrogen and oxygen, usually used when the exact composition is unknown

nitroso a chemical prefix indicating an electrically charged combination of a nitrogen and an oxygen atom; as used in this book, nitroso group combines with various organic compounds to form substances that are known to cause cancer (see entries for **Nitrates, Nitrites,** and **Nitrosamines**)

no observed effect level (NOEL) the highest dose level for which no effects have been observed; most testing of toxics is concerned with determining whether a substance causes no adverse effects, so the term no observed adverse effect level (NOAEL) is sometimes used instead

nuclear wastes the radioactive debris left over in a nuclear reactor after most of the original fuel has undergone fission and released its energy

nucleus (1) in physics, the heavy, central portion of atoms; (2) in biology, the part of the cell that contains the genes

Occupational Safety and Health Administration (OSHA) a U.S. agency responsible for health and safety conditions in the workplace

oncogen a substance capable of producing either cancerous or benign (noncancerous) tumors

organic (organic matter) of biological origin; containing a high proportion of carbon atoms

organically grown food food grown and prepared without synthetic chemicals

organic growers farmers who grow foods without pesticides or other man-made chemicals

organochlorines a group of organic chemicals to which varying amounts of chlorine have been added; organochlorine pesticides can also contain oxygen and sulfur

organophosphate a diverse group of organic chemicals containing phosphorus, oxygen, and sometimes sulfur; because these chemicals interfere with nerve signal transmission, they have been used as pesticides and in chemical weapons

osteoporosis loss of bony tissue resulting in bones that are brittle and susceptible to fracture; occurs in the elderly, particularly in women after menopause

outgas the passage of a gas from a solid to the atmosphere

oxidant an agent capable of causing oxidation

oxidation the process of adding oxygen to a chemical; technically, the process of stripping electrons from molecules, thereby changing their properties and altering chemical reactions and bonds

particulate a small, solid piece of matter that is easily lifted into the air, such as dust or ash; smaller, fine particulates are more hazardous than larger, coarse ones because they are more easily inhaled deep into the lungs

pathogen a microorganism capable of producing a disease

peroxyacetyl nitrate (PAN) a particularly hazardous oxidant that is a constituent of smog

permissable exposure limit (PEL) an allowable exposure level in workplace air; it generally pertains to the average exposure over an 8-hour shift

persistence the tendency of some substances to remain unchanged in soils, water, or living organisms for extended periods of time; persistent substances typically resist biological, chemical, and physical breakdown to less toxic forms and therefore pose a long-term hazard

person-sievert a unit expressing the total radiation dose received by a group of people equal to the number of persons exposed times the average exposure per person

person-sievert per becquerel a unit expressing the total radiation dose that would be received by a group of people if one becquerel of activity were released from a specified source or were present in their environment; the total dose in person-sieverts can be obtained by multiplying by the number of becquerels of activity

pesticide a general term for any chemical poison that kills or otherwise controls unwanted insects, rodents, weeds, or other pests

pH a measure of the relative acidity of a liquid. The pH scale ranges from 0 (most acidic) through 7 (neutral) to 14 (most basic); the scale is logarithmic so that pH 3, for example, is ten times more acidic than pH 4.

phenylketonuria (PKU) a rare, inherited disease in which the body cannot break down phenylalanine, an amino acid, and can result in brain damage

photochemical reaction a chemical process stimulated by sunlight

pigmentation a deposit of a colored (or pigmented) substance in the skin

plume the mass of pollution in the air as it travels downwind from its source; the term is also applied to the movement of water pollution, as in "thermal plume," which is the mass of heated water that travels downstream in a river from where a power plant or factory discharges heated water

pneumoconiosis a lung disease caused by inhaling dust particles small enough (less than about a micron in length) to penetrate deep inside the lung; symptoms often show up several decades after initial exposure

pneumonia an inflammation of the lung caused by bacteria or viruses in which the air sacs (alveoli) fill up with pus so that air is excluded

polycyclic aromatic hydrocarbons (PAHs) highly reactive compounds consisting of hydrogen and carbon atoms arranged in multiple rings

potentiation an interaction between chemicals in which one enhances the toxicity of another

precipitate *verb*: to fall out from, usually referring either to the descent of rain, snow, or pollution from the atmosphere or the settling out of suspended material from water; *noun*: the material that precipitates

primary air quality standards maximum allowable concentrations set by the EPA to protect human health against primary pollutants; the Clean Air Act regulates six primary pollutants: sulfur dioxide, nitrogen oxides, carbon monoxide, ozone, particulates, and lead; also called National Ambient Air Quality Standards

primary water quality treatment removal of solid and suspended wastes in polluted water by filtration and settling, followed by chlorination to kill pathogens

protons positively charged particles that, along with neutrons, make up the nucleus of an atom

pulmonary edema accumulation of excessive fluid in the lungs which can be caused by infection, injury, organ failure, insufficient oxygen at high elevations, or toxic materials

pulmonary fibrosis development of excessive connective tissue in the lungs, causing thickening and stiffening of the walls and leading to breathlessness

quality factor a number assigned to each type of radiation that expresses its effectiveness at causing biological damage

rad a unit of radiation dose, where 100 rads = 1 gray.

radiation the transfer of energy by means of either electromagnetic waves or particles of radiation such as beta particles and alpha particles

radioactive isotope a radioactive form of an element

radioactivity (radioactive) a property of certain types of matter, characterized by the spontaneous transformation of the nuclei of its atoms and the emisson of radiation

radiolytic products chemicals formed when radiation strikes matter

rainout the removal of substances from the atmosphere in rain or snow (*see* wet deposition)

rem a unit of radiation dose that incorporates a measure of the biological effectiveness of the specific type of radiation

renal relating to the kidneys, as in "renal failure"

residue the amount of a pesticide (or of its breakdown or transformation products) that remains in soil, water, living plants, and animals, or in food for human consumption, following normal exposure to air, sunlight, water, and the action of living organisms

resistance ability of an organism to withstand the toxic effects of a chemical or pathogen

respiratory arrest cessation of breathing, usually caused by damage to the nervous system control over the breathing process (as in carbon monoxide poisoning)

response as used here, the reaction of an organism to a toxic substance

restricted pesticides pesticides not available for household use; they can be obtained and used only by trained personnel

resurgence an increase in the population of a pest species following initial suppression of the pest by the use of pesticides

risk a complex evaluation of both the amount of potential damage and the probability of the damage actually occurring

rodenticide a poison used to kill rodents (such as rats and mice)

roentgen a measure of radiation dose that is for all practical purposes roughly equal to a rad; technically, it is a measure of the ionizing potential of a beam of radiation

saturation effect the gradual leveling off of a dose–response curve at high doses which occurs in animal tests of toxics because at high doses (where a large fraction of the test animals have already exhibited a response to the dose), the response can no longer keep increasing with increasing dose

secondary air pollutants see **hazardous air pollutants**

secondary air quality standards regulations that apply to **hazardous air pollutants**

secondary outbreaks increases in the size of the populations of normally minor pests as a result of inappropriate pesticide use

secondary treatment of water use of biological processes, particularly bacterial transformations, to accelerate the decomposition of organic wastes in polluted water; if used subsequently to primary treatment, the chlorination step in primary treatment must be avoided

selective pesticide one that is effective against a limited number of species and is not toxic to most

sequester to take up and store for a long time

short-term exposure limit (STEL) the maximum concentration to which workers can be exposed for up to 15 consecutive minutes

sick building syndrome buildings whose indoor air is heavily contaminated with pollutants

sievert a unit of radiation dose that incorporates a measure of the biological potency of the specific type of radiation

silicosis pneumoconiosis caused by inhaling fine silica dust

small airway disease inflammation of the smallest airways of the lung (bronchioles), reducing the amount of air reaching the air exchange spaces (alveoli); one of the chronic obstructive pulmonary diseases

smelter (smelting) a factory that extracts a metal from its ore in a roasting process which usually uses coal burning

smog a complex collection of chemicals formed in the atmosphere from reactions between nitrogen oxides and hydrocarbons

sodium hypochlorite the most common form of the active ingredient in bleach

soluble able to dissolve in a liquid

solvent a liquid capable of dissolving other substances

Special Review a process undertaken by the EPA to reevaluate an in-use pesticide as a result of new evidence questioning the safety of the substance

sulfiting agents any of several sulfur-based preservatives added to foods

Superfund a federal trust fund used for cleaning up toxic waste sites

synergism a synergistic interaction of two or more substances

synergistic a reaction in which the effect of two (or more) substances acting together is greater than the sum of their separate effects

systemic refers to the whole body, rather than a single organ or tissue

systemic pesticide one that is taken up by the roots or leaves of plants and then transported to various parts of the plant where it is eventually ingested by the pest

target organ the specific organ or tissue that is harmed by exposure to a toxic substance; it is not necessarily the organ with the highest concentration of the toxic

teratogen a substance that causes birth defects (teratogenicity is the ability to cause birth defects)

tertiary water treatment use of a wide variety of chemical, physical, and biological techniques to remove organic matter, nitrogen, phosphorus, and metals from waste water; in some situations it can produce recycled water fit for direct human use

threshold dose a transition level of a dose; below the threshold, biological damage is slight, while above it, damage increases rapidly with dose

threshold effect an effect that occurs when a toxic causes an especially small response at low doses because the exposed organism can repair the damage from low doses. Above the threshold dose, the response increases more sharply with increasing dose because the repair mechanisms are overwhelmed

threshold limit value (TLV) a concentration of a substance to which most workers can be exposed without adverse effect; may be expressed as a ceiling limit, a short-term exposure limit, or a time-weighted average

time weighted average (TWA) an allowable exposure concentration averaged over a normal 8-hour workday or a 40-hour work week

tolerance (1) the capacity to withstand a toxic dose without adverse effects on normal growth or function; (2) the maximum residue concentration of a pesticide that is legally allowed in raw agricultural products, processed foods, or animal feed products

toxicity (1) the harmful effects produced by a substance; (2) the capacity of a substance to cause any adverse effects, as based on scientifically verifiable data from animal tests or epidemiology

toxicology the scientific study of the adverse effects of chemicals on living systems, usually by controlled laboratory or clinical investigations

translocation the movement of a substance (for example, pesticides, nutrients, or metals) from one part of a plant to another, as from roots to leaves

trihalomethanes (THMs) cancer-causing chemicals formed during the chlorination of water; each contains one carbon atom, one hydrogen atom, and some combination of three halogen atoms (fluorine, chlorine, bromine, or iodine); the most common form is chloroform

ulcer a break in the skin or in the mucous membrane lining the digestive tract that fails to heal (ulceration is the process of ulcer formation)

ultraviolet (UV) radiation (ultraviolet light) a form of high-energy, invisible light; a portion of the electromagnetic spectrum of shorter wavelength than visible light and capable of inflicting tissue damage

volatile easily converted from the liquid state to

the gaseous under ordinary conditions and therefore capable of rapid dispersal

volatile organic compounds (VOCs) carbon-containing substances, released by both natural processes and human activities that readily produce fumes; their reaction with nitrogen oxides in the presence of sunlight produces photochemical smog; sometimes called reactive organic compounds (ROG)

wavelength the distance between two successive peaks in a wave form; in the electromagnetic spectrum, shorter wavelengths correspond to higher energies

welfare used here to mean the protection of harm to soil, water, crops, natural ecosystems, visibility, climate, and materials of human origin

wet deposition rain, snow, hail, or sleet; the removal of pollution from the atmosphere in such precipitation

whole body dose a radiation dose calculated by dividing the energy of radiation deposited anywhere in the body by the mass of the whole body

X-rays a type of radiation; a high-energy component of the electromagnetic spectrum that has many applications in medicine and industry, but is also capable of inflicting biological damage

Commonly Used Abbreviations for Units

Abbreviation	Unit
Length	
km	kilometer
m	meter
cm	centimeter
mm	millimeter
μm	micron
Å	angstrom
Volume	
L (or l)	liter
m^3	cubic meter
ml	milliliter
cm^3 (or cc)	cubic centimeter
Weight or mass	
kg	kilogram
g	gram
mg	milligram
μg	microgram
ng	nanogram
t	ton (English)
T	tonne (metric)
lb	pound
oz	ounce

Abbreviation	Unit
Concentration	
ppth	parts per thousand
ppm	parts per million
ppb	parts per billion
ppt	parts per trillion
mg/L	milligrams per liter
mg/kg	milligrams per kilogram
μg/ml	micrograms per milliliter
μg/m^3	micrograms per cubic meter
ng/cm^3	nanograms per cubic centimeter
mol/L	moles per liter
Radiation dose or activity	
Gy	gray
Sv	sievert
rad	rad
R	roentgen
Bq	becquerel
Ci	Curie
Energy	
MeV	million electron volt
keV	kilo-electron-volt
eV	electron volt

Abbreviations for Environmental Laws and Institutions

ACGIH   American Conference of Governmental and Industrial Hygienists

ASHRAE   American Society of Heating, Refrigerating, and Air-conditioning Engineers

CAA   Clean Air Act

CERCLA   Comprehensive Environmental Response, Compensation, and Liability Act

CPSC   Consumer Product Safety Commission

CWA   Clean Water Act

DOE   U.S. Department of Energy

EDF   Environmental Defense Fund

EPA   Environmental Protection Agency

EPCRA   Emergency Planning and Community Right-to-Know Act

FDA   Food and Drug Administration

FDCA   Food, Drug, and Cosmetic Act

FIFRA   Federal Insecticide, Fungicide, and Rodenticide Act

MPRSA   Marine Protection, Research, and Sanctuaries Act

NAS   National Academy of Sciences

NIH   National Institutes of Health

NIOSH   National Institute of Occupational Safety and Health

NRC   Nuclear Regulatory Commission

NRDC   Natural Resources Defense Council

NTIS   National Technical Information Service

OSHA   Occupational Safety and Health Administration (and the Occupational Safety and Health Act)

OTA   Office of Technology Assessment

RCRA   Resource Conservation and Recovery Act

SARA   Superfund Amendments and Reauthorization Act

SDWA   Safe Drinking Water Act

TSCA   Toxic Substances Control Act

Annotated Suggested Readings

ARBUCKLE, J. G., et al. 1991. *Environmental Law Handbook*. 11th edition. Rockville, MD: Government Institutes Inc.

An excellent summary of the major environmental laws and regulations, with clear and useful explanations of some of the more confusing aspects of these laws.

Earthworks Group, 1989. *50 Simple Things You Can Do To Save the Earth*. Berkeley, CA: Earthworks Press.

For those who want to do something about reducing environmental hazards, this slim and readable book provides sensible suggestions.

EHRLICH, P. R., EHRLICH, A. H., and HOLDREN, J. P. 1977. *Ecoscience*. San Francisco: W. H. Freeman and Co.

This excellent text provides authoritative and detailed discussions of many of the toxic threats facing humanity. It is also a useful introduction to the broader field of environmental science.

FRIBERG, L., NORDBERG, G. F., and VOUK, V. B., editors. 1986. *Handbook on the Toxicology of Metals*. New York: Elsevier.

International experts provide chapters on the metals of their specialty, covering all the metals in this book and many more, as well as providing information on the regulations adopted in most industrialized countries.

GOSSELIN, R. E., SMITH, R. P., and HODGE, H. C., editors. 1984. *Clinical Toxicology of Commercial Products*. 5th edition. Baltimore, MD: Williams and Wilkins.

While somewhat dated, this book is still a rich source of information about exposures and effects of toxic substances as they are found in commercial products (brand names often included). Extensive descriptions of symptoms and treatments are given.

HARTE, J. 1988. *Consider a Spherical Cow: A Course in Environmental Problem Solving*. Mill Valley, CA: University Science Books.

Readers who want to learn how to estimate for themselves the seriousness of a wide range of environmental problems should consult this book. The step-by-step approach to teaching how to make "back-of-the-envelope" calculations will appeal to those who fear math but want to overcome that.

HAYES, W. J., Jr. 1982. *Pesticide Studies in Man*. Baltimore, MD: Williams and Wilkins.

Written by a physician, this book is useful for those who want to know more about how results of laboratory tests provide information on the human health effects of pesticides. Because a considerable amount of information has become available since the 1982 publication date, it should be supplemented by reading more recent studies.

KLASSEN, C. D., AMDUR, M. O., and DOULL, J., editors. 1986. *Casarett and Doull's Toxicology: The Basic Science of Poisons*. 3d edition. New York: Macmillan Publishing Co.

An excellent and comprehensive textbook, covering the general principles of toxicology and the toxic effects of many of the substances discussed in this book—highly recommended.

LAVE, L. B., and UPTON, A. C., editors. 1987. *Toxic Chemicals, Health, and the Environment.* Baltimore, MD: Johns Hopkins University Press.

This book provides a useful overview of how toxic chemicals are managed in the United States: subjects include managing chemicals in the environment, principles of toxicology, toxic waste clean-up techniques, and public policy issues.

MOTT, L., and SNYDER, K. 1987. *Pesticide Alert.* San Francisco: Sierra Club Books.

Derived from a study by the Natural Resources Defense Council, this book gives a concise summary of the pesticides most commonly found in foods.

National Academy of Sciences, 1987. *Regulating Pesticides in Food: The Delaney Paradox.* Washington, D.C.: National Academy Press.

Although narrowly focused on pesticides in food, this book provides good discussions of risk assessment (including the EPA's methods of evaluating risk) and the problems associated with current pesticide use.

SAX, I. N. 1984. *Dangerous Properties of Industrial Materials.* New York: Van Nostrand–Reinhold.

Containing brief descriptions of the toxic properties of thousands of chemicals used in industry, this book is a useful place to go for information about substances not covered here.

VANDER, A. J. 1981. *Nutrition, Stress, and Toxic Chemicals: An Approach to Environmental Health Controversies.* Ann Arbor, MI: The University of Michigan Press.

Using simple but vivid language and real-life examples of health controversies, the author describes the relationship of the human body to its environment, emphasizing the effects of stress, nutrition, and toxic chemicals on the workings of the body.

Sources for Home Testing Equipment

Air

Radon: Test kits are available in many hardware stores, department stores, and even supermarkets. If they cannot be found, contact your state department of environmental protection for a list of companies whose kits have been approved by the EPA. See the article, "Radon: The Problem No One Wants To Face," in the October 1989 issue of *Consumer Reports* for a description of testing procedures and a list of state toll-free numbers. The best time to test is in winter, when the house is closed up.

Asbestos: Contact your state department of environmental protection for a list of state-approved asbestos contractors. While many contractors can identify asbestos by sight, measuring airborne fibers and removing asbestos requires special equipment and training.

Formaldehyde: Contact Air Technology Corporation, 815 Harbour Way South, Richmond, CA 94804, or Dosimeter Corporation, 6106 Interstate Circle, Cincinnati, OH 45242.

Water

See "Fit To Drink?" in *Consumer Reports*, January 1990, for a discussion of water safety, water testing, and water purification equipment.

Local: Consult the Yellow Pages for state-certified water testing laboratories.

Mail-order: Contact WaterTest, 33 South Commercial Street, Manchester, NH 03101 (phone 1-800-426-8378); National Testing Laboratories, 6151 Wilson Mills Road, Cleveland, OH 44143 (phone 1-800-458-3330); or Suburban Water Testing Laboratories, 4600 Kutztown Road, Temple, PA 19560 (phone 1-800-433-6595).

Metals

Lead in ceramic ware: A kit is available from Frandon Enterprises, Inc., 511 North 48th, Seattle, WA 98103.

Hair testing for metals and minerals: Contact American Mineral Society, P.O. Box 35249, Phoenix, AZ 85069.

Sulfites

A portable kit for use in restaurants is available from Center Laboratories, 35 Channel Drive, Port Washington, NY 11050.

National Hotlines

Poison Control Center

Every state in the United States has at least one poison control center that will help during a poisoning emergency. The closest poison control center number is usually listed in the front pages of the local telephone directory. Take the time now to locate this number. Write it down in a place that is visible from the telephone. For future reference, the number can be written down here as well.

Toll-Free Lines

American Chemical
Society   1-800-424-6767

Asbestos Hotline   1-800-334-8571,
                                       ext. 6741

The Asbestos Hotline provides information about asbestos abatement problems. The hotline operates Monday through Friday from 8:15 A.M. to 5:00 P.M. Eastern Standard Time.

Chemical Manufacturers
Association Chemical
Referral Center   1-800-262-8200

This is a telephone referral system, run by the chemical industry that helps callers answer questions about the toxic properties of consumer products. Operators will help callers make contact with chemical manufacturers. The hotline operates from 8 A.M. to 9 P.M. Eastern Standard Time.

Community Right-   1-800-535-0202
to-Know   or 1-202-479-2449

This EPA group responds to questions about community preparedness and chemical accidents, as well as to questions about how to get further information about toxic chemical releases in specific communities.

Consumer Product
Safety Commission   1-800-638-2772
                 Maryland   1-800-492-8363
      Alaska or Hawaii   1-800-638-8333

Food Safety and Inspec-
tion Service Meat and
Poultry Hotline   1-800-535-4555

This hotline is operated by the Food and Drug Administration to answer questions regarding meat and poultry contamination, grading, and recommended storage procedures.

National Pesticides
Telecommunications   1-800-858-7378
Network   1-806-743-3091

The National Pesticides Telecommunications Network provides information about pesticide products, basic safety procedures, basic safety practices, health and environmental effects, and clean-up and disposal practices. Run out of Texas Tech University Health Sciences Center, this hotline operates 24 hours a day, 7 days a week.

RCRA/Superfund   1-800-424-9346
Hotline   1-202-382-3000

This is the EPA's largest and busiest hotline. Call about questions and documentation related to Superfund regulations and clean-up operations. Hours are 8:30 A.M. to 4:30 P.M. Eastern Standard Time.

Safe Drinking Water   1-800-426-4791

This hotline is operated by the EPA to answer questions about water contamination and the laws regulating water pollution.

Toll Hot Lines

Arts, Crafts, and Theater
Safety   1-212-777-0062

This group answers questions about the toxic properties of art and craft materials.

Index

Bold-faced page numbers indicate entry of toxic in Part Two: A Guide to Commonly Encountered Toxics.

Acaricides
definition of, 112
malathion as, 339
types of, 115–118
Acceptable daily intake (ADI), for pesticides, 124–125
Accidents
chlorine spills from, 270–272
deaths caused by, 14
nuclear, 263, 329, 386
pollution released from environmental ones, 23
risk from, 6
Acetic acid, **197–199**
in foods, 197
Acetone, 39, **198–199**
hazards of high concentrations of, 199
as inert ingredient, 67
as solvent, 109
use in fingernail polish remover, 198–199
Acid rain
and aluminum, 210, 213
causes of, 96
chemistry of, 80
damage to materials from, 99
and forest dieback, 96, 99
formation of, 97
as human health hazard, 99
nitric acid in, 366–367
particulate matter and, 381
salamander's sensitivity to, 89
and smokestack plumes, 78
solutions to, 99–100
sulfur dioxide in formation of, 407, 409
Acids
in acid rain, 80, 96
pH of, 98
Acrolein, **200–201**
Acroosteolysis, 431
Active ingredients, definition of, 115
Active transport, definition of, 38
Activity (radiation), definition of, 148
Acute dose
definition of, 16
of radiation, 151
to target organ, 37

Acute effects, definition of, 28–29
Acute exposure, definition of, xi
Acutely Hazardous Materials Risk Management Act, 191
Acute poisoning, by metals, 104
Acute respiratory effects, of air pollution, 47–48
Acute toxicity
of acrolein, 200
of aldicarb, 206
of aldrin/dieldrin, 208–209
of azinophos-methyl, 228
of dichlorvos, 293
of EDB, 304
EPA guidelines of, 31
of HCH/lindane, 337
of heptachlore, 326
of parathion, 376
of 2,4,5-T, 412
of xylene, 435
Adhesives
methyl ethyl ketone in, 344
toluene in, 415
Aerosols
CFCs used as propellants, 266, 267
definition of, 21, 77
methylene chloride as propellant in, 346, 347
trichloroethane as propellant of, 418
Aflatoxins, 62, **201–203**
as natural food contaminant, 64
nutritional causes for susceptibility to, 43
in nuts and grains, 201–202
in peanut butter, 7
potency of, 30
as potent natural carcinogen, 202
Age, and sensitivity to toxics, 41
Agent Orange, used in Vietnam War, 296, 411
Agricultural inspection, to control pest movements, 135–136
Agriculture
and aflatoxin occurrence, 201–202
ammonia use in fertilizers, 214–215
azinophos-methyl use in, 227
captafol use in, 250–251
cultivation techniques to control

pests, 134–135
2,4-D use in, 281
exposure of pesticides to workers in, 121–123
herbicide use in, 118–119
and loss of pest predators by pesticides, 128
nitrogen fertilizers used in, 360
paraquat use in, 375
parathion use in, 376–378
pesticides use in, 127–130
pesticide use in, 112–113
Air
chloroform in, 274
EDB and EDC in, 303–304
lead in, 335
movement of toxics through, 77–81
sound vibrations in, 368
testing equipment for, 453
Airborne toxics, 78–79
Air conditioners, CFCs in vehicular, 266
Air pollution
acute respiratory effects from, 47–48
asthma from, 47
cadmium in, 245
chemistry of, 80–81
chronic respiratory effects from, 48
and deposition of pollutants, 79–80
hazardous, 175
health hazards of, 47–50
lung cancer from, 11, 49
and movement of toxics, 77–81
nonrespiratory effects of, 49
regulation of, 175–176
units of, 21–22
Air pollution (indoor)
and carbon monoxide, 257
from dry cleaning, 413–414
formaldehyde in, 318–319
nitrogen dioxide in, 365
radon in, 391–392
reduction of, 53–54
sources of, 51–53
tetrachloroethylene in, 413
Air pollution (outdoor)
benzene as, 234

carbon monoxide as, 257
chromium as, 276
damage to forests from, 374
nitrogen oxides in, 365–366
particulate matter in, 379–381
reduction of lead in, 333–335
sulfur dioxide in, 407, 408
tetrachloroethylene in, 413
toluene in, 416
vinyl chloride in, 430
Air quality
improvement in, 176
protection of, 175–176
Air Toxic "Hot Spots" Information
and Assessment Act, 191
Alachlor, **203–205**
as human carcinogen, 204
as pesticide, 124
Alar
breakdown to UDMH, 283, 284
as pesticide, 124
use on apples, 283, 284
withdrawal from market of, 284
Alcohol dehydrogenase (ADH),
definition of, 63
Alcoholic beverages
and carbon tetrachloride, 64
deaths caused by, 14
and EBDC toxicity, 301–302
and enzymes, 38, 42
hazards from, 63–64
and sensitivity to toxics, 41–42
and xylene toxicity, 63–64, 435
Aldicarb, **205–207**
environmental effects of, 206–207
use on watermelons, 123
as very toxic pesticide, 205
Aldrin, **207–209**
acute toxicity of, 208–209
as insecticide, 116
Alfalfa, planted to control lygus
bug, 135
Aliphatic compounds, definition of,
108
Alkali disease, 397
Alkaloids, in potatoes, 136
Allergen, definition of, 41
Allergic reaction
definition of, 40
to inert ingredients, 67–68
to permethrin, 389
to sulfites, 406
Alpha rays
definition of, 142
effects on human body of, 144–
145, 148
and quality factor, 148
Aluminum, **210–213**
in acid rain, 99
and Alzheimer's disease, 57, 210,
211–212
in drinking water, 57, 211
environmental levels of, 211, 212
in food, 210

in fosetyl Al, 322
harm to wildlife from, 89
hazards from, 210–213
reducing consumption of, 212–
213
as toxic metal, 104
Alveoli
definition of, 35
particles in, 35
Alzheimer's disease, and aluminum,
57, 210, 211–212
Americium, as radioactive element,
386, 387
Ames, Bruce, 64
Ames test
criticism of, 65–66
definition of, 64
Ammonia, **214–217**
concentrations in various media,
216
hazards of mixing with bleach,
214–215, 271, 272
hazards of mixing with lye, 214–
215
health effects of concentrations
of, 216
as produced by petrochemical
industry, 106
regulated under CWA, 177
spill hazards of, 214–215
transformed in soil, 83
Anemia, and benzene, 234
Aneurysm, 8
Animals
sensitivity to toxics, 89
toxic concentrations build up in,
86–88
See also Wildlife
Antabuse, 300
Antacids, aluminum in, 210
Antarctica, ozone layer depletion
over, 94
Anthropogenic sources, of radiation, 149–150
Antibodies, in allergic reactions, 41
Anticoagulant, 433
Antifreeze, ethylene glycol in, 306–
307
Antioxidant
BHT and BHA as, 241
selenium as, 396
Ants, safe control of in home, 138
Aphids
reproduction of, 129
resistance to pesticides of, 131
Apple juice, Alar concentration in,
283
Apples
Alar use on, 283
pesticides found on, 124
AP seal, 68
Aquatic systems, 2,4,5-T damage
to, 412

Aquifers
definition of, 59
EDB and EDC accumulate in, 303
movement of toxics through, 82–
83
pollution of, 59
Aromatic hydrocarbon
benzene as, 233
definition of, 108, 233
toluene as, 415
xylene as, 435
Arsenic, **217–221**
in air pollution, 49
from arts and crafts, 68
as cause of lung cancer, 11
concentrations in various media,
220
exposure to, 219
in groundwater, 56
and lung and skin cancers, 218,
220
as pesticide, 113
regulation of, 184
as toxic metal, 104
as toxic product of incineration,
165
uses of, 217
Arteries, diseases of, 8–10
Arts
hazards from materials of, 68–69
reduction of hazards from, 68–69
Asbestos, 19, 41, **222–224**
in air pollution, 49
from arts and crafts, 68
cancer risk from, 222–224
as cause of lung cancer, 11, 27–28
as example of epidemiology
study, 27
indoor air pollution from, 51
as regulated by CAA, 175
as regulated by TSCA, 180
test for presence of, 350
and workplace right to know, 189
Asbestosis, definition of, 35, 223
Ash
beryllium in, 239
cadmium in, 244–245
hazards of, 165
Asian restaurants, monosodium
glutamate used by, 351
Aspartame, **225–226**
Asphalt, **226–227**
Aspirin
aluminum in, 210–211
and heart disease, 9
Asthma
definition of, 47
and ozone (pollution), 373
from particulate pollution, 380
from sulfites, 406
from sulfur dioxide, 408, 409
Atherosclerosis
as caused by cigarette smoking,
50

definition of, 8
Atlantic Ocean, PCBs in, 383
Atmosphere
    deposition of pollutants from, 79–80
    movement of toxics through, 77–81
    and protection of air quality, 175–176
Atmospheric chemistry, definition of, 80
Atmospheric inversions
    definition of, 77–78
    nitrogen oxides in, 365
    and ozone, 372
    and plumes, 79
    as trap for pesticide vapors, 122
Atmospheric pollution, see Air pollution
Atomic number, definition of, 141
Atomic weight, definition of, 141
Atoms, definition of, 141
Automobiles
    ethylene glycol use in, 306–307
    units of exhaust from, 22
    vinyl chloride in new, 431
Avicides, definition of, 112
Azinophos-methyl, **227–229**
AZT, 182

B[a]P, see Benzo[a]pyrene
Bacillus thuringiensis, 118, 134, 254
Background radiation
    definition of, 149
    See also Natural background radiation
Background risk
    and cancer, 17
    definition of, 15
Bacon, nitrites in, 360
Bacteria, as contaminants in drinking water, 56
Bactericides, definition of, 112
Bananas, aldicarb banned on, 207
Barbiturates, and alcohol use, 63
Barium, **229–230**
    in groundwater, 56
    muscle effects of, 230
Batteries
    cadmium in, 244, 246
    mercury hazards from, 342
BCEE, 243–244
BCME. See Bis(chloromethyl)ether
Beans, dicamba toxicity to, 290
Becquerel (Bq), definition of, 148
Beer, sulfur dioxide use in, 407
Beets, aldrin/dieldrin in, 209
Behavior, lead effects on, 334
Benefits, versus risk, 6
Benokmyl, as pesticide, 124
Benomyl, **231–232**
    as fungicide, 119
    toxicity to wildlife, 232

Benzene, **233–235**
    from arts and crafts, 68
    as cause of leukemia, 49
    prevention of toxicity from, 43
    as regulated by CAA, 175
    ring structure of, 233
    as solvent, 109
    toluene substitute for, 415
    use in petrochemical industry, 108
    as volatile, 81
Benzo[a]pyrene, **236–238**
    in air pollution, 49, 51
    as cause of lung cancer, 11
    in tobacco smoke, 51
Berylliosis, definition of, 239
Beryllium, **238–240**
    as cause of lung cancer, 104
    concentrations of, 240
    lung hazards from, 239
    as regulated by CAA, 175
    as toxic product of incineration, 165
Beta particles, from strontium-90, 401
Beta rays
    definition of, 142
    effects on human body of, 144–145, 148
    and quality factor, 148
BHA, **241–242**
    as food additives, 62, 241–242
    possible benefits from, 241–242
Bhopal, India, Union Carbide disaster, 190
BHT, **241–242**
    as food additives, 62, 241–242
    possible benefits from, 241–242
Binding, of toxics to blood proteins, 36–37
Bioaccumulation. See Bioconcentration
Bioactivation, 37, 41
    and barbiturates, 63
    definition of, 37
Biocide, chlorine as, 272
Bioconcentration
    of benzo[a]pyrene, 236
    of chlorinated hydrocarbons, 116
    of DDT, 286, 287–288
    definition of, 82, 86
    and food chain, 86–88
    illustrated, 87
    of mercury in fish, 341, 343
    of naphthalene, 353
    of nickel, 356
    of solvents, 111
"Biodegradable" plastics, 168–169
Biodegradable products, 169
Biological control
    of pest species, 133–134
    problems with, 136–137
    use in home gardens, 137–139
Biomagnification
    definition of, 86

    See also Bioconcentration
Biorational control
    of pest species, 133–134
    problems with, 136–137
Biosphere, toxics in, 86–90
Birds
    DDT bioconcentrated in, 88, 286, 287
    diazinon toxicity to, 290
    eggshell thinning from DDT in, 286, 287, 288
Birth defects
    caused by solvents, 110, 111
    EBDCs causing, 301
    from ELF fields, 311
    from malathion, 339
    vinyl chloride as cause of, 431
    warfarin causing, 434
Bis(chloromethyl)ether, **243–244**
Bitumen, definition of, 226
Bladder cancer, 13
Bleach
    chlorine in, 270–271
    dioxin as by-product of, 296–297
    hazards of mixing with ammonia, 214–215, 271, 272
    hazards of mixing with vinegar, 271, 272
    nontoxic types of, 167
Blind staggers, 397
Blood
    filtered by kidneys, 39
    lead effects on, 334
    MSG effects on, 352
    solvents damage to, 110
    toxics in, 36–37
Blood-brain barrier, definition of, 39
Blood clotting, warfarin used to prevent, 433
Bloodstream
    distribution of toxics by, 36–37
    uptake of toxics into, 36
Bodily uptake
    and acute toxicity classification, 31
    of pollutants, 22–23
    of toxics, 34–43
Body. See Human body
Body membranes. See Membranes
Boll weevil, resurgence of, 131
Bollworm
    controlled by IPM, 132
    resurgence of, 131–132
Bologna, nitrites in, 360
Bone
    cadmium hazards to, 246
    plutonium damage to, 387
    storage of toxics in, 37
    strontium-90 in, 401
    vinyl chloride effects on, 431
Bone cancer, from stronium-90, 401
Bone marrow, cesium-137 destruction of, 264

Botanical insecticides
    definition of, 118
    success of, 118
Bottom ash, 165
    PCBs in, 384
Botulism
    definition of, 359
    nitrates/nitrites protection from,
        359, 360
Brain, 39
    aluminum effects on, 212
    carbon monoxide effects on, 258
    lead damage to, 333
    mercury damage to, 341–342
    stimulation by aspartame, 225
Brake fluid, ethylene glycol in, 306–
    307
Breast cancer
    deaths from, 11, 12–13
    and oral contraceptives, 13
    protection from, 12–13
Breast milk
    pesticides in, 120
    strontium-90 in, 401
    toxics that accumulate in, 40
Breathing
    of asbestos fibers, 222
    of toxics, 34–35
    uptake of solvents by, 110
    See also Inhalation
Breeder reactors, 386
British units, examples of, 19–20
Broad spectrum pesticides
    carbaryl as, 253
    damage from, 136
    definition of, 115
Bromine, in TRIS, 423
Bronchitis
    as caused by cigarette smoking, 50
    from particulate pollution, 380
    See also Chronic bronchitis
Burglar alarms, ultrasound used in,
    426
Burning
    benzo[a]pyrene given off by, 236
    carbon monoxide from, 257
    of wastes, 164–165
Burns
    from ammonia, 214–215
    from microwaves and radio
        waves, 348
    from ultraviolet radiation, 429

CAA. See Clean Air Act (CAA)
Cadmium, 37, **244–247**
    in air pollution, 49
    from arts and crafts, 68
    as cause of lung cancer, 11
    concentrations of, 247
    and the kidneys, 104
    nutritional causes for susceptibil-
        ity to, 43
    and prostate cancer, 13
    in tobacco smoke, 51

    as toxic metal, 104
    as toxic product of incineration,
        165
    units in water, 20
    uses of, 244
    in wastes, 163
Caffeine, **248–250**
    and cancer, 249
    during pregnancy, 249
    effect on nervous system, 248
    as food additive, 62
    sleep disturbances from, 248
Caffeinism, definition of, 249
Calabrese, Edward, 43
Calcium, lead binding to, 37
California
    aldicarb use in, 205–207
    DBCP in, 121
    farmworkers exposed to pesticides
        in, 122–123
    overuse of pesticides in, 131–132
    and Proposition 65, 192
    right-to-know innovations in,
        189, 190, 191–192
California Public Interest Research
    Group (CALPIRG), 167
Cancer
    and acrolein, 200
    and aflatoxins, 202–203
    and Alar, 283, 284
    and Ames test, 30, 64–66
    and arsenic, 218, 220
    and benomyl, 231
    and benzo[a]pyrene, 236–237
    and beryllium, 240
    breast, 12–13
    and captan/captafol/folpet, 251
    as cause of death, 10–14
    caused by food, 64–66
    caused by solvents, 110, 111
    in children from ELF fields, 311
    and chloroform, 274–275
    and chromium, 278
    as chronic effect from toxic met-
        als, 104–105
    colon and rectal, 11–12
    cure rate of, 10
    deaths from, 8, 151
    and Delaney Clause, 62, 182
    and dioxin, 297–298
    and EDB, 304–305
    and epidemiology studies, 28
    and ethylene oxide, 308
    and ETU, 301–302
    and food additives, 62
    and formaldehyde, 319–320
    and heptachlor, 326
    linked to pesticide use, 121
    of lungs, 49
    and magnitude of risk, 7
    and methylene chloride, 347
    and natural versus synthetic pes-
        ticides, 65
    and nickel, 355

    and nitrosamines, 359, 363
    and OSHA regulations, 180–181
    from particulate pollution, 380
    and plastic manufacturing, 69
    from plutonium, 387
    prevention of, 10
    and radiation dose, 151
    from radon, 391
    risk of, 5
    and saccharin, 394
    stages of, 10–11
    statistics for United States, 12
    and synthetic food dyes, 316
    and tetrachloroethylene, 414
    time to develop, 41
    and toxic substances, 13–14
    and TRIS, 422–423
    vinyl chloride as cause of, 431
Captafol, **250–252**
    as fungicide, 119
Captan, **250–252**
    as carcinogenic pesticide, 124
    as fungicide, 119
Carageenan, **262**
Carbamate insecticide, 116–118
    aldicarb as, 205
    carbaryl as, 253
    EBDCs as, 300
    environmental effects of, 117–118
    human health effects of, 117
Carbaryl, **253–255**
    toxicity to honeybees, 254
Carbendazim, 232
Carbofuran, 118
Carbon, atom illustrated, 142
Carbon black, **255–256**
    and PAH hazards, 256
Carbon dioxide
    and greenhouse effect, 91
    and indoor air pollution, 51
Carbon monoxide, 21, **257–259**
    as cause of heart disease, 49
    hazards from, 257–258
    methylene chloride decomposes
        to, 346
    as regulated by CAA, 175
    sources of, 257
Carbon tetrachloride, **260–261**
    and alcoholic beverages, 64
    in depletion of ozone layer, 111
    as inert ingredient, 67
Carboxyhemoglobin (COHb),
    257–258
Carcinogen, 28
    in air pollution, 49
    alachlor as, 204
    asbestos as, 223
    benzene as, 234
    definition of in humans, 29, 32
    EPA classification system of,
        31–32
    high risk versus low risk, 182
    no safe dose of, 30
    pesticides as, 124

and Proposition 65, 192
in tobacco smoke, 51
Cardboard
  dioxin in bleached, 296
  recycling of, 168
Cardiovascular diseases, 8–10
Carpet, indoor air pollution from, 51, 53
Carpet cleaner
  tetrachloroethylene in, 413
  trichloroethylene in, 420
Carrier chemicals, definition of, 38–39
Carrots
  aldrin/dieldrin in, 209
  DDT on, 125, 286
Cars. *See* Automobiles
Carson, Rachel, 114
Catalysts, definition of, 80
Category III toxic, definition of, 31–32
Category II toxic, definition of, 31–32
Category I toxic, definition of, 31–32
Category IV toxic, definition of, 31–32
Cathode ray tubes, 310
Caustic chemicals, 34, 36
Caution label, 31–32
Central Valley (California), selenium pollution in, 397
Ceramics
  hazards from glazes of, 68
  lead in, 333
CERCLA, provisions of, 172, 185
Cervical cancer, 13
Cesium-137, **263–265**
  from Chernobyl nuclear accident, 263, 265
  exposure to, 263–265
  as nuclear fission fragment, 146
  released from Chernobyl, 78
CFCs, **265–268**
  Montreal Protocol to limit, 96
  and ozone layer depletion, 95–96, 265–266, 267
  reducing use of, 266–267
  regulation of, 267
  restricted under FFDCA, 182
  as solvent, 109
  in styrene cups, 71
  use of, 95–96
  use in refrigeration, 265–266
Cheeses, aluminum in, 210
Chemical industry. *See* Petrochemical industry
Chemicals
  California regulation of, 191–192
  ethylene glycol to produce, 306
  produced by chemical industry, 108
  regulation by TSCA, 179–180
  xylene used to make, 435

Chemicals and Allied Products Industry, 108
Chemistry
  of air, 80–81
  of elements, 141
  of radioactive isotopes, 141–142, 145
  of water, 83
Chernobyl nuclear accident
  cesium-137 from, 263, 265
  dose to world population from, 148–149
  iodine-131 release from, 329, 331
  plumes from, 78–79
Children
  and aflatoxin poisoning, 202–203
  arsenic exposure of, 218
  arts and crafts hazards to, 68
  asbestos exposure of, 222
  aspartame hazards to, 225–226, 352
  bleach hazards to, 272
  and caffeine, 249–250
  cancer risk from ELF fields, 311
  cigarette smoking by, 50
  ethylene glycol poisoning of, 306–307
  lead hazards to, 49, 58, 105, 333, 334
  mercury hazards to, 342
  MSG effects on, 352
  naphthalene toxicity to, 353
  nicotine hazards to, 358
  particulate matter hazards to, 380
  respiratory infections in, 48
  risk from Alar, 283–284
  saccharin hazards to, 394–395
  sensitivity of toxics to, 41
  of smokers, 51
  sodium hydroxide poisoning of, 399
  sulfur dioxide hazards to, 409
  TRIS used in sleepwear of, 422–423
Chinese restaurants, monosodium glutamate used by, 351
Chinese restaurant syndrome, 351–352
Chloracne, from dioxin, 297
Chloramines, 271
Chlordane, **268–270**
Chlordecone, exposure to, 120
Chlorinated hydrocarbons
  chlorine in, 271
  as insecticides, 116
Chlorinated solvents
  hazards of, 109
  use of, 109–110
Chlorinated water, 271–272
  chloroform exposure from, 273–274
Chlorination
  and PCB toxicity, 383
  to treat water, 56, 57

Chlorine, **270–273**
  altered by burning of, 165
  from arts and crafts, 68
  dioxin as by-product of, 296–297
  as solvent, 109
  substitutes for in bleach, 167
Chlorofluorocarbons. *See* CFCs
Chloroform, **273–276**
  in drinking water, 57
  as narcotic, 274
  restricted under FFDCA, 182
Chlorox, 109
Chocolate, caffeine in, 248
Cholesterol, and cardiovascular disease, 9
Cholinesterase
  azinophos-methyl inhibition of, 228
  carbaryl effects on, 253
  diazinon interference with, 289
  malathion inhibition of, 339
  organophosphate effect on, 117
  parathion inhibition of, 377
Chrome plating, hazards of, 277, 278
Chromium, **276–279**
  from arts and crafts, 68
  environmental levels of, 278
  forms of, 276
Chromium(III)
  benefits of, 276
  in food and water, 277
Chromium(VI)
  and lung cancer, 276, 277–278
  sources of, 277
Chronic beryllium disease, definition of, 239
Chronic bronchitis
  definition of, 48
  See also Bronchitis
Chronic dose
  definition of, 16
  in GI tract, 36
  to target organ, 37
Chronic effects, 28–29
Chronic exposure, definition of, xi
Chronic obstructive pulmonary disease (COPD)
  as caused by cigarette smoking, 50
  definition of, 48
  and ozone (pollution), 373
Chronic poisoning, by metals, 104
Chronic respiratory disease, from particulate pollution, 380
Chronic respiratory effects, 48–49
Chrysanthemums
  causing gorilla extinctions, 390
  as insecticide, 388
Cigarette smoking
  and arsenic, 218, 220
  as benzene source, 233–234
  benzo[*a*]pyrene given off by, 236
  and cadmium, 245

carbon monoxide exposure from, 257–259
as cause of COPD, 48
as cause of lung cancer, 11
deaths from, 50
diseases caused by, 50
hazards of, 65
lung cancer from, 49
nickel in, 355
nicotine and, 358
and nitrosamines, 361
particulate matter hazards from, 381
quitting to avoid cancer, 11
and radon exposure, 149
risk of harm from, 6
and SIDS, 258
toluene in, 416
trends in habits of, 50
Cilia, sulfur dioxide effects on, 408–409
Circle of poison, 126
Clams, chlordane toxicity to, 269
Classification systems of toxics, 31–33
Clean Air Act (CAA), 99
    and CFC phase out, 267
    new amendments to, 176
    provisions of, 172, 175
    success of, 175–176
Clean Water Act (CWA), 121
    1977 amendments to, 174
    problems with, 178
    provisions of, 172, 177
    success of, 177–178
Climate
    altered by nuclear war, 154
    global warming, 91–94
Clinical ecology, 42
Clostridium botulinum, 359
CMME, 243–244
Coal
    beryllium in, 239
    cadmium in, 244
    contribution to greenhouse effect from, 91
    indoor air pollution from, 51
    sulfur dioxide from, 408
Coastal waters, dumping of wastes in, 163–164
Cockroaches
    lindane use on, 336
    safe control of in home, 138
Co-distills, definition of, 83
Coffee, caffeine in, 248
Coliform bacteria, 90
Colon and rectal cancers
    deaths from, 11
    and food preservatives, 12
Color additives, 182
Color Additives Amendment (1960), 61
Community right to know
    and aluminum, 213

and asbestos, 224
and benzene, 235
and captan, 252
and carbaryl, 254
and carbon tetrachloride, 261
and chlordane, 270
and chlorine, 272
and chloroform, 275
and chromium, 279
and creosote, 280
and 2,4-D, 283
and DEHP, 300
and dichlorvos, 293
and dioxane, 295
and EDC, 305
and ethylene glycol, 307
and formaldehyde, 320
and heptachlor, 327
and hydroquinone, 328
and mercury, 344
and methylene chloride , 347
and methyl ethyl ketone, 345
and nickel, 356
and parathion, 378
and saccharin, 395
and selenium, 397
and sodium hydroxide, 400
and styrene, 404
success of, 190–191
tetrachloroethylene as, 415
and toluene, 417
and trichloroethane, 419
and trichloroethylene, 421
and vinyl chloride, 431
and vinylidene chloride, 432
Compact disk players, safety of, 332
Comprehensive Environmental Response, Compensation, and Liability Act, 172, 185
Computers, ELF fields from, 310
Congress
    and Clean Water Act, 177–178
    and reauthorization of Clean Air Act, 176
    and regulation of toxics, 171–174
Congressional Budget Office, 159, 161
Conservation of energy, to reduce toxics source, 167–168
Consumer products
    comparisons of, 69–73
    formaldehyde in, 319
    hazardous wastes from, 70
    less toxic substitutes of, 168–169
    made by petrochemical industry, 106–111
    methylene chloride in, 346
    nickel in, 355
    reducing hazards from, 69–73
    and right to know, 191
    solvents in, 108–111
    styrene in, 403
    toxics in, 67–73
    trichloroethane in, 418

trichloroethylene in, 420
ultrasound uses in, 426
Consumer Product Safety Commission (CPSC), and TRIS controversy, 422–423
Consumer safety, of pesticides, 123–126
Contact insecticide
    chlordane as, 268
    definition of, 115
    parathion as, 377
    pyrethrum as, 388
Cooking
    acrolein in, 200
    microwave radiation in, 348
    and nitrogen oxide exposure, 365–366
Cooking stoves
    gas versus electric, 48
    as source of indoor air pollution, 51, 53
Cookware
    aluminum in, 210
    cadmium in, 245
COPD. *See* Chronic obstructive pulmonary disease (COPD)
Corn, alachlor use on, 203
Coronary thrombosis, 8
Corrosion, of pipes, 56
Cosmetics
    acetic acid in, 197
    ethylene glycol in, 306–307
    regulation of, 182
    saccharin use in, 394
Cosmic rays, tritium produced by, 424
Cotton
    and arsenic exposure, 218
    azinophos-methyl use on, 227–228
    methyl-parathion use on, 377
    pesticide overload on, 131–132
Cotton diapers, versus disposable, 70, 72–73
Cottonseed meal, aflatoxin in, 202
Coumarins, 433
CP seal, 68
Crafts
    hazards from materials of, 68–69
    reduction of hazards from, 68–69
    trichloroethane use in, 418
Creosote, **279–280**
    benzo[*a*]pyrene in, 236
Crop rotation, to control pests, 135
Crop workers. *See* Fieldworkers
Cubic centimeter, definition of, 19–20
Cubic meter, definition of, 19–20
Cultivation techniques
    problems with, 136–137
    success in pest control, 134–135
Cups, paper versus plastic, 70, 71
Curie (Ci), definition of, 148
Curie, Marie, 148

CWA. *See* Clean Water Act (CWA)

2,4-D, **281–283**
  in Agent Orange, 281, 411
  as common weed killer, 281
  as herbicide, 119
Dairy products, heptachlor contamination of, 325
Daminozide, **283–285**
  as pesticide, 124
  use on apples, 283
  See also Alar
Danger poison label, 31–32
Daughter isotope, definition of, 142
DDD, 286
DDE, 286
DDT, **286–288**
  bioconcentration of, 86, 88
  in breast milk, 40
  as carcinogenic pesticide, 124
  on carrots, 125
  control of malaria-carrying mos-
    quitoes, 113, 286–287
  as food contaminant, 65
  health hazards of, 287
  as insecticide, 116
  nutritional causes for susceptibil-
    ity to, 43
  resistance of mosquitoes to, 130
  in soil, 83
  U.S. ban of, 286, 288
  worldwide distribution of, 286
Deafness, caused by noise, 368–369
Death
  and cancer, 10–14
  and cardiovascular diseases, 8
  causes of, 8–14
  from sulfites, 405
Decaffeinated coffee, methylene
  chloride in, 346
Decaying, definition of, 142
Decay products
  definition of, 142
  of radon, 391
Decibel levels
  of sounds, 368–370
  of ultrasound, 427
Deep well injection, as hazardous
  waste disposal, 161
Defoliation, and Agent Orange,
  296, 411
Deforestation, and greenhouse
  effect, 94
DEHP. *See* Di(2-ethylhexyl)phthal-
  ate
Delaney Clause
  controversy over, 62
  definition of, 62
  and pesticides, 125
  and raw versus processed food,
    181–182
Delayed radiation, definition of, 153
Dementia, caused by aluminum,
  210–211

Dental assistants, mercury vapor
  exposure of, 341
Dental caries, fluoride prevention
  of, 313, 314
Dental fluorosis, 314
Dentists
  mercury vapor exposure of, 341
  oxalic acid use by, 370
Dermatitis
  and acetic acid, 197
  and acetone, 199
  caused by solvents, 110
  nickel causing, 354, 355–356
Detoxify
  definition of, 37
  by enzymes, 38
Di(2-ethylhexyl)phthalate, **298–300**
  used to soften plastics, 298–299
Diabetes, acetone poisoning misdiagnosed as, 199
Diapers, disposable versus cotton,
  70, 72–73
Diazinon, **289–290**
  relative safety of, 289
Dibromochloroporpane (DBCP)
  exposure to, 121
  in groundwater, 121
Dicamba, **290–292**
  as alternative to 2,4,5-T, 290
  as herbicide, 119
Dichlorodiphenyltrichloroethane.
  See DDT
Dichloromethane. *See* Methylene
  chloride
Dichlorvos, **292–293**
Dieldrin, **207–209**
  acute toxicity of, 208–209
  as carcinogenic pesticide, 124
Diet
  as cause of colon and rectal
    cancers, 11
  food additives in, 61–66
  and nitrosamines, 361
  saturated fat in, 8–9
  and susceptibility to toxics,
    41–43, 42–43
  zinc in, 436–437
Diet soft drinks
  aspartame use in, 225
  saccharin use in, 394
Diffusion, definition of, 38, 79
Dinoseb, EPA emergency cancellation of, 184
Dioxane, **294–295**
Dioxin, **296–298**
  in air pollution, 49
  broken down by intense sunlight,
    166
  contamination of 2,4-D, 281
  extreme toxicity of, 296, 297
  in food containers, 297
  as insecticide, 116
  regulation of, 180, 184

  as toxic product of incineration,
    165
  units of, 21
Discharge, units of, 19
Disease
  cardiovascular, 8–10
  causes of, 8–14, 27
  occurrence of, 28
Disposable diapers, versus cotton,
  70, 72–73
Disposable economy, 157
Disposal, of wastes, 159–164
Dizziness, 7
DMNA, as dicamba contaminant,
  290, 291
DMSO, and the skin, 36
DNA
  damage from air pollution, 49
  mutations of, 30
  radiation effect on, 144
Domestic produce, pesticides on,
  125–126
Dose
  of cesium-137, 264
  definition of, 15
  of iodine-131, 330–331
  in laboratory testing, 29
  of plutonium, 388
  of radiation, 147–148
  of strontium-90, 402
  of tritium, 426
Dose-response relation (curve)
  definition of, 15–16
  linear, 17, 18
  in toxicology studies, 29
Downwind transport, of toxics,
  78–79
Drain cleaners
  sodium hydroxide in, 398, 399
  trichloroethane in, 418
Drano, 398, 399
Dredge spoils, dumping in oceans,
  163–164
Drinking water
  alachlor in, 204
  aluminum in, 211
  barium in, 229–230
  beryllium in, 238
  biological safety of, 56
  carbon tetrachloride in, 260
  chlorine use in, 271–272
  chloroform exposure from, 273–
    274
  chromium in, 277
  contaminants from home, 57–58
  distribution system contaminants
    of, 56–57
  EDB and EDC accumulate in, 303
  fluoride in, 313–315
  health hazards from, 55–58
  improvement of quality of, 58
  lead in, 335
  nitrates in, 360, 363
  pesticides in, 120

protection of quality of, 177–179
reduction of metal contamination in, 58
regulation of lead in, 187–188
and Safe Drinking Water Act, 178
source contaminants of, 56
supply of, 55
tetrachloroethylene in, 413
toxics in, 81
trichloroethylene in, 420
Drugs
as defined by FFDCA, 182
hazardous wastes from, 70
regulation of, 182–183
sulfites in, 405
Dry cleaning, tetrachloroethylene used in, 53, 413, 414
Dry deposition, definition of, 79
Dumping
in oceans, 163–164, 186–187
of wastes, 159
Dust
amount inhaled, 21–22
as particulate matter source, 379
plutonium in, 387
Dyes, in food, 316–317

Ears, noise damage to, 368–369
Earthworms, chlordane toxicity to, 269
EBDCs, 300–302
as most widely used fungicides, 300–301
as pesticide, 124
Ecological effects, of toxics, 88–90
Ecosystems
hazards from toxics to, 88, 90
natural versus agricultural systems, 128
Ecotoxicology
definition of, 88
goals of, 89–90
EDB. See Ethylene dibromide (EDB)
EDBCs
as fungicide, 119
special review by EPA of, 119
EDC. See Ethylene dichloride (EDC)
Eggshells, DDT thinning of, 286, 287, 288
Electrical capacitors, PCBs used in, 382
Electric blankets, ELF fields from, 310
Electric fields
hazards from, 310–311
in households, 312
Electric power plants
nitrogen oxides from, 365
sulfur dioxide from, 408
Electromagnetic fields, extremely low frequency, 310–312

Electromagnetic spectrum
definition of, 143–144
and microwaves and radio waves, 348
and ultraviolet radiation, 428
Electrons, definition of, 141
Elements, definition of, 141
ELF fields. See Extremely low frequency electromagnetic fields
Emergency Planning and Community Right-To-Know Act (EPCRA), 190
Emission rate, of pollution, 16
Emphysema
as caused by cigarette smoking, 50
definition of, 48
Endangered Species Act, 89
Energy, conservation of, 167–168
Energy formula ($E = mc^2$), 146
Environment
chromium levels in, 278
contamination by hazardous wastes, 161
effects of pesticides on, 127–130
global hazards of pollutants to, 91–100
harmful effects on solvents in, 111
movement of toxics through, 77–85
nickel in, 357
ozone (pollution) damage to, 374
PCBs in, 384–385
protection of marine, 164
and styrene problem, 404
ten ways to reduce toxics in, x
trichloroethylene widespread in, 420
tritium in, 425
Environmental Protection Agency (EPA)
carcinogens categories of, 31–32
and Clean Air Act, 175
and Clean Water Act, 177
emergency cancellation of pesticides, 184
emergency suspension of 2,4,5-T, 412
as federal regulatory agency, 171
and FIFRA, 183–184
guidelines for acute toxicity, 32
management of wastes by, 160–161
and Ocean Dumping Act, 186–187
Environmental Protection agency (EPA), and pesticides on field hands, 122, 123
Environmental Protection Agency (EPA)
and RCRA, 184
and Safe Drinking Water Act, 178
toxics classification of, 31–32
and TSCA, 179–180

Enzymes
altering of chemical structure by, 37–38, 41
and detoxification of alcoholic, 38, 42
lack of, 41
and metabolism of toxics, 38
organophosphate effect on, 117
that breakdown alcohol, 63–64
zinc requirements of, 437
EPA. See Environmental Protection Agency
Epidemiology
and cancer, 28
definition of, 27
limitations of, 28
Erg, definition of, 147
Escherichia coli, 90, 177
Eskimos, and cesium-137 bioconcentration, 263
Esophagus
nitrosamines causing cancer in, 363
sodium hydroxide effects on, 399
Ethanol
hazards from, 63–64
See also Alcoholic beverages
Ethylenebisdithiocarbamates. See EBDCs
Ethylene dibromide (EDB), 303–305
acute toxicity of, 304
carcinogenicity of, 304–305
EPA emergency cancellation of, 184
as food contaminant, 65
as fumigant, 118
Ethylene dichloride (EDC), 303–305
Ethylene glycol, 306–307
ethylene oxide used to manufacture, 308
as poison, 306
Ethylene oxide, 308–309
Ethylene thiourea. See ETU
Ethyl-parathion. See Parathion
ETU
distribution of, 301
hazards of, 301
Exercise
and cardiovascular disease, 9
and ozone exposure, 373
and particulate matter in air, 381
and sulfur dioxide poisoning, 409
Exhalation, toxics removed by, 39
Exposure
background radiation, 149–150
to pesticides, 120–123
protection from in workplace, 180–181
and regulation of toxics, 179–184
versus response, 17
versus risk, 15–16
Extremely low frequency elec-

tromagnetic fields, **310–312**
definition of, 143
hazards from, 311
regulation of, 311
Exxon tanker *Valdez,* 188
Eyes
acetic acid effects on, 197
ammonia hazards to, 215
bis(chloromethyl)ether hazards
to, 243
effects from acrolein, 200
ethylene glycol effects on, 306
formaldehyde effects on, 319
laser light effects on, 332
microwave radiation effects on,
348
mineral fibers effects on, 350
sodium hydroxide effects on, 399
ultraviolet radiation effects on,
429
xylene effects on, 435

False negative result, definition of,
29
Farm animals, selenium poisoning
of, 395, 397
Farmworkers
alachlor exposure of, 203–204
pesticides exposure of, 121–123
Fasting, 37
Fat (body)
and BHA and BHT, 241–242
HCH/lindane stored in, 337
storage of toxics in, 37
Fat (dietary), 8–9
and benzene toxicity, 43
and cancer, 11, 12–13
Di(2-ethylhexyl)phthalate con-
tamination of, 298–299
Fat-soluble molecules, 38
FDA. *See* Food and Drug Adminis-
tration (FDA)
Feces, toxics removed in, 39
Federal Cancer Policy, 180
Federal Drug Administraion (FDA),
and food color regulation, 316–
317
Federal Food, Drug, and Cosmetic
Act (FFDCA)
problems with, 181–182
provisions of, 172, 181
Federal Insecticide, Fungicide, and
Rodenticide Act (FIFRA), 125,
183–184
Federal regulations, governing
toxics, 171–188
Federal Water Pollution Control
Act, 177
Fertilizers
ammonia use in, 214–215
nitrates in, 359, 360
Fiberglass, 350–351
Fieldworkers
aldrin/dieldrin exposure of, 208

parathion poisoning of, 376, 377–
378
pesticides exposure of, 121–123
FIFRA. *See* Federal Insecticide,
Fungicide, and Rodenticide Act
(FIFRA)
Fingernail polish remover, 198–199
Fireplaces, indoor air pollution
from, 51
Fire retardant
PBBs used as, 382
TRIS as, 422–423
Fires
carbon monoxide from, 257
from nuclear war, 153
as particulate matter source, 379
Fish
captafol toxicity to, 252
cesium-137 in, 263–264
in contaminated lakes, 82
DDT bioconcentration in, 287–
288
EBDC toxicity to, 302
lindane toxicity to, 338
mercury in, 341, 343
parathion toxicity to, 378
PCBs contamination of, 383, 384
2,4-D toxicity to, 281, 282
zinc hazards to, 438
Fission. *See* Nuclear fission
Fission fragment, definition of, 146,
147, 153
Flame retardant, TRIS as, 422–423
Flea collars, dichlorvos use in, 292
Flea powder, carbaryl in, 253
Flies
lindane use on, 336
safe control of in home, 138
Fluoridation, of public water, 313–
315
Fluoride, **313–315**
controversy over, 313
damage from, 314
in drinking water, 57
health benefits of, 314
Fluorocarbon propellants, carbon
tetrachloride in, 260
Fluorosis, 314
Flushing, of lakes, 81–82
Fly ash, 165
PCBs in, 384
Foam
CFCs used in, 265, 266–267
urea-formaldehyde insulation, 318
Foam cushions, as source of indoor
air pollution, 51, 53
Folpet, **250–252**
as carcinogenic pesticide, 124
as fungicide, 119
Food
aluminum in, 210
arsenic in, 217–218
barium in, 229
beryllium in, 238

BHA and BHT in, 241–242
cadmium in, 245
carageenan in, 262
color additives to, 316–317
Di(2-ethylhexyl)phthalate contamination of, 298–299
dioxin in containers of, 297
irradiation to preserve, 151–153
lead in, 333
monosodium glutamate use in,
351–352
nickel in, 354–355, 357
nitrates naturally in, 359–361
nitrites used to preserve, 359–360
regulation of safety of, 181–182
selenium in, 395
SST on, 286
vinyl chloride in, 430–431
vinylidene chloride in, 432
zinc in, 436–437
Food additives
BHA and BHT as, 241
cancer causing, 62
carrageenan as, 262
definition of, 61
examples of, 62
and health, 61–66
nitrites as, 360
regulation of, 181–182
sulfites as, 405
versus naturally harmful substances, 64–65
Food Additives Amendment (1958),
61
Food chain
and bioconcentration, 86–88
mercury bioconcentration in, 341
PCBs accumulate in, 382
Food colors, **316–317**
amount used in United States, 317
cancer causing, 62
definition of, 61
health effects of very high doses
of, 317
regulation by FDA, 316–317
Food and Drug Administration
(FDA), 152, 181–183
Food, Drug, and Cosmetics Act, 61
Food irradiation
benefits of, 153
misconceptions about, 152
risks of, 152–153
Food preservatives. *See* Food additives; Preservatives
Food production, pesticide use in,
113
Forest dieback, and acid rain, 96, 99
Forests
2,4-D use on, 281
and greenhouse warming, 93
ozone (pollution) damage to, 374
Formaldehyde, **318–321**
from arts and crafts, 68
and bis(chloromethyl)ether, 243

in foam, 170
indoor air pollution from, 51, 53
regulation of, 320, 321
restricted under FFDCA, 182
in smog, 80
widespread occurrence of, 318
Formalin, 318
Fosetyl Al, **322–323**
relatively low risk from, 322–323
Frankfurters, nitrites in, 360
Freckle cream
hydroquinone in, 327
oxalic acid in, 370
Frequency, definition of, 143
Fruits
captan used on, 250
EBDCs used on, 300–301
lindane used on, 336
pesticides used on, 124, 181–182
sulfites in, 405
Fuel reprocessing, definition of, 152
Fumigant
EDB and EDC as, 303
ethylene oxide as, 308
lindane as, 336
sulfur dioxide as, 407
Fumigants
carbon tetrachloride in, 260
definition of, 118
human health hazards from, 118
Fungi, use of fungicides on, 119
Fungicides
benomyl as, 231
captafol as, 250
captan as, 250
definition of, 112
development of systemic types of,
130
EBDCs as, 300
folpet as, 250
fosetyl Al as substitute for, 322
regulation of, 183–184
types of, 119–120
use of, 119–120
Furans, 296
Furniture finish strippers, methyl
ethyl ketone in, 344
Fusion. See Nuclear fusion

Galvanized containers, zinc in, 436–
437
Gamma rays
definition of, 142, 143
and quality factor, 148
used to preserve foods, 152
Garbage
burning of, 164–165
categories of materials in, 158
as hazardous, 161–162
increase in, 157–159
Gardening
diazinon use in, 289
glyphosate use in, 323–324
list of garden pests in, 139

pesticide use in, 113
pyrethrum use in, 388
safe pest control in, 137–139
Garlic solution, as pesticide substitute, 137
Gas. See Natural gas
Gasoline
benzene in, 233
lead in, 175–176, 333
toluene in, 415
Gas stoves
nitrogen dioxide produced by,
365–366
respiratory infections and, 366
Gastrointestinal (GI) tract
arsenic effects on, 220
caffeine effects on, 249
chemicals in, 35–36
EDB and EDC effects on, 304
sodium hydroxide effects on, 399
Gene pool, harm to, 89
Generally recognized as safe
(GRAS), 181
carageenan as, 262
definition of, 61
nickel as, 356
origin of list of, 61–62
Germany, forest dieback in, 96, 99
GI tract. See Gastrointestinal (GI)
tract
Glass wool, 350–351
Global climate
hazards to, 91–94
See also Climate
Glue
acetone in, 198
toluene in, 415
vinylidene chloride in, 432
Glutamate levels, MSG effects on,
352
Glyphosate, **323–325**
relative low toxicity of, 324
used on marijuana, 375
Government Accounting Office
(GAO), 183–184
Grains, hazard from aflatoxins in,
201–203
Gram, definition of, 20
Grapes, sulfur dioxide use on, 407
GRAS. See Generally recognized as
safe (GRAS)
Gray (unit), definition of, 147–148
Great Lakes, PCBs in, 383
Greenhouse effect
definition of, 91
evidence of, 92–93
future problems from, 93
illustrated, 92
and rainfall changes, 91–92
reducing severity of, 94
Greenhouse gases
and CFCs, 265, 267
definition of, 91
Green tobacco sickness, 358

Grocery bags, paper or plastic question, 69–70
Groundwater
alachlor in, 204
aldicarb in, 206
benzene in, 233
carbon tetrachloride in, 260
contamination of, 160–161, 178–
179
definition of, 58
and disposable diaper problem,
70–71
EDB and EDC accumulate in, 303
methylene chloride in, 347
movement of toxics through, 82–
83
new legislation on, 188
pollution in, 58–59
quality of, 56, 177–179
and Safe Drinking Water Act,
178–179
selenium in, 397
trichloroethylene in, 420
Group A (human carcinogen), 32
Group B (probable human carcinogen), 32
Group C (possible human carcinogen), 32
Group D (not classifiable as to
human carcinogenicity), 32
Group E (evidence of noncarcinogenicity for humans), 32
Guthion, 227
Gypsy moth, 135–136
carbaryl use on, 253, 254

Hairspray, methylene chloride in,
346, 347
Half-life
of aldicarb, 206
definition of, 142–143
of iodine-131, 329
of plutonium, 386
and potential for damage, 145
of strontium-90, 401
Halogens
definition of, 109
use in petrochemical industry, 108
Halons, 265
Ham, nitrites in, 360
Hanford, Washington, radioactive
leaks from sites at, 162
Hardening of the arteries, 8–10
Hazard Communication Standard,
189
Hazardous air pollutant, 175
acrolein as, 201
asbestos as, 223
cadmium as, 247
captan as, 252
carbaryl as, 254
carbon tetrachloride as, 261
chlordane as, 270
chlorine as, 272

chloroform as, 275
chromium as, 279
creosote as, 280
2,4-D as, 283
DDT as, 288
DEHP as, 300
dichlorvos as, 293
dioxane as, 295
dioxin as, 297–298
EDC as, 305
ethylene glycol as, 307
formaldehyde as, 320
heptachlor as, 327
hydroquinone as, 328
mercury as, 343
methylene chloride as, 347
methyl ethyl ketone as, 345
nickel as, 356
parathion as, 378
PCBs as, 385
plutonium as, 387
selenium as, 397
styrene as, 404
tetrachloroethylene as, 415
toluene as, 417
trichloroethane as, 419
trichloroethylene as, 421
vinyl chloride as, 431
vinylidene chloride as, 432
Hazardous and Solid Waste Amendment (HSWA), 173, 184
Hazardous wastes
    bis(chloromethyl)ether in, 243
    cleanup of sites of, 160–161, 185
    definition of, 158
    land disposal of, 160–162
    management of, 158–159
    new processing technologies for, 165–166
    regulation of, 184–187
Hazards
    of air pollution, 47–50
    to body from metals, 104–105
    from consumer products, 67–73
    determination of, 31
    ecological versus human, 88–90
    and exposure level, 16–17
    to global environment, 91–100
    from municipal garbage, 161–162
    risk of harm from, 5–6
    from solvents, 110–111
    in the workplace, 189–190
HCH. See Lindane
Headaches, caused by aspartame, 225
Head lice, lindane use on, 337
Health hazard. See Hazard
Health and Human Services (HHS), radon guidelines of, 392, 393
Hearing loss, caused by noise, 368–369
Heart, carbon monoxide effects on, 258
Heart attacks, deaths from, 8

Heart disease
    and aspirin, 9
    as caused by cigarette smoking, 50
    protection against, 9
Heavy metals
    definition of, 103
    See also Toxic metals
Heptachlor, **325–327**
    and chlordane, 268
    environmental damage from, 326–327
    as insecticide, 116
    in milk, 123
Heptachlor epoxide, persistence of, 326
Herbicide
    alachlor as, 203–205
    definition of, 112
    dicamba as, 290
    dioxin as, 296
    2,4-D as most extensively used, 281
    glyphosate as, 323
    organic types, 119
    paraquat as, 375
    rate of use of, 113
    systemic type, 115
    2,4,5-T as, 411
    use of, 118–119
Herpes, BHT and BHA as self-treatment for, 241, 242
Hexachlorocyclohexane (HCH). See Lindane
High blood pressure, 8–9
High-density lipoproteins (HDLs), 9
High-level wastes, definition of, 162
High-voltage transmission lines (HVTLs)
    ELF fields in, 310–311
    hazards from, 311
    regulation of, 311–312
Hiroshima, radiation dose in, 151
Hobbies
    hazards from materials of, 68–69
    reduction of hazards from, 68–69
Home
    asbestos hazards in, 223
    captan use in, 250
    diazinon use in, 289
    dichlorvos use in, 292–293
    drinking water quality in, 58
    electric fields in, 312
    ELF field hazards in, 311
    formaldehyde in, 318
    magnetic fields in, 312
    malathion use in, 339
    microwave radiation in, 348
    pyrethrum use in, 388
    radon hazards in, 187, 391–392
    safe pest control in, 137–139
    sodium hydroxide hazards in, 399
    sources of air pollution in, 52

testing equipment sources, 453
    warfarin use in, 433
Honeybees
    carbaryl toxicity to, 254
    killed by pesticides, 127, 130
    parathion toxicity to, 378
    sensitivity to carbamates, 117
Hospitals, ethylene oxide use in, 308
Hotlines, 455
Hot pepper solution, as pesticide substitute, 137
Household cleaners, oxalic acid in, 370
House plants, to decrease indoor air pollution, 54
Houston, Texas, vinyl chloride exposure in, 430
Human body
    effect of insecticides on, 116–117
    harm from chemicals in, 34–43
    hazards from metals, 104–105
    hazards from solvents, 110–111
    nitrates converted to nitrites in, 361
    radiation penetration into, 144–145
    toxics exiting from, 39–40
    zinc needed by, 437
    See also Bodily uptake
Human carcinogen
    asbestos as, 223
    bis(chloromethyl)ether as, 243
    chromium(VI) as, 278
    nickel subsulfide as, 355
    nitrosamines as, 363
    passive smoke as, 51
    See also Carcinogen
Human risk, versus ecological risk, 88–89
HVTLs. See High-voltage transmission lines (HVTLs)
Hydraulic fluid, PCBs used in, 382
Hydrocarbons
    definition of, 108
    role in forming smog, 80
Hydrochloric acid, **270–273**
    and bis(chloromethyl)ether, 243
    use in petrochemical industry, 108
Hydrogen, tritium as radioactive form of, 424, 425
Hydrogen chloride, **270–273**
    health effects of, 272
Hydrologic cycle, 55
Hydrolysis, of parathion, 377
Hydroquinone, **327–328**
    from arts and crafts, 68
Hydrosphere, definition of, 81
Hyperactive airways, caused by air pollution, 47
Hypertension, 8–9
Hyperthyroidism, iodine-131 use for, 329
Hypochlorite, **270–273**
    health effects of, 272

Immune system, beryllium effects
  on, 239
Imported produce, pesticides on,
  125–126
Incineration
  and PCBs, 384
  special hazards of, 165
  toxic products of, 165
  of wastes, 159, 164–165
Industry
  petrochemical, 106–109
  recycling in, 166–167
  reduced use of toxics in, 167
  xylene use in, 435
Inert ingredients
  definition of, 67
  lack of tolerances for, 125
  in pesticides, 115
  as solvents, 110–111
  as toxic, 67–68
  trichloroethylene as, 420
Infants
  aspartame hazards to, 225–226,
    352
  carbon monoxide effects on, 258
  chromium in formula of, 277
  and drinking during pregnancy,
    63
  exposure to toxics in breast milk,
    40
  harmed by mother's smoking, 50
  harm from toxic metals, 105
  mercury hazards to, 342
  MSG effects on, 352
  naphthalene toxicity to, 353
  nitrites effects on, 359
  sensitivity to toxics of, 41
Infectious diseases, control of, 8
Ingredients, inert toxic, 67–68
Inhalation
  of asbestos fibers, 222
  of ethylene oxide, 308
  of formaldehyde, 318
  of mercury vapors, 342
  of methylene chloride, 346
  of naphthalene, 353
  of toxics by, 34–35
  of trichloroethylene, 421
  of xylene, 435
Inorganic compounds
  definition of, 108
  examples of, 109
Inorganic pollution, of water, 56
Insect growth regulators (IGRs),
  134
Insecticides
  DDT as, 286
  definition of, 112
  nicotine used as, 358
  rate of use of, 113
  regulation of, 183–184
  systemic type, 115
  types of, 115–118

See also Organophosphate
  insecticide
Insects, EDB and EDC use on, 303
Insulation, mineral fibers in, 350–
  351
Integrated Pest Management (IPM)
  azinophos-methyl use in, 227
  and cotton disaster, 131–132
  definition of, 132
  EBDCs used in, 300–301
  home garden application of, 137–
    139
  problems of, 136–137
  success of, 132–133
International Agency for Research
  on Cancer, 31
Inversions. See Atmospheric
  inversions
Iodine-131, **329–331**
  damage to thyroid gland from,
    145
  as nuclear fission fragment, 146
  released from Chernobyl, 78
Ionization, definition of, 83
Ions, definition of, 83
IPM. See Integrated Pest Management (IPM)
Irradiation, of food, 151–153
Irritant, definition of, 36
Isomers
  lindane as, 336
  of PCBs, 382
Isotopes
  cesium-137 as, 263
  definition of, 141–142
  effects on human body of, 144–
    145
  half-life of, 142–143, 145
Itai-itai disease, 246

Japanese
  low incidence of atherosclerosis
    of, 8
  PCBs poisoning of, 382
  radiation and cancer studies of,
    151
Japanese restaurants, monosodium
  glutamate used by, 351
Juvenile hormone, 134

Kepone, exposure to, 120
Keshan disease, 396
Ketone, methyl ethyl ketone as,
  344, 345
Kidney dialysis
  and aluminum hazards, 210–211
  DEHP exposure from, 299
Kidneys, 34, 39
  aluminum hazards to, 211
  and cadmium, 104, 245–246
  and cancer, 13
  carbon tetrachloride effects on,
    260–261

chloroform effects on, 274
dioxane effects on, 294
ethylene glycol effects on, 306
fosetyl Al effects on, 322
lead effects on, 334
oxalic acid effects on, 371
solvents damage to, 110
tetrachloroethylene effects on,
  413–414
toxic chemicals in, 35
Kilns, hazards from, 68
Kilogram, definition of, 20

Labeling
  about sulfites, 405, 406
  requirements on drugs, 182–183
  as warning, 31–32
Laboratory animals
  results of studies from, 33
  used to predict human response,
    29–30
Laboratory testing
  high doses used in, 17, 29
  problems with, 29–30
  of toxics, 27–30
Lactose
  intolerance to, 41
  and lead, 42
Lakes
  improvement in, 177
  pollution in, 81–82
  protection of quality of, 177–179
  water layers in, 81–82
Landfills
  burial of ash in, 165
  categories of materials in, 158
  and disposable diaper problem,
    70, 72–73
  hazardous waste in, 161
  overfilling of, 159–160
  regulation of, 185
  styrene in, 404
Laser light. **331–332**. See also Ultraviolet radiation
  intensity of, 331–332
Laser printers, safety of, 332
Lawn mowers, manual versus
  power, 169
LD_{50}, definition of, 29, 31
Lead, 30, 42, **333–336**
  in acid rain, 99
  from arts and crafts, 68
  blood levels of, 335
  in breast milk, 40
  concentration in environment,
    333–335
  in dishware, 181
  in drinking water, 187–188
  EDB use with, 303
  in gasoline, 103
  hazard to children, 49, 58, 105
  health effects of, 334, 335
  in milk, 42

minimizing the toxic effects of, 42
new legislation on, 187
nutritional causes for susceptibility to, 43
poisoning, 58
reduction in gasoline, 175–176
as regulated by CAA, 175
risk from, 16
stored in bones, 37
as toxic product of incineration, 165
Lead poisoning, 104
Leafy vegetables, iodine-131 in, 329–330
Leather, hazardous wastes from, 70
Leavening agents, aluminum in, 210
Legislation
abbreviations of laws, 450
new or proposed, 187–188
on toxics, 172–174
Length, metric units of, 20
Lesions, definition of, 36
Lettuce, mevinphos on, 125
Leukemia
and benzene, 234
from plutonium, 387
and radiation, 145, 151
Life expectancy, 8
Lifespan, increase in, 8
Lifestyle, and sensitivity to toxics, 41
Light
dual nature of, 143
laser, 331–332
and ultraviolet radiation, 428
Lindane, 336–338
as insecticide, 116
Linear dose-response relation, 17
of cancer and radiation, 151
Liter, definition of, 19–20
Liver, 34, 39
cancer from aflatoxins, 202–203
carbon tetrachloride effects on, 260–261
chloroform effects on, 274
DEHP effects on, 299
dioxane effects on, 294
harm from alcohol, 63
Kepone effects on, 120
methylene chloride effects on, 346–347
plutonium damage to, 387
solvents damage to, 110
tetrachloroethylene effects on, 413–414
toxic chemicals in, 35
vinyl chloride effects on, 431
Los Angeles
air pollution in, 47
air quality improvements in, 176
atmospheric inversions in, 78
benzene in air of, 49
nitrogen oxides in air of, 365

smog in, 80, 365
Loudness levels, of hazardous noises, 369
Love Canal, 157, 160, 184, 185
Low-density lipoproteins (LDLs), 9
Low frequency electromagnetic fields, 310–312
L-tryptophan, FDA recall of, 182
Luminous dials, tritium in, 424
Lung cancer
and air pollution, 49
from arsenic, 218, 220
asbestos as cause of, 27–28, 223–224
and benzo[a]pyrene related deaths, 237
and beryllium, 239–240
and bis(chloromethyl)ether, 243
and cadmium, 245
and chromium, 276, 277–278
cigarette smoking as cause of, 11, 27–28
deaths from, 11, 14, 50
increase in rate of, 10–11
from particulate pollution, 380
from radon, 391
Lungs
air pollution damage to, 48
ammonia hazards to, 214–215
asbestos hazards to, 222–224
beryllium effects on, 238–240
bis(chloromethyl)ether hazards to, 243
effects on growth of, 48–49
function of, 35
nickel effects on, 355
nitrogen dioxide effects on, 365–366
paraquat damage to, 375
particles in, 35
particulate matter damage to, 379, 380–381
plutonium damage to, 387
radon damage to, 151, 391
sulfur dioxide effects on, 408–409
Lye, 398–400
hazards of mixing with ammonia, 214–215
Lygus bug
cultivation techniques to control, 135
overuse of pesticides on, 131–132

Magnetic fields
hazards from, 310–311
in households, 312
Malaria
controlled by DDT, 113, 286–287
controlled by lindane, 337
controlled by malathion, 339
Malathion, 339–340
relative safety of, 339–340
toxicity ranking of, 31

Malnutrition, 42
Mancozeb, 300–302
as fungicide, 119
Maneb, 300–302
as fungicide, 119
Marijuana, paraquat used on, 375
Marine Protection, Research, and Sanctuaries Act (MPRSA), 173, 186–187
Material Safety Data Sheets (MSDS)
on solvent exposure, 110
and worker right to know, 190
Meat products
monosodium glutamate use in, 351–352
nitrites in, 359–360
selenium in, 395
Medicine
ethylene oxide use in, 308
ultrasound applications in, 426
warfarin uses in, 433
Mediterranean fruit fly, 136
MEK. See Methyl ethyl ketone
Melanoma, 10
and ozone layer protection, 94
and PCBs, 384
and ultraviolet radiation, 13, 429
Membranes
as barriers to toxics, 39
movement of chemicals through, 38–39
Mercury, 341–344
environmental hazards of, 343
in fish and seafood, 341–343
as pesticide, 113
as pollution in water, 83
as regulated by CAA, 175
restricted under FFDCA, 182
toxic effects of, 342–343
as toxic product of incineration, 165
in wastes, 163
Mesotheliomas, definition of, 223
Metabolism, 36
of alcohol, 63–64
definition of, 37
Metabolite, 41
definition of, 37, 121
Metal
beryllium in alloys of, 239
chromium as, 276
exposure routes to body, 104
hazardous wastes from, 70
lead as, 333
mercury as, 341
mobilized in environment, 103–104
nickel as, 354
properties of, 103
selenium as, 395
sources of, 103
testing equipment for, 453
toxic, 103–105

trichloroethylene as degreaser of, 420
See also Toxic metals
Metal fume fever, definition of, 437
Metastasis, in cancer, 10–11
Methemoglobinemia, definition of, 363
Methylene chloride, **346–347**
  from arts and crafts, 68
  as inert ingredient, 67
  as solvent, 109
Methyl ethyl ketone, **344–345**
  as inert ingredient, 67
  as solvent, 109
Methylmercury, 341–345. *See also* Mercury
Methyl mercury, as pollution in water, 83
Methyl-parathion, **376–379**
Metiram, **300–302**
  as fungicide, 119
Metolachlor, 204
Metric system, definition of, 19
Metric ton, definition of, 20
Mevinphos, on lettuce, 125
Mexico
  DDT from, 287
  paraquat used in, 375
Mice, used in laboratory testing, 29
Microbial insecticides, success of, 118, 134
Microgram
  definition of, 20
  example of, 21
  per liter equivalents, 20–21
Micron, definition of, 79
Microsomal ethanol oxidizing system (MEOS), definition of, 63
Microwave ovens, radiation from, 348
Microwave radiation, **348–349**
  effects of, 349
  sources of, 349
Migrant workers, exposure to pesticides of, 121–123
Mildew, use of fungicides on, 119
Milk
  aflatoxin in, 202
  dioxin in containers of, 297–298
  heptachlor in, 123, 325
  iodine-131 in, 329
  strontium-90 in, 401
Milligram, definition of, 20
Mineral fibers (nonasbestos), **350–351**
Mixing rates, of lake water, 81–82
Mobile homes, formaldehyde in, 318
Mold
  aflatoxin producing, 201–203
  as natural food contaminant, 64
  use of fungicides on, 119
Mongoose, and sugarcane disaster, 136

Monocultures, definition of, 128
Monosodium glutamate (MSG), **351–352**
  as food additive, 62
Montreal Protocol, and CFC phase out, 96, 267
Mosquitoes
  controlled by DDT, 113, 286–287
  controlled by lindane, 337
  DDT resistance in, 130
  use of pesticides for, 113
Moth balls, 353–354
Mother's milk. *See* Breast milk
Moths, safe control of in home, 138–139
Motor vehicles
  harm of noise from, 369
  nitrogen oxides from, 365
  toluene from, 416
  See also Automobiles
Mouth, uptake of toxics through, 35–36
Mouthwash, fluoride in, 313
MPRSA. *See* Marine Protection, Research, and Sanctuaries Act (MPRSA)
MSG. *See* Monosodium glutamate (MSG)
Mucous membranes
  chlorine effects on, 271
  sodium hydroxide effects on, 399
Municipal wastes
  as hazardous, 161–162
  land disposal of, 159–160
  management of, 158–159
Muscles
  barium effects on, 230
  ethylene glycol effects on, 306
Mutagen
  definition of, 30
  ethylene oxide as, 308
  lindane as, 337–338
  pesticides as, 124
  and saccharin, 394
  testing of, 30–31
  trichloroethane as, 418
  TRIS as, 423
  vinyl chloride as, 431
Mutations
  and benomyl, 231–232
  definition of, 30
  produced by toxic metals, 105

Nagasaki, radiation dose in, 151
Nanogram, definition of, 20
Naphthalene, **353–354**
  as fumigant, 118
Narcotic
  chloroform as, 274
  EDC as, 303
  trichloroethylene as, 421
Nasal passages
  chromium(VI) effects on, 277–278

nitrosamines causing cancer in, 363
  particles trapped in, 35
National Academy of Sciences, studies on pesticides, 124
National Aeronautics and Space Administration (NASA), 54
National Ambient Air Quality Standards (NAAQS), 175
National hotlines, 455
National Institute of Occupational Safety and Health (NIOSH), 180
National Water Quality Inventory, 177
Natural background radiation, definition of, 149
Natural enemies, of pest species, 133–134
Natural gas
  contribution to greenhouse effect from, 91
  use in petrochemical industry, 106
Natural Resources Defense Council (NRDC), pesticide report of, 123–124
Negligible risk, 182
  and food color, 316–317
Nematicides, definition of, 112
Nervous system
  acetone depression of, 199
  aldrin/dieldrin effects on, 208–209
  aluminum effects on, 212
  arsenic effects on, 220
  carbaryl effects on, 253
  carbon monoxide effects on, 258
  CFCs effects on, 266
  DDT effects on, 287
  disorder of caused by Kepone, 120
  lead effects on, 334
  mercury effects on, 342
  stimulated by caffeine, 248
  tetrachloroethylene effects on, 413–414
Neurotoxin
  insecticides as, 116
  mercury as, 341
Neutrons, definition of, 141
Newspaper
  carbon black in, 255
  recycling of, 168
New York Bight, ocean dumping in, 164
Nickel, **354–357**
  in environment, 357
  in food, 354–355, 357
  in tobacco smoke, 51
  widespread occurrence of, 355
Nickel carbonyl, definition of, 354
Nickel contact dermatitis, 354, 355–356
Nickel-electroplating, saccharin use in, 394

Nickel subsulfide
  as cancer causing, 355
  definition of, 354
Nicotine, 358–359
  as botanical insecticide, 118
  as pesticide, 112
NIMBY, and radioactive wastes,
  162
NIOSH. *See* National Institute of
  Occupational Safety and Health
  (NIOSH)
Nitrates, 359–364
  conversion to nitrites in body, 361
  distribution of, 360–361
  exposure to, 362
  as food additive, 62
  in groundwater, 56, 58
  in infants, 40
  in soil, 83
Nitric acid, in acid rain, 366–367
Nitric oxide, 365
Nitrites, 359–364
  conversion from nitrates, 361
  distribution of, 360
  exposure to, 362
  health hazards of, 363
  in soil, 83
Nitrogen dioxide, 365
  health effects of, 367
  and indoor air pollution, 51
  as oxidant, 365
  role in smog formation, 372
Nitrogen oxides, 365–367
  in acid rain, 80, 96
  nutritional causes for susceptibil-
    ity to, 43
  outdoor air concentrations of, 366
  as regulated by CAA, 175
Nitrosamines, 359–364
  cancer caused by, 359, 363
  carbamates converted to, 117
  as cause of lung cancer, 11
  concentrations of, 362
  exposure to, 362
  nutritional causes for susceptibil-
    ity to, 43
  production in stomach of, 361
  in tobacco smoke, 51
NOAEL, definition of, 30
Noise, 368–370
  health problems caused by, 368–
    369
  regulation in workplace of, 369
  ultrasound as form of, 426
Noise Control Act (1972), 370
Noncarcinogen, safe doses of, 30
Nonfood items, as defined by
  FFDCA, 182
Nonhazardous wastes, land disposal
  of, 159–160
No observed adverse effect level
  (NOAEL), definition of, 30
No observed effect level (NOEL),
  for pesticides, 124–125

No-Pest Strip, 292–293
Norwegians, and food color ban, 62
"Not in my backyard" (NIMBY),
  and radioactive wastes, 162
NOX. *See* Nitrogen oxides
Nuclear accident, with plutonium,
  386, 387
Nuclear fission
  and Chernobyl accident, 78–79
  definition of, 145–146
  harmful radiation from, 146
  illustrated, 147
Nuclear fusion
  definition of, 146
  tritium as fuel in, 424
Nuclear power plants
  and cesium-137, 263, 264
  iodine-131 from, 329
  nuclear fission in, 146
  plutonium from, 386
  strontium-90 from, 401
  tritium from, 424–425
  wastes from, 162
Nuclear war, destruction from, 153–
  154
Nuclear wastes. *See* Radioactive
  wastes
Nuclear weapons, 146, 153–154
  cancer caused by testing of, 387
  cesium-137 from testing of, 263,
    264
  iodine-131 from testing of, 329
  plutonium released from testing
    of, 386
  strontium-90 released from testing
    of, 401
Nuclear winter, 154
Nucleus, definition of, 141
Nutrasweet, 225–226
Nutrients, transport across membranes, 39
Nutrition
  and reduced risk from lead, 42
  and susceptibility to toxics, 42–43
Nuts, hazard from aflatoxins in,
  201–203

Occupational Safety and Health Act
  (OSHA)
  problems with, 180–181
  provisions of, 173, 180
Occupational Safety and Health
  Administration (OSHA)
  function of, 53
  noise regulation by, 369
Ocean dumping
  regulation of, 164, 186–187
  of wastes, 163–164
Ocean Dumping Act
  problems with, 186–187
  provisions of, 186–187
Office of Technology Assessment
  (OTA), 185

Oil
  beryllium in, 239
  contribution to greenhouse effect
    from, 91
  hazardous wastes from, 70
  regulation of, 185
  spills, 82, 188
  See also Petroleum
Oil Pollution Act, 188
Oil spills
  cleanup of, 188
  new legislation on, 188
Olney, John, and MSG, 352
Oncogens, definition of, 124
OPs. *See* Organophosphates (OPs)
Oral contraceptives, link to breast
  cancer, 13
Orchard crops
  azinophos-methyl use on, 227–
    228
  daminozide (Alar) use on, 284
Organic compounds
  definition of, 108
  examples of, 109
Organic growers, definition of, 132
Organic pollution, in water, 56
Organochlorines
  aldrin as insecticide, 207–209
  chlordane as, 268
  DDT as insecticide, 286
  dieldrin as insecticide, 207–209
  heptachlor as pesticide, 325
  as insecticides, 116
  lindane as insecticide, 337
  PCBs as, 382
Organophosphate insecticide
  azinophos-methyl as, 227
  diazinon as, 289
  dichlorvos as, 292
  fosetyl Al as, 322
  malathion as, 339
  parathion as, 376
Organophosphates (OPs)
  human health hazards of, 116–117
  as insecticides, 116–117
Organotin, new legislation on, 187
OSHA. *See* Occupational Safety
  and Health Administration
  (OSHA)
Osteoporosis, and fluoride, 314
Overweight, and chloroform effects,
  275
Oxalic acid, 370–371
Oxidant
  definition of, 80
  nitrogen dioxide as, 365
  ozone as, 372
  sources of precursors of, 373
Oxidation, definition of, 80
Ozone (pollution), 28, 47, **372–374**
  acetic acid in, 197
  chemistry of, 372
  environmental damage from, 374
  health effects of, 373

nitrogen oxides forming, 365
nutritional causes for susceptibil-
    ity to, 43
as oxidant, 80
as regulated by CAA, 175
in smog, 80
toluene in formation of, 417
and ultraviolet radiation, 429
versus ozone layer, 94
Ozone hole, 94. *See also* Ozone
    layer
Ozone layer
cause of depletion of, 13, 95–96
CFCs depletion of, 95–96, 265–
    266, 267
definition of, 94
depletion over Antarctica, 94
depletion by solvents, 111
effect of nuclear war on, 153
illustrated, 95
and Montreal Protocol, 96

Packaging, avoiding excessive, 169
PAHs. *See* Polycyclic aromatic
    hydrocarbons (PAHs)
Paint
benzene in oil-based, 234
carbon black in, 255
hazardous wastes from, 70
lead in, 333, 334
toluene in, 415
xylene in oil-based, 435
Paint remover, methylene chloride
    in, 346
Pajamas, TRIS used in children's,
    422–423
PAN. *See* Peroxyacetyl nitrates
    (PAN)
Pancreas, and cancer, 13
Paper
dioxin in bleached, 296
recycling of, 168
Paper pulp mills, dioxin from, 298
Paper versus plastic question, 69–70
Paralysis, from parathion, 377
Paraquat, **375–376**
as herbicide, 119
use on marijuana plants, 375
Parathion, **376–379**
as carcinogenic pesticide, 124
poisoning of fieldworkers by,
    376, 377
toxicity ranking of, 31
Particle board, formaldehyde degas-
    sing from, 319
Particulate matter, **379–381**
and acid rain, 381
in air pollution, 47
definition of, 21, 77
and indoor air pollution, 51
nitrogen dioxide in, 365
and radioactive isotopes, 145
as regulated by CAA, 175

size classification of, 379
sources of emissions of, 380
Parts per billion
as air pollution unit, 22
definition of, 21
Parts per million
as air pollution unit, 22
definition of, 21
Parts per trillion, definition of, 21
Passive smoke
hazards from, 51
nicotine in, 358
Pathogenic bacteria, 57
PBBs, **382–385**
animal feed contaminated by, 382
PCB Regulatory Improvement Act,
    187
PCBs, **382–385**
in breast milk, 40
in environment, 384–385
as insecticides, 116
new legislation on, 187
prohibited from land disposal, 161
regulated by TSCA, 180
regulation of, 184
toxicity of, 383
widespread use of, 382
PCE. *See* Tetrachloroethylene
Peanut butter, hazard from afla-
    toxins in, 201–203
Peanuts, daminozide (Alar) use on,
    284
Peas, dicamba toxicity to, 290
Pectin, 43
Permethrin, **388–390**
as botanical insecticide, 118
as carcinogenic pesticide, 124
as pyrethrum synthetic substitute,
    389
Peroxyacetyl nitrates (PAN), in
    smog, 80
Persistence
of chlordane, 268
of chlorinated hydrocarbons in
    environment, 116
of DDT, 286, 287
of dicamba, 291
of dieldrin, 207, 209
of EDB, 305
of lindane, 337
of parathion, 377
of PCBs, 382
of tetrachloroethylene, 413
of trichloroethane, 419
Person-sievert, definition of, 148–
    149
Person-sievert per becquerel, defini-
    tion of, 149
Peru, pesticide overuse on cotton
    in, 131
Pesticides
agricultural effects of, 113–115
alachlor as most widely used,
    203–205

aldicarb as, 205
alternatives to use of, 132–137
arsenic in, 217–218
carbaryl as, 253
chlordane as, 268
classification of, 115–120
consumer safety of, 123–126
2,4-D as, 281
daminozide as, 283
DDT as, 286
definition of, 112
describing risk from, 15–16
diazinon as, 289
dichlorvos as, 292
economic contraints of use of,
    130–131
EDB banned as, 303
environmental effects of, 126–130
exposure to, 120–123
farmworkers exposed to, 121
hazardous wastes from, 70
history of use of, 112–115
human health effects of, 120–123
on imported produce, 125–126
natural versus synthetic, 65
overuse on cotton, 131–132
patterns of use of, 115–120
perceived risk from, 7
production graph of, 114
reducing exposure to, 126
regulation of, 181–182, 183–184
synthetic organic types, 113–115
tolerance level of, 124–125
units of, 21
used on fruits and vegetables, 124
See also Herbicide; Insecticides
Pesticide strips, dichlorvos use in,
    292
Pest species
alternative control of, 132–137
behavior and growth control reg-
    ulators of, 134
control by mechanical and cultiva-
    tion, 134–135
control by natural enemies, 133–
    134
effect of pesticides on, 127–130
genetic and reproductive manipu-
    lations of, 134
increase in secondary, 128–129
regulatory control of, 135–136
resurgence of primary, 128–129
Petrochemical industry
definition of, 106
hazards from, 108
illustrated, 107
raw materials used in, 106–107
regulation by TSCA, 179–180
wastes from, 159
xylene use in, 435
Petrochemicals
definition of, 106
sources and products of, 106–108

See also Chemicals; Petrochemical industry
Petroleum
  benzene in products, 234–235
  underground storage tanks, 179
  use in petrochemical industry, 106
Pets, ethylene glycol poisoning of, 306–307
Pewter, lead in, 333
Pharmaceuticals, xylene used to make, 435
Phenylketonuria (PKU) disease, and aspartame, 225
Pheromones, in insects, 134
Photochemical oxidants, **372–374**
Photochemical reaction
  definition of, 80
  nitrogen dioxide formed by, 365
  and ozone (pollution), 372
Photographic developer, hydro-quinone in, 327–328
Photons, definition of, 143
pH scale
  definition of, 96–97
  illustrated, 98
Phytoplankton, PCB sensitivity of, 384
Pill, (the), link to breast cancer, 13
Pineapples, fosetyl Al use on, 322
Pipes
  lead solder joints in, 58
  metals released upon corrosion of, 56
Placenta, 39
Planetary warming, 91–94
Plant growth regulators, 134
Plants
  ozone (pollution) damage to, 374
  sulfur dioxide damage to, 409
Plasma, definition of, 37
Plasma torch, used to destroy toxics, 166
Plastic
  acetone in, 198
  carbon black in, 255
  Di(2-ethylhexyl)phthalate added to, 298–299
  hazardous wastes from, 70
  recycling of wastes, 167
  styrene in, 403
  vinyl chloride in, 430
  xylene used to make, 435
Plastic bags, versus paper, 69–70
Plastic cups, versus paper, 70–71
Plastic food wrap
  DEHP contamination of food from, 299
  vinylidene chloride in, 432
Plumes
  and atmospheric inversions, 79
  course of, 78–79
  definition of, 78
  deposition from, 79–80
Plutonium, **386–388**

lung cancer caused by, 387
radioactive isotopes of, 386–387
radioactive wastes from, 162–163
Plutonium-239, effects on human body of, 144–145
Plywood
  formaldehyde degassing from, 319–320
  indoor air pollution from, 51
Pneumoconiosis, definition of, 35
Pneumonitis, chemical, 239
Point Reyes Bird Observatory, iodine-131 harm to, 330
Point source pollution, 178
Poison control centers, 455
Poisoning, 34
  acute, 104
  by aldicarb, 205
  by arsenic, 218
  by azinophos-methyl, 228
  by carbon monoxide, 257–258
  chronic, 104
  by diazinon, 289
  by dichlorvos, 293
  by EDC and EDB, 304
  by ethylene glycol, 306
  by formaldehyde, 319
  by lead, 333, 334
  by lindane, 337
  by mercury, 341, 342
  by paraquat, 376
  by pesticides, 122, 123–124
  by warfarin, 434
Pollutants. *See* Pollution
Pollution
  concentration units of, 19–22
  describing risk from, 15–16
  discharge units of, 19
  units in air, 21–22
  units in human body, 21
  units in water, 19
  See also Air pollution; Water pollution
Pollution emission rate, definition of, 16
Polonium, half-life and damage to body from, 145
Polybrominated biphenyls. *See* PBBs
Polychlorinated biphenyls. *See* PCBs
Polycyclic aromatic hydrocarbons (PAHs)
  and carbon black hazards, 256
  regulation of, 237
Polyvinyl chloride (PVC)
  industrial recycling of, 166
  pipes made of, 430
  vinyl chloride in, 430, 431
Populations
  study of disease in, 27
  versus species protection, 89
Possible human carcinogen
  definition of, 32

lindane as, 337
paraquat as, 375
parathion as, 378
permethrin as, 389
styrene as, 404
Potassium iodide, for protection from iodine-131, 330
Potatoes
  aldicarb banned on, 207
  aldrin/dieldrin in, 209
  alkaloids in, 136
  chlordane on, 269
  DDT on, 286
  pesticides found on, 124
Potency, of carcinogen, 30
Potentiation, caused by OPs, 117
Pots, hazards from aluminum, 211, 213
Pottery, lead in, 333, 334
Precipitate, definition of, 81
Predatory insects, to control pest species, 133–134, 137–139
Pregnancy
  and caffeine, 249
  carbon monoxide effects on, 258
  danger from lead during, 37
  and drinking, 63
  and ELF field hazards, 311
  and lead poisoning, 334
  mercury hazards during, 341–342
  and PCBs, 384
  and smoking, 51
  ultrasound used during, 426
  and warfarin hazards, 434
Premanufacture notices (PMNs), 179
Preservatives
  BHA and BHT as, 241–242
  and colon and rectal cancers, 12
  food irradiation as alternative to, 152–153
  hazards from, 61–62
  nitrites as, 360
  regulation of, 181–182
  risk of harm from, 6
  sulfites as, 405
Primary air quality standards, 175
Probability
  as basis of risk, 5–6
  misunderstanding of, 17
Probable human carcinogen
  alachlor as, 204
  aldrin/dieldrin as, 208–209
  benomyl as, 231
  benzo[*a*]pyrene as, 236–237
  beryllium as, 240
  cadmium as, 245
  captafol as, 251
  captan as, 251
  carbon tetrachloride as, 261
  chlordane as, 269
  chloroform as, 275
  creosote as, 280
  DDT as, 287

definition of, 32
dioxane as, 295
EBDCs as, 301
EDC as, 304
folpet as, 251
formaldehyde as, 319–320
heptachlor as, 326
methylene chloride as, 347
PCBs as, 384
tetrachloroethylene as, 414
trichloroethylene as, 421
Processed food
Alar use on, 283
BHA and BHT in, 241–242
carageenan in, 262
hazards from, 62
monosodium glutamate use in, 351–352
sulfites in, 405
Products. See Consumer products
Prompt radiation, definition of, 153
Proposition 65 (California)
limitation of, 192
provisions of, 192
Prostate cancer, 13
Protons, definition of, 141
Prussian blue, and cesium-137, 264
Public health and safety, protection of, 179–184
Pulmonary fibrosis, 104
and aluminum dust, 211
Pure Food and Drug Act, 61
Pyrethrins, 390
Pyrethroids, 388–390
as botanical insecticide, 118
Pyrethrum, 388–390
as botanical insecticide, 118
causing gorilla extinctions, 390
as natural insecticide, 388
as pesticide, 112
as safe for home gardens, 137

Quality factor, of radiation, 148
Quicksilver, 341

Rad, definition of, 147
Radar signals, radio frequency radiation from, 348
Radiation
anthropogenic sources of, 149–150
background levels of, 149–150
and cesium-137, 263–265
definition of, 142
doses to body of, 147–148
effects on human body of, 144–145
estimating risk of, 150–151
food preserved by, 151–153
hazardous wastes from, 162–163
human sensitivity to, 88–89
and iodine-131, 329
nature of, 141–145

produced in fission process, 146
prompt versus delayed, 153
and radon, 391–393
standards of, 149–150
and strontium-90, 401
and tritium, 424–425
units of, 146–149
Radioactive, definition of, 142
Radioactive isotope
americium-241 as, 386
iodine-131 as, 329
plutonium-239 as, 386
released from Chernobyl, 78
strontium-90 as, 401
Radioactive wastes
land disposal of, 162–163
long half-lives of, 162–163
ocean dumping of, 186–187
as regulated by CAA, 175
and risk-benefit comparisons, 6
special dangers of, 163
Radioactivity
nature of, 141–143
See also Isotopes; Radiation
Radio frequency radiation, 348–349
Radiolytic products, definition of, 152
Radio waves. See Radio frequency radiation
Radon, 391–393
as cause of lung cancer, 11, 49
half-life and damage to body from, 145
in homes, 187
as indoor air pollution, 391–392
leaks into home, 53
lung cancer from, 391
lung damage from, 151
measurement of, 392
as natural background radiation, 149–150
new legislation on, 187
Rain
changes in due to greenhouse effect, 91–92
deposition of air pollutants by, 80
Rainout, definition of, 79
Rash, 36
and chromium, 278
from nickel contact, 355
Rats
barium as poison for, 229
used in laboratory testing, 29
warfarin as poison for, 433
Raw food, regulation of, 181–182
Raw materials, of petrochemical industry, 106–107
RCRA. See Resource Conservation and Recovery Act (RCRA)
RDAs. See Recommended Daily Allowances (RDAs)
Reagan administration, and workplace right to know, 189

Recipes, for safe pest control in gardens, 137
Recommended Daily Allowances (RDAs), 42
Rectal cancer, deaths from, 11
Recycling
centers, 168
by consumers, 168
in industry, 166–167
of paper and cardboard, 168
of plastic wastes, 167
to reduce hazardous wastes, 162
to reduce source of toxics, 166–169
of tires, 167
of wastes, 185
Red No. 40, 316
Reentry intervals, into pesticide treated fields, 122–123
Refrigerators, CFCs used in, 265, 266
Regulation
abbreviations of laws and institutions, 450
of air quality, 175–176
of chemicals, 179–180
and controls on pest species, 135–136
controversy over, 7–8
of cosmetics, 182
of drugs, 182–183
federal, 171–188
of food safety, 181–183
new or proposed laws, 187–188
of permissible radiation dose, 150
of pesticides, 122, 183–184
problems with, 171, 174
state, 191–192
of toxics in California, 192
of wastes, 184–187
of water quality, 177–179
of workplace exposure, 180–181
Regulatory control, of pest species, 135–136
Rem, definition of, 148
Reprocessing, definition of, 162
Reproductive system
lead effects on, 334
PCB effects on, 383
Resistance
to benomyl, 232
to DDT, 288
increase in, 129–130
of pest species, 127–130
of rats to warfarin, 433, 434
Resource Conservation and Recovery Act (RCRA)
provisions of, 173, 184
and radon regulation, 187
Respiratory effects
acute, 47–48
chronic, 48–49
Respiratory infections, and gas stoves, 366

Respiratory system
  chromium(VI) effects on, 277–278
  sulfites effects on, 406
Response
  definition of, 15, 16
  versus dose, 17
Restaurants, sulfites used in, 405
Restricted pesticide, definition of, 122
Resurgence
  agricultural loses from, 129–130
  of pest species, 127–130
RF radiation. *See* Radio frequency radiation
Rhodophycae, 262
Rhubarb, oxalic acid in leaves of, 370
Right to know
  community, 190–191
  federal programs, 189, 191
  growth of movement of, 188–189
  problems with, 191
  and solvents regulation, 111
  state programs, 191–192
  in workplace, 189
  See also Community right to know
Risk
  of cancer, 11
  of cancer from asbestos, 222–224
  of chemicals to human health, 179
  control of, 7
  definition of, 5
  and Delaney Clause, 181–182
  ecological versus human, 88–89
  in epidemiology studies, 27–28
  estimates of, 16–18
  of hazardous wastes, 161
  inherited, 6–7
  language of, 15–23
  of lung cancer from plutonium-239, 388
  of lung cancer from radon, 393
  magnitude of, 7
  misunderstandings about, 5–8
  of radiation, 150–151
  reduction of, 170
  scientific description of, 15–18
  and toxic sensitivity, 40
  versus exposure, 15–16
Risk-benefit comparisons, 6
Rivers
  dieldrin in, 208
  nitrates in, 360
  toluene in, 416
Road workers, asphalt hazards to, 226–227
Rock wool, 350–351
Rocky Flats plutonium plant accident, 386, 387
Rodenticides
  definition of, 112
  regulation of, 183–184

warfarin as, 433
Roofers, asphalt hazards to, 226–227
Roots, uptake by aldicarb, 206
Roundup, 323–325
Roundworms, dichlorvos use on, 292
Rubber
  carbon black in, 255
  styrene in, 403

Saccharin, **394–395**
  replaced by aspartame, 225
  in toothpaste, 394
Safe Drinking Water Act (SDWA), provisions of, 174, 178
Safe Drinking Water and Toxic Enforcement Act (California), 192
Safe levels, of carcinogens versus noncarcinogens, 30
Salad bars, sulfites used in, 405
Salting, nitrates used in, 359, 360
Salt mines, as nuclear waste disposal sites, 162
SARA. *See* Superfund Amendments and Reauthorization Act (SARA)
Saturated fat, 8–9
Saturation effect, definition of, 17–18
Sausage, nitrites in, 360
Savannah River reactor
  radioactive leaks from, 162
  tritium from, 425
Schools, asbestos use in, 222
Scrubbing, definition of, 99
SDWA. *See* Safe Drinking Water Act (SDWA)
Seafood
  cadmium in, 245
  mercury in, 341–342
Sea level rise, due to greenhouse effect, 92, 93
Seaweed, monosodium glutamate in, 351
Secondary outbreaks
  agricultural loses from, 129–130
  of introduced predator insects, 136
  of pest species, 127–130
Secondary treatment, of sewage, 178
Second-hand smoke. *See* Passive smoke
Selenium, **395–398**
  anticancer role of, 396
  harm to wildlife from, 89, 90
  and human nutrition, 396
  natural source of, 396
  poisoning of farm animals by, 397
  to prevent benzene toxicity, 43
  in soil, 83
  as toxic product of incineration, 165
Sensitive groups, 40–42

Sensitivity
  and age, 41
  definition of, 41
  and lifestyle, 41
  to toxics, 40–42
  of wildlife to toxics, 89
Sewage
  chlorine use in treatment of, 271–272
  regulated under CWA, 177
  secondary treatment of, 164, 178
  tertiary treatment of, 178
"Shakes," caused by Kepone, 120
Showers, chloroform from, 274
Sick building syndrome, definition of, 53
Sievert (Sv), definition of, 147–148
Silent Spring, and pesticide use, 114
Silica fibers, 350–351
Silicosis, definition of, 35
Silverfish, safe control of in home, 138
Silvex, 296–297
  EPA emergency cancellation of, 184
Skeletal fluorosis, 314
Skin
  ammonia hazards to, 215
  arsenic effects on, 220
  benzo[a]pyrene effects on, 236
  bis(chloromethyl)ether hazards to, 243
  captafol effects on, 251
  creosote effects on, 280
  dioxane effects on, 294
  dioxin effects on, 296–297
  formaldehyde absorbed through, 318–319
  laser light effects on, 332
  mineral fibers effects on, 350
  naphthalene exposure to, 353
  oxalic acid effects on, 371
  sodium hydroxide effects on, 399
  solvents hazards to, 110
  ultraviolet radiation effects on, 429
  uptake of toxics through, 36
  xylene effects on, 435
Skin bleach
  hydroquinone as, 327–328
  oxalic acid in, 370
Skin cancer, 13. *See also* Melanoma
  increase due to ozone layer depletion, 95
  from ultraviolet radiation, 429
Sleep disturbances, from caffeine, 248
Sleepwear, TRIS used in children's, 422–423
Sludge, dumping in oceans, 163–164
Small airway disease, 48
Small intestine, toxic chemicals in, 35

Smog
    definition of, 80
    formation of, 372
    health effects of, 373
    nitrogen dioxide in, 365
    sulfur dioxide in, 407, 408
    toluene in formation of, 417
Smokestacks
    and arsenic exposure, 218
    gaseous emissions from, 165
    plumes from, 78–79
    scrubbing of, 99
    sulfur dioxide from, 408
Smoking. *See* Cigarette smoking;
    Passive smoking
Snow blindness, from ultraviolet
    radiation, 429
Soap solution, as pesticide substi-
    tute, 137
Sodium fluoride, 313
Sodium hydroxide, **398–400**
    household hazards of, 399
    severe corrosive hazards of, 399
Sodium monofluorophosphate, 313
Soft drinks
    aspartame use in, 225
    caffeine in, 248, 249
    chloroform in, 274
    saccharin use in, 394
Soil
    cadmium in, 244–245
    chemistry of, 83–84
    chlordane in, 268
    movement of toxics through,
        83–84
    PCBs in, 383
    radon in, 391
    selenium in, 396
Solar energy, used to destroy toxics,
    165–166
Solid wastes, definition of, 158
Solvent
    acetone as, 198
    benzene in oil-based, 234
    carbon tetrachloride in, 260
    definition of, 108–109
    dioxane as, 294
    EDC as, 303
    environmental effects of, 111
    ethylene glycol as, 306
    human health effects of, 110–111
    methyl ethyl ketone as, 344
    trichloroethane as, 418
    trichloroethylene as, 420
    types of, 109–110
    xylene used to make, 435
Soot
    as catalysts, 80
    deposition of, 79
Sounds
    decibel levels of various, 368
    frequency of, 426
    intensity of, 370, 426
    See also Noise

Soviet Union, Chernobyl accident,
    78–79
Soybeans, alachlor use on, 203
Special review
    of alachlor, 204
    of aldicarb, 207
    of captan/captafol/folpet, 252
    of 2,4-D, 283
    of daminozide (Alar), 285
    of diazinon, 290
    of dichlorvos, 293
    of EBDCs, 302
    of formaldehyde, 320
    of pesticides by EPA, 183–184
Species, versus population protec-
    tion, 89
SPF, and ultraviolet radiation pro-
    tection, 429
Spills
    of chlorine, 270–272
    of hydrochloric acid, 270–272
    of oil, 82, 188
Spray cans, risk of harm from, 5
Spraying of pesticides. *See* Pesticides
Stannous fluoride, 313
Statistical tests, limitations of, 28
Steel
    sulfur dioxide corrosion of, 409
    zinc to galvanize, 436
Sterilization, by ethylene oxide, 308
Stomach
    nitrosamines production in, 361
    problems in women factory work-
        ers, 42
    sodium hydroxide effects on, 399
    toxic chemicals in, 35
Stomach cancer, 10
Storage batteries, lead in, 333
Stratosphere, definition of, 94
Stratospheric ozone
    depletion of, 94–96
    See also Ozone layer
Stress, caused by noise, 368
Strokes, deaths from, 8
Strontium-90, **401–402**
    and becquerel unit, 148
    as nuclear fission fragment, 146
Styrene, **403–404**
    in plastic cups, 71
    use in plastics, 403–404
Styrofoam
    CFCs in, 267
    styrene in, 403
    use of pellets, 169
Subchronic effects, 28–29
Suicides, carbon monoxide used in,
    257, 258
Sulfates, **407–410**
    in air pollution, 47
Sulfites, 28, **405–407**
    allergic reaction to, 40
    asthmatic reaction to, 406
    as food additive, 62
    as food preservatives, 405

testing equipment for, 453
Sulfur, as produced by petrochemi-
    cal industry, 106
Sulfur dioxide, 21, 28, **407–410**
    in acid rain, 80, 96
    in air pollution, 47
    from arts and crafts, 68
    in atmospheric inversions, 78
    concentrations from various loca-
        tions, 408
    health effects from, 408–409
    long-term solutions to problem
        of, 409
    as regulated by CAA, 175
    in sulfites, 405
Sunbathing, hazards of, 429
Sunburn, from ultraviolet radiation,
    429
Sun protection factor. *See* SPF
Suntan lotion
    hydroquinone in, 327–328
    and ultraviolet radiation, 429
Superfund Amendments and Re-
    authorization Act (SARA)
    problems with, 186
    provisions of, 186
Superfund law
    problems with, 185–186
    provisions of, 172, 179, 185
Superfund sites, cleanup of, 185–186
Swallowing
    and ethylene glycol damage, 306
    of toxics, 35–36
Sweat, toxics removed in, 40
Sweet-N-Low, 394
Swimming pools
    chlorine use in, 271–272
    chloroform exposure from, 273
Synergist
    definition of, 388
    in pesticides, 115
Synergistic effect, definition of, 28
Synthetic materials, indoor air pol-
    lution from, 51, 53
Synthetic pesticides
    production of, 114
    use of, 113–115
Systemic
    benomyl as, 231
    definition of, 36
    glyphosate as, 323
    herbicides, 115
    insecticides, 115
Systemic poison, definition of, 205

2,4,5-T, **411–412**
    dioxin as by-product of, 296–297
    EPA emergency cancellation of,
        184
    as exported pesticide, 125–126
    as herbicide, 119
Talc, 68
Tanning, hazards of, 429
Tar, definition of, 226

Target organ, 38, 42
  definition of, 34
  dose to, 36–37
TCA. *See* Trichloroethane
TCDD, 296–298. *See also* Dioxin
TCE. *See* Trichloroethylene
Tea
  caffeine in, 248
  fluoride in, 313
Teeth, mottling of by fluoride, 314
Television, radio frequency radiation from, 348
Termites
  chlordane use on, 268
  dieldrin use on, 207, 209
  heptachlor use for, 326
Tertiary treatment, of sewage, 178
Test animals. *See* Laboratory animals
Testicular injury, from DEHP, 299
Testing. *See* Laboratory testing
Tetrachloroethylene, 413–415
  as chlorinated solvent, 109
  dry cleaning use of, 53, 413–414
  as inert ingredient, 67
Tetrahydrothalimide, 251
Textiles, hazardous wastes from, 70
Thalidomide, 250
Theoretical maximum residue contribution (TMRC), for pesticides, 125
Thermometers, mercury in, 341
Thiabendazole, 232
Thickener, carageenan as, 262
Thiophanate-methyl, 232
Three Mile Island nuclear accident, iodine-131 release from, 329
Threshold dose, versus safe levels, 30
Threshold effect
  definition of, 17–18
  of radiation, 151
Thrift shops, 168
Thule, Greenland, nuclear weapons crash, 386, 387
Thyroid gland, iodine-131 in, 145, 329–330
Tin-based chemicals, new legislation on, 187
Tires
  carbon black in, 255
  recycling of, 167
  styrene in, 403
Tobacco budworm, secondary outbreak of, 131
Tobacco leaves, nicotine in, 358
Tobacco smoke, 13–14. *See also* Cigarette smoking
  acrolein in, 200
  carcinogens in, 51
  nickel in, 355
  nicotine in, 358
  particulate matter hazards from, 381

as source of toxic metals, 105
Tobacco water, as pesticide substitute, 137
Toilet bowl cleaner, naphthalene in, 353
Tolerance
  and Delaney Clause, 181–182
  of EBDCs, 302
  level of pesticides, 120
  for pesticides on foods, 124–125
Toluene, 415–417
  from arts and crafts, 68
  as gasoline additive, 415
  health effects of, 416
  reduction of hazards from, 416–417
  as solvent, 109
  use in petrochemical industry, 108
  as volatile, 81
  in workplace, 53
Tooth decay, fluoride prevention of, 313, 314
Toothpaste
  fluoride in, 313
  saccharin in, 394
Total suspended particulates (TSP), definition of, 380
Toxicity
  of hydroquinone, 327–328
  of PCBs, 383
  See also Acute toxicity; Chronic toxicity
Toxicity testing, 28–30
  high doses used in, 17, 29
Toxic metals
  aluminum as, 210
  beryllium as, 238
  cadmium as, 244
  and cancer, 104–105
  chromium as, 276
  exposure routes to body, 104
  half-lives of, 163
  hazards to humans from, 104–105
  lead as, 333
  mercury as, 341
  mobilized in environment, 103–104
  nickel as, 354
  reduction of exposure to, 105
  selenium as, 395
  significance and sources of, 103–104
  in soil, 84
  as water pollution, 83
  See also Metals
Toxicology, 28–30
  definition of, 27
Toxic pathways, 85
Toxics
  activities to avoid use of, 169
  in air, 47–54
  in biosphere, 86–90
  and cancer, 13–14
  in consumer products, 67–73

downwind transport of, 78–79
EPA classification of, 31–33
exit from body, 39–40
in food, 61–66
in the human body, 34–43
language of, 15–23
metabolism of, 37–38, 41
movement through body, 38
movement through environment, 77–85
in nature, 64–66
radioactive types of, 141–154
recycling to reduce source of, 166–169
reduction of use in industry, 167
regulation of, 171–192
risk of harm from, 5–8
ten ways to reduce in environment, x
terminology of, xiv
testing of, 27–31
units of, 18–23
versus toxins, xiv
in water, 55–59
ways to consume less, 167–169
in the workplace, 189–190
Toxics Release Inventory (TRI), 190
Toxics Substances Control Act, 29
Toxic Substances Control Act (TSCA)
  problems with, 179–180
  provisions of, 174, 179
Toxic wastes
  definition of, 159
  extent of problem of, 185
  new processing technologies for, 165–166
  regulation of, 184–187
  See also Hazardous wastes; Wastes
Toxins, versus toxics, xiv
Trace metals
  definition of, 103
  See also Toxic metals
Traffic, carbon monoxide from, 257
Transformers, PCBs used in, 382
Transmission lines, ELF fields in, 310–312
Trap planting, definition of, 135
Trash. *See* Garbage; Wastes
Trees, ozone (pollution) damage to, 374
Trichloroethane, 418–419
  as chlorinated solvent, 109
  vinyl chloride used to make, 430
Trichloroethylene, 420–422
  potency of, 30
  as solvent, 109
Trihalomethanes (THMs)
  and bladder cancer, 13
  definition of, 57
TRIS, 422–423
  ban of, 423
  cancer caused by, 422–423

in pajamas, 168
use in children's sleepwear, 422–423
Tritiated water, definition of, 424
Tritium, **424–426**
relative safety of, 424–425
Trout, mercury sensitivity to, 343
Tumors, cancerous, 10–11
Turbulence, definition of, 79

Ultrasound, **426–428**
definition of, 426
Ultraviolet light, in destruction of ozone layer, 80
Ultraviolet radiation, **428–430**
absorbed by skin, 428, 429
from arts and crafts, 68
and melanoma, 13
and ozone layer, 94
skin hazards of, 429
three types of, 430
wavelengths of, 143
Underground petroleum storage tanks
benzene in, 233
regulation of, 59, 179, 186
Unique radiolytic products (URPs), definition of, 152
United States
coal-burning plumes in, 79
garbage in, 157
harmful effects of ozone layer depletion in, 94–95
herbicides use in, 118–119
high-fat diet in, 8–9
insecticides use in, 115–116
ozone (pollution) problem in, 372–373
pesticides use in, 112–113
radiation dose regulation in, 150
regulation of toxics in, 171–188
regulatory control of pest species in, 135–136
sulfur dioxide emmissions in, 408
urban air pollution in, 22
use of British units, 19–20
U.S. Forest Service
dicamba use by, 291
2,4-D use by, 283
U.S. Nuclear Regulatory Commission, 150
U.S. Product Safety Commission, 68
Units
abbreviations of, 449
of air pollution, 21–22
of concentration, 19–22
definition of, 19
of discharge, 19
for nonradioactive toxics, 18–23
of pollution in human body, 21
for radioactive toxics, 146–149
Upholstery cleaner, tetrachloroethylene used in, 413

Upper respiratory system, 200
ammonia hazards to, 214–215
formaldehyde effects on, 319
Uptake, of pollutants into body, 22–23, 34
Upwelling, of air to remove pollution, 78
Uranium-235, use in bombs, 145
Uranium-238
definition of, 141
half-life of, 143
Uranium-239, plutonium from, 386
Urban air
and carbon monoxide, 257–258
methylene chloride in, 346
nitrogen oxides in, 365, 366
ozone in, 372–373
pollution in United State, 22
sulfur dioxide in, 408
tetrachloroethylene in, 413
trichloroethane in, 418
trichloroethylene in, 420
Urea-formaldehyde foam insulation (UFFI), 318
Urine, toxics removed in, 39
Utah, beryllium mined in, 239
UV. *See* Ultraviolet radiation
UV-A radiation, 429, 430
UV-B radiation, 430
UV-C radiation, 430

VCM. *See* Vinyl chloride
Vegetables
EBDCs used on, 300–301
iodine-131 in, 329–330
lindane used on, 336
as nitrate source, 361, 363
pesticides used on, 124, 181–182
sulfites in, 405
Ventilation
to decrease indoor air pollution, 53
to flush out radon, 392
Vietnam War, and Agent Orange, 296, 411
Vinegar, 197
hazards of mixing with bleach, 271, 272
Vinyl chloride, **430–431**
from breakdown of trichloroethylene, 420
as cancer cause, 431
DEHP contamination of water from, 299
EDC used to produce, 303
industrial control of, 166
as regulated by CAA, 175
regulated by TSCA, 180
restricted under FFDCA, 182
in soil, 111
and workplace right to know, 189
Vinylidene chloride, **432–433**
Vitamin C, as nitrosamine inhibitor, 361, 364

Vitamin D, and ultraviolet radiation, 428
Vitamin E, as nitrosamine inhibitor, 361, 364
Vitamin supplements, 42
zinc in, 437
Volatile, definition of, 81
Volatile organic compounds (VOCs), role in smog formation, 365, 372
Volume, metric units of, 19–20

Warfarin, **433–434**
household use of, 433–434
Warning label, 31–32
Waste crisis
definition of, 157
overview of, 157–159
Waste disposal
on land, 159–164
in ocean, 163–164
Wastes
benzene in household, 234
bis(chloromethyl)ether in, 243–244
crisis of, 157–159
hazardous, 160–162
land disposal of, 159–163
management of, 184–187
municipal, 159–160
new processing technologies for, 165–166
nonhazardous, 159–160
ocean dumping of, 186–187
processing of, 164
radioactive, 162–163
recycling of, 185
reduction of, 185
treatment of, 164
See also Hazardous wastes; Solid wastes
Water
barium in, 229–230
chemical processes in, 83
chloroform exposure from, 273–274
flow and mixing of pollution in, 81
fluoride in, 313–315
in ground, 59
quality of, 55, 177–179
and regulation of ocean dumping, 186–187
testing equipment for, 453
tritium in, 424
units of toxics in, 20–22
zinc in, 436
See also Drinking water
Watermelons, aldicarb use on, 123
Water pollution, 55–59. *See also* Drinking water
bacteria as cause of, 56
chlorination to treat, 56, 57
concentration units of, 19–21

improvements in, 177–178
and movement of toxics, 81–83
and reduction of metal contamination, 58
regulation of, 177–179
sources of contaminants, 56–58
Water purification devices, 58
Water-soluble molecules, 38
Wavelength
definition of, 143
of ultraviolet radiation, 428
Weed killer
2,4-D as, 281
glyphosate as effective, 323
paraquat as, 375
2,4,5-T as, 411
Weeds, use of herbicides on, 118–119
Weevils, safe control of in home, 138
Weight, metric units of, 20
Well water
and concentration of pollutants, 19
nitrates in, 360, 363–364
Wet deposition, 79
Whole body dose, definition of, 147
Wildlife
benomyl toxicity to, 232
noise harm to, 369
parathion toxicity to, 376, 377
selenium poisoning of, 395, 397
toxic threat to, 86–90

warfarin poisoning of, 434
See also Animals
Wind, and movement of toxics, 78–79
Window cleaner, dioxane in, 294
Windscale fuel reprocessing plant
accident at, 387
tritium from, 425
Wine
sulfites in, 405
sulfur dioxide use in, 407
Wood, formaldehyde in products of, 319
Wood preservatives
arsenic in, 217–218
creosote as, 279–280
Woodstoves, benzo[a]pyrene given off by, 236
Workplace
air pollution in, 53
asbestos hazards in, 223
benzene in, 234
beryllium exposure in, 239–240
bis(chloromethyl)ether in, 243–244
dioxane in, 295
ELF field hazards in, 311
exposure to acetic acid in, 197
formaldehyde in, 318
inhalation of toxics in, 34
methyl ethyl ketone in, 345
nickel in, 355
noise regulation in, 369

and OSHA, 180–181
right to know, 189
styrene in, 403
World Health Organization (WHO), 31

X-rays, 143, 153
and ultrasound hazards, 427
Xylene, **435–436**
and alcohol use, 63
from arts and crafts, 68
as inert ingredient, 67
as solvent, 109
use in petrochemical industry, 108

Yellow No. 5
allergy to, 317
widespread use of, 316

Zinc, **436–438**
from arts and crafts, 68
deficiency versus overload, 437
and human nutrition, 436–437
nutritional causes for susceptibility to, 43
relation to cadmium, 244
sulfur dioxide corrosion of, 409
in tobacco smoke, 51
Zinc chloride, 436, 437
Zinc oxide, 436, 437
Zinc toxicosis, definition of, 437
Zineb, **300–302**
as fungicide, 119

Designer: Linda M. Robertson
Compositor: Prestige Typography
Text: 10/12 Stempel Garamond
Display: Helvetica/Stempel Garamond
Printer: Malloy Lithographing, Inc.
Binder: John H. Dekker & Sons, Inc.